Preadjusted Edgewise Fixed Orthodontic Appliances

Preadjusted Edgewise Fixed Orthodontic Appliances

Principles and Practice

Edited by

Farhad B. Naini
BDS (Lond.), MSc (Lond.), PhD (KCL), FDS.RCS (Eng.), M.Orth.RCS (Eng.),
FDS.Orth.RCS (Eng.), GCAP (KCL), FHEA, FDS.RCS.Ed
Consultant Orthodontist
Department of Orthodontics
Kingston Hospital NHS Foundation Trust
St George's University Hospital NHS Foundation Trust
London, UK

Daljit S. Gill
BDS (Hons), BSc (Hons), MSc (Lond.), FDS.RCS (Eng.), M.Orth.RCS (Eng.),
FDS (Orth) RCS (Eng.), FHEA
Consultant Orthodontist
Department of Orthodontics
Great Ormond Street Hospital NHS Foundation Trust and UCLH Eastman Dental Hospital
London, UK

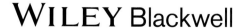

Registered Offices
John Wiley & Sons, Inc., 111 River Street, Hoboken, NJ 07030, USA
John Wiley & Sons Ltd, The Atrium, Southern Gate, Chichester, West Sussex, PO19 8SQ, UK

Editorial Office
9600 Garsington Road, Oxford, OX4 2DQ, UK

For details of our global editorial offices, customer services, and more information about Wiley products visit us at www.wiley.com.

Wiley also publishes its books in a variety of electronic formats and by print-on-demand. Some content that appears in standard print versions of this book may not be available in other formats.

Library of Congress Cataloging-in-Publication Data

Names: Naini, Farhad B., editor. | Gill, Daljit S., editor.
Title: Preadjusted edgewise fixed orthodontic appliances : principles and
    practice / edited by Farhad B. Naini, Daljit S. Gill.
Description: First edition. | Hoboken, NJ : Wiley-Blackwell, 2022. |
    Includes bibliographical references and index.
Identifiers: LCCN 2021014308 (print) | LCCN 2021014309 (ebook) | ISBN
    9781118817698 (paperback) | ISBN 9781118817582 (adobe pdf) | ISBN
    9781118817599 (epub)
Subjects: MESH: Orthodontic Appliances, Fixed
Classification: LCC RK521 (print) | LCC RK521 (ebook) | NLM WU 426 | DDC
    617.6/43–dc23
LC record available at https://lccn.loc.gov/2021014308
LC ebook record available at https://lccn.loc.gov/2021014309

Cover Design: Wiley
Cover Image: (Top) Courtesy of Richard Cousley; (Bottom) Courtesy of Farhad B. Naini

Set in 9.5/12.5pt STixTwoText by Straive, Chennai, India

Printed in Singapore
M085743_140921

To our families and our profession

Contents

Preface *xxi*
Acknowledgements *xxiii*
Contributors *xxv*
Introduction: What is the Preadjusted Edgewise Appliance? *xxix*

Farhad B. Naini and Daljit S. Gill

What Does 'Edgewise' Mean *xxix*
What Does 'Preadjusted' Mean *xxxiv*
  The Three Orders of Tooth Movement *xxxiv*
  The Six Keys to Normal Occlusion *xxxv*
  Customisation and Preprogramming of Brackets *xxxvii*
  Prescription *xxxviii*
  Expression *xxxviii*
Preadjusted Edgewise Appliance Components *xxxix*
  Brackets *xxxix*
  Tubes/Bands *xxxix*
  Archwires *xxxix*
  Other *xl*
Bracket Design Features *xl*
  Horizontal Slot, Clearance and Bearing Points *xl*
  Tie-wings *xlii*
  Stem *xlii*
  Base *xlii*
  Identification Mark *xlii*
  Additional Components *xlii*
  Extent of Preadjustment (Preprogramming) *xliii*
Bracket Positioning *xliii*
Stages of Treatment *xliv*
Conclusion *xliv*
References *xliv*

Part I   **Principles** *1*

1   **Principles of Treatment Planning** *3*

Farhad B. Naini and Daljit S. Gill

Introduction *3*
Patient Concerns *4*
Patient Motivation and Compliance *4*

Handling Patient Expectations *4*

Medical History *6*

General Dental Health *6*

Previous Orthodontic Treatment *7*

Treatment Timing: When Should Treatment be Undertaken? *7*

   Teasing and Bullying *7*

   Dental Health Problems and Habits *8*

   Relevance of Growth and Growth Estimation *8*

Problem List *9*

Treatment Aims *11*

   Aesthetic-Centred versus Occlusion-Centred Planning *11*

   Static and Functional Occlusion, Stability and Health *13*

Presenting the Treatment Options *14*

   No Treatment *15*

   Treatment with Limited Objectives *15*

   Orthodontics Alone *15*

   Orthodontics in Association with Multidisciplinary Care *15*

How do we decide whether or not to Extract Teeth? *15*

Space Analysis and Space Planning *17*

Informed Consent *21*

What Should be Included in a Treatment Plan *23*

Treatment Mechanics *23*

References *26*

2   Principles of Orthodontic Biomechanics *29*

Farhad B. Naini and Daljit S. Gill

Introduction *29*

Basic Concepts and Principles *30*

   Spatial Planes and Axes of Rotation as a Frame of Reference *30*

   Force *30*

   Centre of Resistance *33*

   Moment *34*

   Couple *35*

   Centre of Rotation *37*

   Pure Rotation *37*

   Retraction and Protraction *37*

   Retroclination and Proclination *38*

   Tip *38*

   'Tipping' *38*

   Torque *38*

Newton's Laws of Motion and Static Equilibrium *38*

Displacement of Rigid Bodies *39*

   How do Teeth Translate with Edgewise Fixed Appliances? *40*

Control of Tooth Movement *41*

   Extension Hooks and the Centre of Resistance *41*

   Moment-to-Force Ratios and Controlling Root Position *42*

Types of Tooth Movement *44*

   Simple ('Uncontrolled') Tipping *46*

   Controlled Tipping *46*

   Translation (Bodily Movement) *46*

   Root Movement *46*

Pure Rotation *47*
Clinical Applications and Relevance *47*
One-Couple Force System *48*
Two-Couple Force System *48*
Space Closure *49*
Space Closure with Sliding Mechanics *49*
Space Closure with Closing Loop Mechanics *52*
Conclusion *54*
References *55*

3   Anchorage *57*

Zaid B. Al-Bitar

Introduction *57*
Terminology *58*
Anchorage Value *59*
Force Levels and Pressure Distribution in the Periodontal Ligament *59*
Quality of the Supporting Structures *60*
Occlusal Intercuspation *60*
Facial Growth and the Vertical Dimension *60*
Root Morphology *61*
Interproximal Contacts *61*
Assessment of Anchorage Need *61*
Classifications of Anchorage *61*
Classification of Anchorage According to the Site of Anchorage *61*
Classification of Anchorage According to the Anchorage Need (Anteroposterior Plane) *61*
Classification According to the Plane of Anchorage *62*
Anchorage Control with Fixed Appliances *62*
Intermaxillary Anchorage *62*
Increasing the Number of Teeth in the Anchorage Unit *63*
Controlling Pressure Distribution in the Anchorage and Active Units *64*
Extraoral Anchorage *66*
Avoiding or Reducing Forces on the Anchorage Unit *66*
Utilising Intraoral Musculature *71*
Occlusion *71*
Maintaining the Arch Length *71*
Bone Anchorage *72*
Adjunctive Methods for Anchorage Control *73*
Anchorage Creation *73*
Headgear *73*
Intraoral Distalising Appliances *74*
Direct Bone Anchorage *74*
Anchorage Loss *74*
References *75*

4   Consent *79*

Gavin J. Mack

Introduction *79*
Types of Consent *80*
Implied Consent *80*
Verbal Consent *80*

Written Consent *80*

Valid Consent *80*

Withdrawal of Consent *81*

Treatment Options *81*

Avoiding Orthodontic Treatment *81*

Orthodontics with Limited Objectives *81*

Comprehensive Orthodontics for Occlusal Correction *81*

Key Factors to be Communicated with Patients *82*

Treatment Duration *82*

Expected Compliance *82*

Retention Protocol *82*

The Costs of Treatment *82*

Treatment Benefits *83*

Enhanced Smile Aesthetics *83*

Enhanced Dental Health *83*

Enhanced Occlusal Function *84*

Psychosocial Benefits *84*

Unfounded Claims for the Benefits of Orthodontic Treatment *84*

Treatment Risks *84*

Damage to Teeth *84*

Damage to the Periodontium *85*

Pain and Discomfort during Treatment *86*

Rare and Unusual Injuries *87*

Relapse *87*

Effective Communication *88*

Patient Information Leaflets *88*

Websites *88*

Clinical Predictions *89*

Involvement of Family and Friends *89*

Conclusions *89*

References *90*

5   Dentolegal Aspects of Orthodontic Treatment *93*

Alison Williams

Introduction *93*

Advertising *94*

The Initial Consultation *94*

Recording the Patient's Concerns *94*

Pretreatment Orthodontic Examination *95*

Dental Health Assessment *95*

Taking Radiographs as Part of the Orthodontic Assessment *96*

Pretreatment Records *97*

Storage of Records *98*

Dentolegal and Ethical Issues that may Arise During Treatment Planning *99*

Obtaining Consent *100*

Who is Able to Provide Consent? *102*

Dentolegal Issues Arising During Active Orthodontic Treatment *102*

Transfers *105*

Non-compliance *105*

Non-attendance *105*

Non-payment of Fees *106*

Supervision of Orthodontic Therapists   *106*
Retention   *106*
Relapse   *107*
Duty of Candour   *107*
Responding to a Complaint   *108*
References   *109*

Part II   **The Preadjusted Edgewise Appliance**   *111*

6   **Bracket Design**   *113*

Chris D. Donaldson

The Origins of Fixed Appliance Bracket Design   *113*
   Le Bandeau   *113*
   Appareil de Schangé   *114*
   Edward Angle and his Appliances   *114*
   Begg Appliance   *117*
   Tip-Edge Appliance   *117*
   Further Appliance Improvements   *117*
Preadjusted Edgewise Straight-wire Appliance   *117*
   Andrews Straight-wire Appliance   *118*
Straight-wire Appliance: Bracket Prescriptions   *121*
   Non-customised   *123*
   Semi-customised   *127*
   Fully Customised   *128*
   Optimal Bracket Positioning   *128*
Straight-wire Appliance: Bracket Modifications   *129*
   Bracket Material   *129*
   Slot Dimensions   *132*
   Auxiliary Slots   *132*
   Bracket Base   *132*
   Standard, Auxiliary, Headgear and Lip Bumper Tubes   *133*
   Tie-wings   *133*
   Archwire Ligation   *134*
Acknowledgements   *135*
References   *135*

7   **Bracket Placement**   *137*

Hemendranath V. Shah, Daljit S. Gill, and Farhad B. Naini

Introduction   *137*
Design Features of Preadjusted Edgewise Appliance Brackets   *137*
   Primary Design Features   *138*
   Slot Siting Features   *138*
   Auxiliary Features   *139*
   Convenience Features   *140*
Direct versus Indirect Bonding   *140*
   Advantages of Direct Bonding   *141*
   Disadvantages of Direct Bonding   *141*
   Advantages of Indirect Bonding   *141*
   Disadvantages of Indirect Bonding   *141*

Direct Bonding Technique *141*
　Localising the FA Point *141*
　Measuring the Distance from the Incisal Edge *141*
Indirect Bonding Technique *142*
　Stages of Indirect Bonding *142*
Banding Molars and Premolars *143*
　Separators *143*
　Banding Technique *145*
Tips for Bracket Selection in Certain Situations *145*
References *146*

8　Bonding in Orthodontics *147*

Declan Millett

History *147*
Bonding Procedure *148*
　Bracket Types and Bonding *148*
　Enamel Preparation *148*
　Bonding Process after Enamel Etching *150*
Bonding to Artificial Substrates *151*
Indirect Bonding *151*
Bonding Adhesives *152*
Health Risks Associated with Bonding *154*
　Blue Lights *154*
　Cytotoxicity of Adhesives *154*
Effectiveness of Adhesives *154*
　Factors Affecting Clinical Bond Failure *154*
　Bonding of Orthodontic Brackets *154*
　Rebonding a Debonded Attachment *154*
　Bonding of Molar Tubes *154*
　Effectiveness of the Light-curing Units *155*
Debonding *156*
　Patient Appraisal *156*
　Procedure and Enamel Damage *156*
　Risks *156*
　Tooth Colour Change *156*
　Management of Demineralisation Lesions Post Debond *156*
Bonded Retainers *157*
　Types and Bonding *157*
　Adhesives for Bonding of Fixed Retainers *157*
Additional Uses of Bonding in Orthodontics *158*
Future Possibilities of Orthodontic Bonding *158*
Summary *158*
Acknowledgements *159*
Further Reading *159*
References *159*

9　Debonding *165*

Lucy Davenport-Jones

Introduction *165*
Preparation *166*
Stainless Steel Brackets *166*

Ceramic Brackets *166*
  Polycrystalline Alumina Brackets *167*
  Monocrystalline Alumina Brackets *167*
  Bracket Fracture *167*
Self-ligating Brackets *168*
Lingual Appliances and Bite Turbos *168*
Solvent Use *168*
  Organic Solvents *168*
  Peppermint Oil *168*
Electrothermal Debonding *168*
Laser Debonding *168*
Band Removal *169*
Composite Resin Removal *169*
  Multifluted Tungsten Carbide Bur *169*
  Diamond Finishing Bur *169*
  Scalers *169*
  Lasers *169*
Finishing Techniques *169*
  Enamel *169*
  Composite *170*
  Porcelain *171*
Iatrogenic Damage *171*
  Burns *171*
  Enamel Fractures and Tear-out Injuries *171*
  Pulpal Injury *171*
  Debanding Injuries *171*
Particulates *171*
Conclusions *172*
References *172*

10   Archwires *175*

Leila Khamashta-Ledezma

Introduction *175*
Properties of Archwires *176*
  Stress–Strain Curves and Physical Properties *176*
  Cantilever and Three-point Bending Tests *178*
  Effects of Changing the Diameter or Length of Archwires *178*
  Other Laboratory Tests and Physical Properties *179*
Archwire Shape and Arch Form *179*
Archwire Materials *180*
  Precious Metal Alloys *180*
  Stainless Steel *180*
  Cobalt Chromium *181*
  Nickel Titanium *181*
  Beta-Titanium *184*
Aesthetic Archwires *185*
  Coated Metal Archwires *185*
  Fibre-reinforced Composite Archwires *186*
Fatigue *187*
Corrosion of Metal Alloys *188*
  Types of Corrosion *188*

Clinical Significance of Corrosion *190*

Methods to Reduce Corrosion *190*

Which is the Best Aligning Archwire or Archwire Sequence? *191*

Pain from Initial Archwires *192*

Pharmacological Management *192*

Non-pharmacological Management *193*

Root Resorption from Different Archwires *194*

Is there Evidence that Different Archwires Cause Different Amounts of Root Resorption? *194*

Allergy to Nickel *195*

Pathological Process *195*

Signs and Symptoms and Management *195*

When and How Much Nickel is Released from Appliances? *196*

Allergies to Other Metals *197*

Acknowledgements *197*

References *197*

11 The Use of Auxiliaries in Orthodontics *203*

Andrew T. DiBiase and Jonathan Sandler

Introduction *203*

Anchorage and Space Management *203*

Intermaxillary Traction and the Use of Elastics *203*

Palatal Arches *204*

Lingual Arches and Space Maintainers *205*

Headgear and Extraoral Traction *207*

Class II Correction *208*

Herbst Appliance *209*

Fixed Class II Correctors *211*

Tooth Movement *211*

Nickel Titanium Coil Springs *211*

Closing Loops *212*

Utility and Intrusion Archwires *212*

Sectional Archwires *214*

Torquing Spurs *214*

Hooks *216*

Piggyback Archwires *216*

Ballista Spring *217*

Conclusion *217*

References *218*

12 Optimising Fixed Appliance Treatment with Orthodontic Mini-implants *219*

Richard R. J. Cousley

Introduction *219*

OMI Advantages *220*

Flexible Timing of Anchorage *220*

No Additional Requirements for Patient Compliance *220*

Predictable Treatment Outcomes and Reduced Treatment Times *220*

Enhanced Control of Target Teeth Movements *220*

Effective Anchorage in all Three Dimensions *220*

OMI Disadvantages *220*

OMI Failure *220*

Root/Periodontal Damage *220*

Pain *221*

Perforation of Nasal and Maxillary Sinus Floors *221*

Damage to Neurovascular Tissues *221*

Mini-implant Fracture *221*

Soft Tissue Problems *221*

Mini-implant Migration *221*

Where Does OMI anchorage Come From? *221*

Anchorage Options: Direct Versus Indirect *223*

Key Clinical Steps Involved in OMI Usage with Fixed Appliances *226*

Clinical and Radiographic Planning *226*

Root Divergence *226*

Pre-insertion Preparation *226*

OMI Insertion *226*

Force Application *227*

Explantation *227*

Three-dimensional Anchorage Applications *228*

Anteroposterior Anchorage *228*

Vertical Anchorage *228*

Transverse Anchorage *231*

References *231*

13 Care of Fixed Appliances *235*

Nazan Adali, Daljit S. Gill, and Farhad B. Naini

Introduction *235*

Before Fixed Appliance Treatment *236*

During Fixed Appliance Treatment *237*

Dental Plaque Biofilm Control Methods *238*

Strengthening of the Enamel Surfaces *241*

Dietary Control *244*

Management of Orthodontic Discomfort *244*

After Fixed Appliance Treatment *245*

Conclusions *245*

References *245*

Part III Stages of Treatment with Preadjusted Edgewise Appliances *247*

14 Alignment and Levelling *249*

Farhad B. Naini and Daljit S. Gill

Introduction *249*

Anchorage Requirements and Preparation *250*

Anchorage Reinforcement with Headgear *252*

Arch Form *255*

Tooth Movement with Preadjusted Fixed Appliances *256*

Alignment *257*

Bracket Positioning Variations *258*

Initial Alignment *258*

Choice of Archwire Size and Material *263*

Placement of Lacebacks *264*

Methods of Archwire Ligation *267*

Cinching versus Bend Backs *269*
Step-by-Step Archwire Placement *271*
Archwire Removal *273*
Space Creation and Redistribution *277*
Crossbite Correction *282*
Ectopic and Impacted Canines and Incisors *283*
Impacted Mandibular Second Molars *286*
Intrusion of Overerupted Maxillary Second Molars *286*
Diastema Closure and Frenectomy *287*
Wire Bending *288*
Pain from Initial Archwires *291*
Accelerated Tooth Movement *292*
Levelling *293*
Conclusion *294*
References *294*

15 Controlled Space Closure *297*

Daljit S. Gill and Farhad B. Naini

Introduction *297*
At Completion of Alignment and Levelling *298*
Objectives during Space Closure *298*
Classification of Anchorage *299*
Types of Space Closure *299*
Sliding Mechanics with the Preadjusted Edgewise Appliance *300*
The 0.018-inch versus 0.022-inch Slot *300*
Working Archwires *300*
Method of Force Application *303*
Force Levels *304*
Incorporation of Second Molars *304*
Two-stage Space Closure versus En Masse Retraction *305*
Frictionless Mechanics with the Preadjusted Edgewise Appliance *306*
Generation of Forces *306*
Generation of Moments *307*
Loop Designs *307*
T-Loop *307*
Segmented Arch Mechanics *308*
Monitoring Space Closure *308*
Conclusion *309*
References *309*

16 Finishing *311*

Mohammad Owaise Sharif and Stephen M. Chadwick

Introduction *311*
Aims and Objectives of Orthodontic Treatment *312*
Common Errors Encountered at the Finishing Stages of Treatment *312*
Alignment *312*
Marginal Ridge Discrepancies and Occlusal Contacts *313*
Interproximal Contacts (Spacing) *314*
Centreline (Dental Midline) *314*
Root Angulation *315*
Buccolingual Inclination *316*
Occlusal Relationship and Overjet *317*

Efficient Finishing: the Importance of Diagnosis and Treatment Planning *317*
    Tooth Size Discrepancies *317*
    Bracket Alterations to Maximise the Efficiency of Treatment and Finishing *318*
    Personalisation of Appliances *318*
    Indirect Bonding *318*
    Incisal Edge Recontouring and Interproximal Reduction *318*
Conclusion *318*
References *318*

17   **Retention** *321*

Simon J. Littlewood

Introduction *321*
Historical background *322*
Aetiology of Post-treatment Changes *323*
    Post-treatment Changes due to Relapse *323*
    Post-treatment Changes due to the Ageing Process *323*
    Consent and Retainers *323*
    Third Molars and Relapse *324*
Reducing Relapse During Treatment *324*
Choice of Retainers *324*
Fixed Retainers *324*
    Placement of a Fixed Retainer *325*
    Problems and Complications with Bonded Retainers *326*
    Maintenance of Bonded Retainers *326*
Removable Retainers *327*
    How Often Should they be Worn? *327*
    Adherence with Removable Retainers *327*
    Hawley-type Retainer *327*
    Clear Plastic Retainers *328*
    Positioners *328*
Responsibilities in Retention *329*
    Responsibilities of the Orthodontist *329*
    Responsibility of the Patient *329*
    Responsibility of the General Dentist *329*
Conclusions *329*
Acknowledgements *329*
References *329*

Part IV   **Management of Malocclusions with Preadjusted Edgewise Appliances** *331*

18   **Management of Class II Malocclusions** *333*

Martyn T. Cobourne and Mithran S. Goonewardene

Introduction *333*
Management Options *334*
    Growth Modification *334*
    Orthodontic Camouflage *335*
    Orthodontics and Orthognathic Surgery *336*
Growth Modification *336*
    Removable Functional Appliances *336*
    Fixed Functional Appliances (Class II Correctors) *338*
Orthodontic Camouflage *342*
    Molar Distalisation Strategies *344*

Orthodontics and Orthognathic Surgery *356*
References *356*

19   Management of Class III Malocclusions *359*

Grant T. McIntyre

Introduction *359*
Treatment Timing for Class III Malocclusion in Relation to Facial Growth *360*
Comprehensive, Camouflage or Compromise Treatment for Class III Cases *362*
  Comprehensive Treatment *362*
  Camouflage Treatment *364*
  Compromise Treatment *366*
Managing the Class III Surgical/Orthodontic Patient with Fixed Appliances *366*
  Interceptive Treatment for Surgical/Orthodontic Cases *367*
Class III Malocclusion Occurring with Cleft Lip and/or Palate *370*
References *370*

20   Management of Deep Incisor Overbite *371*

Farhad B. Naini, Daljit S. Gill, and Umberto Garagiola

Introduction *371*
Aetiology *372*
  Skeletal *373*
  Soft Tissue *373*
  Dental *373*
Indications for Treatment *373*
Considerations in Treatment Planning *374*
  Age *374*
  Upper Lip to Maxillary Incisor Relationship *374*
  Incisor Relationship *374*
  Vertical Skeletal Discrepancy *375*
Methods of Overbite Reduction *375*
  Relative Intrusion of the Incisors *375*
  Absolute Intrusion of the Incisors *375*
  Proclination of the Incisors *375*
Appliances and Techniques for Overbite Reduction *376*
  Removable Appliances *376*
  Functional Appliances *376*
  Fixed Appliances (Continuous Arch Mechanics) *377*
  Fixed Appliances (Segmented Arch Mechanics) *378*
  Auxiliaries *380*
  Headgear *380*
  Absolute Anchorage *381*
  Orthognathic Surgery *381*
  Segmental Surgery *381*
  Conservative Management *382*
Stability of Overbite Correction *382*
Conclusion *384*
References *384*

21   **Management of Anterior Open Bite**   *385*

Chung H. Kau and Tim S. Trulove

Introduction   *385*
Prevalence and Incidence   *385*
Aetiology   *385*
    Skeletal Origins   *386*
Characteristics   *388*
    Increased Lower Face Height: Long Face Syndrome   *388*
    Anterior Open Bite   *389*
Clinical Treatment   *389*
    Concepts   *389*
    Primary Dentition/Mixed Dentition   *389*
    Late Mixed Dentition/Early Permanent Dentition   *389*
    Late Permanent Dentition   *390*
Retention and Stability   *394*
Conclusion   *394*
References   *394*

22   **Management of the Transverse Dimension**   *397*

Lucy Davenport-Jones

Introduction   *397*
Crossbites   *398*
Indications for Maxillary Expansion   *398*
Removable Appliances   *399*
    Upper Removable Appliance   *399*
    Coffin Spring   *399*
Functional Appliances   *400*
Aligners   *400*
Fixed Appliances   *400*
    Headgear with Fixed Appliances   *400*
    Archwires and Auxiliaries   *401*
    Transpalatal Arch   *401*
    Lingual Arch/Utility Arch   *401*
    Cross Elastics   *401*
    W-Arch/Porter Appliance   *401*
    Quadhelix (Bihelix/Trihelix)   *403*
    NiTi Expanders   *404*
Mid-Palatal Suture   *404*
    Protraction Headgear   *404*
    Rapid Maxillary Expansion   *405*
Surgical Expansion   *409*
    Surgically Assisted Rapid Palatal Expansion   *409*
    Segmental Maxillary Surgery   *410*
Retention   *411*
References   *411*

Part V   Appendices *413*

Appendix 1   Orthodontic Instruments *415*

Farhad B. Naini and Daljit S. Gill

Appendix 2   Orthodontic Elastics and Elastomeric Materials *423*

Farhad B. Naini and Daljit S. Gill

Introduction *423*
Intraoral Elastic Configurations *423*
   Intra-arch Elastics *423*
   Inter-arch Elastics *423*
Points of Application *424*
Instructions for Use of Intraoral Elastics *424*
Elastomeric Materials *425*
   Elastomeric Modules *425*
   Elastomeric Chain *425*
   Elastomeric Thread/String *425*
   E-links *425*

Index *427*

Preface

'We find that the very principle upon which teeth are made to grow irregularly is capable, if properly directed, of bringing them even again. This principle is the power which many parts (especially bones) have of moving out of the way of mechanical pressure.'

John Hunter (1728–1793), Chapter VI,
Irregularities of the teeth, History of the Human
Teeth *(1771)*

Sustained mechanical pressure will move teeth that are not ankylosed. Needless to say, placing a fixed appliance, ligating an archwire and watching the teeth move over time may appear relatively easy to the uninitiated. However, planned and guided movement of teeth into their ideal aesthetic, functional and stable positions, whilst mitigating the undesirable effects of treatment, and achieving this in a reasonable time frame with minimum patient discomfort, is far from easy.

Dental students and orthodontic trainees in their early years will often observe their teachers assessing a patient's teeth intently, deep in thought. It is no coincidence that orthodontics has long been known as the 'thinking person's specialty', and is, in fact, the first established specialty in dentistry and one of the first throughout medicine. Orthodontics is a complex and multifaceted specialty, requiring, amongst other things, a thorough understanding of normal and aberrant craniofacial growth and development, dentofacial aesthetics and function, and the biomechanical principles and utilisation of a variety of appliances. As such, learning orthodontics requires dedication and hard work – there is no effortless path and no available shortcuts.

Most credible graduate orthodontic specialty training programmes now run over three years full-time (this has been the UK model for many years), or a part-time equivalent. In the UK, those desiring to learn more about multidisciplinary care, orthognathic surgery, and cleft and craniofacial surgery require an additional two years of full-time training and further examinations. First-year graduate trainees in orthodontics often feel like outsiders, overwhelmed by the highly esoteric and technical language being used around them, new concepts and even new instruments. Confusion is the order of the day. It takes sustained effort to assimilate and grasp the significance of all the factors required in orthodontic treatment, particularly with fixed appliances. However, over time, and usually by the middle to the end of the second year, through practice and immersion, the language becomes comprehensible, the concepts understandable, and the invisible connections between the various aspects of orthodontics become visible.

Modern preadjusted edgewise bracket designs can trace their ancestry to the original edgewise appliance, designed by Dr Edward H. Angle, and first introduced on 2 June 1925 at the Fourth Annual Meeting of the Edward Angle Society of Orthodontists. Interestingly, initially Angle did not name the appliance. The term 'edgewise' refers to the archwire, meaning that a rectangular archwire is placed into a horizontal bracket slot via its narrower edge, such that it has a larger buccolingual dimension compared with its occlusogingival dimension. A number of important advances in orthodontics followed; however, from a technical perspective, the next notable advance was the introduction, by Dr Lawrence Andrews, of preadjusted brackets to be used with straight wires. Added to this was the development of the acid-etch bonding technique and its subsequent application in orthodontics, together with developments in archwire materials, all of which have advanced fixed appliance therapy significantly.

Preadjusted edgewise orthodontic appliances provide the clinician with the unique ability to control tooth movement reliably, in the three planes of space and round the three axes of rotation. This three-dimensional control over tooth movement requires expertise, discretionary judgement and finesse, and is subject to misapplication in untrained hands.

Didactic teaching of orthodontics can only be delivered in segments, each of which, metaphorically speaking, is analogous to the fragments of a jigsaw puzzle. No matter in which order the segments are presented to the student, until all the segments have been positioned accurately, the full picture will not be apparent or completely coherent. The purpose of this book is specific: it is to cover comprehensively the information required to understand and use preadjusted edgewise appliances. It is our intention that having read all the chapters in this book, together with practical chairside training, the reader will view the whole picture of preadjusted edgewise fixed appliance treatment with complete clarity.

The book comprises 22 chapters separated into four sections. Although most of the chapters can be read independently, the ideas have been presented in an order chosen with some care. Section I (Principles) covers the principles of treatment planning, orthodontic biomechanics, anchorage, consent and dentolegal considerations. Section II (The Preadjusted Edgewise Appliance) provides an in-depth description of the appliance systems, including bracket design, bracket placement, bonding, debonding, archwires, the use of orthodontic auxiliaries, mini-implants (temporary anchorage devices) and care of fixed appliances. Section III (Stages of Treatment) provides a comprehensive, step-by-step account of the four stages of treatment, with separate chapters on alignment and levelling, controlled space closure, finishing and retention. Section IV (Management of malocclusions) covers the treatment of each major category of malocclusion, with separate chapters on the management of Class II malocclusions, Class III malocclusions, deep bite malocclusions, anterior open bite malocclusions, and malocclusions with transverse problems. The two appendices at the end cover orthodontic instruments and orthodontic elastics.

Many of the authors invited to contribute chapters to this book are internationally renowned leaders in orthodontics. The contributing authors have provided comprehensive and practical chapters, analysing the scientific literature and providing their technical expertise, all complemented with sound judgement. They have described the rationale for their decisions based on up-to-date evidence and long-term clinical experience. The editors' desire is that the chapters in this book will be used by the spectrum of clinicians, from junior trainees through to qualified orthodontists at all levels.

There is a simple rule for clinical practice: excellent clinicians produce consistently excellent results, and 'bad workmen blame their tools'. There is a vast array of bracket designs and fixed appliance systems, and proponents of each extol their virtues whilst trivialising the limitations. This is to be expected in the marketplace, but has no place in a scientifically based clinical endeavour such as orthodontics, where the dominating value is the ability to achieve reliably excellent results for consecutive patients. The development of orthodontic materials and refinements in techniques will no doubt continue, but none will replace sound clinical judgement based on a comprehensive understanding of biological principles, the biomechanical foundations of fixed appliance treatment, and the arduous task of obtaining and cultivating technical ability and thereby gaining legitimate experience. The best clinicians are those who can identify the problems, judge and plan the appropriate treatment together with the patient, and apply selectively the appropriate appliance and mechanics to deal with the patient's presenting problems.

Orthodontics is a beautiful specialty. Unlike most of medicine, our patients do not just need treatment, they desire it, making the ability to undertake orthodontic treatment for patients a distinct privilege.

Farhad B. Naini and Daljit S. Gill

Acknowledgements

The influence of great teachers always remains with their students. We owe a debt of gratitude to our teachers in orthodontics. We were very fortunate to undertake our specialty training at a time when our teachers were at their peak; many were pioneers in the introduction, development and use of preadjusted edgewise appliances in the UK. Most are now retired and some are, sadly, no longer with us, but their influence remains through their students and the continuing excellence of their departments.

Thank you to the staff at the Archives Center, National Museum of American History, Smithsonian Institution, Washington, DC for the superb picture of Dr Edward Angle that appears in the Introduction. Our sincere thanks also to Professor James L. Vaden, Mrs Bonnie Shewairy and the Charles H. Tweed International Foundation for Orthodontic Research and Education for the picture of Dr Charles Tweed, which also appears in the Introduction.

Our sincere thanks to Mr Allan Thom, Professor Roberto Justus and Dr David Birnie for their kindness and help as we were obtaining permission for some of the images used in the book. A special thank you is required to Professor Lee W. Graber and the World Federation of Orthodontists for the picture of Professor Charles Burstone that appears in Chapter 2.

Our thanks also to Dr David Spary, Dr Elif Keser and James Green for a number of images, and to Professor Theodore Eliades for advice on materials. Our sincere thanks to Dr Rob Chate for his advice and kindness, extending over many years. Thank you to Miss Sarah Al-Bitar for her excellence in graphic design and working with her father to create the images in Chapter 3. Our thanks also to Matron Helen Holland and senior orthodontic nurses Janet Barnes and Sonia Steer, and to our trainees, particularly Drs Reem Al-Hadhoud, Serena Amin, Chris Donaldson, Emily Hooper, Georgina Kane, Claudia Lever, Ahmed Omran, Rachel Peacock, Jaya Pindoria and Samuel Reeves for their help in the taking of some of the photographs in this book. Our thanks also extend to Tanya McMullin and the team at Wiley-Blackwell for their support in the development of this book.

Farhad B. Naini and Daljit S. Gill

To my parents and brother, who introduced me to the importance of attempting to understand the world, with gratitude, admiration and love.

As ever, I am indebted to my wife, Hengameh, for her unyielding support. As well as being a graphic designer, Hengameh is a consultant in animal behaviour and welfare and head veterinary nurse in a busy veterinary surgery in Kent, the 'Garden of England'. This book was completed during the time of a global pandemic. During this difficult time, she refused to stay away from work, and worked tirelessly to care for sick, injured and vulnerable animals. Yet, she made time to create the illustrations for my chapters. I am forever humbled by her intellect, compassion and dedication. She demonstrates, every day, that it takes a lot more courage and strength of character to stand against the crowd and show that kindness and compassion to non-human animals, with whom we share this small planet, are far more important than antiquated attitudes, unjustifiable habits and the excuse of 'tradition'. This book would not have been possible without her enthusiasm and commitment.

Farhad B. Naini

There are a great list of people and institutions who I would like to thank, ranging from the National Health Service, which has provided the opportunities and infrastructure to learn orthodontics, Universities and individual people who have inspired me with their teaching, dedication and love for orthodontics, dentistry and medicine. In particular, the late Professor Crispian Scully who was always inspirational, from the time of being a dental student to becoming a Consultant in Orthodontics, because of his prolific nature and his love and dedication towards his profession. My father, Dr Gurmail Gill, who has always given me his wisdom in logical and scientific thought. My mother, Jasvir Gill, who has given love, dedication and a home. I would also like to thank my grandparents, sister (Sumanjit) and friends for their love and guidance, and finally my wife (Balpreet) and my children, Aran and Anika, for their love and support. May they, and all other children, be given the same opportunities that I have been fortunate to have received.

Daljit S. Gill

We are donating the royalties for this book to animal welfare charities chosen by Hengameh Naini.

Contributors

Nazan Adali, MSc, BDS(Hons), BSc, FDS.RCS(Orth), M.Orth.RCS(Eng), MFDS.RCS(Eng), FHEA
Consultant Orthodontist and Cleft Lip and Palate Lead
Maxillofacial Centre
Luton and Dunstable University Hospital NHS Foundation
   Trust
Visiting Postgraduate Lecturer, King's College London
London, UK

Zaid B. Al-Bitar, BDS, MSc, MOrth.RCS (Eng.)
Professor of Orthodontics
Vice Dean for Graduate Affairs
Faculty of Dentistry, University of Jordan
Senior Consultant Orthodontist
University of Jordan Hospital
Amman, Jordan

Stephen M. Chadwick, FDSRCS, MSc, MOrthRCS, MA, FDS(Orth)RCS, FDS(Orth)RCPS
Consultant Orthodontist
Countess of Chester Hospital NHS Foundation Trust
Chester, UK

Martyn T. Cobourne, BDS (Hons), FDS.RCS (Eng.), FDS.RCS (Ed.), MSc, MOrth.RCS (Eng.), FDS.Orth.RCS, PhD, FHEA
Professor and Honorary Consultant in Orthodontics
Academic Head of Orthodontics
Centre for Craniofacial and Regenerative Biology
Faculty of Dental, Oral and Craniofacial Sciences
King's College London
Guy's Hospital
London, UK

Richard R.J. Cousley, BSc, BDS, MSc, FDS, MOrth, FDS(Orth) RCS
Consultant Orthodontist
The Priestgate Clinic, Peterborough and Honorary Consul-
   tant Orthodontist at Peterborough City Hospital
Peterborough, UK

Lucy Davenport-Jones, BDS (Hons), MSc, MFDS.RCS (Edin.), M.Orth.RCS (Edin.), FDS.Orth.RCS (Edin.)
Consultant Orthodontist
St George's University Hospital and Kingston Hospital
Clinical Lead for Dentistry
St George's University Hospital
London, UK

Andrew T. DiBiase, BDS (Hons), FDS.RCS (Eng.), MSc, M.Orth.RCS (Eng.), FDS.Orth.RCS
Consultant Orthodontist
East Kent Hospitals University NHS Foundation Trust
Canterbury, UK

Chris D. Donaldson, MBBS (Lond.), BDS (Lond.), MFDS.RCS (Ire.), MSc (KCL), M.Orth.RCS (Edin.)
Senior Specialist Registrar
Department of Orthodontics
King's College Hospital and St George's Hospital
London, UK

Umberto Garagiola, DDS, PhD
Professor of Orthodontics
Biomedical Surgical and Dental Department
Maxillo-Facial and Odontostomatology Unit
Fondazione Cà Granda IRCCS
Ospedale Maggiore Policlinico
School of Dentistry
University of Milan
Milan, Italy

Daljit S. Gill, BDS (Hons), BSc (Hons), MSc (Lond.), FDS.RCS (Eng.), M.Orth.RCS (Eng.), FDS (Orth) RCS (Eng.), FHEA
Consultant Orthodontist
Department of Orthodontics
Great Ormond Street Hospital NHS Foundation Trust and
   UCLH Eastman Dental Hospital
London, UK

Mithran S. Goonewardene, BDSc(Hons), Cert.Ortho., MMedSc, FICD, FADI, FPFA
Head of Orthodontics
UWA Dental School
Faculty of Health and Medical Sciences
Oral, Developmental and Behavioural Sciences
University of Western Australia
Perth, Australia

Chung H. Kau, BDS, MScD, MBA, PhD, MOrthEdin, FDS-Glas, FDSEdin, FFDIre (Ortho), FICD, FACD, FAMS(Ortho), Cert (Ortho), ABO
Professor and Chairman
Department of Orthodontics
School of Dentistry
University of Alabama
Senior Scientist
Global Center for Craniofacial, Oral and Dental Disorders, University of Alabama
Director
UAB Craniofacial Disorders Clinic in Collaboration with Children's Rehabilitation Services of Alabama, University of Alabama
Birmingham, Alabama, USA

Leila Khamashta-Ledezma, BDS (Lond.), MJDF.RCS (Eng.), MSc (KCL), M.Orth.RCS (Edin.), FDS.Orth.RCS (Edin.), GCAP (KCL), FHEA
Specialist Orthodontist
Wetzikon, Switzerland
Former Consultant Orthodontist
Department of Orthodontics
Guy's and St Thomas' NHS Foundation Trust
London, UK

Simon J. Littlewood, BDS, MDSc, FDS(Orth)RCPS(Glasg), MOrthRCS(Edin), FDSRCS(Eng)
Consultant Orthodontist and Specialty Lead
Orthodontic Department
St Luke's Hospital
Bradford, UK

Gavin J. Mack, BDS (Hons), MSc, MFDS.RCS(Eng), M.Orth.RCS, FDS.Orth.RCS(Eng)
Consultant Orthodontist
Department of Orthodontics
King's College Hospital London
London, UK

Grant T. McIntyre, BDS, FDS.RCPS, M.Orth.RCS, PhD, FDS.Orth.RCPS
Consultant Orthodontist
Professor of Orthodontics
Dundee Dental School and Hospital
Dundee, Scotland

Declan Millett, BDSc, DDS, FDS.RCPS (Glasg.), FDS.RCS (Eng.), DOrth.RCS (Eng.), M.Orth.RCS (Eng.), FHEA
Professor and Head of Orthodontics
Orthodontic Unit
Cork University Dental School and Hospital
University College Cork
Cork, Ireland

Farhad B. Naini, BDS (Lond.), MSc (Lond.), PhD (KCL), FDS.RCS (Eng.), M.Orth.RCS (Eng.), FDS.Orth.RCS (Eng.), GCAP (KCL), FHEA, FDS.RCS.Ed
Consultant Orthodontist
Department of Orthodontics
Kingston Hospital NHS Foundation Trust
St George's University Hospital NHS Foundation Trust
London, UK

Jonathan Sandler, BDS (Hons), MSc, PhD, FDS.RCPS, M.Orth.RCS
Consultant Orthodontist
Chesterfield Royal Hospital
Professor of Orthodontics
University of Sheffield
Sheffield, UK

Hemendranath V. Shah, BDS (Bris), MFDS.RCS(Eng), PG Cert Med Ed (Bris), MOrth.RCS(Ed), DDS (Bris), FDS.Orth.RCS(Eng)
Consultant Orthodontist
Royal Berkshire Hospital NHS Foundation Trust
Reading, UK
Specialist Practitioner
Staines-Upon-Thames and Watford, UK

Mohammad Owaise Sharif, BDS (Hons), MSc (Merit), MJDF.RCS (Eng), MOrth.RCS.Ed, FDS(Orth)RCS (Eng), FHEA
Clinical Lecturer/Honorary Consultant Orthodontist
UCL Eastman Dental Institute
London, UK

Tim S. Trulove, DMD, MS
Adjunct Full Professor
Department of Orthodontics
School of Dentistry
University of Alabama, Birmingham, Alabama, USA
Director, American Board of Orthodontics

Alison Williams, BDS, MSc, PhD, FDS, M.Orth, FDS(Orth) RCS (Eng.), LLM
Specialist Orthodontist
Part-time Clinical Dental Advisor to the General Dental
  Council (UK)
Bank Orthodontic Advisor to the NHS Business Services
  Authority
London, UK

Introduction: What is the Preadjusted Edgewise Appliance?

Farhad B. Naini and Daljit S. Gill

CHAPTER OUTLINE

What Does 'Edgewise' Mean, xxix
What Does 'Preadjusted' Mean, xxxiv
  The Three Orders of Tooth Movement, xxxiv
  The Six Keys to Normal Occlusion, xxxv
  Customisation and Preprogramming of Brackets, xxxvii
  Prescription, xxxviii
  Expression, xxxviii
Preadjusted Edgewise Appliance Components, xxxix
  Brackets, xxxix
  Tubes/Bands, xxxix
  Archwires, xxxix
  Other, xl
Bracket Design Features, xl
  Horizontal Slot, Clearance and Bearing Points, xl
  Tie-wings, xlii
  Stem, xlii
  Base, xlii
  Identification Mark, xlii
  Additional Components, xlii
  Extent of Preadjustment (Preprogramming), xliii
Bracket Positioning, xliii
Stages of Treatment, xliv
Conclusion, xliv
References, xliv

The remit of this book is to describe fixed appliance orthodontic treatment with the preadjusted edgewise appliance. The purpose of this introduction is to set the scene for the book. All the information presented here will be explored in greater depth in the following chapters. Inevitably, the first step is to describe precisely what is meant by a preadjusted edgewise appliance.

What Does 'Edgewise' Mean

Edward Hartley Angle (1855–1930) (Figure 1) is considered to be the pioneer of modern orthodontics, particularly because most modern bracket systems are variations of designs he introduced.[1–4] He had modified the round labial expansion arch of Pierre Fauchard (1678–1761) (Figure 2),

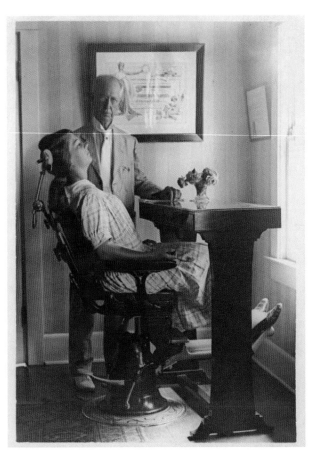

Figure 1 Edward Hartley Angle (1855–1930). Angle was born on 1 June in the town of Herrick, Bradford County, Pennsylvania, USA. His father was of Dutch descent and his mother was born in Ireland. He was the fifth of six children and called 'Hart' by family and friends from a young age. He demonstrated a knack for invention and mechanics from a young age and was gently coaxed towards dentistry at the age of 18 by his mother Isabel, securing an apprenticeship to a local dentist. A few years later he enrolled to study dentistry over two years at the Pennsylvania College of Dental Surgery in Philadelphia. Upon qualifying, he spent three years in dental practice and developed an interest in 'tooth regulation', i.e. the alignment of misplaced teeth, and also in the correction of deformities of the jaws.[1] However, Angle abandoned dentistry due to ill health and chronic respiratory problems (possibly resulting from tuberculosis) and decided to move to a better climate and try his hand at sheep farming in Montana. A blizzard wrecked the ambition for sheep farming and Angle moved to Minneapolis and back to dentistry. By his mid-thirties he was appointed Professor of Orthodontia at the University of Minnesota. He eventually resigned from this and other university positions to concentrate on his practice and the development of *orthodontia* (the term used by Dr Angle throughout his life); in 1892 he announced that he would practice orthodontia solely, thereby becoming the first specialist in what would become dentistry's first specialty. In 1908, having divorced his first wife, Angle married Anna Hopkins (Anna began as Angle's secretary but went on to qualify in dentistry from the University of Iowa), who was to become his closest ally, and moved to New York. Angle popularised the term 'malocclusion', and his classification of malocclusion is still widely used.[2–4] His most enduring contributions were his innovative development of fixed orthodontic appliances and most modern bracket systems are variations of designs he introduced. He created the Angle School of Orthodontia to advance the science and the specialty. In 1922 he began the Angle College of Orthodontia in Pasadena, entirely free of charge for students and patients, with financial support from his grateful alumni. Edward Angle is widely regarded as the pioneer of modern orthodontics. Source: Dr. Edward H. Angle Orthodontics Papers. With kind permission of the Archives Center, National Museum of American History, Smithsonian Institution, © Smithsonian Institution, Washington, DC, 2020.

first described in the early eighteenth century, which evolved through a number of modifications until Angle's **ribbon arch** appliance, described in 1915 (Figure 3). The ribbon arch bracket had a vertical slot. The ribbon archwire was rectangular in cross-section, but with the occlusogingival dimension being longer than the buccolingual. It was formed from gold–platinum and its edges were gently rounded. When the ribbon archwire was seated in the vertical bracket slot, it was held in place by a lock pin. This design was a significant improvement on former designs, but still did not provide the control of root positioning that Angle desired.

A decade later, Angle described the **edgewise arch**, which he believed combined the best features of his former appliances. In a presentation given at the fourth annual meeting of the Edward H. Angle Society of Orthodontists on 2 June 1925, in Berkeley, California, Angle introduced the edgewise arch as 'The Latest and Best in Orthodontic Mechanism'.[5] As with previous appliances, the brackets were all soldered to bands. The vertical slot used with the ribbon arch was reorientated to the horizontal, and placed in the face of the bracket (Figure 4). The initial appliance had two types of brackets. Angle described the **alignment bracket** as his 'Stradivarius', as he felt its form to be extremely efficient (Figure 5).[5] This bracket was intended for use on the incisors and canines only. The other type of brackets, originally designed for use on the premolars, were termed **tie brackets**, but were eventually applied to all the teeth, obviating the need for the alignment brackets (Figure 6). The shape of these tie brackets was very similar to cleats used on sailing vessels for rope fastening. The rectangular slot had its greatest dimension in the horizontal plane. Its height and depth dimensions were 0.022 × 0.028 inches, respectively (Figure 7a). A twin or *Siamese* bracket followed (Figure 7b), which is the precursor to the modern bracket design.

The original **edgewise archwire** was made of gold alloy rolled into a rectangular shape, measuring 0.022 × 0.028 inches (or sometimes 0.022 × 0.025 inches), with squared corners (unlike the ribbon arch, which had rounded corners). The edgewise archwire was named because, unlike the ribbon archwire, it would be seated horizontally with its long dimension being the buccolingual (i.e. rotated by 90° to the orientation it had with the ribbon arch appliance), thereby seating into the bracket slot with its narrower edge, hence the term 'edgewise' (Box 1). It is the edgewise archwire that gave the name to what eventually developed into the **standard edgewise appliance and technique** (Figure 8).[6–9]

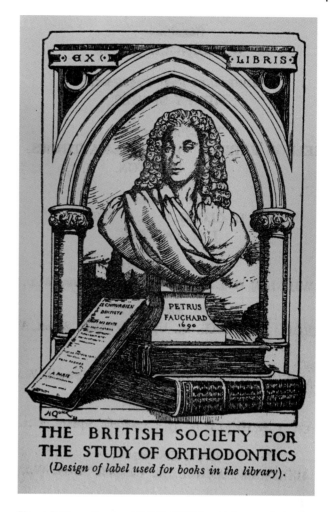

Figure 2 Pierre Fauchard (1678–1761) is widely regarded as the pioneer of modern dentistry. Fauchard was born in a very modest home in Saint-Denis-de-Gastines, in north-western France, in 1678. At the age of 15 he joined the French Royal Navy where he developed an interest in diseases of the mouth and teeth in sailors during long voyages. Once he left the navy he practiced medicine at Angers University Hospital. He described himself as a 'Chirugien Dentiste' (surgical dentist), which was unusual as most dentists at the time just extracted teeth, rather than treating disease. In addition to introducing many instruments and techniques, Fauchard also began to develop appliances to move the teeth (see Chapters 3 and 6). Fauchard eventually moved to Paris and there realised that medical libraries lacked textbooks on dentistry. This prompted his decision to write *Le Chirugien Dentiste*, first published in 1723 and eventually published as two volumes in 1728. The book is regarded as the first complete scientific description of dentistry. The English translation had to wait for over two centuries, eventually being published in 1946. Source: frontispiece to the *Transactions of the British Society for the Study of Orthodontics*, published in 1923. Courtesy of the British Orthodontic Society.

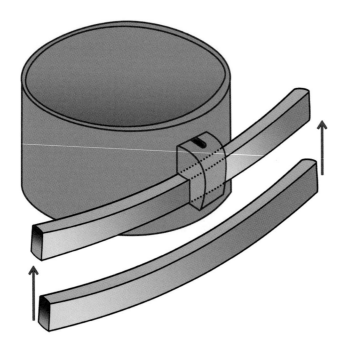

Figure 3 Edward Angle's ribbon arch appliance, described in 1915. The ribbon archwire was rectangular in cross-section, but had its greatest dimension in the vertical (occlusogingival) plane. It had rounded corners. It was named for its resemblance to a decorative ribbon tied round the hair or waist. The ribbon archwire was seated vertically into the bracket slot. The bracket slot had its greatest dimension in the vertical plane. Such ribbon-wise archwires are re-emerging for use in some contemporary lingual orthodontic bracket systems.

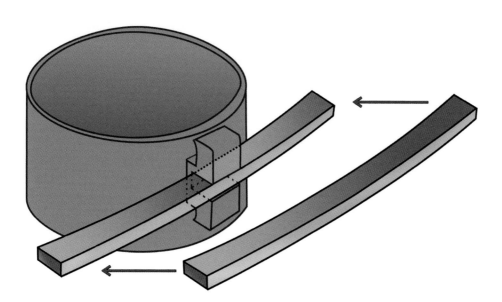

Figure 4 Angle's edgewise arch and bracket. The vertical slot used with the ribbon arch was reorientated to horizontal, and placed in the face of the bracket. This rectangular slot had its greatest dimension in the horizontal plane. Angle turned the ribbon archwire through 90° and inserted it from its narrower edge, i.e. 'edgewise', into the horizontal rectangular slots in the faces of the brackets.

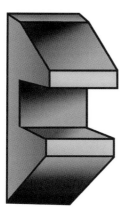

Figure 5 The original alignment bracket was intended for use on the incisors and canines only. Eventually, Angle abandoned these in favour of tie brackets.

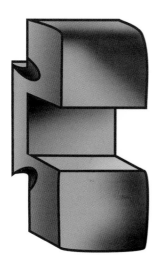

Figure 6 The tie brackets were originally intended for use on the premolar teeth, but eventually became the bracket design of choice for all the teeth. Their shape was very similar to cleats used on sailing vessels for rope fastening.

Box 1 Etymology and Meaning of the Term 'Edgewise'

The term *edgeways* (US *edgewise*) means with the edge forwards or sideways, for example 'we carried the piano in edgeways'. It implies moving forward horizontally in the direction of the edge of the moving object. In the UK, the use of the adjective *edgeways* dates back to 1566, and *edgewise* to 1715. As such, the etymology of the term *edgewise* in relation to orthodontics centres on the use of American English, being an American-derived fixed appliance system, courtesy of Dr Angle. A number of words

that in the UK are considered to be 'English' words that have been Americanised in fact turn out to be early seventeenth-century English words that were in common usage in Britain and which were transported to the then colonies by the Pilgrim Fathers, words such as 'gotten', the 'Fall' and 'sidewalk'. These words remained frozen and unaltered in America, while in Britain they changed to become 'got', 'autumn' and 'pavement', respectively. The same is true for the word 'edgewise'. In the UK, when we say, 'I couldn't get a word in edgeways', the Americans will say 'edgewise'. It signifies through the narrowest gap, or the narrowest edge, i.e. in a rectangular archwire it is the narrow 'edgewise' aspect that faces towards the front of the bracket slot, not the broader 'flatwise' aspect that is perpendicular to it. Hence the names 'edgewise archwire' and eventually 'edgewise fixed appliance'.

In describing his new appliance, Dr Angle wrote[5]:

'It will be noted that the rectangular arch is applied edgewise to the brackets instead of sidewise or flatwise, as in its use in the ribbon arch mechanism. For this reason, it will hereinafter be designated the edgewise arch, to distinguish it from the ribbon arch which also is rectangular in form. Used in this novel manner, the arch is more delicate and graceful in appearance, besides having greater power under certain conditions and far greater elasticity or range of operating force under others, as in widening dental arches, effecting some forms of root movement, tipping teeth into their correct upright axial relations, etc.'

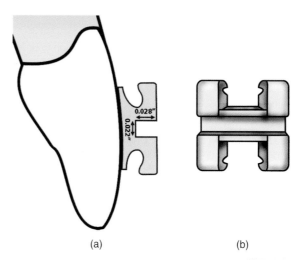

(a)   (b)

Figure 7 (a) The rectangular slot had its greatest dimension in the horizontal plane. Its height and depth dimensions were 0.022 × 0.028 inches, respectively. (b) Twin or Siamese edgewise brackets were like having two adjoining narrow single-width edgewise brackets on one bracket base.

What Does 'Preadjusted' Mean

Angle used the same bracket on all the teeth. Therefore, archwire bends had to be placed in relation to the **three orders of tooth movement**. What does this mean? The three orders of tooth movement and their relationship to archwire bends are described in the following sections.

The Three Orders of Tooth Movement

- **First-order tooth movement**: teeth crowns are of different thicknesses in the buccolingual dimension, therefore horizontal/radial **first-order bends (in–out bends)** were required to compensate for this in the buccolingual dimension.
- **Second-order tooth movement**: teeth tend to have varying degrees of mesiodistal angulation or **tip**, so

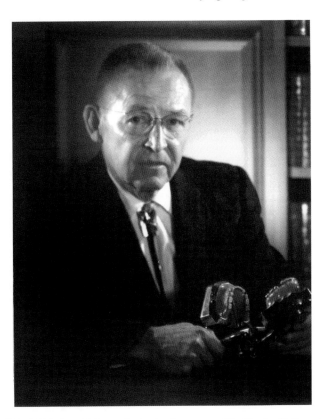

Figure 8 Charles Henry Tweed (1895–1970). In addition to Dr Angle, the name of Dr Charles H. Tweed is the most intimately related to the development of the edgewise appliance. Dr Tweed was born and practiced dentistry in Phoenix, Arizona, before he was accepted to be taught orthodontics by Dr Angle, although his initial training was under a number of Dr Angle's previous students in Pasadena, California.[6] For the last two years of his life, Angle worked closely with Tweed, as he regarded him as one of his best students. Tweed would use the edgewise appliance to treat his patients in his practice in Phoenix and every four months, over a period of two years, would take progress records (and sometimes the patients) to Angle in Pasadena, who acted as the supervisor. It was Angle who advised Tweed that to be proficient in orthodontics and the edgewise appliance, he had to dedicate his life's work to it as a specialist. Dr Tweed duly complied, and his practice in Phoenix was dedicated to orthodontic treatment with the edgewise appliance. The term 'edgewise appliance' rather than just 'edgewise arch' may well have been first used in the personal correspondence between Dr Angle and Dr Tweed. Following the passing of Angle, Tweed continued using the edgewise appliance with Angle's authoritative and inflexible doctrine of non-extraction treatment for all patients. The unquestioned assertion that non-extraction treatment always provides the best aesthetic results was followed by Dr Angle's disciples. However, after about half a decade, Tweed found that a large number of his treated cases presented with dentoalveolar protrusion. He went on to re-treat 300 of his cases that he found to have developed dentoalveolar protrusion with non-extraction treatment, and undertook this second course of treatment with premolar extractions. He found that the aesthetic results improved.[7–9] As such, he realised that some cases required dental extractions to provide the best results and prevent excessive dental protrusion. However, he was met with extreme resistance from the devotees of Dr Angle. Dr Tweed developed one of his most famous phrases at this time: 'Just put your plaster on the table', i.e. let the treatment result speak for itself. As clinicians saw his results, views gradually changed. Dr Tweed brought four important parameters to the fore of the specialty: the importance of facial aesthetics as a defining goal for orthodontic treatment, the importance of the post-treatment stability of the dentition, the health of the periodontium, and the importance of occlusal function. Dr Tweed eventually moved his orthodontic practice to Tucson in Arizona, which is now home to the Charles H. Tweed International Foundation for Orthodontic Research and Education. It is often said that although Dr Angle gave orthodontics the edgewise bracket and archwire, it was Dr Tweed who showed orthodontists how to use it. Source: with kind permission of the Charles H. Tweed International Foundation for Orthodontic Research and Education.

second-order bends had to be placed in the archwire to obtain correct tooth angulation.

- **Third-order tooth movement**: the buccolingual inclination of each tooth had to be correctly achieved, hence **third-order (torquing) bends** were placed in the archwire. The orthodontic use of the term 'torque' (derived from the Latin *torquere*, to twist) refers to a square or rectangular archwire **stressed in torsion** (Figure 9); when engaged in an edgewise bracket, this leads to a change in the inclination of the tooth. As an orthodontic colloquialism or shorthand this is often referred to as 'torquing the tooth', although the torque is in fact the rotational force that is applied to the tooth through the engagement of the archwire and bracket slot.

Therefore, with the standard edgewise appliance, the in–out, tip and torque of the teeth had to be achieved by wire bending and then duplicated or altered in successive archwires. This meant a great deal of wire-bending skill was required with the standard edgewise technique.

In 1952, in an attempt to overcome this problem, Reed Holdaway suggested that in the initial bracket placement, some brackets may be placed angulated by a small degree relative to the standard positioning employed in the standard edgewise appliance set-up in order to reduce the wire bending requirements:[10]

> *'The reason artistic positioning bends are necessary at any time is due to the malposition acquired when brackets are positioned parallel with the long axis of the tooth. … it is just as easy to hook the case up with brackets angulated … and thus eliminate further those arch wire bends in the vertical plane. … If, in conventional bracket placement, it is desirable in the later stages of treatment to place artistic positioning bends to secure an angulation of the teeth which is pleasing, is it not better right from the beginning to have all bracket action gradually align the teeth in correct positions? … through angulation of the edgewise brackets, even though the degree may be slight, many troublesome problems solve themselves. … It is easier to prevent problems by anticipating them in the initial hook-up than to bend arch wires into all sorts of complicated designs to correct them later on.'* [Emphasis added. Note that 'hook-up' refers to the placement of the fixed appliances.]

The Six Keys to Normal Occlusion

However, the next major leap in fixed appliance orthodontic treatment occurred in 1970 when Dr Lawrence F. Andrews developed a new fixed orthodontic appliance with bracket modifications such that *specific brackets were customised for each tooth*.[11] This was based on the analysis of the dental study models of 120 non-orthodontically treated individuals obtained by Andrews from other orthodontists, general dentists, university faculty and students, with 'naturally excellent occlusions' and teeth that were 'straight and pleasing in appearance'.[12] Andrews undertook a detailed study of the relationships and positions of

Figure 9 A rectangular archwire stressed in torsion, i.e. torque has been applied to the archwire.

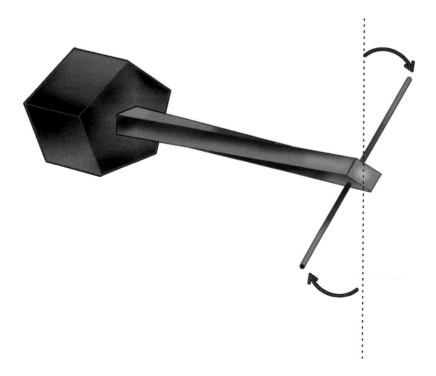

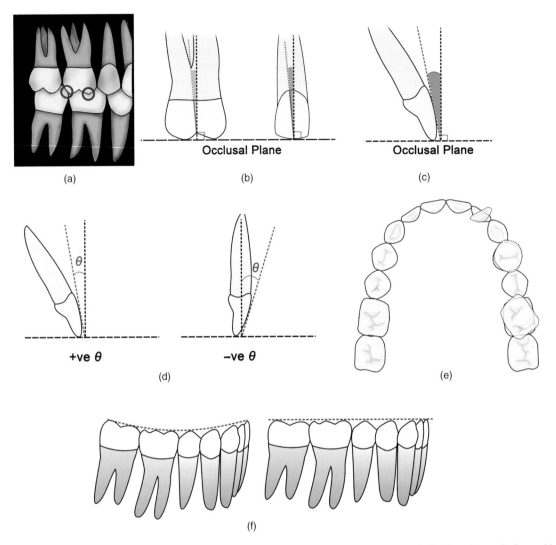

Figure 10 (a) Key I: molar relationship. (b) Key II: crown angulation. Crown angulation or tip was defined as the angle formed by the facial axis (long axis) of the clinical crown and a line perpendicular to the occlusal plane, for all the teeth except the molars. The buccal groove was used as the reference for the long axis of molar teeth. Most of the teeth have a natural mesial angulation of their crowns. (c) Key III: crown inclination. This was defined as the angle between a line perpendicular to the occlusal plane and a line that is parallel and tangential to the long axis of the clinical crown at its midpoint. (d) Crown inclination that is lingual/palatal relative to a perpendicular from the occlusal plane is designated as positive torque. Crown inclination that is labial/buccal relative to a perpendicular from the occlusal plane is designated as negative torque. (e) Key IV: no rotations. Rotation of incisor teeth tends to occupy less space. Rotation of premolar teeth (unless they are very round in shape) and molar teeth tend to occupy more space and may affect normal occlusal relationships. Key V: tight interdental contacts. As demonstrated on the right side of this maxillary occlusal view, if there are no tooth size discrepancies, interdental contact points should be tight, with no interdental spaces. (f) Key VI: the mandibular sagittal occlusal curve (curve of Spee) is measured from the most prominent cusp of the mandibular second molar to the mandibular central incisor crown tip. A relatively flat curve of Spee is required for a normal dental–occlusal relationship.

the tooth crowns in these study models, thereby identifying *consistent characteristics* in them, which prompted his description of the **Six Keys to Normal Occlusion** (in this case, the word 'normal' implies an optimal occlusion).

1. Molar relationship (Figure 10a): the distal surface of the distobuccal cusp of the maxillary first permanent molar occludes with the mesial surface of the mesiobuccal cusp of the mandibular second molar. The mesiobuccal cusp of the maxillary first permanent molar falls within the buccal groove situated between the mesial and middle cusps of the mandibular first permanent molar. The mesiolingual cusp of the maxillary first molar seats in the central fossa of the mandibular first permanent molar.

2. Crown angulation (mesiodistal 'tip') (Figure 10b): the gingival portion of the long axis of each crown is distal

to the occlusal/incisal portion. The degree of this mesial crown tip varies with each tooth type.

3. Crown inclination (labiolingual or buccolingual 'torque') (Figure 10c): crown inclination is the angle formed between a line 90° to the occlusal plane, and a line tangent to the middle of the labial or buccal clinical crown. The long axes of the incisor crowns are labially inclined. In the maxillary arch, there is a relatively constant palatal crown inclination from the canines through to the premolars, slightly increasing with the molars. In the mandibular arch, there is a progressively increasing lingual crown inclination from the canines through to the second molars. If the crown inclination is lingual/palatal relative to a perpendicular from the occlusal plane, it is designated as positive torque (e.g. +7° of torque). If the crown inclination is labial/buccal relative to a perpendicular from the occlusal plane, it is designated as negative torque (e.g. −7° of torque) (Figure 10d).

4. No rotations (Figure 10e).

5. No interdental spaces; there are tight contacts between adjacent teeth (Figure 10e).

6. A relatively flat curve of Spee (Figure 10f).

Customisation and Preprogramming of Brackets

The purpose of the *preprogrammed brackets* and appliance described by Andrews was to eliminate or at least reduce the requirement for complex wire bending in relation to all three orders of tooth movement and to achieve the Six Keys as an end result for the majority of patients.[13–16] As such, varying the bracket thickness compensated for the first-order or **in–out** archwire bends (Figure 11). Additionally, the molar tubes, particularly the second molar tubes, were **offset** to prevent their rotation (Figure 12).

The angulation of the teeth was achieved with **mesiodistal tip** built into the bracket for each tooth by angulation of the slot relative to the long axis of the crown (Figure 13). It should be noted that with many bracket systems, the mesiodistal tip is now built into the angle formed between the lateral edges and the upper and lower edges of brackets, with the slot parallel to the upper and lower edges (Figure 14). The angles are relative to perpendiculars to the occlusal plane.

Finally, the inclination of each tooth was achieved by preprogramming the **buccolingual torque** (i.e. the final buccolingual inclination) of each tooth into its specific bracket. This could be achieved in two ways. If the bracket slot was cut into the bracket face at an angle, such that placing a rectangular archwire would automatically lead to torsional forces to the tooth, this was termed having **torque in the face** of the bracket (Figure 15a). Alternatively, the bracket base could be contoured, such that its placement on the tooth and the subsequent seating of a rectangular

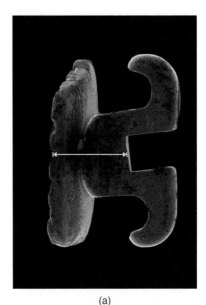

(a)

(b)

Figure 11 (a) In–out bracket thickness. The buccolingual (labiopalatal) thickness of brackets varies from the base of the bracket slot to the posterior aspect of the bracket base, where it meets the enamel surface; effectively, variation in the length of the bracket stem affects the 'in–out' position of the teeth. (b) Brackets with different in–out thicknesses.

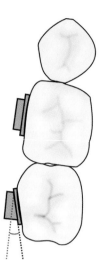

Figure 12 Second molar tube offsets.

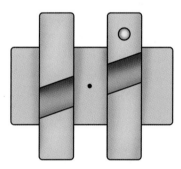

Figure 13 The original Andrews bracket had the mesiodistal crown tip built into the angulation of the slot of each bracket. The central black circle is the slot point, which, if extended lingually, would lie over the facial axis (FA)-point on the enamel surface.

archwire into the slot would automatically place torsional forces onto the tooth; this was termed having **torque in the base** of the bracket (Figure 15b). Andrews favoured the latter approach in his original appliance because it allowed a level slot line-up (Figure 16). However, both methods are employed depending on the manufacturer of contemporary bracket systems, which use CADCAM (computer-aided design and computer-aided manufacturing) systems such that modern brackets may have torque in the base, torque in the face or a combination of the two.

Therefore, the term **preadjusted appliance** means that the in–out, tip and inclination are built into each bracket, rather than having to be bent into the archwire as with the standard edgewise appliance. Andrews named his original preadjusted edgewise appliance the *straight-wire appliance*; in this context, the term 'straight wire' means a length of

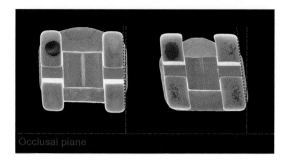

Figure 14 With many modern bracket systems, the tip is now built into the angle formed between the lateral edges and the upper and lower edges, with the slot parallel to the upper and lower edges. The mesiodistal tip angles are relative to perpendiculars to the occlusal plane. The figure demonstrates two brackets with different degrees of mesiodistal tip.

wire in the shape of an approximate dental arch form, but with *no* in–out, tip or torque bends incorporated in the wire itself. This was an idea whose time had come, and which transformed modern fixed appliance orthodontic treatment (Table 1).

Prescription

Inevitably, opinions regarding the ideal amount of tip and torque for each bracket and tooth in each bracket system vary not because Andrews' 120-norms data is incorrect but because compensations need to be placed into the brackets for biomechanical inefficiencies of each appliance in achieving the desired results. The tip and inclination values of the brackets for the individual teeth built into each bracket system are referred to as the appliance's **prescription**. Each appliance prescription is argued to position the teeth with greater precision and improve treatment efficiency, but all are in relation to the positioning of average teeth of average morphology. Additionally, some types of treatment (e.g. extraction versus non-extraction treatment) or some malocclusions (e.g. Class II division 2 malocclusions) may require different degrees of incisor torque to achieve the best results. However, as the morphology of teeth vary from the average, sometimes quite considerably, a variable amount of wire bending is inevitable for some patients, particularly during the final finishing stages of treatment.

Expression

The ability of an archwire engaged in a bracket to express the preprogrammed final position of a tooth in relation to its in–out position, crown tip and crown inclination is referred to as the **expression** of the prescription. For example, clinicians will use the following phrases: 'I need to ligate a full-thickness archwire to express the torque in the maxillary incisors', or 'the mandibular canine tip hasn't been fully expressed', etc.

Table 1 Design features of the Andrews straight-wire appliance (the original preadjusted edgewise appliance).

- Customised brackets for each individual tooth type
- Pre-angulated slots to obtain mesiodistal tooth tip. Brackets could be placed 'squarely' on the crowns of teeth, instead of being angulated. This prevented rocking of the brackets
- Bracket bases were inclined for each tooth type ('torque in the base') to achieve correct tooth inclination or 'torque'. The centre of each slot was at the same height as the middle of the clinical crown
- Bracket bases were compound contoured, i.e. contoured vertically as well as horizontally, to permit good bracket-to-tooth fit and a reproducible location of the bracket slot in relation to the crown. (Standard edgewise brackets were only contoured horizontally)
- The distance from the enamel surface of the bracket base to the base of the bracket slot varied for each tooth, allowing correct in–out requirements
- Accuracy in bracket siting was of paramount importance; if a bracket was not located correctly, the preprogrammed prescription would be proportionally altered. An oft-quoted orthodontic mantra for preadjusted appliance systems, still heard today, is that 'finishing' a case begins the moment brackets are placed
- Wire bending was still possible if required, particularly in the finishing stage of treatment, but the requirement would be far reduced and potentially obviated in many cases
- Each bracket had its own identification feature as to tooth type
- The Six Keys to Normal Occlusion were preprogrammed in the appliance

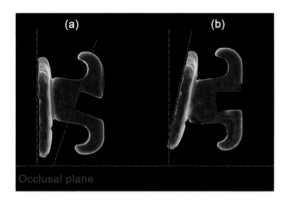

Figure 15 (a) Torque in the face of a bracket. (b) Torque in the base of the bracket.

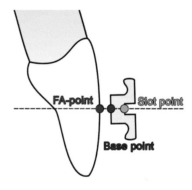

Figure 16 Andrews favoured torque in the base of the bracket as it allowed a level slot line up. The facial axis (FA)-point on the crown surface, the base point of the bracket base and the slot point on the slot base were thereby on the same horizontal plane.

Preadjusted Edgewise Appliance Components

The basic components of preadjusted edgewise appliances are described in the following sections (Figure 17).

Brackets

With the introduction of the acid-etch technique, brackets are now bonded to the labial surface enamel of the teeth in a predetermined position (see following sections). Variations in bracket design, dimensions and prescriptions have resulted in the availability of numerous bracket systems (see Chapter 6).

Tubes/Bands

Tubes may be bonded to the buccal surface of molar teeth, or may be available as an attachment on bands, which are cemented to teeth. The tubes carry the ends of an archwire, and have hooks; some designs can be converted into brackets and additional (double or triple) tubes may be available in some designs, such as headgear tubes on maxillary first permanent molar bands or an auxiliary archwire tube for double archwire techniques (e.g. Burstone and Ricketts mechanics). Bands with brackets may be used for any other tooth if the tooth surface does not allow bonding, for example severe enamel hypoplasia (see Chapter 8).

Archwires

These are available in different materials (e.g. nickel–titanium alloy, titanium–molybdenum alloy, stainless steel, etc.), cross-sectional shapes and sizes (Figure 18) (see Chapter 10). Archwires are either obtained with a preformed arch shape, known as the arch form of the

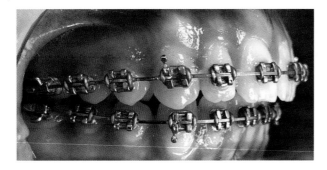

Figure 17 Modern preadjusted edgewise systems predominantly use twin brackets on the incisor, canine and premolar teeth, and either bonded tubes or bands on molar teeth. The upper right lateral incisor bracket has been inverted.

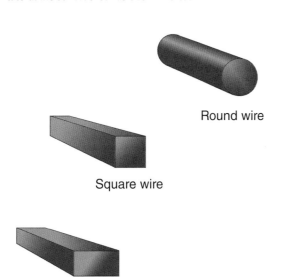

Round wire

Square wire

Rectangle 'edgewise' wire

Figure 18 Archwire cross-sections commonly used with preadjusted edgewise appliances.

archwire, or may be available on a reel, in which case the wire needs to be shaped to the ideal arch form by the clinician. Archwire cross-sectional dimensions in imperial and metric units are shown in Table 14.3.

Other

These include components for placement of the brackets and bands (e.g. bonding agents and cements, respectively), various elastomeric and steel ligatures, crimpable or soldered archwire hooks, elastomeric chains, nickel–titanium space-closing coils, space-maintaining closed coils, separating elastics and intraoral elastics.

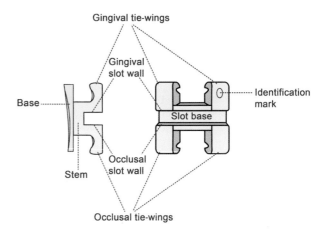

Figure 19 Components of modern preadjusted edgewise brackets. Lateral and frontal view of a maxillary left central incisor bracket is shown.

Bracket Design Features

The basic design of a preadjusted edgewise bracket consists of a number of components, each relevant to the correct functioning of the appliance (Figure 19).

Horizontal Slot, Clearance and Bearing Points

The horizontal slot is rectangular in cross-section and located in the face of the bracket, into which the archwire seats. The **slot base** is the lingual wall of the slot. The slot also has an occlusal and a gingival wall.

An important concept to consider is the **clearance** between an archwire and a bracket slot, sometimes referred to as **play**. Clearance may be defined as the excess space left in a bracket slot when an archwire has been seated. It depends on the relative difference in size between the archwire and the bracket slot, i.e. the larger the archwire dimensions, the less the clearance between the archwire and slot and, thereby, the less play or freedom for the archwire to move in the slot.

A distinction is made between clearance in the first-, second- and third-order. **First-order clearance** is the vertical clearance between an archwire and a bracket slot, measured as the distance between the archwire, when it is resting against the bracket slot's occlusal or gingival wall, and the bracket slot's opposing wall (Figure 20a and Table 2).

Second-order clearance is the angle through which an archwire may be angulated within a bracket slot, relative to the horizontal axis of the slot, before contacting diagonally

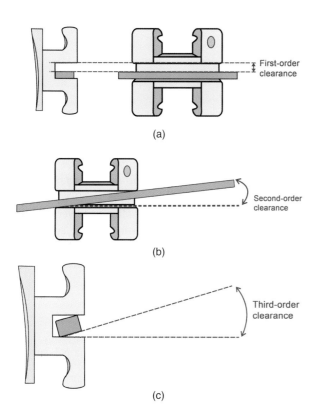

(a)

(b)

(c)

Figure 20 Bracket clearance (play): (a) first-order clearance; (b) second-order clearance; (c) third-order clearance.

Table 2 Vertical clearance between archwires of different dimensions and an 0.022 × 0.028-inch bracket slot.

Archwire dimensions (inches)	Vertical clearance (inches)	Vertical clearance (mm)
Round		
0.012	0.010	0.25
0.014	0.008	0.20
0.016	0.006	0.15
0.018	0.004	0.10
0.020	0.002	0.05
Square		
0.016 × 0.016	0.006	0.15
0.018 × 0.018	0.004	0.10
0.020 × 0.020	0.002	0.05
Rectangular		
0.016 × 0.022	0.006	0.15
0.017 × 0.025	0.005	0.13
0.018 × 0.025	0.004	0.10
0.019 × 0.025	0.003	0.08
0.021 × 0.025	0.001	0.03
0.0215 × 0.028	0.0005	0.01

the most mesial and distal aspects of the occlusal and gingival walls of the slot (Figure 20b). Second-order clearance is also referred to as the **contact angle**, or sometimes as **second-order slop**.

Third-order clearance is the angle through which a square or rectangular archwire may be rotated round its long axis, i.e. 'torque' placed, before its diagonally opposing edges contact the occlusal and gingival walls of the bracket slot (Figure 20c). The third-order clearance angle is sometimes referred to as the **torsional play angle** or, more commonly, as **third-order slop**. For example, there is 7° to just over 10° of torsional play or slop between a 0.019 × 0.025-inch archwire and a 0.022 × 0.028-inch bracket slot,[17] although the amount may be even greater due to manufacturing imprecisions in archwire and bracket slot dimensions.[18] Therefore, the larger the cross-sectional dimensions of a rectangular archwire, the greater its capacity to fully express the bracket's built-in torque.

The points at which an active archwire contacts the bracket slot walls in the second or third order are referred to as **bearing points** (Figure 21). Therefore, the bearing points are the points at which an archwire imparts forces

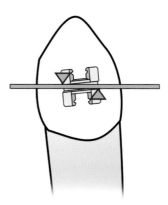

Figure 21 The bearing points are the points at which an archwire transmits forces onto the bracket.

onto the bracket. Increasing the distance between the bearing points reduces the play between the archwire and bracket. For example, the mesiodistal play for a wide twin bracket will be less than a narrower bracket (Figure 22).

The third-order clearance between an archwire and bracket slot indicates how many degrees the archwire must be rotated within the slot before its edges contact the slot's

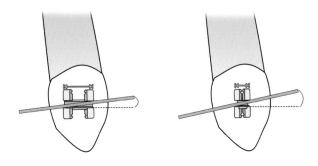

Figure 22 The mesiodistal play for a wide twin bracket will be less than for a narrower bracket.

occlusal and gingival walls, thus enabling it to transmit third-order information to the tooth. The degree of play depends on the slot height and the archwire dimensions and morphology (e.g. bevelling of the archwire edges). However, both bracket slot sizes and archwire dimensions may differ considerably from their manufacturer's stated dimensions. Such imprecisions in manufacture inevitably affect the play between the archwire and slot and therefore the torque expression capacity of an appliance system.[19-23]

Therefore, although the appliance prescription (tip and torque values in each bracket) are very important when choosing an appliance to treat a patient, what is far more important is the individual patient's *response* to the brackets and archwires used. Because of inherent variations in tooth morphology, periodontal response and bone biology, there will inevitably be some variation in response between different patients. *No bracket prescription or appliance system will suit every patient perfectly.* As such, this makes the clinician's observational ability in assessing dental and smile aesthetics of paramount importance,[24, 25] particularly in the finishing stages of treatment. Inevitably, a variable amount of artistic wire-bending may be required for ideal finishing (see Chapters 14 and 16).

Tie-wings

Occlusal and gingival to the slot, the bracket extends to form the tie-wings, round which elastic or steel ligatures may be placed to secure an archwire in position. The most commonly used brackets have four tie-wings, two occlusally and two gingivally positioned, separated by the horizontal slot and a vertical groove or slot in the middle of the bracket. These are known as twin or Siamese brackets. They are useful in permitting partial ligation of severely malaligned teeth. The vertical slot is very useful in the initial placement and positioning of the bracket, as the middle of the vertical slot may be aligned with the long axis of the clinical crown (LACC). An alternative design is referred to as solid brackets, which have only two tie-wings, one

occlusal and one gingival to the horizontal slot, but twin brackets are more commonly used. Another variation is to have three tie-wings, which still permits partial ligation.

Stem

This joins the bracket face, slot and tie-wings to the bracket base. Ideally, the occlusogingival height of the bracket stem should be less than the combined height of the tie-wings; the tie-wings thereby curve over the stem and provide the undercuts required to tie the ligatures used to secure an archwire into the bracket slot. The width of the stem should also be mesiodistally narrower than the bracket base, which permits ligatures to rest against the bracket base and thereby prevents them from resting on the adjacent enamel surface, potentially reducing the risk of enamel demineralisation.

Base

This holds the bracket stem onto the enamel surface. Brackets are usually bonded to the enamel surface, and such bracket bases usually have some form of mechanically retentive base that may interlock with the bonding agent (see Chapter 8). In order for the bracket prescription to work effectively, it is imperative that the bracket base fits onto the enamel surface as precisely as possible. The shape of the bracket base is thereby curved in the vertical and horizontal dimension, which is described as **compound contouring** or **compound curvature**.

Identification Mark

Unlike standard edgewise brackets, which were the same for all the teeth, preadjusted edgewise brackets are individualised for each tooth. Therefore, it is important for the clinician to be able to easily identify each bracket and to orientate it correctly. To facilitate this, most manufacturers place an identification mark, usually on the face of the distogingival tie-wing. Steel brackets may have this mark cast onto the bracket, which is often also painted a specific colour denoting each tooth.

Additional Components

Some brackets will have integrated hooks, which permit the attachment of elastics or active springs. Self-ligating brackets have various designs for engagement of an archwire without the need for other types of ligation (see Chapter 6).

Extent of Preadjustment (Preprogramming)

Some older brackets were only **pre-angulated**, i.e. the bracket slot was angulated relative to the horizontal axis of the bracket and thereby with respect to the plane in which the archwire would seat. Therefore, the mesiodistal (second-order) angulation of the tooth was built into the bracket and would express when a straight wire was engaged. Some brackets were **pre-torqued**, i.e. the bracket slot was rotated round its horizontal axis, relative to the bracket base. Therefore, engagement of a large rectangular or square archwire would provide the pre-programmed buccolingual (third-order) inclination of the tooth. Modern brackets are fully preprogrammed, i.e. they are pre-angulated and pre-torqued and have built-in insets and offsets to accommodate differences in buccolingual crown thicknesses between adjacent teeth.

Bracket Positioning

In order to reach the preprogrammed treatment desti-nation, it is imperative that the brackets are accurately positioned on each tooth crown. This requires an easily identifiable location for siting brackets on the clinical crowns of each tooth. Andrews advised bracket placement at the midpoint of the LACC. The term 'facial axis of the clinical crown' (FACC) is also used (Figure 23).[13–15] This is on the long axis of the crown of a tooth, midway between its mesial and distal surfaces. For molars, the LACC is identified by the dominant vertical mid-buccal groove in the maxillary arch and by the anterior buccal groove in the mandibular arch. It should be noted that the LACC is *not* the same as the long axis of the tooth.

In terms of the vertical position of a bracket on each tooth, Andrews described the long axis (LA)-point, also termed the **facial axis (FA)-point**, which should be at the midpoint of the crown in the vertical dimension, i.e. it is the midpoint of the labial/buccal face of the clinical crown. Andrews explained that trained clinicians can consistently place brackets at the FA-point by eyeballing, as the human eye is good at finding the centre of objects. On positioning brackets, the centre of the bracket slot should overlie the FA-point, with the mesial and distal sides of the bracket parallel with and evenly straddling the LACC. The LACC and FA-points may be marked up on a duplicate set of a patient's dental study models at the chairside prior to bracket placement, which helps guide bracket positioning.

Therefore, in summary, bracket placement consists of placing the vertical guidelines parallel to the LACC and then moving the bracket up and down vertically until the midpoint of the slot is at the same height as the FA-point. As such, the use of bracket positioning gauges as an aid to positioning the brackets was not deemed necessary.

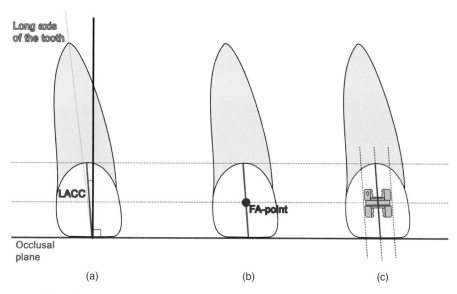

(a) (b) (c)

Figure 23 The facial axis (FA)-point and the long axis of the clinical crown (LACC). A maxillary right central incisor is shown in this example. (a) The LACC is on the long axis of the crown of a tooth, midway between its mesial and distal surfaces. The crowns of teeth tend to have a natural mesial angulation, which varies depending on the tooth. Therefore, the LACC has varying mesial angulation, depending on the tooth in question. The long axis of the tooth (drawn from tip to apex, shown as a dotted green line) does not necessarily correspond to the LACC. (b) The FA-point should be at the midpoint of the crown in the vertical dimension, i.e. it is the midpoint of the labial/buccal face of the clinical crown. The LACC is shown (purple line). (c) On positioning brackets, the centre of the bracket slot (slot point) should overlie the FA-point, with the mesial and distal sides of the bracket parallel with and evenly straddling the LACC.

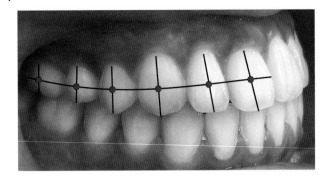

Figure 24 Andrews plane. Assuming a level sagittal occlusal curve (relatively flat curve of Spee), the Andrews plane is an imaginary plane that would intersect the crowns of correctly positioned teeth at the FA-points (red circles), separating the occlusal and gingival portions of each crown. The LACC of each maxillary tooth on the right side are also shown.

However, it should be noted that some contemporary bracket systems judge vertical bracket position relative to the incisal/occlusal edge of teeth and, as such, bracket positioning gauges may be used with these systems by some clinicians (see Chapter 7).

Andrews also described an imaginary plane, the **Andrews plane**, which, assuming no curve of Spee, would intersect the crowns of properly positioned teeth at their FA-points, separating the occlusal and gingival portions of each crown (Figure 24). As such, at the end of successful treatment, the bracket slots should form a straight line (along the Andrews plane), in which an unbent rectangular archwire could be placed without bends or torsion, or, if already in place, it would be passive.

Stages of Treatment

After diagnosis and treatment planning, the approximately successive stages of treatment with preadjusted edgewise appliances include:

- alignment and levelling
- controlled space closure
- finishing
- retention.

These are described in detail in the successive chapters in Section III.

Conclusion

As mentioned previously, the purpose of this introduction is to provide a brief overview of the preadjusted edgewise appliance. This information will be covered in detail in the following chapters.

References

1 Naini FB. Historical evolution of orthognathic surgery. In: Naini FB, Gill DS (eds). *Orthognathic Surgery: Principles, Planning and Practice*. Oxford: Wiley Blackwell, 2017.

2 Hahn GW. Orthodontic profiles: Edward Hartley Angle (1855–1930). *Am. J. Orthod.* 1965;51:529–535.

3 Peck S. A biographical portrait of Edward Hartley Angle, the first specialist in orthodontics. Part 1. *Angle Orthod.* 2009;79:1021–1027.

4 Peck S. A biographical portrait of Edward Hartley Angle, the first specialist in orthodontics. Part 2. *Angle Orthod.* 2009;79:1028–1033.

5 Angle EH. The latest and best in orthodontic mechanisms. *Dent. Cosmos* 1928;70:1143–1158.

6 Vaden JL. Charles H. Tweed, 1895–1970. *Am. J. Orthod. Dentofacial Orthop.* 2015;147:S171–S179.

7 Tweed CH. Indications for the extraction of teeth in orthodontic procedures. *Am. J. Orthod. Oral Surg.* 1944;30:405–428.

8 Brandt S. JPO interviews Dr Charles H. *Tweed. J. Pract. Orthod.* 1967;1:142–148.

9 Brandt S. JPO interviews Dr Charles H. *Tweed. J. Pract. Orthod.* 1968;2:11–19.

10 Holdaway RA. Bracket angulation as applied to the edgewise appliance. *Angle Orthod.* 1952;22:227–236.

11 Andrews LF. *The straight-wire appliance concept. Bull. Pacific Coast Soc.* Orthodont. 1970.

12 Andrews LF. The six keys to normal occlusion. *Am. J. Orthod.* 1972;62:296–309.

13 Andrews LF. *The Straight-Wire Appliance: Syllabus of Philosophy and Techniques (revised edn)*. San Diego, CA: Lawrence F. Andrews, 1975.

14 Andrews LF. The straight-wire appliance, origin, controversy, commentary. *J. Clin. Orthod.* 1976;10:99–114.

15 Andrews LF. The straight-wire appliance. *Explained and compared. J. Clin. Orthod.* 1976;10:174–195.

16 Andrews LF. *Straight Wire: The Concept and Appliance*. San Diego, CA: LA Wells, 1989.

17 Meyer M, Nelson G. Preadjusted edgewise appliances: theory and practice. *Am. J. Orthod.* 1978;73:485–498.

18 Dalstra M, Eriksen H, Bergamini C, Melsen B. Actual versus theoretical torsional play in conventional and self-ligating bracket systems. *J. Orthod.* 2015;42:103–113.

19 Kusy RP. A review of contemporary archwires: their proprieties and characteristics. *Angle Orthod.* 1997;67:197–208.

20 Sifakakis I, Pandis N, Makou M, et al. Torque expression of 0.018 and 0.022 inch conventional brackets. *Eur. J. Orthod.* 2013;35:610–614.

21 Meling TR, Ødegaard J. On the variability of cross-sectional dimensions and torsional properties of rectangular nickel-titanium arch wires. *Am. J. Orthod. Dentofacial Orthop.* 1998;113:546–557.

22 Cash AC, Good SA, Curtis RV, McDonald F. An evaluation of slot size in orthodontic brackets: are standards as expected? *Angle Orthod.* 2004;74:450–453.

23 Arreghini A, Lombardo L, Mollica F, Siciliani G. Torque expression capacity of 0.018 and 0.022 bracket slots by changing archwire materials and cross section. *Prog. Orthod.* 2014;15:53.

24 Naini FB, Gill DS. Smile aesthetics. In: *Naini FB. Facial Aesthetics: Concepts and Clinical Diagnosis.* Oxford: Wiley Blackwell, 2011.

25 Naini FB, Gill DS. Dentogingival aesthetics. In: *Naini FB. Facial Aesthetics: Concepts and Clinical Diagnosis.* Oxford: Wiley Blackwell, 2011.

Section I

Principles

1

Principles of Treatment Planning

Farhad B. Naini and Daljit S. Gill

CHAPTER OUTLINE

Introduction, 3
Patient Concerns, 4
Patient Motivation and Compliance, 4
Handling Patient Expectations, 4
Medical History, 6
General Dental Health, 6
Previous Orthodontic Treatment, 7
Treatment Timing: When Should Treatment be Undertaken?, 7
  Teasing and Bullying, 7
  Dental Health Problems and Habits, 8
  Relevance of Growth and Growth Estimation, 8
Problem List, 9
Treatment Aims, 11
  Aesthetic-Centred versus Occlusion-Centred Planning, 11
  Static and Functional Occlusion, Stability and Health, 13
Presenting the Treatment Options, 14
  No Treatment, 15
  Treatment with Limited Objectives, 15
  Orthodontics Alone, 15
  Orthodontics in Association with Multidisciplinary Care, 15
How do we decide whether or not to Extract Teeth?, 15
Space Analysis and Space Planning, 17
Informed Consent, 21
What Should be Included in a Treatment Plan, 23
Treatment Mechanics, 23
References, 26

Introduction

Comprehensive clinical diagnosis of the craniofacial complex and the analysis of diagnostic records have been described elsewhere (presented in detail in *Facial Aesthetics: Concepts and Clinical Diagnosis* and chapters 5 and 6 of *Orthognathic Surgery: Principles, Planning and Practice*).[1,2] The reader is directed to these sources for the required systematic clinical evaluation leading to clinical diagnosis, which is beyond the scope of this chapter. The purpose of this chapter is to describe the principles of treatment planning for orthodontic patients, specifically in relation to preadjusted edgewise appliances.

There are numerous skills that a clinician embarking on fixed appliance orthodontic treatment must acquire, including diagnosis, treatment planning, technical expertise in the use of a variety of removable, functional and fixed appliances, and an understanding of multidisciplinary care. Of these skills, competence in logical treatment planning is often the most difficult and the slowest to acquire as it requires judgement as well as skill.

A methodical approach to the collection and analysis of information from the patient interview and clinical evaluation is the precondition to successful treatment planning. The treatment planning process follows a logical sequence, from clinical diagnosis through to the synthesis of the definitive treatment plan and the proposed sequencing of mechanics required to accomplish the plan (Figure 1.1).

Patient Concerns

The most important question to have answered from the patient interview is to elicit the patient's actual concern(s). This becomes fraught with potential misunderstandings due to either the clinician misinterpreting the patient's terminology, or patients misusing clinical terminology, both carrying the risk of not addressing the patient's actual concerns. For example, a patient may complain of 'the space between my teeth' and present with a maxillary dental midline diastema of 3 mm and a 10 mm anterior open bite. Without accurate questioning, it would be easy enough for the clinician to misinterpret the patient's concern to mean their open bite, even though the patient's only concern may be their diastema. Therefore, an initial open question, such as 'What are your concerns?' may be followed by specific closed questions such as 'Which space are you referring to?'

Younger patients may use contemporary colloquialisms, such as describing a significant Class II division 1 incisor relationship as having 'goofy teeth', whether due to prominent or proclined maxillary incisors or normally positioned maxillary incisors on a Class II skeletal pattern with mandibular retrognathia. Alternatively, the term 'wonky' may be used by patients to describe dental crowding, rotations, crossbites or even spacing. The patient's exact meaning should be deciphered. Adult patients may use more descriptive terminology but with a different perception of the word from its clinical meaning, for example patients often use the term 'overbite' when they mean incisor overjet.

With children, it is also important to ascertain whether the patient's concerns match those of their parents. This is also true of adult patients presenting with their partners or family members. Where concerns differ, this should be explored and discussed further, and will be particularly relevant when obtaining consent.

The referring dentist's concerns are also part of the equation. It is important to ascertain whether the impetus for the referral was from the patient, or whether the dentist felt that treatment was required; the patient-driven referral may mean a greater degree of motivation and cooperation with proposed treatment, whereas the dentist-instigated referral may be an issue in terms of patient motivation for treatment that potentially they did not desire.

Patient Motivation and Compliance

The patient's motivation for treatment is invariably correlated with their potential compliance with proposed treatment. Asking a patient to rate their level of distress regarding their presenting malocclusion on a scale from 0 (no concern) to 10 (extreme concern) may be a useful starting point. It is important to ascertain whether their concern is primarily aesthetic, functional, or both. It is also important to ascertain whether a patient demonstrates **external (extrinsic) motivation**, when the motivation is from the urging of others or based on unrealistic expectations of the impact of the treatment result on their external life and circumstances (e.g. the desire to obtain a promotion or find a partner), or **internal (intrinsic) motivation**, i.e. the desire for an improved dentofacial appearance or occlusal function, or both, because of the patient's own desire for treatment. Externally motivated patients are less likely to be happy with the results of treatment, regardless of the quality of the result.

The dental health and aesthetic components of the Index of Orthodontic Treatment Need (IOTN) may be useful for patient and parent counselling, particularly when they present with excessive concerns regarding minor aesthetic or occlusal discrepancies.[3]

If a patient persistently focuses on a minor or potentially imperceptible 'deformity' and their level of dissatisfaction and concomitant anxiety exceeds what would be considered justifiable, both socially and clinically, the patient may have a **body image disorder**, such as body dysmorphic disorder (BDD).[4] In such circumstances, the patient should be informed in a polite and straightforward manner that they may benefit from a consultation with an appropriately trained clinical psychologist or liaison psychiatrist.

Handling Patient Expectations

Socially well-adjusted patients with relatively stable lives and realistic expectations are likely to benefit from treatment. This relates to the attitudes of adult patients and to those of young patients *and* their parents. Patients, or parents, with unrealistic expectations, in terms of both the potential aesthetic treatment results and the potential effects of treatment on their life (e.g. the assumption that they will get a promotion if their teeth are aligned, or that their child will win a talent show) will inevitably be unhappy with the results of treatment.

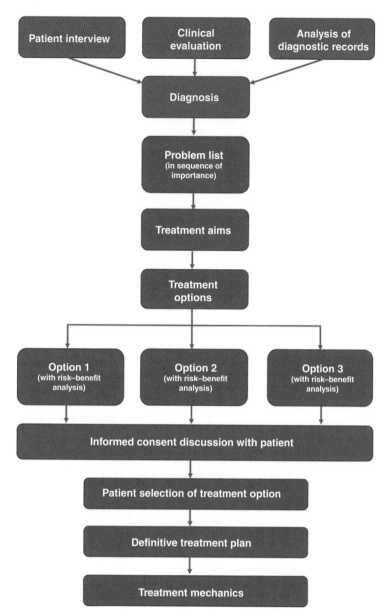

Figure 1.1 Algorithm for devising a definitive treatment plan. The adage 'If you don't know what's wrong, you can't fix it' is rather apt in this context. If the 'knowing what is wrong' applies to clinical diagnosis, the strategy of 'how to fix it' is the purpose of treatment planning. Clinical diagnosis involves the collection of factual information based on the patient interview, a methodical, accurate and thorough clinical evaluation of dentofacial aesthetics and dental-occlusal function, and the analysis of the diagnostic records (shown in green). Unlike diagnosis, which is essentially a fact-finding procedure, treatment planning requires judgement, as not every plan will be ideal for every patient. Even a set of identical twins may choose different treatment options for the same problem, and each may well be right depending on their reasoning. Once the clinical diagnosis has been reached, the first formal step in the treatment planning process following this is the development of a **problem list**. In reality, at this stage there may be two problem lists. The first is simply an ordered list of the presenting problems that are a concern for the patient, in order of what is most important for the patient to what is least important. The second is a logically sequenced list based on factors identified by the diagnosing clinician as needing to be dealt with in the treatment plan. Ideally the two lists should tally; when discrepancies exist, it is important to discuss the reasons why until a consensus is reached. Having established the ordered problem list, the next stage is to identify the **treatment aims** (what the patient and clinician would like to achieve). When the aims of treatment have been determined, the next step is to decide on the available **treatment options** that may be presented to the patient for their consideration, together with a jargon-free discussion of the risk/cost/harm versus benefit analysis of each option. This forms the **informed consent discussion** with the patient, following which they should be given time to contemplate the information provided so that they can select their preferred option, which becomes the **definitive treatment plan**. The final stage of treatment planning involves the formation of a step-by-step (i.e. visit-by-visit) list of the **treatment mechanics**, i.e. what will be done at each visit (bearing in mind that some changes are inevitable), and with what mechanics these movements will be achieved, including the archwire placed and the required mechanics to provide the desired tooth movements.

Clinicians should never over-promise a result, or downplay the length of treatment or its potential complications (e.g. root resorption, decalcification, pulp devitalisation, fenestration or dehiscence of alveolar cortical plates, alveolar bone loss, ankylosis), or social costs, i.e. the inconveniences and sacrifices required of the patient in undergoing treatment. Patients must understand their role in treatment progress. Lack of patient cooperation, whether in maintaining oral hygiene, keeping appointments or wearing elastics as instructed, is likely to lead to unsuccessful treatment.

Medical History

A thorough medical history is mandatory. Standardised self-administered questionnaires may be helpful in encouraging more truthful responses to sensitive questions. Patients may complete such a questionnaire prior to their consultation, but the responses should be double-checked by the clinician.

The majority of patients presenting for orthodontic treatment are fit and healthy. However, certain medical conditions may affect the provision and outcome of orthodontic treatment. When previously diagnosed, a history of allergies or allergic reactions must always be ascertained prior to instigating treatment. Patients with type IV delayed hypersensitivity reactions to nickel may require nickel-free brackets and archwires. For patients with type I immediate natural rubber latex allergies, latex gloves or elastics must be avoided. Many manufacturers now avoid latex in such products for all patients.

Patients at risk of developing infective endocarditis no longer require antibiotic prophylaxis.[5] However, an excellent level of pretreatment oral hygiene, and its maintenance throughout treatment, is even more important in such patients, to reduce the potential for bacteraemia. It may also be better to use bonded molar tubes rather than bands, to aid in the maintenance of optimal oral hygiene.

Removable appliances, particularly those made of acrylic, are contraindicated in patients with poorly controlled grand mal epilepsy, to avoid their potential fracture during a seizure and subsequent aerodigestive injury, swallowing or inhalation. Headgear is also contraindicated in these patients due to the risk of eye or facial injury.

Adult orthodontics is now far more common and adults may present with more complicated medical histories or on multiple medications. The use of bisphosphonates for osteoporosis has become commonplace, and as well as the potential obviation of dental extractions, such medications may affect orthodontic tooth movement through suppression of osteoclastic activity.

Another category that may have added difficulties for clinicians is **special needs orthodontics**. Some patients may have practical physical problems making access more demanding, for example patients with spinal abnormalities, such as scoliosis, may find it difficult to lie flat in a dental chair for an extended period of time, and patients with cerebral palsy may lack the manual dexterity required for maintenance of oral hygiene or placement of orthodontic elastics. However, such potential difficulties are not valid reasons to withhold treatment that would otherwise be beneficial for a patient. Nowhere is this more true than in the management of patients with Down syndrome or those on the autistic spectrum. The most important quality for a clinician undertaking special needs orthodontics is patience. Each patient should be given time to get used to the clinical team and the clinical environment. Parents and carers are also invaluable, and a team approach is required. When trust develops, special needs patients, even those who initially may not even sit in the dental chair, can be excellent and compliant patients. There is very little to compare with the satisfaction of achieving a good orthodontic result and thereby improving the quality of life for special needs patients.

The treatment of special needs patients may require some common-sense modifications of the average appointment, the most obvious being to book longer appointments in order not to rush a patient getting used to the team and the environment. It is also useful for the clinical staff to wear clear masks (Figure 1.2), which negates some of the problems with communication during appointments for patients on the autistic spectrum and those with learning difficulties, and makes it easier for patients with hearing loss as they can still lip read and see facial expressions.

General Dental Health

A high standard of oral and dental health is a prerequisite for fixed appliance orthodontic treatment. Poor oral hygiene increases the risk of gingivitis and periodontal problems, and a high frequency of sugar in the diet can lead to enamel decalcification around the fixed appliance brackets. Consumption of acidic drinks, particularly those with high sugar levels, will have erosive effects on the enamel.

Insufficient improvement in oral hygiene prior to treatment after appropriate oral health education in an otherwise competent patient is usually a reliable indicator of poor compliance with orthodontic treatment.

A patient's past dental history may be relevant to future behaviour.[6] Patients who regularly attend their dentist and

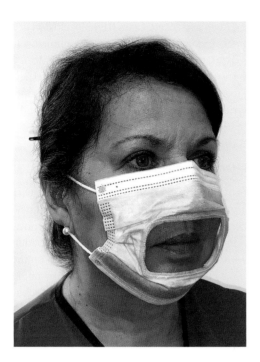

Figure 1.2 Clear masks negate some of the problems with communication during appointments for patients on the autistic spectrum and those with learning difficulties, and makes it easier for patients with hearing loss as they can still lip-read and see facial expressions.

act on advice regarding oral hygiene and diet are more likely to comply with orthodontic treatment. Casual attenders to their dentist may have poor compliance with subsequent orthodontic treatment. However, a high dental caries rate and a heavily restored dentition, even in good attenders, is a cause for concern. Patients who ignore their dentist's advice, such as reducing the frequency of sugar intake, are also likely to ignore their orthodontist's instructions during treatment.

Patients with high levels of anxiety about dental treatment may find complex prolonged orthodontic treatment difficult. It may be better to delay complex orthodontic treatment until overall dental anxiety has been reduced using techniques such as systematic desensitisation. This will make future orthodontic treatment easier for the patient and the clinician.

A history of previous dental trauma should always be taken, even if such trauma occurred years previously. Evidence of previous trauma is not always evident on clinical examination, but such teeth may be at greater risk of pulpal necrosis or root resorption with fixed appliance orthodontic treatment. Pretreatment radiographs should always be checked for signs of caries, alveolar bone loss, and short, blunt or thin root morphology which may be a risk factor for root resorption.

Previous Orthodontic Treatment

A history of previous orthodontic treatment may be a useful guide to potential patient cooperation with treatment. Failure to complete previous treatment with another clinician, particularly in teenage patients when the referral is instigated by the parents, is likely to result in continued lack of cooperation from the patient. Alternatively, adult patients often attend, having failed to cooperate with orthodontic treatment in their teenage years. These patients may well be motivated and cooperate with treatment. However, a full discussion of what is realistically achievable is required, for example if the teenage failed treatment was with functional appliances. Adults may also seek treatment for relapse following poor retainer wear, where previous orthodontic treatment was successful. The implications of prolonged retainer wear must be explored at length, as a second course of treatment is again likely to be unstable without long-term retention.

Another potential complication of previous treatment includes previous dental extractions, when the extraction space has been closed or otherwise lost, and where space is now required to correct the presenting malocclusion. In such situations, further dental extractions may not be possible, and alternative methods of space creation may be required (see later sections on teeth extraction and space analysis). A second course of fixed appliance orthodontic treatment may also increase the risk of root resorption.

Treatment Timing: When Should Treatment be Undertaken?

Teasing and Bullying

The psychosocial importance of dentofacial appearance cannot be underestimated.[7] Difficulties can arise for patients if they desire treatment when they are not yet at the right age to obtain treatment. Desire for orthodontic treatment may arise in early adolescence, often as a result of negative comments, teasing or bullying in the school environment.

The bully attempts to harm or intimidate their victim, often repeatedly, and physical appearance is one of the main targets for teasing and bullying. Unfortunately, bullying has not reduced, despite purported social progress. If anything, the now commonplace use of social media for schoolchildren (and adults) has given rise to a new and potentially more pervasive source of bullying with mass online teasing and victimisation. Prolonged exposure to bullying may lead to anxiety, depression, low self-esteem and even suicidality, particularly in more vulnerable adolescents.[8]

A cross-sectional study of adolescents aged 10–14 years attending UK hospital orthodontic departments for potential orthodontic treatment found the prevalence of bullying to be nearly 13%.[9] Being bullied was significantly associated with a Class II division 1 incisor relationship, increased overjet, and a high need for orthodontic treatment assessed using the Aesthetic Component of the IOTN. Bullied participants also reported lower levels of social competence, physical appearance-related self-esteem and general self-esteem, and higher levels of oral symptoms, functional limitations, emotional and social impact from their oral condition, resulting in a negative impact on overall oral health-related quality of life (OHRQoL). A follow-up study to measure the self-reported frequency and severity of bullying in these patients, after they had commenced interceptive orthodontic treatment, found that undergoing orthodontic treatment may in itself have a positive effect on adolescents experiencing bullying related to their malocclusion and their OHRQoL.[10]

Another study assessed 920 children from randomly selected schools and in the school environment, investigating the experience of bullying in a representative sample of Jordanian schoolchildren.[11] The prevalence of bullying was found to be 47%, with the percentage subjected to name-calling nearly 41%. A significantly greater proportion of victims of bullying reported playing truant from school and disliking school compared with those who were not bullied. Teeth were the number one feature targeted for bullying, followed by strength and weight. The three most commonly reported dentofacial features targeted by bullies were spacing between the teeth or missing teeth, shape or colour of the teeth, and prominent maxillary incisors.

When viewed from the broad context of overall psychosocial and emotional development, visually obvious dentofacial traits, such as prominent maxillary incisors, and the negative response of others to them, may be viewed as **handicapping malocclusions**,[12] as the malocclusion may markedly restrict the individual's ability to function socially, as well as physically (the term 'handicapping' should not be used in the presence of patients, for obvious reasons). Therefore, these can significantly affect psychosocial and emotional development, and social interaction, particularly of more vulnerable children. The relevance of the stage of dental development to issues related to handicapping malocclusions is an important consideration. Some patients may benefit from early interceptive treatment, for example to retrocline maxillary incisors or align impacted maxillary incisors, and where such treatment is deemed appropriate, and in the patient's best interest, it should be carried out. However, occasionally active treatment cannot be undertaken despite the patient's concerns, such as a severe Class III malocclusion in a growing patient. In such circumstances, the clinician may act somewhat akin to a counsellor. Explaining to a patient that future treatment is available may in itself help the patient to cope, and sometimes upper arch alignment may be undertaken earlier, if deemed appropriate and helpful for the patient.

Dental Health Problems and Habits

As already described, orthodontic treatment with fixed appliances should not be undertaken until oral health has been achieved and oral hygiene is optimal. The only potential caveat is the treatment of special needs patients and those with learning difficulties if achieving optimal oral hygiene may not be possible, but the patient would benefit from some form of orthodontic treatment, albeit with limited objectives. In such situations, the clinician should work closely with parents/carers and ideally an experienced dental hygienist, in order to carry out treatment in the best interests of the patient. Concerted pretreatment efforts and continuous attempts during treatment should be made to improve oral hygiene and treatment duration kept as short as reasonably achievable.

Digit sucking habits should ideally have stopped by the primary dentition stage at least, and is often followed by spontaneous reduction in the severity of a resulting malocclusion. A digit sucking habit that has continued into the permanent dentition stage must cease prior to fixed appliance treatment. These habits can be difficult to give up as they provide comfort, particularly at night. As such, if all else fails, a fixed thumb guard may be fitted for approximately six months prior to instigating fixed appliance treatment (see Chapter 11, Figures 11.7 and 11.8). Nail biting habits can potentiate orthodontically induced root resorption and should also cease prior to active treatment.

Relevance of Growth and Growth Estimation

Prior to fixed appliance treatment, some patients may benefit from functional and dentofacial orthopaedic appliances, which are growth-dependent and ideally should be timed to coincide with the maximal pubertal growth spurt (Figure 1.3). For most patients, simple questions about potentially recent rapid growth in height, an increase in size of clothes and shoes, and standing height compared to siblings and parents provide an idea of their likely position on the growth curve. Alternatively, this may be achieved by plotting standing height measurements on a gender-specific **growth chart**, or by using the **cervical vertebral maturation (CVM) method**, which involves examining the patient's lateral cephalometric radiograph

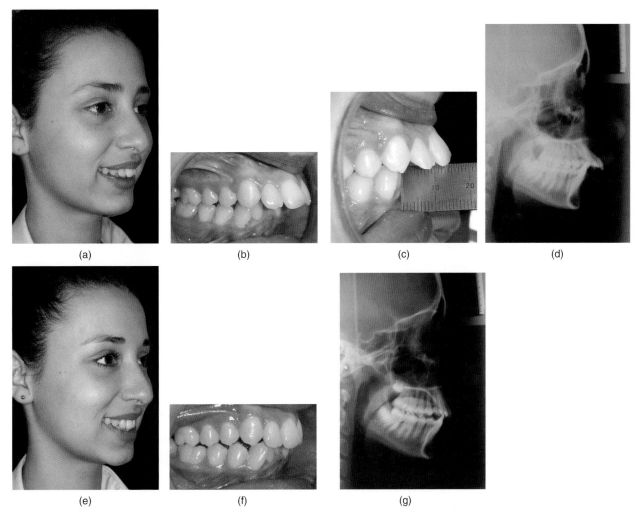

Figure 1.3 (a–d) Pretreatment photographs and lateral cephalometric radiograph of a patient with a Class II division 1 incisor relationship on a moderate Class II skeletal pattern, with proclined maxillary incisors, Class II canine and buccal segment relationships, and a 14-mm incisor overjet. (e–g) After 12 months of functional appliance treatment (12 months full-time wear and 3 months part-time nights-only wear), demonstrating an improved sagittal dental arch relationship towards Class I incisor and buccal segment relationships.

for a change in the morphology of the second and third cervical vertebrae, specifically for the caudal surfaces to progress from a flat to concave morphology.[13] In addition, the rapid adolescent growth may well facilitate tooth movement with fixed appliances.

Problem List

The problem list is simply a logically ordered list of the presenting problems that are a concern for the patient and those identified by the diagnosing clinician as needing to be dealt with in the treatment plan and corrected. The information required to generate a problem list is derived from three sources (Table 1.1):

- the patient interview/consultation
- clinical evaluation of the patient

- analysis of diagnostic records (e.g. radiographs, scans, clinical photographs, and dental study models, including space analysis and space planning).

Where possible, the problems should be noted quantitatively, such as a reduced upper lip height of 15 mm (average 20 mm for age and sex of the patient), or exact degree of crowding. Alternatively, some problems may be classified as mild, moderate or severe. The benefit of this very basic classification is to allow the clinician to begin to form an idea of whether treatment can be undertaken with orthodontics alone (e.g. a mild Class II skeletal pattern), whether other forms of treatment may be required (e.g. a moderate Class II skeletal pattern requiring dentofacial orthopaedic appliances or orthodontic camouflage treatment), or whether complex multidisciplinary treatment is required (e.g. a severe Class II skeletal pattern). The clinical

Table 1.1 Information required to generate a problem list for a standard orthodontic patient contemplating fixed appliance orthodontic treatment[a].

Diagnostic information source	Information required to generate a problem list
Patient interview	• Presenting complaint(s), in order of priority for the patient. Does it match the order of priority for the clinician? • Patient's perception: does it tie in with the clinician's evaluation? • Motivation: internal or external? High or low? • Expectations: realistic or unrealistic? • Cooperation and potential compliance • Medical history • Dental history (e.g. regular or casual attender to dentist) • Family history (e.g. siblings having orthodontic treatment; are family supportive?) • Social history (e.g. smoking, history of truancy from school)
Pathology evaluation (clinical and radiographic)	• Is there any pathology (e.g. dental caries, gingivitis, periodontal disease, alveolar bone loss)? • Is there any pain, noises or limitation of movement related to the temporomandibular joints (TMJs)? • Previous trauma to the teeth (history or signs)
Clinical evaluation	
Soft tissue evaluation	• Nasolabial angle, specifically lower component (i.e. upper lip inclination in profile view) (Figure 1.4). If the upper lip is inclined backwards as part of an obtuse nasolabial angle, avoid maxillary incisor retraction. Alternatively, a proclined upper lip may be due to proclined maxillary incisors (Figure 1.5) • Is the lower anterior face height (LAFH) reduced, average or increased in proportion to the facial proportions. If increased, may need to avoid posterior dental extrusive movements • Upper lip height: is it short, average or increased? • Maxillary incisor exposure in relation to upper lip at rest (Figure 1.6a). If there is reduced incisor exposure, avoid maxillary incisor intrusion. Also assess incisor and gingival exposure on smiling (Figure 1.6b) • Maxillary dental midline in relation to the mid-philtrum of the upper lip and facial midline: is it coincident, and are the incisors correctly angulated mesiodistally?
Skeletal evaluation	• Is the maxilla and associated dentoalveolus sagittally prominent, average or retrusive? • Is the mandible and associated dentoalveolus sagittally prominent, average or retrusive? • Is the maxillary–mandibular planes angle increased, average or reduced? • Is the maxillary occlusal plane level in frontal view, or is there a transverse cant (Figure 1.7)? If there is a cant, can it be corrected orthodontically, can it be accepted, or is surgery potentially required?
Dental evaluation	• What is the inclination of the labial crown face of the maxillary incisors in profile smiling view? A tangent to the labial face should be approximately parallel to the true vertical, with the patient in natural head position (Figure 1.8).[1, 14] If the crown face is proclined or retroclined, it is likely to require correction • Is the mandibular dental midline coincident with the maxillary dental midline and facial midline (Figure 1.9)? • Are the incisors correctly angulated mesiodistally (Figure 1.10)? • Are the dental arch forms symmetrical? • What is the overall shape of the dental arch forms? • What is the incisor overjet? • What is the incisor overbite? • Is there an anterior open bite (AOB)? If so, is it predominantly skeletal, soft tissue or habit-related in aetiology? • What is the degree of crowding, spacing or rotations? • Are there missing teeth, extra teeth (supernumerary or supplemental), crossbites, premature contacts with displacements, impacted or ectopic teeth? • Are there any overerupted or infraoccluded teeth? • Is the gingival morphology thin or thick biotype (Figure 1.11)? • Is there any gingival recession (Figure 1.12)?
Analysis of diagnostic records	
Panoramic radiograph	• Overall dental assessment and comparison of left–right symmetry
Cephalometric analysis	• Particularly if skeletal deviations from the average are evident, or if significant change in incisor positions is planned. Mandatory if orthognathic surgery is contemplated

Table 1.1 (Continued)

Diagnostic information source	Information required to generate a problem list
Study models	• Evaluation of dental arch symmetry • Space analysis and space planning (see below)
Other	• Serial height measurements • Cone beam computed tomography (CBCT), e.g. evaluating positions of difficult impacted teeth, or significant facial asymmetry potentially requiring surgical correction • Maxillary occlusal radiograph: to assess root morphology and for localisation of impacted canines using the parallax method

(a) More complex treatment, such as orthognathic surgery, requires more than the basic information provided in this table. For further information, see chapters 5 and 6 of *Orthognathic Surgery: Principles, Planning and Practice*.[2]

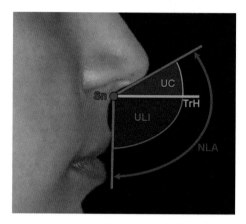

Figure 1.4 The nasolabial angle (NLA) may be divided into an upper component (UC) and a lower component, which is effectively the upper lip inclination (ULI), by a true horizontal line (TrH) passing through subnasale (Sn, defined as the deepest midline point where the base of the nasal columella meets the upper lip), with the patient in natural head position. Source: modified from Naini FB. *Facial Aesthetics: Concepts and Clinical Diagnosis*. Oxford: Wiley Blackwell, 2011, used with permission.

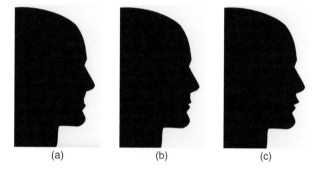

Figure 1.5 (a) Retroclined upper lip, which is usually a sign of lack of support for the upper lip, from a retruded maxilla/maxillary dentoalveolus or retruded/retroclined maxillary incisors. (b) Normal upper lip inclination. (c) Proclined upper lip, which may be due to proclined maxillary incisors.

diagnosis is based on a synthesis of the salient information collected from the above, which leads to the formation of the patient-specific problem list.

Treatment Aims

If the problem list has been accurately compiled to identify the problems requiring correction, the aims of treatment usually follow seamlessly from the list. In this context, because the clinical diagnosis described above leads to the formation of a problem list, treatment planning therefore becomes a problem-solving exercise. The aims of treatment should consider:

- addressing the patient's concerns
- improving or at least not deteriorating facial and smile aesthetics
- establishing and maintaining a functional and stable dental occlusion

- prioritising and determining the sequence of the planned stages of treatment.

It is important that the aims of treatment are logically ordered. For example, growth-related treatment requiring functional appliances takes precedence over incisor alignment in a patient near their pubertal growth spurt, or implementing treatment to arrest the trauma associated with a deep incisor overbite would need to be at the top of a list of aims.

If there is inconsistency between the order of priorities of the patient/parents and the clinician, as occasionally happens, a frank discussion is required to explain why a certain part of the treatment may need to be the initial focus (e.g. if it is growth related and time is running out). It is important that the patient/parents agree with the proposed steps in the planned treatment.

Aesthetic-Centred versus Occlusion-Centred Planning

In the early stages of orthodontic fixed appliance development at the beginning of the twentieth century, orthodontic treatment aimed to improve the dental occlusion; this was based on the conviction that well-aligned teeth in a Class I occlusion, with all the teeth present, would automatically

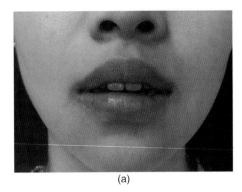
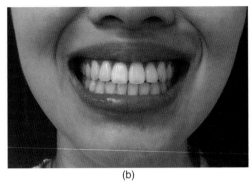

(a)   (b)

Figure 1.6 (a) Maxillary incisor exposure in relation to the upper lip in repose tends to be most attractive at approximately 2–5 mm, usually more in women than men. (b) On smiling, most of the maxillary incisor crowns and possibly 1–2 mm of the labial gingivae are evident.

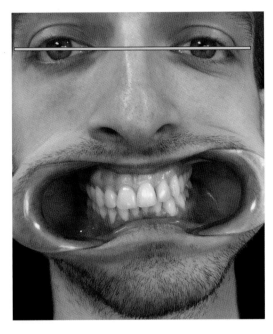

Figure 1.7 A maxillary occlusal plane cant, which is down on the patient's right side. In patients with level eye positions, the maxillary occlusal plane is usually approximately parallel to the interpupillary line.

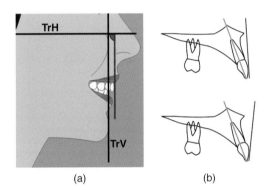

(a)   (b)

Figure 1.8 (a) The inclination of the labial crown face of the maxillary incisors should be evaluated in profile smiling view. A tangent to the labial face should be approximately parallel to the true vertical, with the patient in natural head position. (b) The inclination of a tangent to the labial crown face of the maxillary incisor (purple line) is more important than the inclination of the entire tooth (green line), as it is the incisor crown that is aesthetically visible. These two parameters are not directly related. Source: (a, b) Naini et al. The maxillary incisor labial face tangent: clinical evaluation of maxillary incisor inclination in profile smiling view and idealized aesthetics. *Maxillofac. Plast. Reconstr. Surg.* 2019; 41: 31–38.

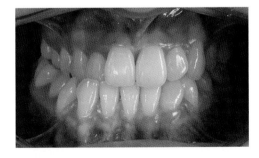

Figure 1.9 Mandibular dental midline is significantly to the right of the maxillary dental midline. Mandibular right canine was ectopic and unerupted. The mesiodistal angulation of the incisors is normal. There is a right-sided posterior crossbite. With unilateral posterior crossbites the clinician must always check for a lateral mandibular displacement.

lead to an 'ideal' facial aesthetic result. As is so often the case, untested beliefs were promoted as irrefutable facts for a few decades. However, evaluation of case results over time demonstrated this view to be inaccurate, with many cases resulting in extreme dentoalveolar protrusion or prone to significant relapse. Towards the middle of the twentieth century, outlooks shifted towards treating to arbitrary cephalometric *hard tissue* standards, particularly in relation to the sagittal position of the mandibular incisors, predominantly because cephalometric analysis was poorly understood and thereby often misapplied in clinical practice.[15] Opinions and outlooks continued to wax and wane for a number of decades. Parallel to, but separate

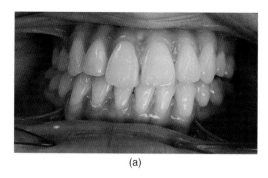 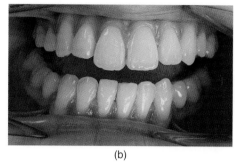

(a) (b)

Figure 1.10 (a) Mandibular incisor mesiodistal angulation is significantly angulated to the patient's left. (b) This is even more evident on slight opening of the mouth.

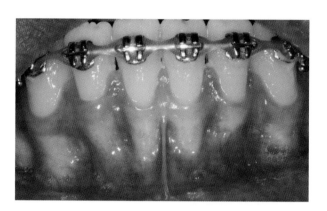

Figure 1.11 Patients with a thin gingival biotype often present with a 'washboard' appearance of the anterior tooth roots, particularly in the mandibular incisor and canine region.

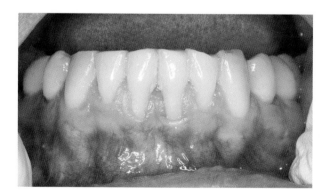

Figure 1.12 Gingival recession evident in the central incisor region and buccal segments.

from, the development of orthodontics was the development of orthognathic surgery; contrary to orthodontic planning, many of the early pioneering surgeons were promoting the importance of the facial soft tissue aesthetic result as the most important consideration.[16]

Within modern orthodontics, an **aesthetic-centred** approach to treatment planning, with emphasis on the most aesthetic relationship of the maxillary incisor position within the face, in repose and in animation, has now superseded earlier **occlusion-centred** approaches, based around the lower incisor position and static occlusal goals.[17] This is particularly important if **orthodontic camouflage** treatment is being planned; this refers to the treatment of a malocclusion where the skeletal discrepancy is not corrected, but the teeth are repositioned through their supporting alveolar bone in order to improve the dental occlusion. Undertaken incorrectly, orthodontic camouflage treatment may worsen facial appearance; for example, in a Class II malocclusion predominantly due to mandibular retrognathia, with the maxillary incisor sagittal position essentially normal, any retraction of the maxillary incisors to reduce the incisor overjet to a Class I incisor relationship (an occlusion-centred approach) may have significant detrimental facial aesthetic effects, such as reducing support for the upper lip and creating an obtuse nasolabial angle. In such patients, an aesthetic-centred approach would suggest that consideration is given to aligning the teeth and either maintaining or only partially correcting the incisor overjet.

Static and Functional Occlusion, Stability and Health

The other aims of orthodontic treatment are to obtain a well-interdigitated and well-functioning dental occlusion, a relatively stable result (or at least avoiding unstable movements) and an improvement in the patient's health-related quality of life.

The Six Keys to Occlusion described the morphological characteristics of an 'ideal' **static occlusion**: correct molar relationship, correct crown angulation (mesiodistal 'tip'), correct crown inclination (buccolingual or labiolingual inclination), no rotations, no interdental spaces, and a flat or very mild curve of Spee.[18] A seventh key was later added, that of correct relative tooth sizes. Achievement of a well-interdigitated dental occlusion is an aim of orthodontic treatment with fixed appliances (Figure 1.13).

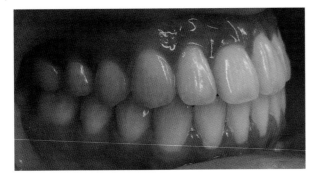

Figure 1.13 A relatively well-interdigitated dental occlusion.

In addition, improved **functional occlusion** is also an aim of treatment, referring to the dynamic relationship of the maxillary and mandibular teeth during dentally guided mandibular movements (e.g. lateral and protrusive movements), away from and towards maximum intercuspation, without occlusal interferences and providing protection and health of the periodontium and ideally well-functioning temporomandibular joints.

The most stable dental–occlusal outcome is an important aim of treatment. Depending on the original malocclusion and the dental movements undertaken, some may be inherently predicted as being unstable, for example closing a large maxillary midline diastema or correcting severe dental rotations. However, the biological variability and response to treatment between different patients means that it is not possible to predict accurately the degree of stability of standard orthodontic treatment with fixed appliances. Therefore, long-term wear, albeit often night-time wear of removable retainers, is deemed mandatory for patients desiring to maintain their treatment result.[19] Patients at greater risk of relapse may require bonded retainers in addition to removable retainers.

The definition of health provided by the World Health Organization (WHO), which has not been amended since 1948, is that 'health is a state of complete physical, mental and social well-being and not merely the absence of disease or infirmity'. A primary focus of modern healthcare is on the effects of treatment on a patient's quality of life, with OHRQoL defined as a multidimensional construct that includes a subjective evaluation of the individual's oral health, functional well-being, social and emotional well-being (which incorporate positive health states such as happiness and confidence), expectations and satisfaction with care, and sense of self.[20] It is an integral part of general health and well-being. Oral health can affect anyone's life,[21] but the importance of children's oral health to their overall health and well-being has been highlighted, together with the profound impact that oral health can have on children's quality of life.[22, 23] Orthodontic treatment deals with physical well-being by focusing on dental–occlusal function, and with mental and social well-being by focusing on improving dentofacial aesthetics. Evidence for the improvement in quality of life from orthodontic treatment and orthognathic surgery is increasing.[24]

Presenting the Treatment Options

Having established the aims of treatment, the next step is to decide on the available treatment options, which may deal with only some, most or all of the treatment aims. Depending on the complexity of the case, this will often result in a number of treatment options of ascending complexity that may be presented to the patient for their consideration. The treatment plans should be unambiguous and not unnecessarily ambitious for the orthodontist, particularly when addressing the patient's concerns does not require such treatment. If a specific treatment option is more appropriate for a patient, then that should be discussed, as should the reasons for the degree of appropriateness (e.g. considering factors such as the patient's motivation, ability to comply with the treatment, or medical history). Treatment planning should be undertaken in collaboration with the patient and where appropriate the interaction of parents/carers, in order to do what is best for that individual patient at the most appropriate time.

Occasionally, a patient's **mental capacity** can become a cause for concern if it becomes difficult for the clinician to assess whether the patient understands and desires treatment or if the motivation for treatment is parentally driven. Mental capacity may be defined as the ability to make one's own decisions. An individual lacking mental capacity (e.g. due to learning difficulties or mental health problems) may find it difficult to:

- understand the information given to them
- retain the information for long enough to enable their decision-making
- weigh up the information provided to reach a decision
- communicate their decision.

In such situations sound judgement from the clinician is paramount, and in some circumstances treatment may need to be delayed and advice sought from the appropriate medical or mental health professionals (see Chapter 5).

When explaining to patients that there are different treatment options, clinicians should beware that patients often misinterpret the presentation of choice, and may think that the clinician is either uninformed or lacks the judgement to reach a decision. This possibility may be negated by clearly explaining that there is good information about how these treatment options differ and that you will discuss the pros and cons of each approach with them.

Generally speaking, there are four potential orthodontic treatment options:

- No treatment
- Treatment with limited objectives
- Orthodontics alone
- Orthodontics in association with multidisciplinary care.

No Treatment

For a patient presenting with a malocclusion, there are two important questions to be answered. The first question is 'Does the patient need treatment?' If the answer is yes, the second question is 'Does the patient desire treatment?' If the impetus for referral is either from the referring dentist or possibly parents, and the patient does not desire treatment, this may well affect their compliance with any treatment and thereby its potential success or failure.

Orthodontic treatment should not be considered in patients with potential BDD; for those with malocclusions combined with excessive levels of anxiety, treatment should not be considered unless the patient is first assessed by an appropriately trained mental health clinician.[4]

Treatment with Limited Objectives

The three overriding aims of orthodontic treatment are 'ideal' dentofacial aesthetics, 'ideal' occlusal function and 'ideal' stability of the obtained result. Realistically, even with highly experienced clinicians, these are not always achievable due to patient-related factors. For a variety of reasons, a patient may not desire or be able to tolerate long and complicated treatment, or may prefer to avoid multidisciplinary treatment, or may prefer a more aesthetic result even if it might compromise stability. The clinician's judgement remains paramount in deciding which compromises are feasible in order to obtain the result most favoured by the patient. Therefore, treatment with limited objectives is effectively an agreed trade-off between what the clinician could achieve despite lengthy and/or complex treatment versus what the patient can realistically tolerate to achieve an acceptable, albeit compromise in the treatment result. With appropriate concessions and cooperation from the patient/parents/carers, and realistically achievable aims, a successful outcome is more likely. Clearly, treatment should only be undertaken if the clinician considers it to be in the patient's best interest.

Treatment with limited objectives should never be undertaken due to lack of experience on the part of the clinician. In such circumstances, appropriate referral to a more experienced clinician should be instigated without hesitation.

Orthodontics Alone

For many patients, fixed appliance orthodontic treatment in the hands of an appropriately trained clinician can provide exemplary results. Difficulties may arise when patients present with underlying skeletal problems. In growing patients, the decisions are whether a malocclusion is amenable to a functional appliance, orthopaedic headgear or facemask treatment and, if so, whether the patient will wear such appliances. In older patients, the question is essentially one of orthodontic camouflage treatment versus orthognathic surgery, as previously discussed.

For patients with a Class I malocclusion on a skeletal Class I pattern, treatment planning is generally undertaken in the lower dental arch, with preservation of the sagittal position of the mandibular incisors and the intercanine width. This is based on consideration of the development of the teeth within the zone of neutral pressure between the lips/cheeks and tongue. Although maintenance of these parameters does not automatically confer stability, in the absence of other reliable predictors, it is considered clinically advisable. Maxillary arch mechanics to achieve a Class I incisor and canine relationship follow.

However, when Class II or III skeletal discrepancies are evident, the treatment approaches include either growth modification/dentofacial orthopaedics in growing patients, orthodontic camouflage treatment, or orthognathic surgical correction.

Orthodontics in Association with Multidisciplinary Care

Orthodontic treatment may have to be considered in conjunction with other dental, surgical or medical specialties as required, depending on the requirements of each specific case. These include maxillofacial surgery for orthognathic patients, oral surgery for patients requiring exposure of impacted/ectopic teeth, frenectomies or other oral surgical procedures, restorative dentistry for patients with hypodontia, and cleft or craniofacial teams. In such situations the clinician will require the appropriate training.

With any of the options described, the risk/cost/harm versus benefit considerations must be discussed in full, allowing the patient to make an informed decision regarding their choice of treatment (see section Informed Consent).

How do we decide whether or not to Extract Teeth?

The debate between extraction and non-extraction treatment is almost as old as the orthodontic profession.

However, a practical and common-sense approach with sound judgement is the main requirement in the decision-making process. The obvious perceived disadvantage for the patient of dental extractions is the loss of the permanent teeth involved. The other disadvantage is the potential detrimental facial soft tissue aesthetic changes from excessive retraction of the incisor teeth leading to retrusion of the lower face in profile view (sometimes referred to as 'dishing-in' of the profile), resulting from reduced dentoalveolar support for the labial soft tissues. The latter is essentially an issue related to incorrect planning, poorly controlled mechanics, or both. Other possible disadvantages of dental extractions are the potential complications of surgery, poor patient experience, the anxiety involved for some patients, and the unattractive appearance of some extraction spaces, although this is usually short term.

The advantages of dental extractions are to provide space for other teeth in the presence of crowding severe enough not to be amenable to other forms of space creation, to allow incisor retraction in cases of excessive protrusion, or in Class II or Class III camouflage treatment. Dental extractions may also be necessary for other reasons, such as surgical removal of extremely ectopic teeth not amenable to alignment, or broken down/carious/hypoplastic teeth. Appropriately undertaken dental extractions may even be beneficial in terms of facial aesthetics; for example, maxillary first premolar extractions providing space to retrocline and retract excessively prominent maxillary incisors can improve labial competence and reduce labial prominence.

There are a number of methods of gaining space available in orthodontics (discussed in more detail in Chapter 14). Of these, extractions should be at the bottom of the list, which means that if the treatment plan calls for dental extractions, other possibilities have been exhausted and it is in the best interests of the patient.

In some 'borderline' patients, it may not be obvious at the outset whether treatment can be successfully carried out on a non-extraction basis by expansion of the dental arches or other forms of space creation. In such situations, treatment may be undertaken with a **therapeutic diagnosis** approach, i.e. begin non-extraction and reassess during treatment. If the incisors begin to appear excessively prominent and the patient agrees with the finding, dental extractions may be undertaken. If this approach is contemplated, it should be discussed in full at the planning and consent stages of treatment.

The idea that extraction treatment automatically leads to retrusion of the labial part of the facial profile or that non-extraction treatment always leads to protruded incisors and broad dental arches is inaccurate and misleading. The outcome of treatment is dependent on correct treatment planning by a competent clinician, combined with logical mechanics based on a thorough understanding of anchorage (e.g. how to close space with mesial movement of buccal segments as opposed to excessive retraction of incisors) and competent handling of the chosen appliance.

The decision of whether dental extractions are required should never be taken lightly, and should always take into consideration the following.

- **Lip–incisor relationship**: this important aesthetic relationship is the foundation stone of dentofacial aesthetics in treatment planning.[1] The best possible sagittal, vertical and transverse position and inclination of the maxillary central incisors is the main target for the end of treatment. If the maxillary incisor labial crown face is relatively parallel to the true vertical line in a smiling profile view of a patient in natural head position, any proclination will likely be detrimental to smile aesthetics.[1, 14]

- **Facial soft tissue form and thickness**: the presenting facial soft tissue form and likely change with extraction versus non-extraction treatment are important. For example, thin retrusive lips can tolerate incisor proclination or protraction from expansion treatment, and any further labial retraction from extraction treatment should be avoided if possible, or if extractions are required, space closure should be controlled to reduce incisor retraction as far as possible. Conversely, in patients with thick flaccid lips, there may be very little effect on the lip posture or prominence in relation to sagittal movement of the incisor teeth.

- **Stability**: the potential stability of the result is an important parameter; for example, excessive proclination of the teeth into the labial soft tissues may lead to greater risk of relapse, particularly in the lower arch. However, retroclined teeth may have a greater ability to be proclined, albeit avoiding dehiscence of thin labial alveolar bone and potential gingival recession.

- **Space analysis**: occlusal factors should be evaluated methodically, ideally with a formal and thorough space analysis (see following section).

When dental extractions are required, the choice of teeth will depend on a number of factors:

- **Degree and site of crowding**: if crowding is severe enough to warrant extractions, in an otherwise healthy dentition, the teeth usually planned for removal are the premolars. As a general guideline, the further a tooth is situated from the site of crowding, the less space will be available for tooth alignment. Therefore, the greater the degree of labial segment crowding (usually equating to dental arch crowding of anything more than 8–9 mm), the more likely that first premolar extractions will be required. In growing patients with erupting canines that are short of space, appropriately timed first premolar extractions may allow the eruption of the canines and some spontaneous relief of crowding. If space requirements are less (between 5 and 8 mm), consideration should be given to second premolar extractions.

- **Type of malocclusion**: in *Class I malocclusions* requiring premolar extractions, the decision to extract is first made in the lower arch. The corresponding extraction is undertaken in the upper arch, for example if mandibular first premolars are to be extracted, the extraction pattern in the maxilla is also the first premolars. This helps to correct or maintain a Class I buccal segment relationship. In a *Class II malocclusion* requiring incisor relationship correction as well as relief of crowding, the space requirements will usually be greater in the maxillary arch. If first premolar extractions are required for relief of crowding in the mandibular arch, the corresponding teeth will usually be extracted in the maxillary arch. If the space requirements are less in the mandibular arch, a common extraction pattern is the extraction of upper first and lower second premolars. This aids buccal segment correction, as it reduces the tendency for forward movement of the upper molars and allows greater forward movement of the lower first molars, which moves the molar relationship towards Class I. Alternatively, if there is mild crowding in the lower arch, it may be treated on a non-extraction basis, extracting premolars in the upper arch only, finishing to a Class II molar relationship. This extraction pattern helps maintain the sagittal position of the lower incisors, which forms the limit to maxillary incisor retraction, reducing the likelihood of their excessive retraction. In *Class III malocclusions*, the converse is true, in that the mandibular incisors usually need to be moved lingually, potentially increasing the space requirement in the lower arch. As such, the usual extraction pattern is mandibular first premolars and maxillary second premolars. Alternatively, if the maxillary arch is well aligned or only mildly crowded and the sagittal incisor position acceptable, the maxillary arch may be treated on a non-extraction basis, finishing to a Class III molar relationship.
- **Presence of teeth**: in patients with hypodontia, if one maxillary lateral incisor is congenitally missing, in the presence of crowding, consideration may be given to removal of the contralateral lateral incisor (particularly if it is diminutive in form) in order to avoid the requirement for future prosthetic tooth replacement and to provide symmetry to the dental arch and final aesthetic result. Factors that need to be considered with

this approach include the degree of gingival exposure on smiling and the size, shape and colour of the maxillary canines.[25] The canines may eventually require some lateralisation, which refers to modification to their shape (usually by enamel removal at the tip, and sometimes addition of composite resin mesial and distal to the tip) to appear more like lateral incisors (Figure 1.14). If both lateral incisors are severely crowded, and erupted lingually/palatally, their extraction can simplify treatment and reduce treatment time, so long as the canines make suitable substitutes, i.e. are of suitable morphology to mimic or be modified as lateral incisors. Severely ectopic canines may be considered for surgical removal; although removal of canines is not commonly undertaken, in appropriately selected cases it may significantly reduce treatment time, and the lateral incisor–first premolar contact can be aesthetically and occlusally satisfactory.

- **Health of the teeth**: compromised teeth (carious, heavily restored, hypoplastic or previously traumatised) with a poor long-term prognosis should always be considered during treatment planning when extractions are required. Even if the teeth are not those usually selected to correct the presenting malocclusion, nevertheless with appropriate anchorage management and carefully planned mechanics, their extraction may be in the patient's best interests. However, if treatment time would be significantly increased, this would need to be discussed with the patient. Caries and hypoplasia often affect the first permanent molar teeth, as these are the first molar teeth to erupt, and their extraction may help create space for second and sometimes even third molar teeth (though third molar eruption and position is unpredictable). Maxillary central incisors are the usual teeth to be involved in trauma and if extraction is unavoidable, consideration should be given to either maintain the space for a prosthetic replacement or, occasionally, to removal of both central incisors and modification of the lateral incisors as central incisors. The latter approach is uncommon and would need to be planned carefully with restorative dental specialists from the outset.

Space Analysis and Space Planning

Space analysis of the dental arches may be defined as the assessment of the amount of space required for alignment and occlusal correction and the space creation and utilisation planned to achieve those aims.[26, 27] As such, in terms of occlusal parameters, orthodontic treatment may

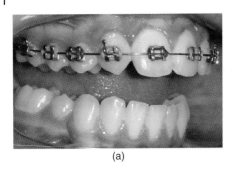 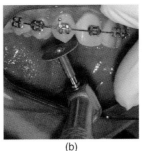 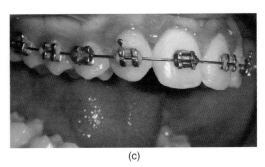

(a) (b) (c)

Figure 1.14 (a) Missing maxillary lateral incisors, with treatment undertaken by space closure, positioning the canines adjacent to the central incisors. (b) Lateralisation of the canines may be undertaken with enameloplasty of prominent canine tips. The authors favour the use of flexible contouring discs (beginning with the coarse abrasive grade for reshaping of the enamel, followed by the finer grades for polishing) mounted on a mandrel in a slow-speed contra-angle handpiece. (c) Canine tip has been reshaped. If the patient desires, composite may be added to the mesial and/or distal of the canine tip in order to mask its appearance further.

be viewed as the **redistribution of space**. Although a number of methods of space analysis have been described, we favour the comprehensive space planning system developed for the permanent dentition at the Royal London Hospital over many years (described in detail in chapter 10 of *Orthodontics: Principles and Practice*).[28]

In our view, the absolute measurements and values derived from space analysis are perhaps not as important as the systematic nature of the assessment. It is very easy for an inexperienced clinician to view a set of orthodontic study models and just 'see' crowding or spacing, and not consider all the other parameters that are relevant to space requirements and space utilisation. For example, a crowded dental arch may be treated on a non-extraction basis if the plan requires transverse arch expansion and incisor proclination. Alternatively, a well-aligned dental arch may require extractions if significant incisor retraction is planned. A logical order to case assessment and space analysis means it is less likely for the clinician to miss something or make an error in the planning process. The methodical approach of this system helps to develop ordered thinking, and is particularly helpful for those in training. It is important to reiterate that space planning for the dentition should always be undertaken with due consideration for dentofacial aesthetics, particularly regarding the position of the incisor teeth in relation to the face, and of the stability of the end result.

The Royal London Hospital space analysis consists of two parts, summarised as follows.

1. Assessment of the space requirements in each dental arch (Table 1.2).
2. Planning the creation and utilisation of space, i.e. how the space will be created and used in treatment.

Of the factors assessed, crowding and incisor sagittal retraction have the most significant space implications,

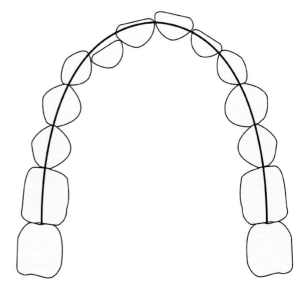

Figure 1.15 Dental arch crowding should be measured in relation to the arch form that best reflects the majority of the teeth. The ideal labiolingual position of the incisors should be considered, which is not necessarily the most prominent incisor.

with levelling, arch width and incisor inclination changes affecting space by no more than 2–3 mm per arch.

Once the space requirements in each dental arch have been calculated, space creation and space utilisation are planned. The following parameters should be considered.

- **Tooth reduction and enlargement**: the amount of tooth material in both dental arches should be in proportion for a good occlusion. Disproportion between the sizes of individual teeth in a patient is termed a **tooth size discrepancy**. The most common tooth size discrepancy is narrow maxillary lateral incisors (normal-width upper lateral incisors are usually approximately two-thirds the width of the central incisors and should always be wider than the mandibular lateral

Table 1.2 Summary of space requirements in space analysis.

Space requirements	Assessment method	Notes[a]
Crowding and spacing (Figure 1.15)	Study models	Crowding should be quantified in relation to an arch form that reflects the majority of the teeth, usually established as passing through the majority of the buccal cusps and incisor tips (avoiding individual teeth displaced from the arch form)
		Measure mesiodistal widths of the teeth (using a clear ruler) that do not lie on the selected arch form anterior to the first molars in each arch. Crowding is calculated by subtracting the space available in each arch
		The incisors which contribute to the arch form should be the same as those which will be traced on the lateral cephalometric radiograph (see below)
Levelling occlusal curve (Figure 1.16)	Study models	Increased occlusal curves are due to slipped contacts in the vertical plane. Levelling the occlusal plane involves restoring the contact point relationships
		The sagittal curve of the occlusion is assessed in relation to a flat plane from the distal cusps of the first molars to the incisal edges. The depth of the curve is measured from the premolar cusps to the flat plane
		Only one value is provided for each arch
		For the lower dental arch: • No space allowance for a depth of <3 mm • Allow 1 mm of space for 3 mm depth of curve • Allow 1.5 mm of space for 4 mm depth of curve • Allow 2 mm of space for a 5 mm depth of curve
		For the upper dental arch: • 1 mm space is recorded in Class II division 2 cases with a significant sagittal occlusal curve
Arch width change	Study models	Allow 0.5 mm space for each millimetre posterior arch width change (0.7 mm/mm expansion if using rapid maxillary expansion)
		The overall effect of 1 mm expansion across the upper intermolar width is 0.6 mm of space creation, e.g. 5 mm expansion will result in approximately 3 mm of additional space in the arch
		Arch width contraction reduces the available space in the same proportion. Arch contraction has a space requirement, i.e. all else being equal, space would need to be created by interdental enamel reduction, extraction or incisor protrusion
Incisor sagittal position change (bodily retraction or protraction) (Figure 1.17)	Lateral cephalometric radiograph[b]	Allow 2 mm of space for each 1 mm of planned incisor retraction, i.e. for each 1 mm of planned retraction of the maxillary incisors, 1 mm of space will be required per side
		Conversely, protraction (bodily advancement) of the upper incisors by 1 mm will create 1 mm of space distal to the incisors per side (i.e. 2 mm per arch)
		This is evaluated in relation to the planned target incisor overjet (usually 1.5–4 mm)
Incisor inclination change (Figure 1.18)	Lateral cephalometric radiograph[b]	Applies only to the maxillary incisors
		Allow 1 mm space for every 5° change affecting all four incisors, and 0.5 mm space if only two incisors affected
Incisor mesiodistal angulation change (Figure 1.19)		Applies only to the maxillary incisors
		Although 0.5 mm space is appropriate for correction of each parallel-sided vertical tooth, no allowance is usually given as angulation corrections tend to be included in the crowding assessment

(a) In our view, the figures quoted should be seen as guidance and should not be viewed as absolute or prescriptive.
(b) We suggest that this assessment is supplemented with clinical evaluation of the maxillary incisor crown face inclination in a profile smiling view of the patient in their natural head position.

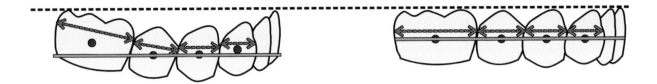

Figure 1.16 Increased occlusal curves are due to slipped contact points in the vertical plane. Levelling the occlusal plane involves restoring the contact point relationships. This requires space if arch lengthening by incisor proclination is to be avoided.

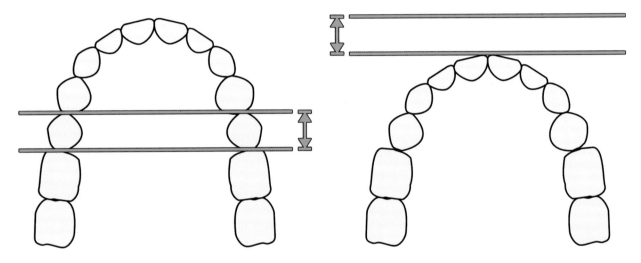

Figure 1.17 Bodily incisor retraction by a distance requires the same amount of space in each buccal segment. In this example, the space required for incisor retraction has been achieved by mid-arch premolar extractions.

incisors), although premolar size may also be variable. When individual teeth are of reduced size/width relative to the others, it may be necessary to create space around them for eventual enlargement in order to achieve a good dental occlusion (e.g. restorative building up of narrow maxillary lateral incisors). Conversely, if a tooth is unusually wide, the mesiodistal width may be reduced by interproximal enamel reduction. In an intact dental arch, there are 11 contact areas mesial to the first molars, and removal of 0.5 mm of enamel per contact point (i.e. 0.25 mm per tooth surface) can provide approximately 5.5 mm of space, provided that there is enough enamel thickness and tooth morphology of anterior teeth is favourable (triangular incisors are amenable to interproximal enamel reduction, whereas narrow parallel-sided incisors may be unsuitable).

- **Missing teeth**: the decision to open space for prosthetic replacement of missing teeth is similar to the principle of building up narrow teeth discussed above.

- **Extractions**: the mesiodistal width of permanent teeth to be extracted is recorded. For example, extraction of maxillary first premolars, each 7 mm in width, will create 14 mm of space.

- **Molar distal movement**: this results in an increase in arch length. For example, 2 mm of molar distal movement per side results in 4 mm increase in overall arch length. This was particularly applicable to the maxillary dental arch with headgear used for distal movement, but the use of temporary anchorage devices (TADs) permits distal movement in the mandibular arch in selected cases.

- **Molar mesial movement**: the space gained from dental extractions is not entirely available for relief of anterior crowding or incisor retraction as some of the space will be 'lost' by forward movement of the posterior teeth. This is significant when decisions regarding the requirement for **anchorage reinforcement** are being considered, for example significant incisor retraction will lead to

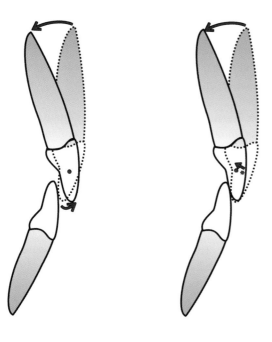

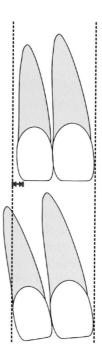

Figure 1.18 Correcting the inclination of retroclined maxillary incisors requires space if an increase in the incisor overjet is to be avoided. Superimposition of maxillary incisors by registration on the contact point (*left*) demonstrates an increase in the overjet after palatal root torque. However, registration on the point of occlusal contact with the mandibular incisor (*right*) demonstrates a gingivopalatal movement of the contact point after palatal root torque. Either way, additional space is required in the arch to accommodate for palatal root torque.

Figure 1.19 Teeth that are angulated tend to occupy slightly more space in the arch.

greater forward movement of the posterior dentition. A very approximate percentage estimation is that 60% of mandibular first premolar space is available for labial segment alignment without anchorage reinforcement, reducing to 40% if second premolars are extracted. The space available from similar extractions in the maxillary arch is lower, as there is a greater tendency for maxillary molar mesial movement. If forward movement of the molars is not desired, anchorage reinforcement should be planned, by adding intraoral anchorage reinforcement (e.g. Nance palatal arch), extraoral anchorage such as headgear, or TADs.

- **Growth considerations and space**: provision should be made for the potential effects of differential mandibular growth in growing patients. Growth estimation is unpredictable, but must be considered. Mandibular growth usually exceeds maxillary growth in the sagittal plane by a few millimetres between the ages of 9 and 16 years. This may be beneficial in Class II cases and detrimental in Class III cases. If Class III growth is likely, additional space will be required for dental compensation and retroclination of the mandibular incisors.

If space analysis is carried out accurately, with due consideration of the treatment aims, the balance of space required and how this is created and utilised should equal zero. If not, the process should be reviewed, including the treatment aims, to assess whether they are achievable, or whether appropriate modifications are required, such as different extraction pattern or greater anchorage reinforcement. This is very useful for the clinician and in terms of patient information for informed consent.

The information acquired from the space planning process should be integrated with the information gathered from the patient interview, clinical evaluation and analysis of other diagnostic records in order to formulate the treatment plan.

Informed Consent

From a modern and ethical standpoint, medical treatment is viewed as something done for the patient with their involvement in the decision-making process, rather than something done to the patient because the clinician has deemed it necessary and in their supposed best interests. The latter approach, termed the **paternalistic model**, is no longer justified, and is deemed unethical and legally indefensible in most situations, particularly for elective treatment. The former or **autonomous model** is the preferred approach in most societies, and the clinician responsible for obtaining consent should act with sensitivity and mindfulness of each patient's particular needs.

If a patient is to have autonomy in their choice of treatment, they must be provided with sufficient information using easily understandable, jargon-free terminology that will allow them to make an informed decision. During the informed consent discussion, the clinician should discuss and explain the following.

- **Patient's presenting complaint**: the patient's presenting problems need to be fully explained to the patient, to ensure that patient and clinician are not unwittingly misunderstanding each other. It is easier than one might think for patient and clinician to be talking at cross purposes; for example, the patient with a midline diastema and an anterior open bite who complains of 'the space between my teeth' may only be referring to one or other of the spaces. It is important to ensure that the clinician has identified the patient's main concern(s), and that the treatment plan will address those concerns.
- **Alternative treatment options**: these must be discussed, and the advantages, disadvantages and potential outcomes of each approach considered, including that of no treatment. It is no longer justified to provide only a written information sheet or to ask the patient to sign a consent form (often containing medical jargon), neither of which constitutes valid consent.
- **Treatment time**: the likely average length of treatment should be discussed for each option, and *never* underestimated. Patients should also be aware that treatment sometimes takes longer than expected, particularly if the teeth move more slowly than expected, or if patients continuously damage their appliances, do not maintain a high standard of plaque control, continuously miss appointments or do not comply with instructions, such as requirements for intraoral elastic wear. Patients should also be made aware of the risks of discontinuation of treatment before its completion against the clinician's advice, resulting for example in extraction spaces remaining.
- **Compromises**: if compromises are unavoidable, they must be discussed with the patient, with reasonable explanations provided.
- **Consequences of no treatment**: the potential consequences of not undergoing treatment, including not undergoing treatment at that time, should be discussed (e.g. if functional appliances or other growth-related treatments are being considered).
- **Need for retention**: the long-term requirement for retainer wear, the type of retainers required, and their long-term management must all be discussed and agreed.
- **Risk/harm/cost versus benefit considerations**:[29] these should be discussed for each option. Clinicians should always remember that what you tell a patient before treatment is sound professional advice; what you tell them after treatment is viewed as an excuse. The clinician should be absolutely candid and unambiguous about the details and potential risks of treatment, even if such information causes the patient to decline treatment. The patient should be fully aware of the potential **risks** or **harms** associated with both the orthodontic treatment (e.g. decalcification, root resorption) and any concomitant multidisciplinary care. The **cost** of treatment does not equate to monetary cost in the UK National Health Service (except for long-term costs of replacing retainers, and the potential financial implications of parents taking time off work to accompany their children to appointments), but to the imposition of treatment on a patient's daily life (see 'treatment burden' in following paragraphs); in other words, the **inconveniences** and **sacrifices** required of the patient in undergoing treatment, both in terms of **social costs (**e.g. time off school, university or work, the potential social impact of having fixed orthodontic appliances on a long-term basis, the extra effort required in maintaining a very high standard of oral hygiene, and avoidance of certain dietary products due to having an orthodontic appliance) and **emotional costs** (e.g. the effect of initial worsening of the appearance with some forms of treatment such as Class III preparation for orthognathic surgery, or possible psychological effects such as the potential anxiety of having treatment). Only when the balance between risks/costs and benefits has been discussed unequivocally with the patient and the proposed treatment has a high likelihood of success should treatment proceed.
- **Shared decision-making**: this concept refers to an approach where clinicians and patients share the best available evidence when faced with the task of making decisions, and where patients are supported to consider options in order to achieve informed preferences.[30] This concept rests on supporting a process of deliberation for the patient, and on understanding that decisions

should be influenced by exploring and respecting what matters most to patients as individuals. It also rests on the clinician accepting the core principle that individual self-determination is a desirable goal in which clinicians need to support their patients. This makes good communication skills mandatory as patients' abilities to assimilate potentially esoteric information or conceptualise different outcomes from different treatment approaches will be variable. The process of shared decision-making is difficult for many reasons, including limitations of the evidence base, challenges in comparing diverse outcomes, and the time needed to have these discussions. The wide spectrum of harms and benefits of importance to a patient should be discussed, including **treatment burden**. Treatment burden, sometimes referred to as 'patient burden',[31] is a concept initially described in relation to respondents involved in health survey research.[32] In the context of orthodontics, treatment burden may be defined as the patient's subjective experience of hardship from the psychological, physical, and economic effects of undergoing treatment. Occasionally, in their desire to do the best for patients, and with clinical experience of successful comparable treatment on previous patients, clinicians may inadvertently bias the patient's decisions by emphasising the uncertainty related to risks/harms while implying certainty around benefits. This may contribute to a tendency for patients (and sometimes clinicians) to perceive treatment predominantly in terms of benefits, with reduced emphasis of potential risks. However, the purpose of shared decision-making combined with patient autonomy is missed if patients are not provided with accurate unbiased information. The language used by a clinician will guide the patient's decision, and behavioural science has demonstrated that even minor changes in language or framing can significantly alter judgements and decisions.[33] Therefore, it is incumbent upon clinicians to avoid medical jargon when communicating with patients, and to discuss the pros and cons of any viable option carefully. 'True consent' has been defined as 'the informed exercise of choice, and that entails an opportunity to evaluate knowledgeably the options available', which includes 'the degree of harm threatened' and the 'potential benefit of the therapy'.[34]

In orthodontic treatment, involvement of the patient/parents in the decision-making process has the added advantage that the patient will feel that they have some responsibility in the treatment process and the necessary effort required on their part, which may help in compliance with treatment.

Having provided all these explanations, the clinician needs to be certain that the patient has the capacity to provide **valid consent**. It should be evident to the clinician that:

- the patient is able to understand and retain the information provided
- the patient is able to use and weigh the information in the decision-making process.

At this stage it is worth providing the patient and parents with validated information leaflets, such as those designed by the British Orthodontic Society, and giving them time to consider their options. At the following appointment, following further discussion and answering any questions the patient may have, if these conditions have been satisfied and the patient has selected their treatment of choice, their option becomes the **definitive treatment plan**.

What Should be Included in a Treatment Plan

Table 1.3 considers the most pertinent factors to be included in the definitive treatment plan.

Treatment Mechanics

The approximate sequencing of the treatment and technical details (e.g. archwire sequencing, tooth movements and mechanics required to achieve them at each visit) constitutes the final stage of treatment planning. This is a very important exercise, particularly for trainees. It forms the step-by-step framework that the clinician will follow, and is able to refer back to, throughout the treatment process. As with any specialty dealing with human biology, alterations may be required during treatment; for example, a plan to align an impacted maxillary canine will change if the tooth becomes ankylosed during treatment. Nevertheless, a well thought out and logical plan can usually be followed reasonably well, albeit with some modifications, throughout the treatment process.

Table 1.3 What to include in the definitive treatment plan.

Factors	Relevance
Resolving dental health issues	This should be undertaken prior to instigating orthodontic treatment: • Oral hygiene and gingivitis • Periodontal problems • Dental caries • Trauma, e.g. vitality testing, root canal treatment if required • Cessation of habits (e.g. digit sucking, nail biting)
Aims of treatment	Facial aesthetic aims: • Effect of molar extrusion/intrusion on lower anterior face height • Effect of incisor protrusion/retrusion or proclination/retroclination on sagittal lip prominence and lip posture • Comprehensive aims will be discussed for orthognathic treatment Smile aesthetic aims: • Inclination of the maxillary incisor labial crown face tangent (in profile smiling view and frontal view) • Lip–incisor relationship: particularly if intrusion of the maxillary incisors is contemplated, as incisor exposure will reduce Dental–occlusal aims: • Incisor relationship • Canine relationship • Buccal segment relationship • Arch forms Dental aesthetic aims: • If tooth morphology is to be altered (e.g. lateralisation of maxillary canines, or build-ups of narrow maxillary lateral incisors) • Any required restorative/prosthodontic treatment (e.g. prosthetic replacement of missing maxillary lateral incisors)
Growth estimation and treatment timing	If growth-dependent treatment is planned (e.g. functional and dentofacial orthopaedic appliances), these should be timed to coincide with the maximal pubertal growth spurt (see section Relevance of Growth and Growth Estimation)
Methods of space creation	Increasing arch length: • Incisor protrusion or proclination • Distal movement of molars/buccal segments Transverse arch expansion Interdental enamel reduction Dental extractions: which teeth and why, based on dentofacial aesthetics and dental–occlusal space analysis
Timing of extractions	If dental extractions are planned, should they be removed before placement of fixed appliances, ensuring minimal or planned space loss? Is anchorage reinforcement required prior to dental extractions? Is therapeutic diagnosis planned, i.e. begin alignment on a non-extraction basis and decide on necessity of dental extractions during treatment?
Type of appliance(s)	Removable appliances: • Anterior bite plane to aid bonding of the lower arch in deep overbite malocclusions • Expansion of the maxillary dental arch Functional appliances: • For sagittal dental arch improvement as an aid to the proposed fixed appliance treatment Fixed appliances: • Labial (stainless steel, ceramic, gold) • Self-ligating • Lingual • Other (e.g. Begg or Tip-Edge appliances)

Table 1.3 (Continued)

Factors	Relevance
Bracket prescription	Which bracket prescription is planned for use, and why?
	Advantages and disadvantages in relation to the particular case?
Bracket variations	Are any bracket variations planned, and if so, why? For example:
	• Inverting maxillary lateral incisor brackets if in-standing • Contralateral mandibular canine brackets in Class III camouflage cases
	Additionally, will a particular bracket from another appliance or prescription be required for a specific task?
Archwire sequence	The approximate archwire sequence should be planned, including the aims of treatment with each wire (e.g. alignment, sliding mechanics, retraction vs. retroclination, space closure)
Special mechanics	Examples include the use of:
	• Orthodontic mini-implants/ temporary anchorage devices (TADs) • Headgear • Sectional mechanics, e.g. Burstone or Ricketts arches
Retention (type and duration)	Type:
	• Removable retainers (e.g. Hawley, Essix-type vacuum-formed, Begg, Barrer spring-loaded) • Fixed (bonded) retainers, which teeth and in which arch? Why is a fixed retainer required? Usually provided for tooth movements known to be prone to relapse, and are usually in addition to, not instead of removable retainers
	Duration:
	• How long full-time wear is required • When part-time wear may be instigated • Overall duration of wear (usually advised long-term wear will be required)
Regular dental and hygiene visits during treatment	This should be agreed with the patient and dentist/hygienist prior to instigating treatment. Patients must understand the importance of regular monitoring of dental health by their dentist throughout orthodontic treatment, as occasionally patients incorrectly assume that dental check-ups are not required when they are undergoing orthodontic treatment
Oral hygiene	Maintenance of oral hygiene at a high level is expected throughout treatment, and its importance must be relayed to the patient
	The outcome of poor oral hygiene, including potential early cessation of treatment, should be explained to the patient and parents/carers
Timing of input from other specialists	The timing should be considered prior to instigating fixed appliance treatment, ideally by seeing the patient jointly with the appropriate specialist. Examples include:
	• Combined orthodontic–restorative/prosthodontic treatment for missing teeth • Combined orthodontic–periodontal/implantologist treatment (e.g. creating ridge thickness for placement of dental implants) • Combined orthodontic–endodontic treatment to aid either specialist • Combined orthodontic–oral surgical treatment (e.g. surgical removal of teeth, surgical exposure of teeth, frenectomies) • Combined orthodontic–maxillofacial surgical treatment for orthognathic patients
Multidisciplinary care	Complex treatments requiring multidisciplinary care (e.g. orthognathic, cleft or craniofacial care) must be with an appropriately trained multidisciplinary team, and the input from each specialist should be planned prior to treatment
Limiting factors to treatment	Patient-related limiting factors:
	• Medical problems • Dental health problems • Age: if contemplating dentofacial orthopaedic treatment • Compliance: does the patient desire treatment or are they going along with their parents' wishes? Will they look after the appliances, wear elastics, etc?
	Malocclusion-related limiting factors:
	• Severe skeletal discrepancy in patients not desiring orthognathic surgery may be difficult to correct with camouflage treatment • Tooth size discrepancies, when present, may create difficulties in obtaining an optimal occlusion

(Continued)

Table 1.3 (Continued)

Factors	Relevance
Mouthguards	These are required for anyone playing contact sports, and appropriate sports mouthguards are available that protect the patient's soft tissues during sport but do not interfere with orthodontic tooth movement
Wind/brass instrument players	Wind instrument players may be reassured that orthodontic treatment is possible, but must be made aware that there will be some initial difficulties in creating an embouchure, and they are likely to require wax placement over their appliances, at least initially
	Those playing at a high level or with examinations approaching may wish to delay placement of fixed appliances to a more appropriate time
Correspondence with GDP and GMP	It is important for the clinician to maintain correspondence with the patient's GDP regarding the proposed plan and their part in it (e.g. timing of dental extractions). This is also true for the GMP if there are any underlying medical problems that need to be addressed or kept under observation

GDP, general dental practitioner; GMP, general medical practitioner.

References

1 Naini FB. *Facial Aesthetics: Concepts and Clinical Diagnosis*. Oxford: Wiley Blackwell, 2011.

2 Naini FB, Gill DS (eds). *Orthognathic Surgery: Principles, Planning and Practice*. Oxford: Wiley Blackwell, 2017.

3 Fox N. The index of orthodontic treatment need. In: Gill DS, Naini FB (eds). *Orthodontics: Principles and Practice*. Oxford: Wiley Blackwell, 2011.

4 Naini FB. A surgeon's perspective on body dysmorphic disorder and recommendations for surgeons and mental health clinicians. In: Phillips KA (ed.). *Body Dysmorphic Disorder: Advances in Research and Clinical Practice*. Oxford: Oxford University Press, 2017.

5 National Institute for Health and Care Excellence. *Prophylaxis Against Infective Endocarditis:* Antimicrobial Prophylaxis Against Infective Endocarditis in Adults and Children Undergoing Interventional Procedures. Clinical Guideline CG64. London: NICE, 2008 (last updated July 2016).

6 Chate R. Principles of orthodontic treatment planning. In: Gill DS, Naini FB (eds). *Orthodontics: Principles and Practice*. Oxford: Wiley Blackwell, 2011.

7 Macgregor FC. Social and psychological implications of dentofacial disfigurement. *Angle Orthod.* 1979; 40:231–233.

8 Chou WJ, Wang PW, Hsiao RC, et al. Role of school bullying involvement in depression, anxiety, suicidality, and low self-esteem among adolescents with high-functioning autism spectrum disorder. *Front. Psychiatry* 2020; 11:9.

9 Seehra J, Fleming PS, Newton T, DiBiase AT. Bullying in orthodontic patients and its relationship to malocclusion, self-esteem and oral health-related quality of life. *J. Orthod.* 2011; 38:247–256.

10 Seehra J, Newton JT, Dibiase AT. Interceptive orthodontic treatment in bullied adolescents and its impact on self-esteem and oral health-related quality of life. *Eur. J. Orthod.* 2013; 35:615–621.

11 Al-Bitar ZB, Al-Omari IK, Sonbol HN, et al. Bullying among Jordanian schoolchildren, its effects on school performance, and the contribution of general physical and dentofacial features. *Am. J. Orthod. Dentofacial Orthop.* 2013; 144:872–878.

12 Salzmann A. Definition and criteria of handicapping malocclusion: a progress report. *Am. J. Orthod.* 1966; 52:209–212.

13 Baccetti T, Franchi L, McNamara JA. An improved version of the cervical vertebral maturation (CVM) method for the assessment of mandibular growth. *Angle Orthod.* 2002; 72:316–323.

14 Naini FB, Manouchehri S, Al-Bitar Z, et al. The maxillary incisor labial face tangent: clinical evaluation of maxillary incisor inclination in profile smiling view and idealized aesthetics. *Maxillofac. Plast. Reconstr. Surg.* 2019; 41:31–38.

15 Naini FB. Cephalometry and cephalometric analysis. In: *Naini FB. Facial Aesthetics: Concepts and Clinical Diagnosis*. Oxford: Wiley Blackwell, 2011.

16 Naini FB. Historical evolution of orthognathic surgery. In: Naini FB, Gill DS (eds). *Orthognathic Surgery: Principles, Planning and Practice*. Oxford: Wiley Blackwell, 2017.

17 Naini FB, Cobourne MT, McDonald F, Wertheim D. The aesthetic impact of upper lip inclination in orthodontics and orthognathic surgery. *Eur. J. Orthod.* 2015; 37:81–86.

18 Andrews LF. The six keys to normal occlusion. *Am. J. Orthod.* 1972; 62:296–309.

19 Gill DS, Naini FB, Jones A, Tredwin CJ. Part-time versus full-time wear following fixed appliance therapy: a randomized prospective controlled trial. *World J. Orthod.* 2007; 8:300–306.

20 Mouradian WE. The face of a child: children's oral health and dental education. *J. Dent. Educ.* 2001; 65:821–831.

21 Johal A, Alyaqoobi I, Patel R, Cox S. The impact of orthodontic treatment on quality of life and self-esteem in adult patients. *Eur. J. Orthod.* 2015; 37:233–237.

22 Broder HL. Children's oral health-related quality of life. *Community Dent. Oral Epidemiol.* 2007; 35 (Suppl. 1):5–7.

23 Ferrando-Magraner E, Garcia-Sanz V, Bellot-Arcis C, et al. Oral health-related quality of life of adolescents after orthodontic treatment: a systematic review. *J. Clin. Exp. Dent.* 2019; 11:e194–e202.

24 Phillips C, Magraw C. Patient satisfaction and patient-centred outcome measures in orthognathic surgery. In: Naini FB, Gill DS (eds). *Orthognathic Surgery: Principles, Planning and Practice.* Oxford: Wiley Blackwell, 2017.

25 Brough E, Donaldson AN, Naini FB. Canine substitution for missing maxillary lateral incisors: the influence of canine morphology, size, and shade on perceptions of smile attractiveness. *Am. J. Orthod. Dentofacial Orthop.* 2010; 138:705e1–9; discussion 705–707.

26 Kirschen RH, O'Higgins EA, Lee RT. The Royal London Space Planning: an integration of space analysis and treatment planning. Part I: assessing the space required to meet treatment objectives. *Am. J. Orthod. Dentofacial Orthop.* 2000; 118:448–455.

27 Kirschen RH, O'Higgins EA, Lee RT. The Royal London Space Planning: an integration of space analysis and treatment planning. Part II: the effect of other treatment procedures. *Am. J. Orthod. Dentofacial Orthop.* 2000; 118:456–461.

28 Lee RT, Kirschen RH. Space planning for the dentition (space analysis). In: Gill DS, Naini FB (eds). *Orthodontics: Principles and Practice.* Oxford: Wiley Blackwell, 2011.

29 Naini FB, Gill DS. Patient evaluation and clinical diagnosis. In: Naini FB, Gill DS (eds). *Orthognathic Surgery: Principles, Planning and Practice.* Oxford: Wiley Blackwell, 2017.

30 Elwyn G, Coulter A, Laitner S, et al. Implementing shared decision making in the NHS. *BMJ* 2010; 341: c 5146.

31 Sloan J. Asking the obvious questions regarding patient burden. *J. Clin. Oncol.* 2002; 20:4–6.

32 Bradburn NM. *Respondent burden. Proceedings of the Health Survey Research Methods Second Biennial Conference.* Washington, DC: Department of Health, Education and Welfare, 1977.

33 Morgan DJ, Scherer LD, Korenstein D. Improving physician communication about treatment decisions: reconsideration of 'risks vs benefits'. *JAMA* 2020; 324 (10):937–938.

34 Canterbury v Spence, 464 F2d 772, 775 (DC Cir 1972).

2

Principles of Orthodontic Biomechanics

Farhad B. Naini and Daljit S. Gill

CHAPTER OUTLINE

Introduction, 29
Basic Concepts and Principles, 30
   Spatial Planes and Axes of Rotation as a Frame of Reference, 30
   Force, 30
   Centre of Resistance, 33
   Moment, 34
   Couple, 35
   Centre of Rotation, 37
   Pure Rotation, 37
   Retraction and Protraction, 37
   Retroclination and Proclination, 38
   Tip, 38
   'Tipping', 38
   Torque, 38
Newton's Laws of Motion and Static Equilibrium, 38
Displacement of Rigid Bodies, 39
   How do Teeth Translate with Edgewise Fixed Appliances?, 40
Control of Tooth Movement, 41
   Extension Hooks and the Centre of Resistance, 41
   Moment-to-Force Ratios and Controlling Root Position, 42
Types of Tooth Movement, 44
   Simple ('Uncontrolled') Tipping, 46
   Controlled Tipping, 46
   Translation (Bodily Movement), 46
   Root Movement, 46
   Pure Rotation, 47
Clinical Applications and Relevance, 47
   One-Couple Force System, 48
   Two-Couple Force System, 48
   Space Closure, 49
   Space Closure with Sliding Mechanics, 49
   Space Closure with Closing Loop Mechanics, 52
Conclusion, 54
References, 55

Introduction

Mechanics is the area of physics concerned with the motions of macroscopic objects as a result of the forces acting upon them. A force applied to an object will result in its displacement, i.e. a change in the position of the object relative to its environment. **Biomechanics** is the study of the structure, function and motion of the mechanical aspects of biological systems, at any level from whole organisms to cellular organelles, using the methods of mechanics. **Orthodontic biomechanics** refers to the study of the movement of the teeth resulting from applied

Preadjusted Edgewise Fixed Orthodontic Appliances: Principles and Practice, First Edition. Edited by Farhad B. Naini and Daljit S. Gill.
© 2022 John Wiley & Sons Ltd. Published 2022 by John Wiley & Sons Ltd.

forces generated by orthodontic appliances. It includes the biomechanical principles of tooth movement and the technical aspects and design, construction, operation and application of orthodontic appliances to clinical orthodontics.

Orthodontic biomechanics is usually considered one of the more difficult parts of orthodontics, and perhaps is viewed as more of an academic interest rather than of direct clinical relevance. However, this is far from the truth. Integrating the basics of orthodontic biomechanics into everyday clinical practice will improve treatment efficiency and reduce the unintended and undesirable tooth movements that are so often the cause of extended treatment times.

The clinician should understand and integrate the scientific principles of applied biomechanics to the design and application of orthodontic appliances and how they exert forces onto the teeth, and the probable movements of the teeth that are produced. The exact forces involved and complex mathematical equations are not as important as understanding the underlying principles of orthodontic biomechanics.

The purpose of this chapter is to describe the application of orthodontic biomechanics to the preadjusted edgewise appliance systems.

Basic Concepts and Principles

Technical orthodontics may be thought of as the clinical application of forces to move the teeth. Forces act on bodies based on classical Newtonian principles; however, when describing biomechanical principles in orthodontics, consideration should be given to the fact that the bodies in question, i.e. the teeth, are of different shapes, embedded in variable amounts of alveolar bone and other periodontal supporting structures, and the forces are almost always applied at a distance from where they would produce the ideal desired movement.

In order to describe orthodontic biomechanics, a number of terms first need to be defined and relevant concepts described.

Spatial Planes and Axes of Rotation as a Frame of Reference

The orientation and movement of any object in space may be assessed in relation to the three planes of space and the three axes of rotation.[1] A frame of reference, in this context, refers to the spatial planes and geometrical coordinate axes of rotation in relation to which the position and movement of a tooth can be defined and measured (Figure 2.1) (see section Displacement of Rigid Bodies).

Force

In physics, force is defined as a dynamic physical influence that produces motion or stress in a stationary body, or changes its rate of motion, and is the product of mass and acceleration. In orthodontic biomechanics, it signifies the load applied to the teeth in a given direction, usually in order to change their position. The concept of **optimum** or **optimal force** is often discussed in orthodontics (see Chapter 3, Table 3.1); it refers to the force level that will promote the most efficient tooth movement whilst limiting the unwanted side effects (e.g. pain experienced by the patient, root resorption).[2, 3] The magnitude of optimum forces in orthodontic treatment continues to be under investigation.[4, 5]

Traditionally, in orthodontic biomechanics, force is measured in grams, which is a measure of mass, rather than the more accurate unit of force, the newton. This may be because the concept of a *gram of force* acting on a tooth is clinically easier to comprehend, and appears to be more tangible, and because the acceleration inherent in the definition of force in physics is not clinically relevant. A gram-force may be considered as the force of the earth's gravity acting on a gram:

1 newton = 101.97 grams-force (i.e. ~100 grams-force)
and therefore
1 gram-force = 0.98 centinewtons; i.e. 1 gf = ~1 cN

In fixed orthodontic appliance systems, forces may be produced by the deflection of archwires engaged in brackets, the application of elastics, or the placement of a variety of springs. Any such applied force has four properties.

- **Magnitude**: the size or amount of force, e.g. 1 N or 100 grams-force.[6, 7]
- **Point of application/origin**: refers to where the force is applied (e.g. bracket hook).
- **Direction of movement (sense)**: the orientation of the force in relation to the tooth (e.g. backward or upward).
- **Line of action**: a constructed straight line, extending from the point of application, in the direction of the force.

Changing any of these four properties will affect the efficiency of tooth movement, i.e. an optimum magnitude of force must be applied to the correct point in the desired direction of movement. On a two-dimensional diagram, a force may be represented by an arrow. The tail of the arrow is placed at the point of force application, it is orientated in the direction of movement, which represents its line of action, and its length signifies the comparative magnitude in relation to other forces.

A force is a **vector**, characterised by having *magnitude* as well as *direction* (as opposed to scalars, which have

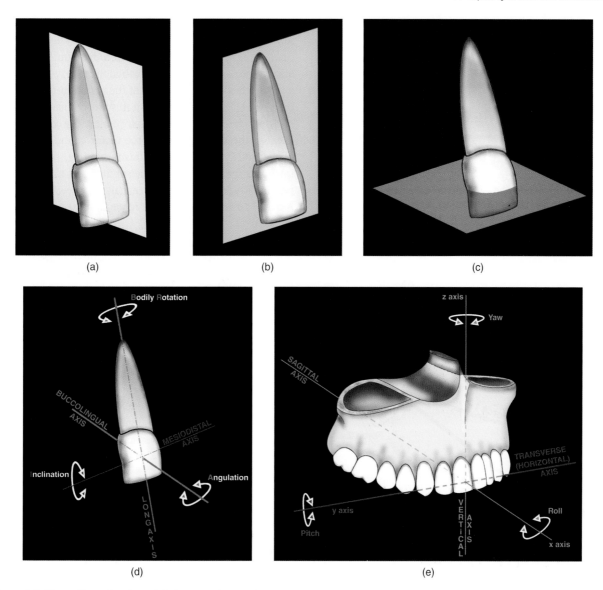

(a) (b) (c)

(d) (e)

Figure 2.1 Three-dimensional spatial planes and axes of rotation as a frame of reference. Translational (bodily) movements may be evaluated in relation to the three planes of space: (a) sagittal (anteroposterior) plane; (b) coronal (facial) plane; (c) transverse (horizontal) plane. Rotational movements may be evaluated in relation to the three axes of rotation (d). (e) Describing the rotation of groups of teeth, the occlusal plane or the jaws is also relative to the three axes of rotation. The terminology used is based on the aviation industry's description of an aircraft, particularly during landing, and is termed *attitude control*. Attitude is the orientation of an aircraft relative to a frame of reference, in this context being the axes of rotation. The terms 'roll', 'pitch' and 'yaw' describe an aircraft's attitude, and may be used to describe rotation of a jaw or occlusal plane. Rotating the aircraft's nose clockwise or anticlockwise is referred to as **roll**, which corresponds with rotation of a jaw round the sagittal or x-axis. Moving the aircraft's nose and tail up and down relative to one another is referred to as **pitch**, which corresponds with rotation of a jaw round the transverse or y-axis. Moving the aircraft's nose left and right is referred to as **yaw,** which corresponds with rotation of a jaw round the vertical or z-axis. The terms pitch, roll and yaw are not used for individual teeth, but they are used for the occlusal plane and jaws and, as such, clinicians should be familiar with their use. Source: Naini FB. *Facial Aesthetics: Concepts and Clinical Diagnosis*. Oxford: Wiley Blackwell, 2011; reprinted with permission.

magnitude but no direction, e.g. weight). Many clinical situations require the addition of a number of forces, a process termed **vector addition**. When multiple force vectors act on a point on a tooth, the sum of these vectors is termed the **resultant force**, which signifies the magnitude of force and the direction of movement. Finding the resultant

force is termed **vector addition**, and is not equivalent to an arithmetical addition unless the forces all act along the same line of action (Figure 2.2), but is a geometrical addition. One way of finding the resultant of multiple vectors is the *parallelogram method*. For example, a maxillary canine hook may have two elastics attached to it, a Class

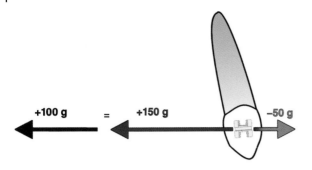

Figure 2.2 Vector addition with forces working along the same line of action. The two applied forces may only be added or subtracted arithmetically, to find the resultant force, if they act along the same line of action.

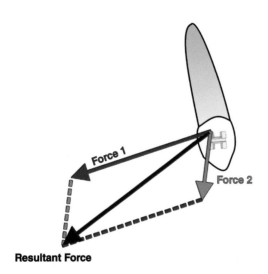

Figure 2.3 Vector addition with forces acting along different lines of action. The resultant force of multiple vectors may be found using the parallelogram method. In this example, a maxillary canine hook has two elastics attached to it, a Class II elastic (Force 1) and an anterior vertical elastic (Force 2). On a diagram, dotted lines may be constructed parallel to Forces 1 and 2, and these are then drawn by placing the origin of each vector at the head of the other, whilst maintaining their length and direction. The actual force vector may then be drawn from the point of force application (in this case the canine hook) to the opposite corner of the constructed parallelogram. This line is the vector sum of Forces 1 and 2, and is the resultant force.

II elastic (Force 1) and an anterior vertical elastic (Force 2) (Figure 2.3). On a diagram, lines may be constructed parallel to Forces 1 and 2, and these are then drawn by placing the origin of each vector at the head of the other, whilst maintaining their length and direction. The actual force vector may then be drawn from the point of force application (in this case the canine hook) to the opposite corner of the constructed parallelogram. This line is the vector sum of Forces 1 and 2, and is the resultant force.

The defining feature of a resultant force is that it has the same effect on a rigid body as the original system of forces. Therefore, by either drawing such a diagram, or by visualising the force vectors, the orthodontist may elect to use a single elastic along the line of the resultant force, rather than two elastics. Alternatively, in some clinical situations, multiple forces may be employed by the orthodontist because the single desired force vector cannot be accomplished due to anatomical constraints (e.g. the desire to intrude a maxillary central incisor along its long axis may require a vertical force and a palatal force, in order to provide a resultant intrusive force along the long axis of the tooth).

In some clinical situations, improved understating of how a single force acts on a tooth requires analysis to identify the direction of its **vector components**. Force vectors may be resolved into components, which is termed **vector resolution**. Separating a force into its components is essentially the opposite of vector addition described above, but may be helpful in undertaking vector addition. More importantly, in clinical practice, determining the various components of a force will aid the clinician's understanding of the direction of tooth movement. For example, a Class II elastic attached to the hook on a maxillary canine will have two vector components, a horizontal (distalising) component and a vertical (extrusive) component (Figure 2.4).

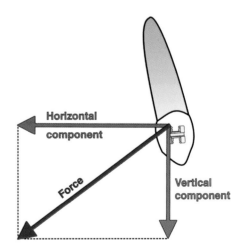

Figure 2.4 Force vector components may be analysed and their directions identified by the process of vector resolution. For example, the single vector force shown here, representing a Class II elastic attached from a mandibular molar hook (not shown) to the maxillary canine, may be divided into its component parts, usually perpendicular to one another. The component directions are usually taken in relation to the occlusal plane, and the magnitude of force in each direction may be approximately determined. Therefore, this Class II elastic force will have a greater distalising component but also an extrusive component.

Centre of Resistance

A robin red breast in a cage

Puts all Heaven in a rage

William Blake (1757–1827) 'Auguries of
Innocence' (c. 1803)[8]

The reader will be forgiven for wondering what this couplet has to do with the biomechanics of tooth movement. The answer lies with Leonardo da Vinci, the inspired artist-scientist who transcended his time, and his interest in mechanics, which he referred to as 'the paradise of the mathematical sciences'.[9] As a young child, Leonardo became fascinated with animals, often holding them in higher regard than humans. Observation of animal slaughter for human consumption prompted him to become a lifelong vegetarian, and in his childhood wanderings through the markets of Vinci he saw caged birds for sale, which he could not tolerate. He would either buy or somehow obtain the birds only to set them free in nearby woods. This simple ethical act prompted his interest in flight. How did birds fly? What was the mechanism that allowed their wings to elevate them into the air, and how, mechanically, did they maintain their flight? This became a lifelong passion, and eventually led to his *Codex on the Flight of Birds* (c. 1505) (Figure 2.5). In this treatise he explained, for the first time, that the centre of gravity of a flying bird does not coincide with its centre of pressure (similar to the aerodynamic centre of an aerofoil), which in biomechanics is called the centre of resistance; this appears to be the first description of the concept. The term itself was popularised in orthodontics by Dr Charles J. Burstone (1928–2015) (Figure 2.6), Professor of Orthodontics at the University of Connecticut, and the pioneer of orthodontic biomechanics.

For a symmetrical free (unconstrained) body in a vacuum, the **centre of mass** is the point within that body where its distribution of mass is concentrated, and where the application of a force will result in bodily movement. In such circumstances, the centre of mass is the same as the centre of resistance (Figure 2.7). In the clinical situation, a tooth is not of uniform and symmetrical shape, and is constrained by its environment, i.e. the alveolar bone and other periodontal support structures. For teeth, the **centre of resistance** may be defined as the point or area where the application of force will result in bodily movement (translation) (Figure 2.8). A red circle is used to represent the centre of resistance of teeth in all the relevant figures in this chapter.

The precise location of the centre of resistance of a tooth cannot be easily identified, but is dependent on the following parameters:

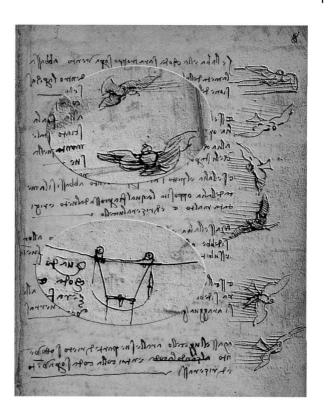

Figure 2.5 Leonardo da Vinci studied the flight of birds in terms of biomechanics and provided the description of the concept of a centre of resistance.

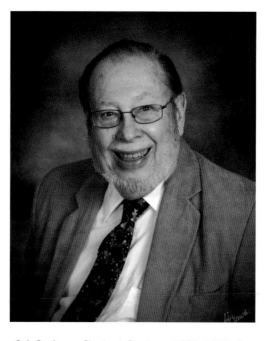

Figure 2.6 Professor Charles J. Burstone (1928–2015). Source: courtesy of the World Federation of Orthodontists.

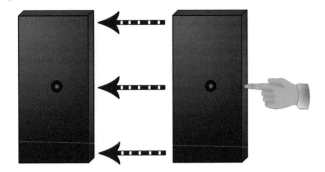

Figure 2.7 A force acting through the centre of mass of a free body in a vacuum will lead to bodily translation. The blue circle represents the centre of mass.

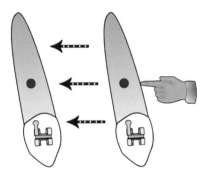

Figure 2.8 In a hypothetical situation, if a single force was able to act directly at the centre of resistance of a tooth, the tooth would bodily translate. The red circle represents the centre of resistance. *Note*: this red circle will be used to represent the centre of resistance of teeth in all the relevant figures in this chapter.

- Root length
- Root morphology
- Number of roots
- Level of alveolar bone and periodontal support.

Although the precise location cannot be accurately determined, analytical investigations have found that for a single rooted tooth with normal alveolar bone and periodontal support, the centre of resistance is located approximately one-third of the distance from the crest of the alveolar bone to the root apex (Figure 2.9).[10–13] For multirooted teeth, it is located approximately in the region of the roots just apical to the furcation. It is important to note that single-rooted teeth, multirooted teeth, segmental groups of teeth connected rigidly as a unit with an orthodontic appliance, each dental arch, and the jaws each have their own centre of resistance. There will also be differences between patients as a result of variation in tooth morphology and periodontal support. In addition, alveolar bone loss or root

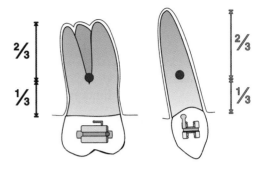

Figure 2.9 Location of the centre of resistance (CR). Analytical investigations have found that for a single-rooted tooth with normal alveolar bone support, the CR is located approximately one-third of the distance from the crest of the alveolar bone to the root apex. For multirooted teeth, it is located approximately in the region of the roots just apical to the furcation.

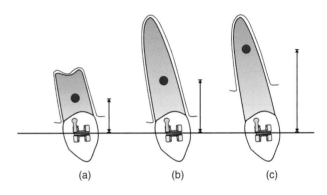

(a)   (b)   (c)

Figure 2.10 Location of the centre of resistance (CR) depends on alveolar bone height and root length. Therefore, root resorption or alveolar bone loss will affect the relative position of the CR of a tooth. (a) Change in position of CR if root resorption has occurred, compared with (b) a normal tooth and (c) with alveolar bone loss. This has clinical implications in fixed appliance orthodontics, as variation in the position of the CR alters the distance from the bracket, where the force is applied, to the CR.

resorption will affect the location of the centre of resistance (Figure 2.10).[14]

Moment

In physics, a moment refers to the turning effect produced by a force acting at a distance on an object, usually defined with respect to a fixed reference point (Figure 2.11). In mechanics, the moment of a force describes the tendency of a force applied to a body to produce rotation. The application of orthodontic forces is typically at the crown of a tooth, and thereby the applied force is not through the tooth's centre of resistance. A force applied at a distance from the centre of resistance will

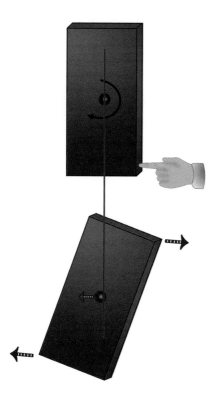

Figure 2.11 A force acting at a distance from the centre of mass of a free body in a vacuum will lead to rotation about the centre of mass, as well as a small amount of bodily translation in the direction of the applied force.

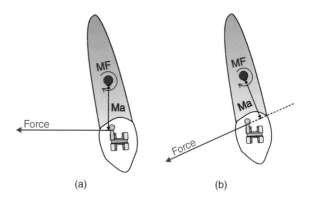

(a)   (b)

Figure 2.12 The moment of a force (MF) is equal to the product of the force magnitude and the perpendicular distance (Ma) from its line of action to the centre of resistance (red circle). The point of force application in both (a) and (b) is the maxillary canine hook, but, for comparative reasons, the forces have different lines of action. The perpendicular distance from the line of action of each force to the centre of resistance is known as the moment arm (Ma).

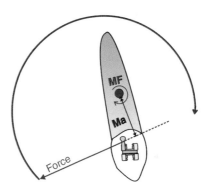

Figure 2.13 The direction of the moment may be found by following the line of action round the centre of resistance towards the point of force application.

not produce bodily movement only, but will also result in rotation. In orthodontic biomechanics, the moment, or more accurately the *moment of force*, describes the tendency of a force applied to a tooth to produce rotation (Figure 2.12).

The magnitude of this rotational effect produced by a force acting at a distance is expressed as the product of the force and the perpendicular distance from the line of action of that force to the centre of resistance. The direction of the moment may be found by following the line of action round the centre of resistance towards the point of force application (Figure 2.13). The perpendicular distance from the line of action of the force from the point of force application to the centre of resistance is termed the **moment arm** (or lever arm) (Figure 2.14). In classical mechanics, the unit is the newton metre (N·m) or newton centimetre (N·cm), but in orthodontics the **gram force-millimetre (gf-mm)** unit is more commonly employed (1 gf-mm = 0.98 N·cm).

The magnitude of the moment of a force may be determined by two variables:

- the magnitude of the force
- the distance from the point of force application to the centre of resistance.

It is within the clinician's capability to manipulate either of these variables in order to achieve the desired tooth movements.

The edgewise orthodontic system can simultaneously deliver forces, moments and counterbalancing moments.

Couple

In mechanics, a couple refers to a pair of equal and parallel forces acting in opposite directions (i.e. opposite lines of action), and tending to cause rotation about an axis perpendicular to the plane containing them. A couple is a moment

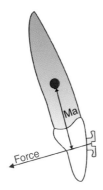

Figure 2.14 The perpendicular distance from the line of action of the force from the point of force application (here the point of force application is the bracket slot) to the centre of resistance is termed the moment arm (Ma), also sometimes referred to as the lever arm.

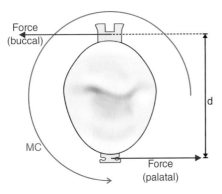

Figure 2.15 The magnitude of a force couple is the product of the magnitude of one of the forces multiplied by the perpendicular distance to the opposite force. For example, the diagram shows the occlusal view of a premolar tooth which is to be rotated using a force couple. If the forces shown are each 60 g (a buccal elastic force applied to the bracket and an equal and opposite palatal force applied to a bonded button), and the distance (d) is 9 mm, the magnitude of the force couple (moment of the couple, MC) would be $60 \times 9 = 540$ gf-mm.

where the sum of the forces is zero. The magnitude of a couple is the product of the magnitude of one of the forces multiplied by the perpendicular distance to the opposite force (Figure 2.15). In order to determine the direction of the rotation, either force may be followed round the centre of resistance and towards the origin of the opposite force.

The moment created by a couple is always round the centre of resistance, *no matter where the pair of forces is applied* (Figure 2.16a,b). As the distance between the two forces of the couple decreases, the overall magnitude of the couple also decreases. *The clinical implication for fixed orthodontic appliances is that no matter where a bracket is positioned on the crown of a tooth, the moment of the couple will lead to rotation of the tooth round its centre of resistance* (Figure 2.16c).

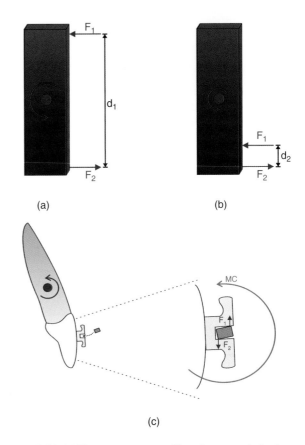

Figure 2.16 (a) The moment created by a force couple is always round the centre of resistance, *no matter where the pair of forces is applied*. A pair of equal and opposite forces is shown acting at a distance on a beam, resulting in rotation round its centre of resistance. (b) As the distance between the forces decreases, the magnitude of the force couple also decreases, but rotation still occurs round the centre of resistance. It should be noted that the pair of forces applied to the beam in this diagram resembles the position of a torquing force couple applied to a bracket on the crown of a maxillary incisor. (c) The clinical implication for fixed orthodontic appliances is that no matter where a bracket is positioned on the crown of a tooth, the moment of the force couple will lead to rotation of the tooth round its centre of resistance. In this diagram, a rectangular archwire with palatal root torque applied is engaged into the bracket slot on a maxillary central incisor. The torsional stress of the engaged archwire places a force couple in the bracket slot. The moment of this force couple (MC) will result in rotation of the maxillary incisor round its centre of resistance and thereby a change in the tooth's inclination.

The magnitude of the couple depends on the magnitude of the forces and the distance between the two forces, with the moment of the created couple being the sum of the moments created by each of the two forces. Where the two forces creating the couple act on effectively opposing sides of the centre of resistance, their effect is additive. This applies to round or rectangular orthodontic archwires changing the angulation of a tooth by engaging in a bracket,

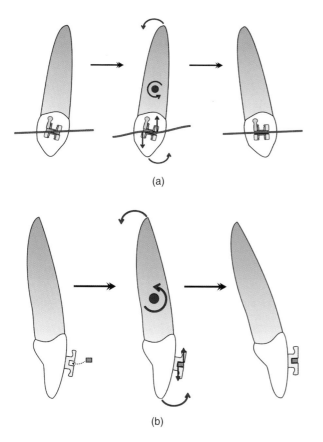

(a)

(b)

Figure 2.17 The magnitude of the couple depends on the magnitude of the forces (shown as two equal and opposite red arrows acting on the bracket) and the distance between the two forces, with the moment of the created force couple being the sum of the moments created by each of the two forces. Where the two forces creating the couple act on effectively opposing sides of the centre of resistance, their effect is additive. This applies to the settings illustrated in (a) and (b). (a) Round or rectangular orthodontic archwires change the angulation of a tooth by engaging in a bracket slot. The expression of mesiodistal tip, i.e. the change in the angulation of the tooth, stops when the archwire becomes passive in the bracket slot. (b) Rectangular archwires change the inclination of a tooth by engaging in a bracket slot. The expression of buccolingual torque, i.e. the change in the inclination of the tooth, stops when the archwire becomes passive in the bracket slot.

and to rectangular archwires changing the inclination of a tooth by engaging in a bracket (Figure 2.17).

Centre of Rotation

This is the point on or outside a body round which all other points on the body rotate. *For a tooth, it is the point round which the tooth actually rotates during movement.* If a force *and* a couple are applied to a bracket on a tooth, this allows control over the location of the centre of rotation and thereby control over the type of tooth movement (see section Types of Tooth Movement). If the

centre of rotation is on a three-dimensional object, it is termed the **axis of rotation** (see Figure 2.1).[1] In rotational movement assessed in two dimensions, the only point on an object that does not move is the centre of rotation. In three-dimensional rotational tooth movement, e.g. retroclination of a proclined maxillary central incisor, the entire tooth rotates round the transverse axis of rotation; therefore, every point on the tooth moves except those located on the axis of rotation.

It is possible to estimate the location of the centre of rotation of a tooth based on the superimposition of pretreatment and end-of-treatment lateral cephalometric radiographs. However, because tooth movements are often not uniform, and may occur incrementally with a variety of inconsistent positional changes over the entire movement, one therefore cannot be certain that rotation occurred exactly round one point or axis over the entire movement. Nevertheless, a retrospective estimation of the centre of rotation can be made (Figure 2.18).

Pure Rotation

This occurs when a force couple is applied such that the rotation of a tooth is with the centre of rotation at the centre of resistance.

Retraction and Protraction

These terms refer to bodily tooth movement (translation) in the labiolingual direction for incisors and the mesiodistal direction for the buccal segments. These terms are *not*

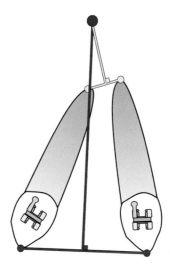

Figure 2.18 Two lines may be constructed from equivalent points of the tooth, e.g. tip and apex, and these connect the pretreatment and end-of-treatment tooth positions. Each line is bisected with a perpendicular, and the point where the two perpendicular lines meet is the centre of rotation (blue circle).

synonymous or interchangeable with retroclination and proclination.[1]

Retroclination and Proclination

These terms refer to the angular deviation of the long axis of a tooth from a line perpendicular to the occlusal plane, in the labiolingual or buccolingual direction, e.g. rotation of an incisor round the transverse axis. These terms are *not* synonymous or interchangeable with retraction and protraction.[1]

Tip

This term refers to active orthodontic forces used to change the angulation of teeth, often by movement of the crown. It also refers to the built-in mesiodistal angulation of preadjusted edgewise brackets, which is part of their prescription.

'Tipping'

This term can, a little confusingly, refer to changes in the angulation or inclination of different teeth, depending on the context in which it is being used. For example, for a maxillary canine, mesial or distal tipping of the tooth refer to a change in its mesiodistal angulation. However, when considering the maxillary incisors, mesial or distal tipping can refer to a change in their mesiodistal angulation (i.e. a rotation round their sagittal axis), whereas the terms 'simple (uncontrolled) tipping' and 'controlled tipping' of the maxillary incisors refer to a change in their labiopalatal inclination, which is a rotation round their transverse axis (see section Types of Tooth Movement). Therefore, it is imperative that the term is defined correctly depending on the context in which it is being used.

Torque

Torque is the force tending to cause rotation and in orthodontics often refers to active orthodontic forces used to change the inclination of teeth, often by root movement. It also refers to the built-in buccolingual inclination of preadjusted edgewise brackets (which is part of their prescription), which generates torque when engaged with a rectangular archwire.

Newton's Laws of Motion and Static Equilibrium

Sir Isaac Newton (1642–1727) (Figure 2.19) is regarded as the most highly gifted pioneer in the fields of mechanics,

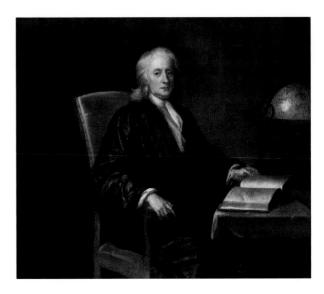

Figure 2.19 Sir Isaac Newton (1642–1727). Source: © National Portrait Gallery, London.

mathematics and physics. In addition to discovering the law of universal gravitation, he also established the three laws of motion, which are relevant to understanding orthodontic biomechanics. **Newton's Laws of Motion** are as follows.[15]

1. **Law of inertia**: every body continues in its state of rest, or of uniform motion in a straight line, unless it is compelled to change that state by forces impressed upon it.
2. **Law of acceleration**: the alteration of motion is ever proportional to the motive force impressed; and is made in the direction of the straight line in which that force is impressed.
3. **Law of action and reaction**: to every action there is always an opposite and equal reaction; or, the mutual actions of two bodies upon each other are always equal, and directed to contrary parts.

The application of these laws to orthodontic biomechanics is important in understanding the working of appliances and their potential unwanted effects. At rest, the sum of all forces on the teeth in the mouth is zero, i.e. they are not moving and may be considered to be in a state of equilibrium (Newton's First Law of Motion). When a force, or a set of forces, is applied to a tooth, the net force will cause the tooth to move (or more accurately 'accelerate', in terms of Newton's Second Law of Motion, though this is not relevant to orthodontics) in the direction exerted by the net force.

Newton's Third Law of Motion may be visualised by thinking of a rowing boat. As the rower pushes the water backwards with her oars, the water simultaneously pushes the boat forward. This Third Law is the most directly relevant to orthodontic biomechanics. For example, imagine a common clinical situation where elastic force is placed from an upper molar to retract an upper canine. The orthodontist wants the canine to move backwards, and the molar not to move forward, or to move only minimally. According to the Third Law, forces occur in pairs; therefore, as the molar exerts a force to retract the canine (the active force), there will be an equal and opposite force protracting the molar (the reactive force). This law forms the basis of the concept of orthodontic anchorage (see Chapter 3).

The term **static equilibrium**, in physics, is defined as a state of rest or uniform (non-accelerating) motion in which there is no resultant force on a body; it is based on Newton's First Law of Motion. In the context of clinical orthodontics, equilibrium refers to the state of non-movement of the teeth, i.e. where the sum of the forces and moments acting on a tooth/group of teeth is zero.[16] To be in a state of equilibrium, there can be no *net force* applied to a tooth in question; any forces on a tooth must be balanced by opposing forces, with their sum being zero. The relevance to orthodontic biomechanics is that the system of forces *acting at any one point in time* may be viewed in relation to the laws of static equilibrium.

Whenever forces or moments are applied to an orthodontic system, if the forces or moments are unequal in magnitude, further forces or moments will occur to oppose them. These latter forces or moments may lead to unwanted movements of teeth in undesirable directions. For example, a two-by-four appliance (a fixed appliance system only engaging the maxillary first molars and incisors), may be used to apply an intrusive force to the maxillary incisors. The opposing force will be an extrusive force on the molars. If the extrusive force is undesirable, which is often the case, then force will be required to prevent such extrusive forces (e.g. from high-pull headgear applied to the molars). Unwanted tooth movements may be predicted and thereby minimised by understanding the concept of equilibrium in any orthodontic system.

Displacement of Rigid Bodies

The physical and geometrical laws governing the displacement of rigid bodies apply *approximately* to the teeth. We must say approximately because teeth are not completely rigid but flex under stress; in addition, the supporting structures of the teeth also flex. However, understanding these laws will help illuminate orthodontic biomechanics.

Newton's discoveries paved the way for scientists who followed him to stand on the shoulders of his incredible intellect, and to further advance science. One of the most important was the Swiss mathematician-scientist **Leonhard Euler** (1707–1783) (Figure 2.20). Euler discovered

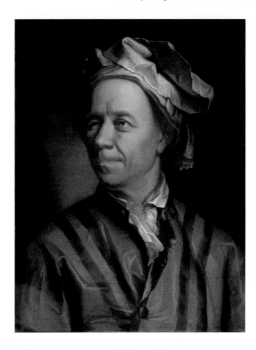

Figure 2.20 Leonhard Euler (1707–1783). Source: Kunstmuseum Basel.

the theorem of pure rotation of a rigid body round a single point, which states that:[17, 18]

> In three-dimensional space, any displacement of a rigid body such that a point on the rigid body remains fixed (the base point) is equivalent to a single rotation about an axis that runs through that point.

Therefore, a rigid body can rotate about a fixed axis, and all the points of the body located on the axis rotate whilst remaining in their position on the axis, whilst all other points on the body rotate round the axis in circular paths. The Euler angles are three angles introduced by Leonhard Euler to describe the orientation of a rigid body with respect to a fixed coordinate system (in this case, the three axes of rotation) (see Figure 2.1d, e). This was built on the previous work of the French mathematician René Descartes (1596–1650) (Latinised name Renatius Cartesius) who pioneered coordinate (analytical) geometry, and after whose Latinised name the **Cartesian coordinate system** is named; this system permitted the location of a point by reference to its distance from coordinate axes (usually denoted the x-axis and y-axis) intersecting at right angles. The addition of a third axis (z-axis) at right angles to the other two axes permits the determination of the position of one or more points in three-dimensional space. This is the origin of the three axes of rotation, based on three mutually perpendicular coordinate axes, and Euler's theorem (see Figure 2.1d,e).

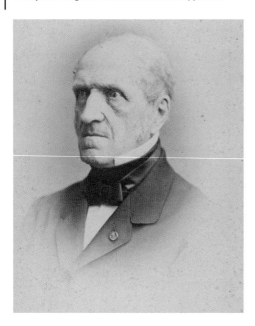

Figure 2.21 Michel Chasles (1793–1880).

After Euler, the French mathematician **Michel Chasles** (1793–1880) (Figure 2.21) discovered the theorem describing the *general displacement of a rigid body*:[19, 20]

> The most general displacement of a rigid body is equivalent to a screw displacement *consisting of a rotation about a fixed axis* [through base point] *plus a translation parallel to that axis*. [Emphasis added]

In other words, the rigid body rotates about an axis through the base point, but the entire body, including base point, translates.

Geometrically, for a given base point, translation and rotation are independent and may take place in any order, or possibly together. The 'base point' in relation to a tooth is the centre of resistance. Therefore, this theorem explains how *a single point force applied to the crown of a tooth, e.g. from a removable appliance spring, can slightly translate the position of the entire tooth, as well as rotating it round its centre of resistance, because all the points of the tooth, including the centre of resistance, move in the direction of the force*. The greatest amount of movement in this situation will be crown movement rotating in the direction of the force, and root movement rotating in the opposite direction, with the entire tooth rotating round its centre of resistance. However, according to Chasles' theorem, the centre of resistance itself will also *translate slightly* in the direction of the force (Figure 2.22). As the location of the force is moved closer to the centre of resistance, the degree of rotation reduces and the degree of translation increases.

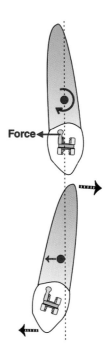

Figure 2.22 A single point force applied to the crown of a maxillary canine (e.g. from an elastic attached to the bracket hook) leads to rotation of the tooth round its centre of resistance, but also to a slight bodily translation of the tooth in the direction of the force.

This concept is very important to understanding how teeth move along an archwire with edgewise appliances, e.g. in sliding mechanics. Teeth do not really 'slide' along an archwire, as one may imagine, when forces are applied.

How do Teeth Translate with Edgewise Fixed Appliances?

Translation (bodily movement) of teeth does not occur by seamless sliding of the teeth along an archwire with edgewise appliance treatment. Fixed orthodontic appliances apply forces to the crowns, not directly through the centre of resistance located in the embedded part of the root. The appliances are also not completely rigid, but will have variable degrees of give. Therefore, fixed orthodontic appliances cannot perfectly translate the position of a tooth through alveolar bone. Nevertheless, translation of teeth does occur when using fixed orthodontic appliances. The question, therefore, is how does translation occur? The answer has been described elegantly by Staley,[21] based on previous work by Bishop,[22] Hixon et al.[23] and Andreasen.[24]

Richard 'Dick' Bishop (1925–1989) was a renowned Professor of Mechanical Engineering at University College London (Figure 2.23). In 1964,[22] he demonstrated how a rigid body could translate (move bodily) by first rotating about one axis and subsequently rotating an equal amount in the opposite direction about a parallel axis. He

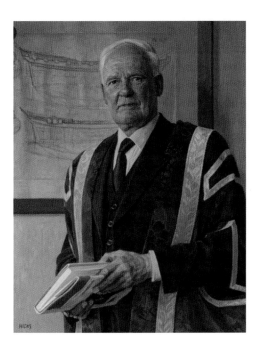

Figure 2.23 Portrait of Professor Richard Evelyn Donohue Bishop (1925–1989). Source: Brunel University London Arts Collection.

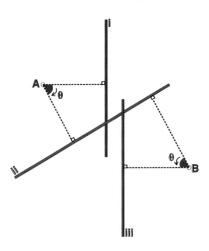

Figure 2.24 Translation (bodily movement) of a rigid body by first rotating about one axis and subsequently rotating an equal amount in the opposite direction about a parallel axis. Bishop illustrated this concept with a line diagram. Line i is rotated through angle θ about an axis at point A, moving it to position ii. An equal and opposite rotation through the same angle θ about an axis at point B moves the tooth to position iii. The line translates in position from i to iii, albeit to a different vertical level. This, effectively, is how teeth translate in the edgewise appliance. The change in the vertical level is controlled in fixed appliance orthodontics by the straight archwire engaged in the brackets. Source: Modified and redrawn from Bishop[22].

illustrated this concept with a line diagram (Figure 2.24). This, effectively, is how teeth translate in the edgewise appliance: they do not bodily 'slide' along the archwire but undergo a series of *ratcheting movements* in the direction of the force, i.e. crown tipping, in the direction of the force, slight translation of the entire tooth (according to Chasles' theorem) in the direction of the force, followed by root uprighting in the direction of the force (Figure 2.25).

Support for this concept of tooth translation with the edgewise orthodontic appliance was provided by Hixon et al.[23, 25] in an investigation of canine retraction along an almost full-thickness 0.0215 × 0.028-inch stainless steel archwire with 0.022 × 0.028-inch bracket slots. They explained that with canine retraction forces of 200 g over a 7-mm span, even such a 'heavy' archwire by clinical standards deflected by approximately 1 mm. Hixon et al.[23] concluded that their findings:

> indicate that retraction, even with conventional arches [archwires], probably consists of initial tipping movements as the arch [archwire] bends, followed by a certain amount of uprighting as the activating force exhausts itself before reactivation. With the Begg technique there is but one large 'tipping' and one 'uprighting' movement, as compared to a series of such movements with conventional [i.e. edgewise] arches. [Words in brackets added]

Bodily tooth movement and space closure with sliding mechanics are discussed further in later sections.

Control of Tooth Movement

For descriptive purposes, let us consider a maxillary central incisor. A single force applied to the labial surface of its crown, e.g. from a spring on an upper removable appliance, will create a moment round the centre of resistance located in the root. If the point of application of a 50-g force is applied to the crown 10 mm from the centre of resistance, this will create a 500 gf-mm moment, with a retroclining effect on the crown, rotating about the centre of resistance (Figure 2.26a). The root apex will rotate in the opposite direction. This works well if the desired movement is retroclination by simple tipping. However, if bodily retraction of the incisor is desired, some form of mechanics will be required to eliminate or at least limit the described moment of the force.

Extension Hooks and the Centre of Resistance

One method of applying a force as close as possible to the centre of resistance of a tooth, in order to reduce the rotational tendency, is to apply the forces to an extension arm/hook (also sometimes termed lever arms, or 'power'

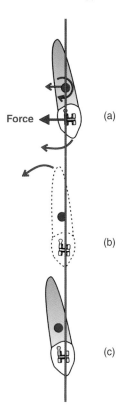

Force ◄———

(a)

(b)

(c)

Figure 2.25 Bodily tooth movement along an archwire with edgewise appliances. The archwire is not shown for clarity. (a) A force is applied to the canine bracket in order to 'slide' the tooth bodily along the archwire in the direction of the force. Initially, the crown tips in the direction of the force and the tooth slightly bodily translates in the direction of the force. (b) Once no further archwire deflection can occur, the crown can no longer move in the direction of the force. At this stage the root uprights in the direction of the force. (c) The tooth has moved bodily from its initial position, in the direction of the force.

arms, though these terms are confusing as they are not acting as levers and have nothing to do with power) integrated to and extending from a bracket on the tooth to the approximate level of the tooth's centre of resistance (Figure 2.26b). A horizontally directed force through the point of application of the extension hook, passing through the centre of resistance, will theoretically lead to bodily tooth movement. However, such attachments are rarely completely rigid and, practically speaking, the extension hook would need to be quite long to approach the centre of resistance of the root, making it potentially hazardous to the soft tissues, potentially unsightly, and an obstacle to the maintenance of oral hygiene. Extension hook designs are available in some bracket systems integrated to the canine brackets, used for canine retraction (Figure 2.27). Extension hooks may also sometimes be crimped or soldered onto a rectangular archwire.

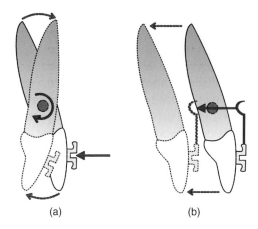

(a)   (b)

Figure 2.26 (a) Simple tipping of the maxillary incisor from a single point force applied to the crown, rotating round the centre of resistance. (b) Theoretically, increasing the length of the extension hook such that the force is applied at the level of, and thereby through, the centre of resistance can result in bodily translation of the tooth. In this case, this is bodily retraction of a maxillary incisor.

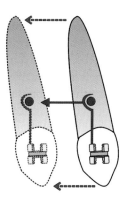

Figure 2.27 Extension hook integrated into a canine bracket. Theoretically, increasing the length of the extension hook such that the force is applied at the level of, and thereby through, the centre of resistance can result in bodily retraction of the canine.

Moment-to-Force Ratios and Controlling Root Position

The second and commonly employed method of controlling tooth movement with fixed appliances is with alteration of **moment-to-force ratios**,[26–28] which is a description of the relationship between the applied force to move a tooth and the counterbalancing force couple (moment) required to prevent the rotational tendency produced as a result of the applied force being at a distance from the centre of resistance.

What does this mean? The force applied to a tooth at the bracket will lead to a moment round the centre of resistance of the tooth; this is called the *moment of the force*, which will be in the direction of the applied force. To counteract the effect of the moment of the applied force, a force couple may be generated at the bracket, creating a new moment, called the *moment of the couple*, which can counterbalance the moment of the force (Figure 2.28). If the moment of the couple is opposite the moment of the force, and equal in magnitude, rotational movement will be prevented, permitting bodily movement.

The ratio of the *moment of the couple* to the *original applied force* will determine the type of tooth movement that occurs; this is the moment-to-force ratio (Figure 2.29). Varying the moment-to-force ratio (by changing the magnitude of the applied force and/or the force couple at the bracket) allows the location of the centre of rotation of a tooth to be altered along its long axis, thereby giving control over the type of tooth movement (see following section).

There is a direct relationship between the magnitude of the applied force and the magnitude of the counterbalancing couple, in that the heavier the applied force to the crown of a tooth, the larger the moment of the force, and thereby the larger the moment of the counterbalancing couple within the bracket required to prevent tipping.

The orthodontic biomechanical mechanism for achieving such a system is a fixed bracket or other attachment on the tooth crown, *constructed such that forces may be applied at two points on the tooth*. This concept was elucidated by Calvin Case in 1921 based on round wires (Figure 2.30).[29] Alternatively, an auxiliary spring may be used together with a round base archwire. The auxiliary spring would be required to place a force on the facial surface of the incisor crown gingival to the bracket, with the force in a palatal direction, causing it to rotate round its transverse axis (which is the usual reason for using such auxiliary springs, i.e. palatal root 'torquing' forces). However, in this situation, this force would need to be opposing the retroclining force at the bracket on the crown, the result being bodily retraction. Such torquing springs are used with traditional Begg appliances, but can be formed for use with some edgewise systems, and are rarely employed for the type of movement described here (Figure 2.31) (see Chapter 11, Figures 11.23 and 11.24), as the use of rectangular archwires has made such complex mechanics unnecessary.

The most common technique and mechanism for the application of a force couple is to use a rectangular archwire ligated into the rectangular edgewise bracket slot in order to generate the moment required to control the incisor inclination during retraction. The two points of contact are the opposite edges of the rectangular archwire within the bracket slot (see Figure 2.17b).

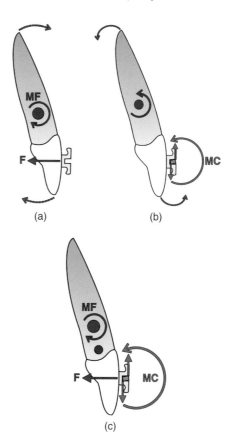

(a)

(b)

(c)

Figure 2.28 Moment-to-force ratios. The force applied to a tooth (F) will lead to a moment round the centre of resistance (CR) of the tooth; this is called the *moment of the force* (MF), which will be in the direction of the applied force. To counteract the effect of the moment of the applied force, a force couple may be generated at the bracket by engagement of an archwire, creating a new moment, called the *moment of the couple* (MC), which can counterbalance the moment of the force. If the moment of the couple is opposite the moment of the force, and equal in magnitude, rotational movement will be prevented, permitting bodily movement. The following examples and Figure 2.29 describe the biomechanics. (a) Application of a single point force (F) to the crown of a maxillary central incisor. This force may be from a labial spring or from a palatally directed elastic; in either case, there is a palatally directed retroclining force on the crown. The moment of the force (MF) will result in rotation round the centre of rotation, which in this situation is almost identical to the CR of the tooth, with the crown moving in the direction of the applied force. (b) If a force couple is applied at the bracket on the crown of the incisor tooth by engaging a rectangular archwire, the tooth will rotate round its CR, leading to a change in the inclination of the tooth. (c) However, if a palatal force is applied, as in (a), and a counterbalancing force couple is applied at the bracket, as in (b), the combination of the applied palatal force (and its moment, MF) and the force couple at the bracket (and its moment, MC) will mean that rotation of the tooth does *not* occur round its CR (red circle). The position of the centre of rotation (blue circle) will alter based on the ratio of the MF in relation to the MC (see Figure 2.29).

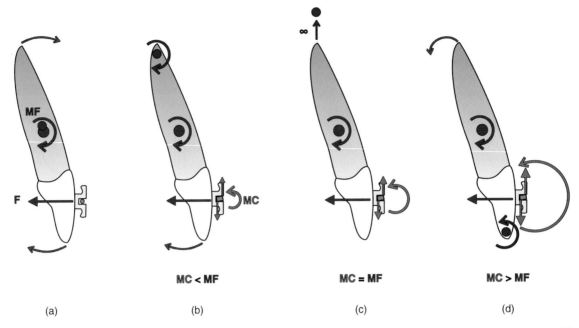

$$MC < MF \qquad\qquad MC = MF \qquad\qquad MC > MF$$

(a)   (b)   (c)   (d)

Figure 2.29 Relationship between moment-to-force ratio and the type of tooth movement. The ratio between the moment of the applied force (MF) and the counterbalancing moment of the couple (MC) determines the type of tooth movement that will occur. This important concept requires further explanation in relation to a common orthodontic situation. Consider the maxillary arch in the space closure stage of fixed appliance treatment. A continuous archwire is in place, and a space-closing force is applied to move the maxillary incisors backwards towards the posterior anchor teeth. This force F is acting at the brackets. The force F will lead to a moment round the centre of resistance; this moment of the force is termed MF. In the following four examples, the magnitude of the force F and the moment of this force, MF, will remain unchanged. (a) If the archwire is a relatively thin round wire, there will be no couple created at the bracket, i.e. MC = 0. The centre of rotation (C_{rot}, blue circle) will be very close to and just apical to the centre of resistance (CR, red circle), and the force F will lead to rotation round C_{rot}. The incisors retrocline by simple tipping, i.e. the crown moves in the direction of the force and the root rotates in the opposite direction. (b) A rectangular archwire is placed in the bracket. The space-closing force F remains the same, and MF thereby remains the same. The rectangular wire in the rectangular slot will lead to the formation of a force couple in the bracket, which is the moment of the couple (MC). If the bracket prescription is with palatal root torque, or if the archwire has palatal root torsional stress applied to it, MC will be the counterbalancing force to MF. As long as MC is less than MF, the tooth crown will still rotate in the direction of the original force F, but because of MC, C_{rot} will move apically. There is less root movement and more crown movement, which is termed controlled tipping. The incisors are still retroclining, but the crowns are moving a greater distance in a palatal direction, with minimal root movement. If C_{rot} moves to the apex, the apex will not move, and the crown will retrocline the greatest distance. (c) If a larger rectangular archwire is placed, or greater palatal torsional root 'torquing' forces are applied, such that MC increases until MC = MF, the tendency to rotation is eliminated; i.e. because MC is the counterbalancing force to MF, the two moments cancel each other, and there is no rotation round CR. C_{rot} moves apically towards infinity, and the effect of the original force F is to bodily translate the incisors in the direction of the force F, i.e. bodily retraction. (d) If even greater torsional forces are placed by the rectangular archwire in the bracket slot, such that MC becomes greater than MF, C_{rot} moves incisally, and there will be greater root movement in a palatal direction. If C_{rot} moves to the incisal tip, the tip will not move, and the root will 'torque' the greatest distance in a palatal direction.

Types of Tooth Movement

When using preadjusted edgewise appliances, the archwires, elastics and springs that deliver forces to the teeth do so via the brackets. Therefore, the application of forces, moments and couples usually occur at the bracket. Predictable tooth movements require an understanding of how applied forces and moments lead to tooth movement.

The range of tooth movements that may occur may be classified into five basic types (Figure 2.32):

- Simple tipping
- Controlled tipping
- Translation (bodily movement)
- Root movement
  - Mesiodistal root 'uprighting'
  - Buccolingual root 'torquing'
- Rotation.

With fixed orthodontic appliances, it is the application of the correct forces and moments that produces the desired tooth movements, i.e. the type of tooth movement that occurs depends on the magnitude, direction and point of application of the applied force and moment. The

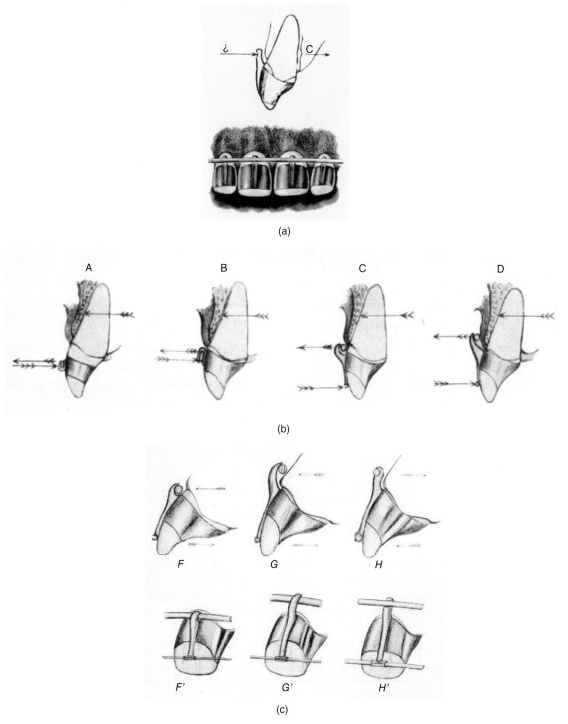

Figure 2.30 The concept of bodily movement from a force couple applied to the crown was described by Calvin Case in 1921. (a) Here, Case is describing a force being applied at point *i*, accomplished by attaching to the crown a rigid 'root-wise extension or bar', in order for the line of force to be sufficiently above the 'point of greatest resistance' at *c*. He suggests that a 'more or less bodily movement' would occur in the direction of the force, but that this would not be with the absolute certainty that would follow the more 'scientific control of the force for this character of movement, described later'. (b) The image marked A represents Edward Angle's method. The force couple is represented by the two arrows at the bracket. The upper arrow represents the 'centre of work' or 'fulcrum' (i.e. centre of resistance). The images marked B–D are Case's gradual modifications of the appliance in order to decrease 'the distance to the area of work or alveolar resistance, both of which greatly increase the mechanical advantage'. (c) Combinations used to create couples for bodily tooth movement. Source: Case CS. *A Practical Treatise on the Technics and Principles of Dental Orthopedia and Prosthetic Correction of Cleft Palate.* Chicago, IL: The C.S. Case co., 1921.

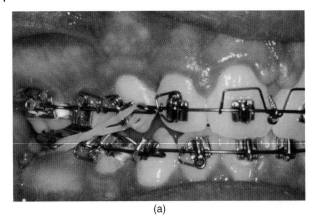

(a)

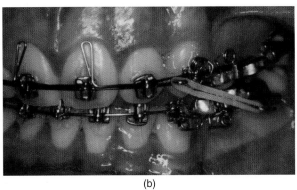

(b)

Figure 2.31 (a, b) Palatal root 'torquing' auxiliaries on the maxillary incisors, being used with a traditional Begg appliance. Source: courtesy of Dr David Spary.

moment-to-force ratio of the applied force and moment will control the location of the centre of rotation and thereby determine the type of tooth movement that occurs (see Figure 2.29). The moment-to-force ratio thereby determines how a tooth, or a segment of connected teeth, will move.

In summary, the centre of resistance of a tooth is anatomically set. The force and moment applied to the tooth, i.e. the moment-to-force ratio, allows the location of the centre of rotation to be determined.[30] The type of tooth movement may be determined by the location of the centre of rotation in relation to the centre of resistance. Controlling the location of the centre of rotation determines the level of control over the type of tooth movement that actually occurs.

Simple ('Uncontrolled') Tipping

This type of tooth movement occurs when a single force is applied to the crown of a tooth, moving the crown in the direction of the force, and the root in the opposite direction. The centre of rotation will be located very close and just apical to its centre of resistance.

This type of movement is useful in converting a Class II division 2 incisor relationship into a Class II division 1 by

simple proclination of the maxillary incisors, or in Class III orthodontic camouflage treatment, where the maxillary incisors are proclined and the mandibular incisors retroclined. When the tooth movements involved are changes in the tooth's labiolingual inclination, the more accurate term is 'simple (uncontrolled) retroclination/proclination'. When the tooth movement involves a change in the tooth's mesiodistal angulation, the term 'simple (uncontrolled) tipping' is accurate. However, the clinician should be aware that the term 'simple tipping' is used in the literature in relation to both angulation and inclination changes.

Controlled Tipping

This type of tooth movement occurs when the centre of rotation is located at (or near) the apex of the tooth; the apex will remain fixed in position as the rest of the tooth moves. It requires a force and a moment (couple) to be placed on the crown. The applied force will move the crown in the desired direction, and the moment prevents the root from moving in the opposite direction.

This type of tooth movement is useful when planning retroclination of proclined maxillary incisors, where their root apices are effectively in the correct position and their crowns are flared labially (which may be more accurately termed 'controlled retroclination'), or in correcting the angulation of mesially or distally angulated canines where the root apex is essentially in the correct position.

Translation (Bodily Movement)

Translation of a tooth occurs when the centre of rotation is located approaching infinity; the direction of movement of the centre of resistance is parallel to the line of action of the force, and every point on the tooth is bodily displaced parallel to the line of action of the force, i.e. the crown and root move in equal amounts in the same direction, with no rotation.

A horizontal force applied at the centre of resistance will result in bodily movement. As this location of applied force is difficult to achieve, simultaneous application of a force and a moment (couple) at the bracket is required, similar to controlled tipping.

Intrusion and extrusion are translational movements that occur in an axial direction, again with the centre of rotation at infinity.

Root Movement

Root movement refers to alteration of the axial inclination of a tooth by moving the root apex whilst maintaining the position of the crown tip. Root movement is made possible when the centre of rotation of a tooth is at (or near) the

Figure 2.32 Types of tooth movement. The centre of rotation is shown as a blue circle. (a) Simple tipping of a maxillary canine. (b) Controlled tipping of a maxillary canine. (c) Translation (bodily movement) of a maxillary canine. The centre of rotation is approaching infinity (∞). (d) Root movement by mesiodistal root 'uprighting' of a maxillary canine. (e) Root movement by buccopalatal root 'torquing' of a maxillary incisor. (f) Rotation of a premolar, shown from an occlusal aspect.

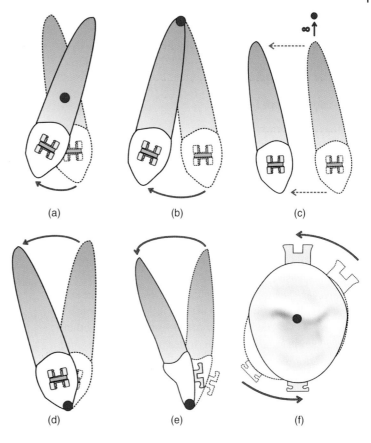

(a) (b) (c)

(d) (e) (f)

crown tip, e.g. incisal edge of a maxillary central incisor, or canine crown tip. The root must move an often significant distance through alveolar bone, which makes this type of movement prolonged and anchorage demanding, although in some circumstances it can be used to provide anchorage; for example, during canine retraction pitted against a molar for anchorage, a force providing mesial root movement of the molar can help resist forward movement of the molar crown.

Root movement in a mesiodistal direction may be referred to as **root uprighting**; it is an important part of the Begg and Tip-Edge appliance systems, but is also used in preadjusted edgewise appliances.

Root movement in a buccolingual direction is referred to most accurately as **changing tooth inclination by root movement**. This is undertaken by the application of torquing forces,[31] from rectangular archwires engaging a rectangular bracket slot (which is why, at the chairside, the orthodontic colloquialism is 'torquing' the incisor root, or 'controlled torquing' of the root).

Pure Rotation

This type of tooth movement occurs when a tooth rotates round its centre of resistance, the centre of rotation (axis of rotation) effectively being the long axis of the tooth.

Clinical Applications and Relevance

In fixed appliance orthodontic treatment, the brackets bonded to the teeth require archwires, elastics or springs to create the forces and moments necessary for tooth movement. In the initial alignment phase of treatment, the brackets are bonded in the most accurate position possible on the crowns of the teeth, but as the teeth are malaligned, the positions of the brackets relative to one another will be out of line. Therefore, engaging the initial aligning archwire will place forces and moments on the teeth via the brackets, leading to movement. In the later stages of treatment, when the brackets are lined up and the teeth aligned on the desired arch form, strategic bends in the archwires can be placed to move individual teeth. Again, these bends engaging the brackets will place forces and moments on the teeth via the brackets, leading to movement. In either of these situations, two kinds of force systems may be generated:

- one-couple force system
- two-couple force system.

Force systems may also be classified as statically **determinate**, which means that the forces and moments can be easily measured and analysed, or as **indeterminate** systems,[32] which are too complex for precise measurements. Essentially, one-couple force systems are determinate, and two-couple systems are indeterminate.

One-Couple Force System

In fixed appliance orthodontic mechanics, one-couple force systems are established when a couple is created only at one end of the system, with only a single force and single point of force application, and thereby no couple, at the other end.[33] One example is a cantilever spring, e.g. to extrude a canine tooth. It is inserted at one end in a molar tube (where the one couple occurs) and at its other end tied to the bracket on the canine (but not engaged into the bracket). The latter application is a single point of contact, with an extrusive force.

However, the more common use of one-couple force systems is with intrusion arches used to intrude incisor teeth (Figure 2.33).[34] The posterior anchor unit is tied together, with a stabilising lingual arch, to form one effective unit. The anterior teeth are also tied together as a segment. The intrusive force is light, therefore the reaction extrusive force on the posterior anchor segment is also light, limiting their unwanted extrusion.

At the chairside, with either of these approaches, the force system from the orthodontic appliance may be

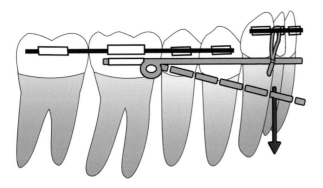

Figure 2.33 Burstone's intrusion arch is an example of a one-couple force system used with preadjusted edgewise appliances. The posterior anchor unit is tied together (including the second molar and premolars) with a heavy rectangular archwire, together with a stabilising lingual arch, to form one effective unit. The anterior teeth are also tied together as a segment. Separate left and right intrusion springs are placed (shown in grey), and tied to the anterior segment archwire (without engaging any brackets). The intrusion springs are tied relatively distally on the anterior segment archwire, so that the line of force is through the centre of resistance of the incisors, to prevent proclination of the mandibular incisors from the intrusive force. The intrusive force is light (it can be measured directly with a force gauge at the chairside), therefore the reaction extrusive force on the posterior anchor segment is also light, limiting their unwanted extrusion.

gleaned by removing the activated wire from its attachment (in both the above situations, this will be the anterior attachment), letting it lie passively, and assessing the position and angle of the wire in relation to the point of application of force on the teeth to be moved.

Two-Couple Force System

When an archwire is engaged between two separate attachments, e.g. between two bracket slots/tubes on different teeth, a two-couple force system is established (i.e. forces and couples occur at both ends). With preadjusted edgewise appliances, the forces and couples may occur in two situations: when a straight archwire is engaged in malaligned brackets (as in the early stages of treatment), or when an archwire with a specified bend is engaged between two brackets on aligned teeth (as in the finishing stages of treatment). Either way, this forms a statically indeterminate system, i.e. too complex for precise determination of the forces and moments on both attachments at any specific time.

When continuous arch mechanics are employed, which is the more common type of mechanics with preadjusted edgewise appliances, the effects of a continuous archwire on a large number of brackets is, to all intents and purposes, almost impossible to accurately analyse,[35, 36] and perhaps not hugely important when taken in the context of overall treatment. What effectively occurs when the initial aligning archwire is engaged in all the brackets is a very complex force system at every bracket, involving forces, moments and counterbalancing couples.[37] As soon as a small degree of movement of even one tooth occurs, the entire force system is likely to change, leading to another complex force system, and so on. However, the teeth are usually moving small distances within the constraints of the appliance, and clinical understanding is used to control and reduce unwanted movements, such as cinching the archwire or adding lacebacks (see Chapter 14).

One of the biomechanical considerations in fixed appliance treatment is **bracket width**. This is particularly relevant when mesiodistal root movement is required for root paralleling, in areas where teeth are excessively angulated, as often happens following space closure (e.g. closing a large midline diastema), or after premolar extraction space closure with sliding mechanics (see subsequent section). The moments required to upright the roots and correct their angulations are easier to generate if the brackets are wider (Figure 2.34).[38] The disadvantage of wider brackets is that the reduced **interbracket span** between adjacent teeth reduces the flexibility and springiness of the archwire, thereby reducing its range of action and making the archwire's ability to align the teeth more difficult.

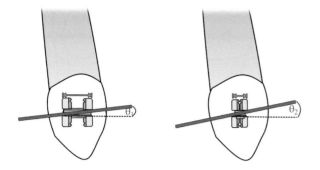

Figure 2.34 Bracket width has important biomechanical considerations for tooth movement. Wider brackets make control of mesiodistal root angulation easier, e.g. root paralleling on either side of an extraction space after space closure, or root uprighting. Bracket width also influences the **contact angle**, which is formed where the wire contacts the corner of the bracket slot. This is relevant to sliding mechanics, as wider brackets reduce the contact angle, which reduces impediments to tooth movement along the archwire. As shown, the contact angle with a wider bracket (θ_1) is less than the contact angle with a narrower bracket (θ_2). However, the disadvantage of wider brackets is a reduction in the length of the archwire in the interbracket span, which reduces the springiness and range of action of the wire, impeding alignment, particularly with initial flexible archwires.

Ideally, the correct balance between bracket width and interbracket span is required. Lack of interbracket span can be compensated for, to a degree, by increasing the flexibility of the aligning archwire, most commonly by choosing a wire of reduced diameter and more flexible material.

The dynamics of this two-couple system are also fundamental to understanding the biomechanical principles governing space closure with sliding mechanics (discussed later).

Space Closure

Space closure is most commonly required in orthodontic treatment following dental extractions for severe crowding and/or retraction of prominent incisor teeth.[39, 40] The planned biomechanics of space closure will depend on the planned final sagittal position of the maxillary incisors in relation to the face (see Chapter 1).[1] There are three potential categories of space closure.

- **Retraction of the incisor segment**: excessive incisor protrusion often means maintaining the posterior dental segment as the anchor unit and, as far as possible, preventing its protraction, and aiming for predominantly incisor retraction. Methods of anchorage reinforcement are discussed in Chapters 3, 12 and 14.

- **Retraction of the incisor segment and protraction of the posterior segment**: simultaneous and relatively symmetrical space closure in this fashion is commonly required during space closure, with approximately equal movement of the anterior and posterior segments for space closure.

- **Protraction of the posterior segment**: in certain situations, such as hypodontia of premolar teeth, when the anterior dental segment is in the correct sagittal position, space closure will be indicated predominantly by protraction of the posterior teeth. In such situations, the anterior dental segment acts as the anchor unit, and anchorage reinforcement may be required (e.g. Class III intermaxillary elastics, temporary anchorage devices or protraction headgear).

In patients with extreme crowding and anteriorly positioned buccal canines, **separate canine retraction** may be required prior to incisor retraction. However, where this is the case, such canine retraction is usually undertaken in the first (alignment and levelling) stage of preadjusted edgewise appliance treatment (see Chapter 14). In the second (space closure) stage of treatment with early standard edgewise appliances, separate canine retraction was usually undertaken prior to incisor retraction, which was thought to help preserve posterior anchorage. However, anchorage loss with this approach tends to be similar to retraction of the canine-to-canine segment.[41] Therefore, with the preadjusted edgewise appliance systems, there are only a few clinical situations where separate canine retraction may be required, e.g. significant midline deviations or very anteriorly positioned buccal canines. In most patients, following alignment and the gathering together of the anterior canine-to-canine segment, the anterior segment is retracted as one unit, termed **en masse retraction**.

There are two basic types of intra-arch space-closing mechanics: sliding mechanics (which involves friction) and loop mechanics. These are discussed in turn.

Space Closure with Sliding Mechanics

For sliding mechanics, the dental arch is first aligned and levelled, and progression through the archwires occurs until a relatively stiff archwire (at least a 0.018-inch round stainless steel archwire in a 0.022 × 0.028-inch slot), usually round or rectangular stainless steel, is in place. *Levelling the arch prior to sliding mechanics is extremely important*, as placement of space-closing forces between the anterior and posterior dental segments when there is still a sagittal curve of the occlusion (curve of Spee) is a mechanically incorrect situation, potentially hindering sliding mechanics (Figure 2.35).

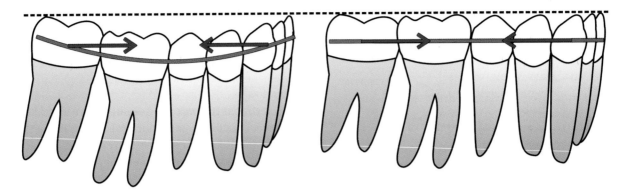

Figure 2.35 Applying space-closing forces by sliding mechanics on an arch that has not yet levelled may lead to a biomechanical impediment to space closure, as the space-closing forces will not be along the archwire and will counteract the levelling forces. Sliding mechanics should begin when the arch has been adequately levelled.

The applied space-closing force may be from elastics, elastomeric chains, elastomeric modules combined with ligature wires, nickel titanium closing coils or other forms of spring. These are stretched and applied horizontally, parallel to the archwire, from the anterior to the posterior dental segment, and the brackets 'slide' along the archwire as space closure takes place.

However, tooth movement along the archwire is not a smooth sliding movement (Figure 2.36). What actually appears to happen is the following: the space-closing force applied to the bracket (parallel to the wire) pulls the tooth, which leads to an initial simple (uncontrolled) tipping movement of the tooth crown towards the direction of the space-closing force. No friction is involved at this stage, and the degree of tipping depends on the clearance between the archwire and the bracket slot, and on the width of the brackets; the larger the archwire dimensions and the wider the brackets, the less tipping occurs. Next, as the bracket continues to tip, it contacts the archwire at diagonally opposite points of the bracket slot (known as **bearing**

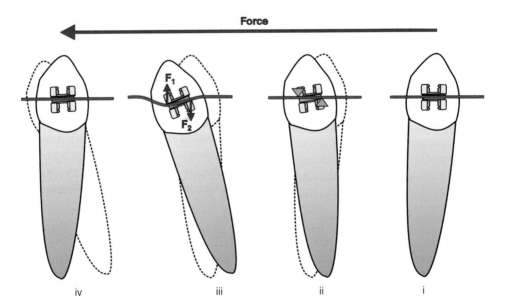

Figure 2.36 Tooth movement along an archwire with sliding mechanics. The diagram demonstrates a mandibular right canine tooth, viewed from the buccal aspect, being retracted along an archwire. (i) The tooth is aligned and levelled. A distal retracting force is applied to the tooth. (ii) The canine tooth undergoes a variable amount of uncontrolled tipping; the crown tips in the direction of the force. The bracket slot's occlusal and gingival walls contact the archwire at the bearing points (the lips of the blue triangles). They begin to deflect the archwire. The amount of crown tipping and the amount of archwire deflection depend on the size and stiffness of the archwire and the width of the bracket. (iii) The tooth translates slightly in the direction of the applied force. When no more archwire deflection is possible, the archwire will put two equal and opposite vertical forces (F_1 and F_2) onto the bracket slot; this is a force couple. (iv) Root uprighting occurs in the direction of the applied retraction force. This process of minute movements repeats over and again, resulting in the apparent distal 'sliding' of the canine along the archwire.

points); at this stage the bracket exerts forces on the wire, and the wire will exert equal and opposite forces on the bracket. The deflection of the archwire and the increased contact between the bracket slot and the archwire trying to move past each other causes friction. The bracket's deflection of the wire continues until the bending moment of the wire is equal to the moment of the applied force. The degree of deflection of the wire is inversely proportional to its stiffness, i.e. the stiffer the wire, the less it will deflect and bend. The tooth translates *slightly* towards the original line of action of the force and then stops as further wire deflection stops. The deflected archwire has now placed two diagonally opposing vertical forces on the bracket slot, leading to a force couple, the moment of which is opposite that of the applied space-closing force. The final phase involves root uprighting in the direction of the space-closing force, although at this stage space-closing crown movement is no longer occurring. These repeated minute tooth movements will move the tooth along the archwire in the direction of the applied force.

At subsequent appointments further activation of the space-closing forces is undertaken, e.g. new elastomeric chains are placed, and the process continues. So, effectively, during sliding mechanics the bracket (and tooth) *walk* along the wire (i.e. in successive steps: crown tipping, slight translation of the entire tooth, and root uprighting, with a wiggle–joggle movement akin to a crown-then-root rocking motion), step by step, rather than freely sliding along the archwire.

The major obstacle to sliding mechanics is the unpredictability of **friction**. Friction is the resistance force encountered when one body moves relative to another body with which it is in contact, i.e. it is the force that resists the relative sliding motion of the two surfaces which are in contact, and it acts tangentially to the two surfaces attempting to move past each other. Friction tends to be highest when attempting bodily movement along an archwire, as in sliding mechanics. The 'sliding' movement of the brackets over the archwire are resisted by friction, and the frictional force is the product of the applied force and the coefficient of friction.[42] The coefficient of friction will vary depending on the two materials in contact and the presence of lubrication. However, and perhaps counterintuitively, the magnitude of the frictional force does *not* depend on the apparent surface area in contact. This is because even smooth surfaces polished to a mirror finish at a macroscopic level are not truly smooth at a microscopic level; the surfaces have irregularities due to surface projections referred to as **asperities** (from Latin *asper*, rough) (Figure 2.37). Actual contact between two surfaces, whether they are being pushed together or with one sliding over the other, only occurs at the peaks of these

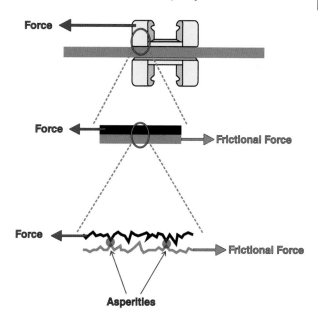

Figure 2.37 During sliding mechanics, when the bracket slots are moving along an archwire, there is relative sliding between the outer surface of the archwire and the inner surface of the bracket slots. However, contact between the wire and bracket slot only occurs at a limited number of peaks of irregular surface projections called asperities.

asperities. When two macroscopically smooth surfaces come into contact, such as an archwire and bracket slot, initially they only contact at the points of some of these surface asperities, which cover only a small proportion of the overall surface area. When the surfaces are subjected to compressive load or shearing forces, the asperities deform, increasing the contact area between the two surfaces. The exact relationship between surface asperities and friction is still poorly understood, and under some circumstances weaker frictional forces may result between macroscopically rougher surfaces while smoother surfaces may exhibit higher levels of friction due to larger levels of actual contact.

In sliding mechanics for space closure, the applied space-closing force is required not only to move the teeth in the active unit, but also to overcome the frictional forces. This places a considerable strain on the anchor unit and may lead to loss of anchorage (Figure 2.38).

The frictional force continues while the two surfaces are in contact, and reduces the effectiveness of the applied force in moving the teeth. Friction is part and parcel of sliding mechanics, but can be reduced by applying lower space-closing forces or reducing the coefficient of friction. Additionally, ensuring adequate clearance, or 'play', between the archwire and bracket slots, adequate levelling of the dental arch prior to instigating space-closing mechanics, using the wire–bracket configurations with

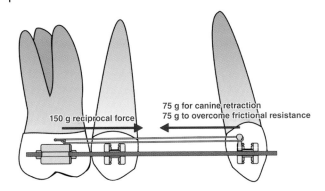

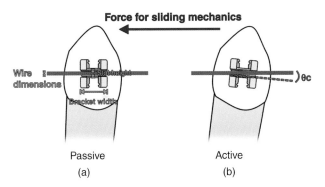

Figure 2.38 In sliding mechanics for space closure, the applied space-closing force is required not only to move the teeth in the active unit (here the active unit is the canine), but also to overcome the frictional forces resisting the tooth movement. Frictional force acts tangential to the common boundary of the two bodies in contact (i.e. the archwire and bracket slot) and resists the motion or tendency to motion of one relative to the other. The exact amount of the frictional force is unknown, and will depend on the number of asperities in contact, the material and other surface qualities of the wire and bracket slot, and the coefficient of friction. Therefore, if 75 g is required to retract a maxillary canine, a considerably larger force will be required to overcome the frictional resistance to the movement of the canine. If a force of 150 g is used (to retract the canine and overcome frictional resistance), this will place a reciprocal protracting force of 150 g on the posterior anchor unit, which can lead to anchorage loss.

Figure 2.39 Critical contact angle for binding (θc). The important parameters during sliding mechanics are the size of the archwire, the bracket slot size, bracket width, and the contact angle between the archwire and bracket slot. (a) Passive configuration in which there is clearance between the archwire and bracket slot and there is excellent alignment and levelling; θc is between 0 and 4.5°. (b) Active configuration during attempted space closure with sliding mechanics, which will be hampered if the critical contact angle for binding (θc) exceeds 5°. If it does, binding will restrict sliding mechanics. Therefore, as long as θc is less than 5°, binding should be minimal and sliding mechanics may still continue relatively unhindered.

the lowest frictional resistance,[43] and reducing the friction in the methods of archwire ligation (e.g. using passive self-ligating brackets, or tying the brackets lightly with steel ligatures) may help (see Chapters 10 and 14). Masticatory forces may also disrupt the contact between wire and bracket slot when the biting forces are applied, perhaps freeing up the system and allowing better movement, although this is somewhat speculative and requires further investigation.

Another important consideration is the **critical contact angle for binding** (**theta c** or **θc**) described by Kusy and Whitley (Figure 2.39).[38, 44] The term **binding** refers to the situation when mesial or distal tipping of a tooth and its bracket results in the bracket slot edges catching against the archwire and impeding sliding of the bracket along the wire. Resistance to sliding increases significantly as the **contact angle (θ)** between an archwire and bracket slot increases. This contact angle depends on three parameters: the size of the archwire, the size of the bracket slot and the width of the bracket. The contact angle beyond which the bracket slot binds against the bracket slot edges is known as the θc. The limits of θc have been found to range between 0 and 4.5°.[44] Therefore, if a clinician wants to use sliding mechanics without any binding, she always has to align and level the teeth within this envelope. If the clinician

exceeds the θc for a given archwire–bracket combination, sliding mechanics will be increasingly compromised as θ increasingly exceeds θc. In conclusion, the maximum value of θc should not exceed approximately 5°, otherwise sliding mechanics will be hampered due to binding.

If differential space closure is required, e.g. predominantly retraction of the anterior canine-to-canine segment as opposed to protraction of the posterior anchor unit, anchorage reinforcement may be required to prevent movement of the posterior segment, e.g. using headgear, intermaxillary elastics, or temporary anchorage devices (see Chapters 3, 12 and 14).[44]

The advantages of sliding mechanics are that it is clinically relatively straightforward, requiring little wire bending and limited chairside time, and the results are relatively predictable as the correct size, shape and material of archwire maintains the occlusal plane and arch form. The disadvantages are the effects of friction and potential loss of anchorage, particularly when mechanics are poorly understood and badly managed.

Further information on sliding mechanics may be found in Chapter 15.

Space Closure with Closing Loop Mechanics

The alternative method to sliding mechanics for space closure is closing loop mechanics.[45] In loop mechanics, there is no 'straight' continuous archwire. The loops are bent into the wires and are subsequently stretched in a mesiodistal

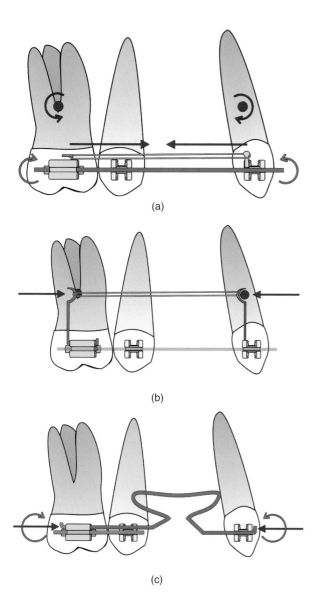

(a)

(b)

(c)

Figure 2.40 Comparison of sliding mechanics and closing loop mechanics for space closure. The examples all consider the bodily retraction of a canine. (a) An active elastic force is applied for sliding mechanics between the molar tube and canine bracket hooks. As this is below the centres of resistance (red circles), there will be moments created round the centres of resistance, tending to tip the crowns towards each other. However, the archwire provides the required counter-moments (shown in grey) to control the tooth movement. (b) If extension hooks are used, such that the line of action of the force passes through the centres of resistance, no moments are produced. As such, theoretically, the main archwire is not required. (c) If closing loop mechanics are used, the closing loop delivers the space-closing forces and the moments required for space closure without a main archwire between the posterior and anterior segments (see Figures 2.41 and 2.42). Friction does not play an appreciable role in closing loop mechanics.

direction for activation prior to being engaged into the relevant brackets either side of the space to be closed. As the activated loop attempts to close, space-closing forces are generated and the teeth are moved towards each other, closing the space. Therefore, friction does not play an appreciable role in loop mechanics (Figure 2.40). The teeth still move through the phases of tooth movement along an archwire as in sliding mechanics, i.e. crown tipping, translation and root uprighting, but the process is claimed to be smoother by some clinicians. However, we are not aware of any randomised controlled trials directly comparing sliding and loop mechanics.

Loop design is an important factor in closing loop mechanics. The ideal closing loop should meet the following criteria:

- Permit a large activation.
- Deliver low continuous forces over the required range.
- Easy chairside fabrication.
- Patient comfort, e.g. not too long and thereby causing irritation to the oral mucosa, or being an oral hygiene hazard.

Standard vertical loop designs are easiest to fabricate at the chairside, but due to the intraoral anatomical restrictions to their height, they will place excessive forces on the teeth, leading to patient discomfort and potentially anchorage loss. The teeth on either side may also excessively tip into the extraction space. The incorporation of additional wire length into the loop design will reduce the applied forces. Because of the aforementioned anatomical restrictions, effective wire length may be increased by using a T-loop design (Figure 2.41). This type of closing loop design, albeit with minor modifications, tends to be favoured. Nevertheless, it is important to note that a considerable variety of loop designs have been described in

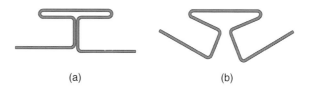

(a)   (b)

Figure 2.41 (a) The T-loop is a favoured closing loop design. Its design permits an increased length of wire to reduce applied force levels whilst simultaneously avoiding encroachment on the patient's soft tissues. (b) Prior to activation, gable bends are placed in the arms of the closing loop adjacent to the closing loop. These will help with control of root position and prevent excessive crown tipping into the extraction space during space closure.

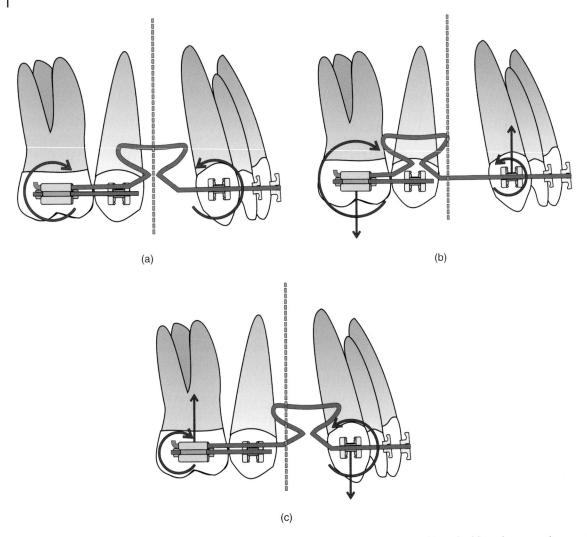

(a)

(b)

(c)

Figure 2.42 (a) When a closing loop is activated and tied into position, if the loop is positioned midway between the anterior and posterior units/segments, the gable bends will provide similar magnitude moments on either side. These permit space closure to progress without the crowns excessively tipping towards one another into the extraction space. (b) If the loop is positioned closer to the posterior unit, the longer anterior leg of the closing loop will have the smaller moment, there will be an extrusive force on the opposite side with the larger moment (the posterior unit), and an intrusive force on the anterior segment. This biomechanical configuration is better in cases with deep incisor overbite. (c) Alternatively, if the loop is positioned closer to the anterior unit, there will be a larger moment on the anterior segment, and an extrusive force on the side of the larger moment (the anterior unit) and an intrusive force on the posterior unit. This configuration is better in cases with reduced incisor overbite.

the clinical literature, but the vast majority have not been tested in laboratory settings or in clinical trials, and in a three-dimensional system can produce unknown forces and unplanned moments with sometimes unpredictable results.

As well as loop design, another important factor to consider in closing loop mechanics is loop position. The mesiodistal position of the loop in the area to be closed will affect the moments on the teeth engaged on either side of the space, and also affect the potential unwanted movements of these teeth.[46] The magnitude of the moments will be greatest at the teeth closest to the loop, as will the

extrusive forces on these teeth, with intrusive forces on the teeth furthest away from the loop (Figure 2.42). This will be relevant if the patient has a reduced or increased incisor overbite.

Further information on closing loops mechanics may be found in Chapter 15.

Conclusion

There are three major components to orthodontic treatment with preadjusted fixed appliances. The first step is clinical diagnosis, which is essentially a collection of factual information, based on the patient interview, clinical evaluation and analysis of diagnostic records. This remains the most important step in any form of dental or medical treatment. The second step is treatment planning, which is extremely important and requires the establishment of accurate aims and objectives towards a planned outcome, but also sound judgement from the clinician. Once these two steps have been accomplished successfully, the final step is the actual technical treatment that is carried out, and this step cannot be accomplished *efficiently* without understanding the principles of orthodontic biomechanics. The chapters in Sections III and IV of this book should be read bearing in mind the information assimilated from this chapter.

References

1 Naini FB. *Facial Aesthetics: Concepts and Clinical Diagnosis.* Oxford: Wiley Blackwell, 2011.

2 Burstone CJ, Koenig HA. Force systems from an ideal arch. *Am. J. Orthod.* 1974;65:270–289.

3 Koenig HA, Vanderby R, Solonche DJ, Burstone CJ. Force systems from orthodontic appliances: an analytical and experimental comparison. *J. Biomech. Eng.* 1980;102:294–300.

4 Smith RJ, Burstone CJ. Mechanics of tooth movement. *Am. J. Orthod.* 1984;85:294–307.

5 Isaacson RJ, Lindauer SJ, Davidovitch M. On tooth movement. *Angle Orthod.* 1993;63:305–309.

6 Pryputniewicz RJ, Burstone CJ. The effect of time and force magnitude on orthodontic tooth movement. *J. Dent. Res.* 1979;58:1754–1764.

7 Nikolai RJ. On optimum orthodontic force theory as applied to canine retraction. *Am. J. Orthod.* 1975;68:290–302.

8 Blake W. *The Pickering Manuscript (c. 1807). Penguin Classics.* London: Penguin Publishing, 1977.

9 Richter JP. *Literary Works of Leonardo da Vinci,* 2nd edn. Oxford: Oxford University Press, 1939.

10 Vanden Bulcke MM, Burstone CJ, Sachdeva RC, Dermaut LR. Location of the centers of resistance for anterior teeth during retraction using the laser reflection technique. *Am. J. Orthod. Dentofacial Orthop.* 1987;91:375–384.

11 Yettram AL, Wright KW, Houston WJ. Centre of loading of a maxillary central incisor under orthodontic loading. *Br. J. Orthod.* 1977;4:23–27.

12 Tanne K, Sakuda M, Burstone CJ. Three-dimensional finite element analysis for stress in the periodontal tissue by orthodontic forces. *Am. J. Orthod. Dentofacial Orthop.* 1987;92:499–505.

13 Andersen KL, Mortensen HT, Pedersen EH, Melsen B. Determination of stress levels and profiles in the periodontal ligament by means of an improved three-dimensional finite element model for various types of orthodontic and natural force systems. *J. Biomed. Eng.* 1991;13:293–303.

14 Geramy A. Alveolar bone resorption and the center of resistance modification (3-D analysis by means of the finite element method). *Am. J. Orthod. Dentofacial Orthop.* 2000;117:399–405.

15 Newton I. *Philosophiae Naturalis Principia Mathematica* (1687). *Trans. Motte A. (1729).* New York, NY: Daniel Adee, 1846.

16 Burstone C. Orthodontics as a science: the role of biomechanics. *Am. J. Orthod. Dentofacial Orthop.* 2000;117;598–600.

17 Euler L. Formulae generales pro translatione quacunque corporum rigidorum (General formula for the translation of arbitrary rigid bodies). *Novi Commentarii academiae scientiarum Petropolitanae* 1776;20:189–207.

18 Shuster MD. A survey of attitude representations. *J. Astronaut. Sci.* 1993;41:439–517.

19 Chasles M. Note sur les propriétés générals du système de deux corps semblables entr'eux. *Bulletin des Sciences Mathématiques, Astronomiques, Physiques et Chemiques* 1830;14:321–326.

20 Peirce B. *A System of Analytic Mechanics.* New York: D. Van Nostrand, 1872.

21 Staley RN. *Orthodontic Laboratory Manual.* Iowa City, IA: University of Iowa, 1987.

22 Bishop RED. Dynamics. In: *Encyclopaedia Britannica,* Vol. 7. London: Encyclopaedia Britannica Ltd, 1964: 822–825.

23 Hixon EH, Aasen TO, Clark RA, et al. On force and tooth movement. *Am. J. Orthod.* 1970;57:476–478.

24 Andreasen GF. *Biomechanical Rudiments.* Iowa City, IA: University of Iowa, 1976.

25 Hixon EH, Atikian H, Callow GE, et al. Optimal force, differential force, and anchorage. *Am. J. Orthod.* 1969;55:437–457.

26 Tanne K, Koenig HA, Burstone CJ, Sakuda M. Effect of moment to force ratios on stress patterns and levels in the PDL. *J. Osaka Univ. Dent. Sch.* 1989;29:9–16.

27 Tanne K, Koenig HA, Burstone CJ. Moment to force ratios and the center of rotation. *Am. J. Orthod. Dentofacial Orthop.* 1988:94:426–431.

28 Cattaneo PM, Dalstra M, Melsen B. Moment-to-force ratio, center of rotation, and force level: a finite element study predicting their interdependency for simulated orthodontic loading regimens. *Am. J. Orthod. Dentofacial Orthop.* 2008;133:681–689.

29 Case CS. *A Practical Treatise on the Technics and Principles of Dental Orthopedia and Prosthetic Correction of Cleft Palate.* Chicago, IL: The C.S. Case co., 1921.

30 Burstone CJ, Pryputniewicz RJ. Holographic determination of centers of rotation produced by orthodontic forces. *Am. J. Orthod.* 1980;77:396–409.

31 Isaacson RJ, Lindauer SJ, Rubenstein LK. Moments with the edgewise appliance: incisor torque control. *Am. J. Orthod. Dentofacial Orthop.* 1993;103:428–438.

32 Choy K, Pae EK, Kim KH, et al. Controlled space closure with a statically indeterminate retraction system. *Angle Orthod.* 2002;72:191–198.

33 Lindauer SJ, Isaacson RJ. One-couple orthodontic appliance systems. *Semin. Orthod.* 1995;1:12–24.

34 Burstone CJ. Deep overbite correction by intrusion. *Am. J. Orthod.* 1977;72:1–22.

35 Drenker E. Calculating continuous archwire forces. *Angle Orthod.* 1988;58:59–70.

36 Rock WP, Wilson HJ. Forces exerted by orthodontic aligning archwires. *Br. J. Orthod.* 1988;15:255–259.

37 Tanne K, Nagataki T, Inoue Y, et al. Patterns of initial tooth displacements associated with various root lengths and alveolar bone heights. *Am. J. Orthod. Dentofacial Orthop.* 1991;100:66–71.

38 Kusy RP, Whitley JQ. Influence of archwire and bracket dimensions on sliding mechanics: derivations and determinations of the critical contact angles for binding. *Eur. J. Orthod.* 1999;21:199–208.

39 Burstone CJ, Koenig HA. Optimizing anterior and canine retraction. *Am. J. Orthod.* 1976;70:1–19.

40 Burstone CJ. The segmented arch approach to space closure. *Am. J. Orthod.* 1982;82:361–378.

41 Heo W, Nahm DS, Baek SH. En masse retraction and two-step retraction of maxillary anterior teeth in adult Class I women. A comparison of anchorage loss. *Angle Orthod.* 2007;77:973–978.

42 Kusy RP, Whitley JQ, Prewitt MJ. Comparison of the frictional coefficients for selected archwire–bracket slot combinations in the dry and wet states. *Angle Orthod.* 1991;61:293–302.

43 Kusy RP, Whitley JQ. Friction between different wire–bracket configurations and materials. *Semin. Orthod.* 1997;3:166–177.

44 Kusy RP, Whitley JQ. Assessment of second-order clearances between orthodontic archwires and bracket slots via the critical contact angle for binding. *Angle Orthod.* 1999;69:71–80.

45 Upadhyay M, Yadav S, Nanda R. Biomechanics of incisor retraction with mini-implant anchorage. *J. Orthod.* 2014;41(Suppl 1):S15–S23.

46 Faulkner MG, Fuchshuber P, Haberstock D, Mioduchowski A. A parametric study of the force/moment systems produced by T-loop activation. *J. Biomech.* 1989;22:637–647.

47 Kuhlberg AJ, Burstone CJ. T-loop position and anchorage control. *Am. J. Orthod. Dentofacial Orthop.* 1997;112:12–18.

3

Anchorage

Zaid B. Al-Bitar

CHAPTER OUTLINE

Introduction, 57
  Terminology, 58
Anchorage Value, 59
  Force Levels and Pressure Distribution in the Periodontal Ligament, 59
  Quality of the Supporting Structures, 60
  Occlusal Intercuspation, 60
  Facial Growth and the Vertical Dimension, 60
  Root Morphology, 61
  Interproximal Contacts, 61
Assessment of Anchorage Need, 61
Classifications of Anchorage, 61
  Classification of Anchorage According to the Site of Anchorage, 61
  Classification of Anchorage According to the Anchorage Need (Anteroposterior Plane), 61
  Classification According to the Plane of Anchorage, 62
Anchorage Control with Fixed Appliances, 62
  Intermaxillary Anchorage, 62
  Increasing the Number of Teeth in the Anchorage Unit, 63
  Controlling Pressure Distribution in the Anchorage and Active Units, 64
  Extraoral Anchorage, 66
  Avoiding or Reducing Forces on the Anchorage Unit, 66
  Utilising Intraoral Musculature, 71
  Occlusion, 71
  Maintaining the Arch Length, 71
  Bone Anchorage, 72
  Adjunctive Methods for Anchorage Control, 73
Anchorage Creation, 73
  Headgear, 73
  Intraoral Distalising Appliances, 74
  Direct Bone Anchorage, 74
Anchorage Loss, 74
References, 75

'Give me but one firm spot on which to stand, and a lever long enough, and I will move the world.'

Archimedes (c. 287–212 BC)[1]

Introduction

Anchorage is considered to be one of the most important and limiting factors in orthodontic treatment. It is an essential part of orthodontic treatment planning, regardless of

Preadjusted Edgewise Fixed Orthodontic Appliances: Principles and Practice, First Edition. Edited by Farhad B. Naini and Daljit S. Gill.
© 2022 John Wiley & Sons Ltd. Published 2022 by John Wiley & Sons Ltd.

the type of appliance or treatment technique used. For this reason, patients also should have some understanding of anchorage considerations, which should form part of any informed consent discussion. Since orthodontists cannot accurately measure the force systems used with fixed orthodontic appliances, anchorage monitoring is essential throughout treatment progress.

In clinical orthodontics, teeth are moved from one location to another within the dental arch via applied forces (through archwires, elastics or springs). The forces used to move a tooth or segments of teeth are usually applied from other teeth (the anchor teeth), either within the same arch or the opposing arch.[2] If the anchor teeth are in the correct position, the clinician will not want them to move. Anchorage is simply the term used to describe the process of ensuring that desired tooth movements occur whilst undesirable tooth movements are controlled and, where necessary, prevented. The anchor teeth, or any other structures providing anchorage, provide resistance to undesired tooth movements.

The importance of anchorage for tooth movement was recognised well before the invention of the modern fixed appliance. Pierre Fauchard (1678–1761), considered by many as the father of modern dentistry, with his of invention of the 'Bandeau' arch in 1728 (Figure 3.1) was one of the pioneers who recognised the need for the provision of adequate anchorage in order to move teeth.[3] This became the basis for Edward Angle's E-arch more than a century later. Recognising the importance of anchorage for his 'edgewise' technique, Angle wrote a whole chapter in his textbook discussing the principles of anchorage and proposed a classification and methods of anchorage management.

During active orthodontic treatment teeth are exposed to forces and moments (see Chapter 2). According to

Newton's Third Law of Motion, also referred to as the law of reciprocal action (Box 3.0), this will always generate reactionary forces in opposite directions.[4] Orthodontic appliances usually have two main parts: the part that is involved directly in tooth movement is referred to as the **active unit** and the part that is involved directly with anchorage, utilising anchor teeth that are not to be moved or to be moved minimally, is referred to as the **reactive (anchor) unit**. It is the duty of the clinician to have a clear understanding of the biomechanics involved in treatment and be equipped with the necessary tools to maximise the desired movements and minimise the unwanted tooth movements. In fact, in many situations, more effort is needed to deal with minimising the reactionary movements than the desired ones. Failure to prevent this undesired movement of the reactive segment is called **anchorage loss**. With the introduction of new fixed appliance techniques and materials, improvement of anchorage control represents one of the main factors that has advanced clinical practice. Traditionally, orthodontists have used the term 'minimise' in relation to anchorage loss, as it was not possible to prevent anchorage loss completely. However, with the advances in bone anchors (termed orthodontic mini-implants, miniscrews or temporary anchorage devices), significant steps towards achieving absolute anchorage have been reached (see Chapter 12).

Box 3.1 Newton's Third Law of Motion

To any action there is always an opposite and equal reaction; in other words, the actions of two bodies upon each other are always equal and always opposite in direction.[4]

In clinical orthodontics, this means that for any action (which refers to the applied force) in a given biomechanical system, there is an equal and opposite reaction force; and that the sum of all the forces and the sum of all the moments in this system will always equal zero.

When talking about anchorage, the anteroposterior plane is what is classically considered. However, the other two planes, i.e. the vertical and transverse planes, should also be considered and are equally important. In fact, treating a malocclusion in one plane could have anchorage implications in the other planes.

Terminology

Prevention of the movement of anchor teeth is termed **anchorage conservation**. Methods of conserving anchorage with fixed orthodontic appliances include involving as

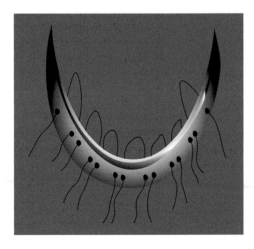

Figure 3.1 Fauchard's 'Le Bandeau' arch.

many teeth as possible in the anchorage unit in order to distribute the force over a larger root surface area, moving teeth separately or in small numbers, using light forces sufficient for desired tooth movement but too small to move the anchor unit, and pitting differential mechanics against one another, e.g. tipping the active unit versus bodily translation of the reactive unit. The **anchorage value** of a tooth, a group of teeth, or an appliance relates to their capacity to resist movement.

Just as an anchor is used to moor a ship to the sea bottom, thus preventing its movement, sometimes **anchorage reinforcement** is required (e.g. Nance palatal arch, headgear, and bone-anchored miniscrews) in order to reduce or eliminate anchorage loss, i.e. the undesirable tooth movement. The term **reciprocal anchorage** refers to situations where equal movement of teeth on either side is desired, e.g. closing a symmetrical maxillary dental midline diastema with elastic force placed between the central incisors.

Anchorage Value

There are many factors that affect the relative ability of a tooth (or a segment of teeth) to act as an anchorage unit in comparison to another. These include the following:

- Force magnitude and pressure distribution in the periodontal ligament
- Quality of the supporting structures
- Occlusal intercuspation
- Facial growth and the vertical dimension
- Root morphology
- Interproximal contacts.

Force Levels and Pressure Distribution in the Periodontal Ligament

Orthodontic tooth movement occurs as a response of the periodontal ligament to mechanical load that results in alveolar bone remodelling. This involves complex molecular and cellular interactions that are still not clearly understood. Important aspects of orthodontic forces to consider in relation to anchorage are force threshold and the rate and type of tooth movement.

In 1932, Schwarz proposed the concept of **optimum force**.[5] An optimal continuous force, according to him, was defined as the 'force leading to a change in tissue pressure that approximated the capillary vessels' blood pressure, thus preventing their occlusion in the compressed periodontal ligament'. Forces well below the optimal level will cause no reaction in the periodontal ligament while forces exceeding this level would lead to

tissue necrosis causing delay in tooth movement. Therefore, the concept of an optimal force level (within a certain range) for tooth movement is based on the hypothesis that a force of a certain magnitude and duration is capable of producing a maximum rate of tooth movement without tissue damage and with the least patient discomfort. This force level may differ for each tooth and each patient. Below this level, the teeth will not move, or not adequately enough for orthodontic treatment. After reaching the threshold for initiation of tooth movement, the rate of movement increases proportionally with increasing force levels until a plateau is reached where further increase in force levels does not augment this rate. In fact, increasing orthodontic force beyond this plateau level results in a reduced rate of tooth movement in addition to risks of tissue damage and root resorption. However, it is the pressure distribution (force per unit area) in the periodontal ligament rather than the absolute force value that is important when considering force levels. Therefore, it is essential when planning for anchorage that the forces per unit area for the active units be within the optimal range, whereas reactive forces should be distributed over a large root surface area within the anchorage unit so that force per unit area lies below the threshold level. This can be accomplished by utilising teeth with larger roots and or increasing the number of anchor teeth compared to the active unit.

The magnitude of this optimum force is different for each type of tooth movement as the distribution of forces within the periodontal ligament are different depending on the ratio of the applied moment relative to the applied force. Approximate values for the forces required to produce different types of tooth movements, based on clinical experience rather than scientific data, are provided in Table 3.1. In a recent systematic review, Theodorou et al.[6] found that the optimal forces for bodily orthodontic movement of teeth with fixed appliances range between 50 and 100 cN ($\sim$50 to 100 g). This was based on measuring forces applied directly to teeth rather than measuring stress and strain levels with the periodontal ligament, which is potentially impossible to perform.

As noted in Table 3.1, among the other types of tooth movement, bodily movement requires the largest force level. As far as anchorage is concerned, more strain on anchor teeth are generated when moving teeth in the active unit bodily as compared with other types of tooth movement. Also, the anchorage value of a tooth that is free to tip is less than a tooth that is restricted in tipping when applying a force couple. Based on this finding, Begg proposed the 'differential force theory', which represents the basic philosophy behind his and the subsequent Tip-Edge appliance techniques. According to Begg, the force applied

Table 3.1 Force levels required for different orthodontic tooth movements (approximate values, based on clinical experience).

Type of movement	Single-rooted teeth (grams of force)	Multirooted teeth (grams of force)
Root uprighting	50	100
Bodily translation	50	100
Tipping	30	60
Rotation	30	60
Extrusion	30	60
Intrusion	10	20

for space closure should be light enough to exceed the 'critical threshold of stress' needed for tooth movement on the active segment of teeth, but should be below this threshold for movement of the anchorage segment. The type of anchorage utilising this theory is called stationary anchorage.

Teeth that have initial angulations or inclinations that are opposite to the direction of applied force usually have better anchorage resistance. For example, during space closure, distally angulated molars have greater anchorage value than molars with mesial angulations. On the other hand, alignment of canines with initial distal angulation will cause greater anchorage strain on the molars compared to canines with mesial angulations.

Many researchers have rejected the optimal force level hypothesis and concluded that there is no relationship between the force magnitude and the rate of tooth movement. They have also shown that the threshold of force level that will start tooth movement is not known, and there is considerable individual variation.[7–10] According to these findings, many clinicians have adopted a different way of anchorage management that will be discussed later in this chapter.[9]

It can be concluded that the relationships between force levels and the threshold or rate of orthodontic tooth movement are not completely understood, and that many additional factors, possibly related to occlusion and facial growth, in addition to other factors, are involved which require further investigation. The majority of studies are based on animal research, which explains the conflicting results within the literature. In spite of this, increasing the anchorage value by increasing the number of teeth and reducing the force levels remains a sound strategy for anchorage management, although this should not be completely relied upon and should be supplemented by other means in cases with increased anchorage demands.

Quality of the Supporting Structures

Teeth with a healthy periodontium offer greater anchorage resistance than teeth with reduced periodontal support. This is because in patients with reduced periodontal support the force levels are distributed over a smaller root surface area.

The quality of the alveolar bone is also an important factor affecting anchorage value. For example, dense bone around mandibular molar teeth results in slower movement of these anchor teeth compared to maxillary molars. This also explains the slower rate of tooth movement into an old extraction space within the mandibular arch.

Occlusal Intercuspation

The effect of occlusion on tooth movement and anchorage has been given more attention in recent years. Dudic et al.[11] found that the rate of orthodontic tooth movement cannot be explained only by force levels; other factors to be considered include inter-arch or intra-arch occlusion and patient age. Teeth within the anchorage unit with good occlusal intercuspation usually have a greater anchorage value and less rate of tooth movement. Occlusal interferences, on the other hand, could impede the movement of the active unit and increase the strain on the anchorage unit.

Facial Growth and the Vertical Dimension

Facial growth can also greatly influence anchorage. Its effect can be favourable if the direction of growth is in the same direction of movement as the active unit. For example, anterior mandibular growth or growth rotation can help with overjet reduction in Class II malocclusions, whereas a posterior growth rotation will have the opposite effect. The same considerations should be taken when treating vertical malocclusions, i.e. deep or open bites in relationship to mandibular growth, and when treating transverse malocclusions, i.e. crossbites and midline shifts. During orthodontic space closure, there is usually more anchorage loss in patients with increased lower anterior face height and maxillary–mandibular plane angles. This may be due to reduced occlusal forces and a more mesial path of eruption in these patients.

Xu[12] has proposed two types of anchorage loss during orthodontic treatment:

1. Mechanical: related to reaction to orthodontic forces.
2. Biological: due to effects of growth and biological forces.

This conclusion was based on the results of his own studies on anchorage loss and from reviews of previous studies on craniofacial growth.[13–17] These studies have shown that in growing subjects, upper molars usually move and tip mesially to a significant extent, which explains anchorage loss even in cases where miniscrews have been used. The other biological forces causing mesial movement of upper molars, according to Xu, were the horizontal component of bite force and the periodontal ligament force.

Root Morphology

Root morphology can also have an effect on a tooth's anchorage value by affecting the force distribution within the periodontal ligament. For example, lower incisors have a flat surface with wider buccolingual dimension. They will, in turn, have less anchorage resistance for labiolingual than mesiodistal movements.

Interproximal Contacts

Teeth with broad and intact contact areas may provide greater anchorage value but this needs to be further investigated.

Assessment of Anchorage Need

As mentioned earlier, anchorage requirements should be assessed during the treatment planning stage. Having a clear vision of treatment goals, type and amount of tooth movement, amount of space needed, a clear understanding of the treatment mechanics involved, and the effects that different components of the appliance have on the different factors affecting the anchorage value will enhance the ability to estimate the anchorage needs of patients. Careful assessment of patient records and applying a comprehensive space analysis method such as the Royal London Space Planning will enable clinicians to objectively assess the anchorage needs.[18, 19] Fiorelli and colleagues[20, 21] introduced computerised methods to predict the force systems for patients with fixed appliances. Although these methods are still not widely used and need further investigation, they could greatly enhance the perfectibility of treatment mechanics and estimation of anchorage requirements in the future. It is usually more prudent to overestimate the anchorage needs as the consequences of underestimations usually have more negative effects on the treatment outcome.

Classifications of Anchorage

Anchorage has been classified in different ways.[22, 23]

Classification of Anchorage According to the Site of Anchorage

Intraoral Anchorage

This type of anchorage is provided by sites located inside the oral cavity. Intraoral anchorage can be further classified as follows.

Source of Anchorage

1. Teeth
2. Soft tissues: anchorage is provided by the actions of intraoral musculature such as cheeks and lips
3. Bone, classified into:
   (a) Direct bone anchorage
       (i) Ankylosed teeth
       (ii) Implants
       (iii) Miniscrews
       (iv) Miniplates
   (b) Indirect bone anchorage.

Jaws Involved

1. **Intramaxillary anchorage**, i.e. provided by the same arch.
2. **Intermaxillary anchorage**, i.e. provided by the opposing arch.

Manner of Force Application

1. **Simple**: resistance to tipping movement where the tooth is free to tip during movement.
2. **Stationary**: resistance to bodily movement where the tooth is permitted to translate only.
3. **Reciprocal**: a situation where movement of a tooth or group of teeth is balanced against movement of another tooth or group of teeth. This movement of the active and reactive units is desirable.

According to the Number of Anchorage Units

1. **Single anchorage**: involves one tooth only.
2. **Compound anchorage**: involves two or more teeth.
3. **Reinforced anchorage**: involves adding non-dental structures to the anchorage unit.

Extraoral Anchorage is Provided by Sites Located outside the Oral Cavity

1. Headgear
2. Facemask.

Classification of Anchorage According to the Anchorage Need (Anteroposterior Plane)

1. **Absolute anchorage**: when all movement is needed only in the active unit with no movement in the anchorage unit.

2. **Maximum (high) anchorage (Type A)**: when the majority of movement is needed in the active unit with minimal movement desired in the anchorage unit.
3. **Moderate anchorage (Type B)**: when equal movement of active and anchorage unit is needed.
4. **Minimal (low) anchorage (Type C)**: when the majority of movement is needed in the anchorage unit.

Clinical experience suggests that, in the anteroposterior plane, if greater than 60% of the space created by dental extraction is required to complete the treatment, it may be considered a high anchorage case, if 30–60% it is medium, and if less than 30% it would be considered a low anchorage case.[23]

It is important to note that anchorage problems can occur not only from insufficient space for the active unit to move into but also from excessive residual space, which requires excessive anchorage loss.

Classification According to the Plane of Anchorage

1. Anteroposterior
2. Vertical
3. Transverse.

Anchorage Control with Fixed Appliances

During treatment with fixed appliances, anchorage can be controlled by affecting the different elements contributing to the anchorage value of both the active and anchorage unit. Different treatment techniques employ a combination of the following methods.

Intermaxillary Anchorage

Intermaxillary anchorage is provided by the opposing arch and can be achieved by the following methods.

Intraoral Elastics

Intraoral elastics can be used for treatment of anteroposterior vertical and transverse malocclusions (Figure 3.2). The anchorage provided by elastics can also be further classified into simple, compound, reciprocal and stationary anchorage. These elastics are usually worn on a full-time basis and changed every 24 hours, so rely on patient cooperation. An important and usually unwanted side effect of using intraoral elastics is their extrusive effect on molars and incisors, which might limit their use in high-angle open bite cases. In

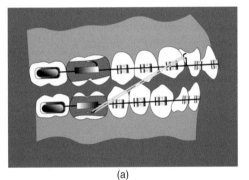
(a)

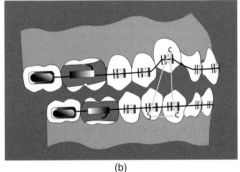
(b)

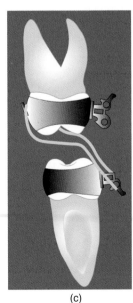
(c)

Figure 3.2 Intermaxillary anchorage can be achieved by using intraoral elastics for the treatment of (a) anteroposterior, (b) vertical and (c) transverse malocclusions.

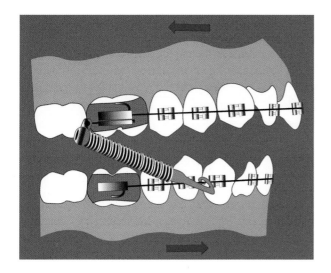

Figure 3.3 Forsus™ appliance, a non-compliance auxiliary, for the treatment of Class II malocclusion.

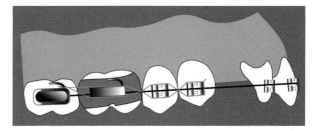

Figure 3.4 A stainless steel ligature wire (in green) can be used to increase the anchorage value of teeth by tying them together.

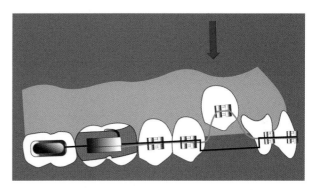

Figure 3.5 Piggyback NiTi wire (in green) to align upper canine.

addition, Class II and Class III elastics can cause mesial tipping and lingual rolling of lower and upper molars, respectively. Prolonged use of Class II or Class III elastics could have adverse effects on the inclination of upper and lower incisors, introduce canting of the occlusal plane and cause root resorption of upper incisors.

Non-compliance Auxiliaries

These auxiliaries are usually indicated for treatment of Class II malocclusions and can be in the form of springs or pistons attached to fixed appliances (Figure 3.3). As their name suggests, they do not rely on patient compliance, contrary to intraoral elastics. These auxiliaries are usually prone to fracture and fatigue and are relatively expensive. However, like intermaxillary elastics, they also cause proclination of lower incisors.[24]

Functional Appliances

Although this subject is outside the scope of this textbook, functional appliances also rely on intermaxillary anchorage for their action. Initial successful treatment of Class II malocclusions with these appliances in growing children usually result in reduced anchorage demands during the second stage of treatment with fixed appliances.

Increasing the Number of Teeth in the Anchorage Unit

Increasing the number of teeth in the anchorage unit, thus increasing the total root surface area of the anchor unit, can be used to increase its anchorage value during the correction of anteroposterior, vertical and transverse malocclusions. There are many ways that this principle may be applied when using fixed appliances.

1. Including the second molars in the anchorage unit.
2. Tying the anchor teeth together as a single unit using stainless steel ligature wires in order to increase their anchorage value (Figure 3.4).
3. Alignment of a severely displaced tooth using a flexible piggyback archwire over a rigid base archwire attached to the rest of teeth as a source of anchorage (Figure 3.5).
4. Using auxiliary wires over a rigid base archwire for tip or torque corrections (Figure 3.6).
5. Extraction pattern: the choice of extraction during orthodontic treatment can affect the number of teeth within both the active and anchorage units. For example, for treatment of Class II malocclusion, the extraction for upper first premolars will result in inclusion of the second premolars in the posterior anchorage unit, thus increasing their anchorage value during treatment. The extraction of lower second premolars will also help with treatment mechanics by limiting the retroclination of lower incisors and helping with correction of molar relationship by mesial movement of lower molars. The reverse extraction pattern (upper second premolars and lower first premolars) can be used in treatment of Class III malocclusions.
6. Subdivision of desired movements: a method of reducing strain on the anchorage unit is to move teeth within the active unit in more than one stage. One of the most common examples is the two-stage treatment of increased overjet starting with the retraction of

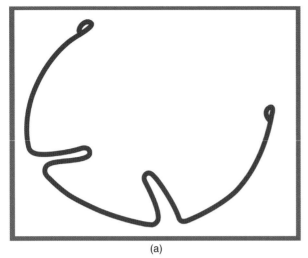

(a)

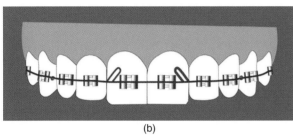

(b)

Figure 3.6 A two-spur torque auxiliary by TP Orthodontics™ (a) can be used to apply palatal toot torque on maxillary central incisors by placing it into bracket slots beneath the main archwire (b).

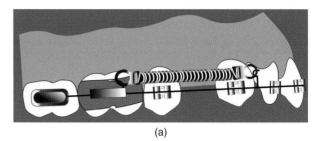

(a)

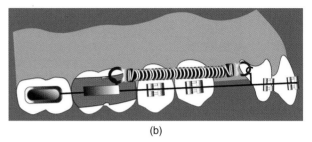

(b)

Figure 3.7 Retraction of upper anterior teeth: (a) en masse retraction; (b) two-step method where upper canines are distalised first.

maxillary canines as a first stage followed by retraction of the incisors. Although the theoretical principle behind this is sound, clinical studies have found no significant difference in anchorage loss with this two-step method compared with moving the canine-to-canine segment en masse (Figure 3.7).[25, 26] This concept is discussed further in Chapter 14.

Controlling Pressure Distribution in the Anchorage and Active Units

Controlling pressure distribution by intentionally angulating specific teeth within the anchorage unit can be used to make them better resist unwanted movement. This can be accomplished by introducing first-, second- or third-order bends in archwires or using specific bracket prescriptions.

First-, Second- and Third-Order Archwire Bends

As mentioned previously, more force is needed for bodily movement of teeth compared with tipping. Anchorage resistance of molar teeth can be increased by applying distal second-order bends (tip-back or anchor bends) thus

committing them to moving only bodily while allowing anterior teeth to tip during space closure and overjet reduction using light forces for both sides (stationary anchorage). Anchorage support using this method, in addition to using intraoral elastics, is the heart of the treatment techniques of Begg and Tip-Edge appliances.

The use of tip-back bends was also an essential component of Tweed mechanics using edgewise brackets. Tweed used the term **anchorage preparation** to describe procedures during which the anchorage value of the upper premolars and molars was increased by tipping them distally before retraction of the anterior teeth. As a general guide, these bends should be very small, i.e. around 30°. It is also important to use light forces that cause movement of the incisors without causing movement of these molars. A common side effect of these bends is the extrusion and distal tipping of molars and proclination and intrusion of the incisors, which might not be desirable in patients with high angle and reduced overbite.

First-order bends can also be used for this purpose. Toe-in bends on molars can be used to prevent mesial rotation during space closure in addition to increasing their anchorage value.

Finally, third-order bends in rectangular or square archwires can also be used to increase the resistance of the anchorage unit. For example, during space closure in the lower arch, over-retraction of the lower labial segment teeth can be reduced by introducing labial crown torque for the lower incisors resulting in space closure by more mesial movement of the buccal segment teeth.

Bracket Prescription

Changing the bracket prescription for individual teeth can be a valuable tool for anchorage control. For example, the MBT bracket prescription has reduced tip values for the upper incisors, canines and premolars compared with the Andrews prescription, in order to reduce strain on molars. This effect has been supported by a randomised clinical trial.[27]

Switching between right and left brackets can also change the second-order prescription of the same tooth. In Class III cases, using contralateral lower canine brackets will change the tip values from mesial to distal, making it easier to tip lower canine crowns distally, rather than distal root tipping, thus helping with lower incisor compensation using lower forces.

Based on the theory of anchorage loss explained earlier, Xu and colleagues have introduced a fixed appliance system called the Physiological Anchorage Spee-wire System (PASS).[28, 29] This system consists of two main components: a special crossed buccal (XBT) molar tube comprising a −7° main tube and a −25° tip-back tube crossing at the mesial end of the molar, and multilevel low-friction (MLF) brackets (Figure 3.8a). During the initial alignment stage using this system, the upper nickel–titanium (NiTi) wire is inserted into the tip-back tube generating a protective moment for the anchor molars from the beginning of treatment in addition to causing upper canines to tip distally at this early stage. According to the authors, this has a significant advantage over the traditional pread-justed edgewise appliance, where upper molars with low tip values were used. In this case, anchorage is usually lost early by their mesial tipping when incisors are engaged into the NiTi wires. By the time tip-back bends are used with stiffer archwires at a later stage, anchorage loss has already occurred, which might be significant especially in high anchorage cases. The other advantage of this system is the control of overbite with the initial archwire in contrast to the conventional system where incisor extrusion and increase in overbite are common side effects (Figure 3.8b). In order to study the clinical effect of the XBT tubes, Chen et al.[28] evaluated the records of 11 patients treated with this system. Linear and angular movements of upper first molars were evaluated via three-dimensional model analysis and cephalometric superimposition, respectively. The average movement of the upper first molars was 1.81° distal tipping and 2.38 mm mesial movement, which could meet the request of maximum anchorage. They concluded that application of XBT

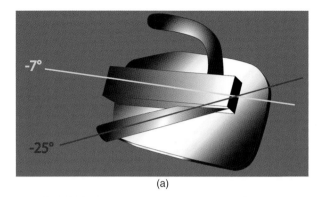

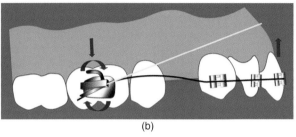

Figure 3.8 The PASS technique. (a) The cross buccal tube. (b) When the archwire is passively engaged into the tipback tube (yellow), it will lie above the anterior brackets. When the archwire is engaged anteriorly (black), a moment on the molar is created to prevent anchorage loss and anterior overbite is maintained.

tubes could be an effective way to preserve molar anchorage without using additional anchorage enhancement appliances.

Variations in bracket torque values can be used for resisting unwanted tooth movements. For example, increased labial root torque value for lower incisors with the MBT system can reduce their proclination when treating Class II malocclusions, especially when Class II elastics are being used. Also, during upper arch expansion using rectangular steel wires, brackets with greater labial root torque on the posterior teeth can be used in order to resist buccal crown flaring and hanging of palatal cusps.

Finally, first-order values of orthodontic brackets, such as anti-rotation values of molars, are helpful in reducing unwanted rotation and anchorage loss, to some extent, during space closure.

Orthodontic Auxiliaries

Different types of auxiliaries can be used to increase anchorage values of teeth, especially during space closure and midline correction. They are more commonly used with the Begg and Tip-Edge systems; for example, sidewinder springs used with the Tip-Edge system produce a mesiodistal root movement that can be used during space closure and correction of midline shift. These are less relevant to preadjusted edgewise systems.

Extraoral Anchorage

Craniofacial and cervical bones can be used as sources of anchorage support during treatment of various malocclusions. The most commonly used extraoral appliances are headgears and facemasks.

Headgears

Headgears can be used to support anchorage of upper posterior teeth by maintaining the molar relationship usually during treatment of crowding and overjet problems. The variables controlling their effect are as follows.

1. **Force magnitude and duration**: anchorage support requires a force level of 250–350 g per side for a minimum of 10 hours per day.
2. **Direction of force in relationship to the occlusal plane**: all headgears have a distal direction of force; however, changing the direction of pull in relation to the occlusal plane will affect the direction of vertical forces on the molars. With **high-pull headgear** the direction of force passes above the occlusal plane and will have an intrusive effect on the upper first molars attached to the facebow via bands. This is usually indicated for high angle and anterior open bite malocclusions, and to resist the extrusive reaction of certain treatment mechanics. **Low-pull (cervical) headgear** has an extrusive effect on the upper molars as the forces will pass below the occlusal plane, and are thus indicated for deep bite, low angle malocclusions. **Straight-pull headgear** has a line of force that is approximately parallel to the occlusal plane and is indicated in malocclusions where no vertical forces on the molars are desired (Figure 3.9).
3. **Direction of force in relationship to the centre of resistance of molars**: bodily movement of molars will occur if resultant forces pass through the centre of resistance of molars, i.e. the trifurcation of their roots. If the resultant forces do not pass though their centre of resistance, tipping movements will occur. This can be controlled by altering the outer facebow length and inclination (see Chapter 14).

Headgear remains a valuable method for anchorage support when treating cases with high anchorage demands, especially in growing children where other effective methods such as direct bone anchorage devices cannot be used.[30] However, excellent patient cooperation is essential for their success. They are also socially limiting and not accepted by adults. More importantly, following the safety guidelines is vital during their wear as there are case reports of serious ocular and other extraoral or intraoral injuries due to the recoil of facebows in cases where these guidelines were not followed.

Facemasks

Facemask, also called reverse-pull or protraction headgear, uses the forehead and chin as a means of anchorage support (Figure 3.10). Although their main indication is the treatment of skeletal Class III malocclusion due to maxillary retrusion during the early mixed dentition stage by protracting the maxilla, they can be used in conjunction with fixed appliances by providing extraoral anchorage for protraction of posterior teeth, especially in hypodontia cases. Potential unwanted side effects of their use include posterior growth rotation of the mandible and the reduction of overbite due to the line of forces in addition to the retroclination of lower incisors. As with traditional headgear, it relies heavily on patient cooperation for success.

Avoiding or Reducing Forces on the Anchorage Unit

Anchorage loss can be minimised by attempting to avoid the application of force, or at least minimising forces, to the teeth that ideally should not move, or only move minimally during treatment. This may be accomplished as follows.

Avoiding Strain on Anchorage Units

This can be accomplished in several ways.

Bonding Rigid Wires Directly to the Anchorage Unit In high anchorage cases, Melsen and Verna[9] recommend delaying alignment of the anchorage unit during space closure. The theory behind this is that periodontal tissues around these teeth are stimulated to remodel long before space closure is initiated, which can result in anchorage loss. This can be done by using rigid wires inserted into molar bands and bonded directly to premolars to establish a passive unit.

Pull and Push Mechanics Applying push mechanics by using open coil springs is an effective method for anchorage preservation that can be used for incisor alignment and the correction of dental midline shifts (Figure 3.11).

Auxiliaries Several auxiliaries can be used for incisor alignment without the need for applying forces on the molars. For example, the Hugo space bar is an auxiliary that is placed on top of the mandibular base archwire and can be used to move the lower incisors laterally thus creating space for lower central incisor alignment (Figure 3.12).[31]

Figure 3.9 (a) High-pull headgear;
(b) low-pull headgear;
(c) straight-pull headgear.

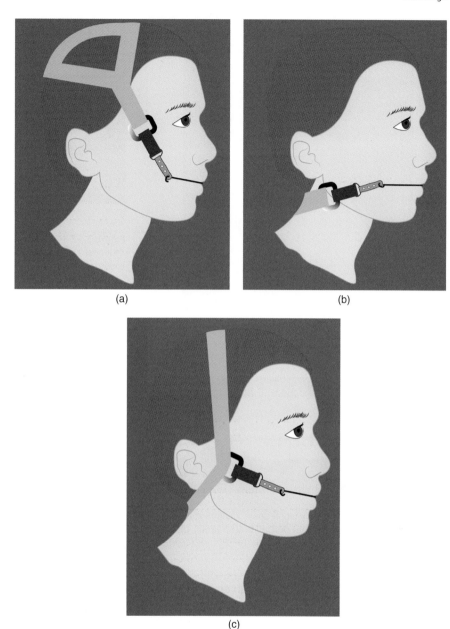

(a)

(b)

(c)

Reducing the Force Level on the Anchorage Unit

The importance of using light forces for differential force mechanics has been explained earlier. With preadjusted edgewise mechanics, there are also several ways to reduce force levels and thus strain on the anchorage unit.

Reducing the Resistance to Sliding Sliding mechanics, which involves movement of brackets along the archwire, is used mainly in the edgewise technique. With this type of mechanics, forces are not only needed for bone remodelling necessary for tooth movement but also to overcome the **resistance to this sliding (RS)** that is generated at

the bracket–wire interface. Increasing the force level will, in turn, have implications for orthodontic anchorage.

Resistance to sliding has been the subject of considerable debate among orthodontists. There is still a lack of understanding of this phenomenon despite a number of studies being published. The reason is the large number of variables affecting RS and the discrepancies among and between both *in vitro* and clinical studies. Savoldi et al.[32] were not able to perform a meta-analysis to study the variables affecting RS due to the incompatibility of experimental parameters, the lack of clear description of study design, materials, and experimental set-up, and the absence of consideration of the normal force (the force

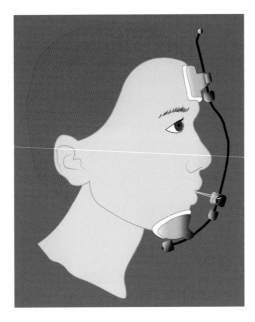

Figure 3.10 Facemask appliance.

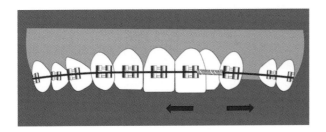

Figure 3.11 Push mechanics by using open coil spring to move upper left canine distally without putting any strain on the posterior anchor teeth.

perpendicular to the sliding) by most studies. They have suggested a protocol in order to achieve more objective evaluations and more relevant applications of *in vitro* findings to clinical treatments.

For a long time, friction has been considered the major cause of RS. **Friction** may be defined as the resistance encountered when one body moves relative to another body with which it is in contact. In clinical orthodontics, this relative movement of two contacting bodies produces a force resisting their relative movement in a direction tangential to the plane of contact. The magnitude of this force (F) is equal to the product of the normal force FN acting perpendicular to the contact surface, multiplied by the frictional coefficient μ ($F = FN \times \mu$). The frictional coefficient depends on the surface roughness and the combination of the materials involved; it is not, however, affected by the surface area of the contacting surfaces.

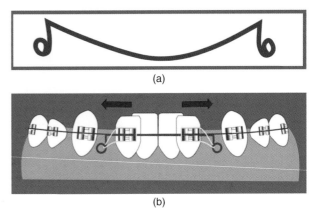

Figure 3.12 Hugo space bar auxiliary (a) can be used to create space for the lower incisors by tying an elastomeric thread from the lateral incisors to the circles of the auxiliary (b).

Several factors have been found to affect frictional forces between brackets and archwires.

Archwire

Material Several studies have shown that frictional forces are least when stainless steel wires and brackets are used together.[33–35] The highest resistance has been found with titanium molybdenum alloy (TMA) archwires. However, this increase in coefficient of friction is related mainly to surface chemistry rather than mechanical friction between the bracket and archwire. Although surface treatment and ion implantation have been suggested to reduce frictional resistance of this wire, this has been shown to be ineffective.[36]

Size and Cross-section Several studies have shown that frictional forces increase as the wire size increases for the same bracket and wire material. Rectangular wires were also shown to have higher values compared to round wires, especially for TMA and NiTi wires.[37, 38] For this reason, dual-geometry wires, such as the Hills dual-geometry wires used with the SPEED™ system, have been introduced by some companies. These wires have a rectangular anterior section that maintains the optimal torque and a round posterior section in order to reduce frictional forces during sliding. The same effect may be clinically performed at the chairside by thinning the sections of a rectangular wire where sliding needs to occur.

Bracket

Material Different brackets have shown variable frictional characteristics due to differences in their chemical and morphological structure. Although ceramic brackets are more aesthetic, studies have shown that they produce nearly twice the friction produced by stainless steel brackets.[39, 40] Incorporating stainless steel slots into ceramic brackets was shown to be effective in overcoming this high frictional force.[41]

Manufacturing Technique Even within the same bracket material, friction differed according to manufacturing technique. Milled stainless steel brackets have been found to have higher friction than sintered and cast brackets.[42, 43] Among different types of ceramic brackets, a study by Cha et al.[44] found that frictional resistance of silica-insert ceramic brackets was comparable to that of conventional stainless steel brackets.

Ligation

Materials Stainless steel ligatures were generally found to cause less friction than elastomeric modules.[45] Several modifications of ligature materials have been suggested to reduce their frictional properties, such as surface coating. This kind of modification has been found to be effective with steel ligatures as Teflon coating was found to reduce their frictional forces.[46] However, contrary to the claims of manufacturers that it reduces friction, polymeric coating of elastomeric modules appears to produce more friction compared with conventional elastomeric ligatures.[47]

Tightness Increasing the tightness of both steel ligatures and elastomeric modules ligated to brackets has been shown to increase frictional forces between the brackets and archwires.[48, 49] Several studies have shown that new designs of non-conventional elastomeric ligatures had lower ligation forces compared to conventional ones.[50, 51]

Self-ligating Brackets Although self-ligation was introduced in 1935, it has gained more interest recently as a means to increase treatment efficiency. Self-ligating brackets have the ability to hold the archwire within the slot by an integral locking mechanism. There are two main categories of these brackets, classified according to their mechanism of closure and interaction with the archwire, i.e. active and passive. **Passive self-ligating brackets** have slides that can be closed without applying active force to the archwire. Conversely, **active self-ligating brackets** have spring clips that press against the archwire. Multiple studies have claimed that self-ligating brackets generate less friction during sliding mechanics,[50, 52, 53] while passively ligated brackets showed less frictional resistance compared with actively ligated systems.[54]

Biological Factors

Saliva There is some controversy in the literature about the effect of saliva on friction. Kusy et al.[55] suggested that the effect of saliva could promote both adhesive and lubricous behaviours depending on the archwire–bracket combination.

Occlusal Forces Occlusal forces during function have been suggested to have a positive effect on reducing friction, although this factor has been found to be inconsistent.[56]

Although the focus of orthodontic research for many years was on controlling friction in order to reduce RS, recent studies have been more doubtful about its impact, stating that it plays only a small role in RS.[57, 58] Researchers have questioned the methodology of previous work, especially since most of our knowledge on this matter is based on *in vitro* studies that do not accurately simulate oral conditions.

According to Kusy and Whitley, two other factors contribute to RS in addition to friction: **binding** and **notching**.[59] Binding occurs when the tipping of a tooth or flexion of the archwire creates contact between the wire and the corners of the bracket (Figure 3.13). This could act as a lock that prevents movement of teeth within the active unit, leading to unwanted movement of the anchorage unit instead. Binding may be affected by the force of contact between the bracket and archwire and the contact angle between them. Increasing bracket width will reduce the binding tendency, as this reduces both the force of contact and the contact angle with the archwire. However, increasing bracket width comes at the expense of reducing the interbracket span, which in turn increases the stiffness of the archwire in this span. However, some *in vitro* studies have reported that narrower brackets are associated with less RS as they offer more clearance for wires during tipping.[35, 60] The addition of rounded bracket slot

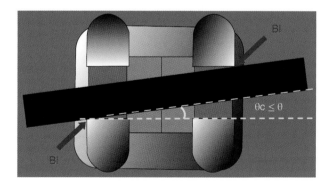

Figure 3.13 Binding of archwire (BI) with the bracket corners starts when the contact angle between the archwire and bracket slot (θ) is equal to the critical contact angle (θc). Binding forces increase further as θ increases.

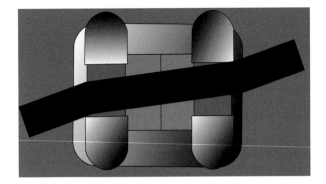

Figure 3.14 When θ is much greater than θc, sliding and tooth movement will stop due to notching of the archwire until this notch is released during function by masticatory forces.

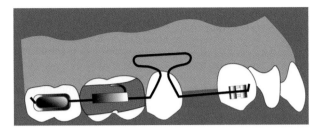

Figure 3.15 Non-sliding mechanics by using T-loop for retraction of upper canine.

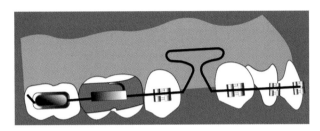

Figure 3.16 Non-sliding mechanics by using T-loops for en masse retraction of upper anterior teeth.

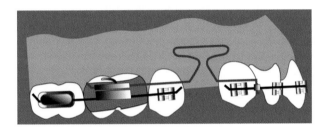

Figure 3.17 Segmental arch mechanics for retraction of upper anterior teeth.

walls has also been shown to reduce the impact of binding on RS but at the expense of control of root position.[61] Notching of wire edges refers to the permanent deformation which occurs at the wire–bracket corner interface (Figure 3.14).

The contribution of these factors on RS has been shown to depend on the stage of active movement of teeth. During the early stages, friction contributes significantly to RS as long as the wire–slot angulation is less than the critical contact angle for binding (θc). As this critical angle is exceeded, binding becomes the major factor affecting RS (Figure 3.13). If the wire–slot angle becomes steeper there will be a risk of wire notching, which, if it occurs, will become the prime source of RS and tooth movement will stop until this notch is released during function by masticatory forces (Figure 3.14).[59, 62]

This recent view may explain the lack of success of measures to control RS that have only targeted friction. Since RS appears to be predominantly due to binding and archwire notching, the use of self-ligating brackets may not be the solution to orthodontic anchorage problems.[63–65] A Cochrane review on the efficiency of self-ligation is currently in progress.

Different treatment methods have been suggested in order to avoid the anchorage problems related to RS, including the following.

1. Differential force mechanics, e.g. the Tip-Edge system.
2. Frictionless mechanics, relying on tooth/teeth movement along with the archwire rather than sliding mechanics. For example:
   (a) Non-sliding mechanics for continuous archwires, with use of closing loops for retraction of a single tooth (retraction spring) or for en masse movement of teeth (Figures 3.15 and 3.16).
   (b) Segmental arch mechanics, where the dental arch is split into two segments: active anterior and anchorage posterior segment. Different types of force systems can be generated by the use of various loops and springs (Figure 3.17).

However, these kinds of mechanics can be complicated, especially for segmental arch mechanics, which also requires more chair time for wire bending, is often more uncomfortable for patients and imposes oral hygiene issues.

Lacebacks Lacebacks are light stainless steel wires placed in the form of figure-of-eight ties that usually extend between the most distal attachments to the canines (see Chapter 14). One of the indications for their use is to apply a light distal force to tip canine crowns distally during the initial alignment stage, which in turn provides space for the alignment of incisors.[66] These forces are usually less than the forces applied by elastics.

Lacebacks are also commonly used during the initial alignment and levelling stage in order to control the arch length between the molars and canines, while the canine tip prescription is being expressed, thus minimising the proclination of incisors. This effect is especially seen in canines that have initial distal angulations. In a systematic review and meta-analysis, Fleming et al.[67] found that the use of lacebacks has neither a clinically nor a statistically significant effect on the sagittal position of the incisors and molars. They also concluded that there is no evidence to support the use of lacebacks for the control of the sagittal position of the incisors during initial orthodontic alignment. However, Long et al.[68] commented on this study: 'with regards to inappropriate statistical pooling and unclear risks of bias in included studies, an alternative conclusion – whether canine laceback is effective in controlling incisor proclination cannot be determined based on current evidence – would be more appropriate'.

Loose Engagement of Severely Displaced Teeth   During initial alignment of severely displaced teeth using NiTi wires, loose engagement of the displaced tooth into the archwire, avoiding full engagement into the bracket slot, will reduce the unwanted reaction on adjacent teeth, especially when no rigid base archwire is being used. This is commonly applied during alignment of high upper canines, where NiTi wire is tied occlusal to the bracket (see Chapter 14, Figure 14.25).

Utilising Intraoral Musculature

The intraoral muscles have been used for anchorage support (Figure 3.18). Forces from lower lip muscles can be used by the lip bumper appliance for lower molar anchorage support. However, common side effects of this appliance include proclination of lower incisors and increase in intercanine width.[69]

Occlusion

Occlusion can have both a positive and negative effect on anchorage when affecting the anchorage and active units.

Anchorage Unit

Fiorelli and Melsen[70] have presented cases where composites onlays have been bonded to the occlusal surface of teeth in order to increase their interdigitation, thus increasing their anchorage value.

Active Unit

The presence of occlusal interferences could impede or slow down the movement of the active unit and also

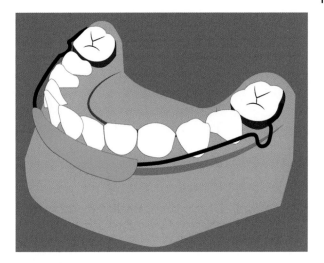

Figure 3.18 Lip bumper appliance.

increase the strain on the anchorage unit. Inaccurate bracket positioning can lead indirectly to this problem. A common example occurs during space closure when lower or upper canine brackets have been placed too far gingivally, resulting in their extrusion and interference with upper canine distalisation and overjet reduction. This effect can also be seen during upper arch expansion when no measures have been taken to disclude the upper posterior teeth by using fixed or removable bite planes. This could cause unwanted expansion of lower arch without improvement of the crossbite correction.

Maintaining the Arch Length

Lingual Arch

Lingual arches have been commonly used for mandibular anchorage support. Forward movement of lower molars can be prevented by maintaining the arch length through close contact of its anterior part with the lingual surfaces of the lower incisors (Figure 3.19). Clinical evidence has shown that they are of limited value for anchorage and could result in significant lower incisor proclination.[71]

Arch Stops

Maintaining arch length can also be accomplished by the use of arch stops in rigid orthodontic archwires (Figure 3.20). These are usually bent just mesial to the first molar bands in a passive manner. They may also be used in treating anterior crossbite cases, when they are used actively by placing the anterior part of the archwire around 2 mm in front of incisor bracket slots in order to provide a force to procline the upper incisors using the first molars as anchorage.

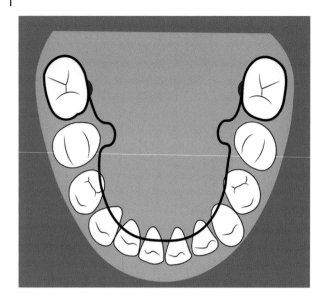

Figure 3.19 Lingual arch appliance.

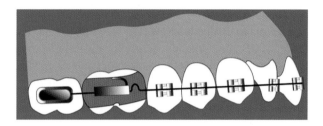

Figure 3.20 Arch stop.

Archwire Cinching

These are bends made on archwires just distal to the last attachment in order to maintain arch length by preventing unwanted proclination of incisors especially during initial alignment (see Chapter 14, Figure 14.26). However, they do not increase the anchorage value of molars.

Bone Anchorage

Indirect Bone Anchorage

Nance Palatal Arch The Nance arch, named after its originator, Hayes Nance, utilises the anterior palate as a source of anchorage (Figure 3.21). It can be most effective in patients with a high anterior palatal vault. Evidence suggests that it can be as effective as temporary anchorage devices and headgear in terms of anchorage support.[30] However, serious problems related to necrosis of palatal mucosa and susceptibility of periodontal disease for maxillary incisors can be found in patients with poor oral hygiene.[72] An important practical consideration is to remove this arch when upper incisors are

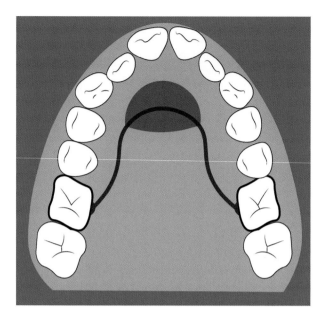

Figure 3.21 Nance palatal arch appliance.

being retracted during overjet reduction, otherwise the acrylic button can become embedded into the palatal tissues.

Cortical Anchorage Ricketts popularised the concept of increasing the anchorage value of molars by torquing their roots against cortical bone. Using this method, tooth movement is slower because of the higher resistance of cortical bone to resorption compared to medullary bone. This technique is no longer recommended as it increases the risk of root resorption. However, reducing the contact of roots with cortical bone within the active unit can be used to reduce anchorage strain, e.g. Bennet and McLaughlin[73] recommend using brackets with reduced labial root torque (zero or +7°) on upper canines instead of −7° in premolar extraction cases.

The transpalatal arch (TPA) has been a very popular method for increasing the anchorage value of molars (see Chapter 14, Figure 14.47). In theory, the effect of a TPA is to prevent movement of molars anteriorly into the narrow part of the tapering palate by the contact of their roots with the buccal cortical bone (cortical anchorage). It also provides anchorage by preventing mesiolingual rotation of molars. However, clinical research has shown that a TPA is not a reliable source for anchorage support in the anteroposterior plane.[74] However, it can be used to provide horizontal and vertical anchorage during alignment of ectopic palatal canines and may be used together with temporary anchorage devices or headgears. The use of a chromosome arch, which is a TPA modified by soldering an extra arch to the second molars, has been claimed to be

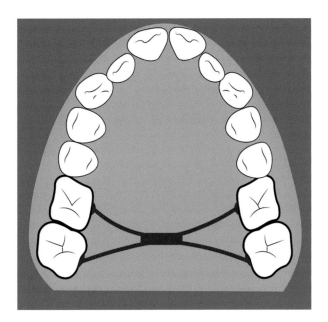

Figure 3.22 Chromosome arch.

much more effective than a TPA and can be used in high anchorage cases (Figure 3.22).[75]

Direct Bone Anchorage

Direct bone anchorage has become an extremely useful method for the management of various malocclusions, bringing orthodontics very close to realising the concept of absolute anchorage. There are advantages over other anchorage reinforcement methods. A more detailed account of orthodontic mini-implants can be found in Chapter 12.

Adjunctive Methods for Anchorage Control

Pharmacological Methods

There has been growing interest in recent years in anchorage management by local application of drugs that affect the activity of cells involved in bone turnover and tooth movement, and this may be a valuable adjunctive approach for orthodontic treatment in the future. Several drugs have been experimentally tested by local delivery adjacent to anchorage teeth to prevent their movement. A systematic review of these drugs found that osteoprotegerin (OPG), a glycoprotein involved in bone metabolism, was the most effective molecule in blocking the action of osteoclasts and thus preventing unwanted tooth movement. However, future studies are necessary to prove its effectiveness in humans.[76]

Surgical Procedures for Accelerating Orthodontic Treatment

Several adjunctive surgical procedures have been used to accelerate orthodontic tooth movement and shorten treatment time. Among these is the alveolar corticotomy procedure, which involves making full-length vertical cuts on the buccal and lingual cortical alveolar bone between teeth, after a mucoperiosteal flap has been lifted, without involving cancellous bone. Additional horizontal osteotomy cuts above the root apices are also involved. This technique has been modified over the years in order to reduce the surgical risks and damage to teeth and bone.[77] Another adjunctive surgical procedure is piezocision, a minimally invasive flapless procedure that uses an ultrasonic piezosurgical knife that makes micro-incisions in the gingiva and cortical alveolar bone.[78]

With regard to their effect on accelerating orthodontic tooth movement, current evidence shows that there is an absence of high-quality and long-term studies to support their claims. However, based on short-term studies, these procedures do appear to show promise as a means of accelerating tooth movement.[79, 80] As for their effect on anchorage, there is conflicting evidence whether they can be of benefit in reducing anchorage demands during orthodontic treatment.[81, 82]

In addition to these surgical procedures, adjunctive non-surgical methods that have been suggested for accelerating orthodontic tooth movement include low-level laser therapy and mechanical vibration. There is very little clinical research concerning their effectiveness for accelerating tooth movement and a literature search showed no data on their effect on anchorage.[83]

Anchorage Creation

In some cases, extraction of teeth and anchorage reinforcement will not be sufficient to achieve the desired treatment goal. In these cases, anchorage creation will be needed by distalisation of the upper posterior teeth. Several methods can be used for this purpose.

Headgear

Headgear can be used as an extraoral traction device of upper molars. This is the same appliance used for anchorage support discussed earlier but with wear time increased to a minimum of 12 hours and force level increased to around 400 g per side. The use of headgear for this purpose can be supported by adding a 'nudger' removable appliance, which includes a spring that prevents mesial movement of molars during the hours when the headgear is not being worn.

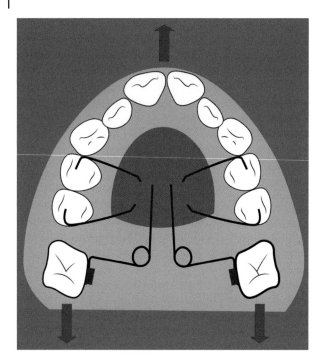

Figure 3.23 Pendulum appliance.

Intraoral Distalising Appliances

Intraoral distalising appliances include a large number of appliances that utilise the palate, teeth or other intraoral structures as the source of anchorage for upper molar distalisation. Commonly used appliances include the pendulum appliance, Jones jig and the distal jet appliances (Figure 3.23). The advantages of these appliances over headgear include less reliance on patient compliance, reduced risk of injury and full-time wear by patients. However, a Cochrane review comparing both appliances concluded that although intraoral appliances were more effective in distalising upper first molars, this effect was counteracted by loss of anterior anchorage, i.e. proclination of upper incisors, which was not found to occur with headgear.[84] However, the review acknowledged that the current evidence is of low or very low quality.

Direct Bone Anchorage

Using direct bone anchorage with implants, miniscrews or miniplates remains the most effective method currently available for distalisation for upper and lower molars. This method shares the same advantages of intraoral distalising appliances, whilst obviating the problems of anterior anchorage loss.[85] In fact, many of the intraoral distalising appliances have been modified to accommodate bone anchorage within their framework in order to overcome their limitations.

Anchorage Loss

It is usually not possible to accurately predict the response of teeth to treatment due to the complexity of the factors affecting the anchorage value of teeth with all the treatment mechanics and biological responses involved and the dependence of many of the anchorage reinforcement methods, such as headgear and elastics, on patient compliance. For this reason, it is essential that anchorage should be continuously monitored and managed during each visit. Anchorage loss occurs when there is undesirable or unexpected movement(s) of the anchorage unit. Failure to detect this at an early stage would usually reduce the scope for correction and leads to a compromised treatment outcome.

One of the easiest methods for monitoring anchorage clinically is the use of pretreatment dental study models. These can be used as a reference for assessing changes in the space available, tooth alignment and occlusion. Study models can provide a more accurate picture of the anchorage situation when treatment involves a single arch only, using the opposing non-treated arch as a relatively stable reference for assessment. However, when treatment involves both arches, a supplemental cephalometric radiograph might be needed in order to accurately assess anchorage loss by comparing with the pretreatment radiograph for incisor inclination and other changes using stable structures for superimposition.

With the introduction of digital study models, there has been a growing interest in looking for stable structures within these models in order to assess tooth movement and occlusal changes, although their current use is mainly for research purposes. The use of the palatal rugae has been proposed for this purpose; however, their positions were found to be affected by facial growth,[86] and alternative methods were suggested for the upper models.[87] As for the lower arch, a recent study has found mandibular tori to be stable structures in adults.[88]

References

1 Jones A. *Pappus of Alexandria. Synagoge ('Collection'). Book 8, proposition 10, section 11.* New York: Springer-Verlag, 1986.

2 Benson PE. Orthodontic anchorage. In: Gill DS, Naini FB (eds) *Orthodontics: Principles and Practice.* Oxford: Wiley Blackwell, 2011.

3 Stoner MM. Past and present concepts of anchorage preparation. *Angle Orthod.* 1958;28(3):176–187.

4 Newton I. *Philosophiae Naturalis Principia Mathematica* (1687) (trans. IB Cohen, AM Whitman, J Budenz of 3rd edition, 1726). Berkeley: University of California Press, 2016.

5 Schwarz AM. Tissue changes incident to orthodontic tooth movement. *Int. J. Orthod.* 1932;18(4):331–352.

6 Theodorou CI, Kuijpers-Jagtman AM, Bronkhorst EM, Wagener FADTG. Optimal force magnitude for bodily orthodontic tooth movement with fixed appliances: a systematic review. *Am. J. Orthod. Dentofacial Orthop.* 2019;156(5):582–592.

7 Brudvik P, Rygh P. The initial phase of orthodontic root resorption incident to local compression of the periodontal ligament. *Eur. J. Orthod.* 1993;15(4):249–263.

8 Owman-Moll P, Kurol J. The early reparative process of orthodontically induced root resorption in adolescents: location and type of tissue. *Eur. J. Orthod.* 1998;20(6):727–732.

9 Melsen B, Verna C. A rational approach to orthodontic anchorage. *Prog. Orthod.* 2000;1(1):10–22.

10 Ren Y, Maltha JC, Kuijpers-Jagtman AM. Optimum force magnitude for orthodontic tooth movement: a systematic literature review. *Angle Orthod.* 2003;73(1):86–92.

11 Dudic A, Giannopoulou C, Kiliaridis S. Factors related to the rate of orthodontically induced tooth movement. *Am. J. Orthod. Dentofacial Orthop.* 2013;143(5):616–621.

12 Xu TM. New concept of physiologic anchorage control. *APOS Trends Orthod.* 2015;5(6):250–254.

13 Iseri H, Solow B. Continued eruption of maxillary incisors and first molars in girls from 9 to 25 years, studied by the implant method. *Eur. J. Orthod.* 1996;18(3):245–256.

14 Xu TM, Zhang X, Oh HS, et al. Randomized clinical trial comparing control of maxillary anchorage with 2 retraction techniques. *Am. J. Orthod. Dentofacial Orthop.* 2010;138(5):544.e1–9.

15 Chen G, Chen S, Zhang XY, et al. Stable region for maxillary dental cast superimposition in adults, studied with the aid of stable miniscrews. *Orthod. Craniofac. Res.* 2011;14(2):70–79.

16 Tsourakis AK, Johnston LE. Class II malocclusion: the aftermath of a 'perfect storm'. *Semin. Orthod.* 2014;20(1):59–73.

17 Teng F, Du FY, Chen HZ, et al. Three-dimensional analysis of the physiologic drift of adjacent teeth following maxillary first premolar extractions. *Sci. Rep.* 2019;9(1):14549.

18 Kirschen RH, O'Higgins EA, Lee RT. The Royal London Space Planning: an integration of space analysis and treatment planning. Part I: assessing the space required to meet treatment objectives. *Am. J. Orthod. Dentofacial Orthop.* 2000;118(4):448–455.

19 Kirschen RH, O'Higgins EA, Lee RT. The Royal London Space Planning: an integration of space analysis and treatment planning. Part II: the effect of other treatment procedures on space. *Am. J. Orthod. Dentofacial Orthop.* 2000;118(4):456–461.

20 Fiorelli G, Melsen B. The '3-D occlusogram' software. *Am. J. Orthod. Dentofacial Orthop.* 1999;116(3):363–368.

21 Fiorelli G, Melsen B, Modica C. The design of custom orthodontic mechanics. *Clin. Orthod. Res.* 2000;3(4):210–219.

22 Rygh P, Moyers R. Force systems and tissue responses to forces in orthodontics and facial orthopedics. In: Moyers RE (ed.) *Handbook of Orthodontics*, 4th edn. Chicago: Year Book Medical Publishers, 1988: 306–331.

23 Naish H, Dunbar C, Williams J, et al. The control of unwanted tooth movement: an overview of orthodontic anchorage. *Orthod. Update* 2015;8(2):42–54.

24 Linjawi AI, Abbassy MA. Dentoskeletal effects of the forsus™ fatigue resistance device in the treatment of class II malocclusion: a systematic review and meta-analysis. *J. Orthod. Sci.* 2018;7:5.

25 Rizk MZ, Mohammed H, Ismael O, Bearn DR. Effectiveness of en masse versus two-step retraction: a systematic review and meta-analysis. *Prog. Orthod.* 2018;18(1):41.

26 Schneider PP, Gandini Júnior LG, Monini ADC, et al. Comparison of anterior retraction and anchorage control between en masse retraction and two-step retraction: a randomized prospective clinical trial. *Angle Orthod.* 2019;89(2):190–199.

27 Talapaneni AK, Supraja G, Prasad M, Kommi PB. Comparison of sagittal and vertical dental changes during first phase of orthodontic treatment with MBT vs ROTH prescription. *Indian J. Dent. Res.* 2012;23(2):182–186.

28 Chen S, Du FY, Chen G, Xu TM. Clinical research of the effects of a new type XBT buccal tube on molar anchorage control. *Chin. J. Orthod.* 2013;20:26–30.

29 Chen S, Chen G, Xu T. Clinical application of the PASS technique. *J. Clin. Orthod.* 2015;49(8):508–515.

30 Sandler J, Murray A, Thiruvenkatachari B, et al. Effectiveness of 3 methods of anchorage reinforcement for maximum anchorage in adolescents: a 3-arm multicenter randomized clinical trial. *Am. J. Orthod. Dentofacial Orthop.* 2014;146(1):10–20.

31 Mizrahi E, Melville R, Padhani F, Hugo A. Auxiliary springs for crown and root movement. In: Mizrahi E (ed.) *Orthodontic Pearls: A Selection of Practical Tips and Clinical Expertise*, 2nd edn. Boca Raton, FL: CRC Press, 2015.

32 Savoldi F, Papoutsi A, Dianiskova S, et al. Resistance to sliding in orthodontics: misconception or method error? A systematic review and a proposal of a test protocol. *Korean J. Orthod.* 2018;48(4):268–280.

33 Garner LD, Allai WW, Moore BK. A comparison of frictional forces during simulated canine retraction of a continuous edgewise arch wire. *Am. J. Orthod. Dentofacial Orthop.* 1986;90(3):199–203.

34 Tidy DC. Frictional forces in fixed appliances. *Am. J. Orthod. Dentofacial Orthop.* 1989;96(3):249–254.

35 Kapila S, Angolkar PV, Duncanson MG Jr,, Nanda RS. Evaluation of friction between edgewise stainless steel brackets and orthodontic wires of four alloys. *Am. J. Orthod. Dentofacial Orthop.* 1990;98(2):117–126.

36 Kusy RP, Whitley JQ, de Araújo Gurgel J. Comparisons of surface roughnesses and sliding resistances of 6 titanium-based or TMA-type archwires. *Am. J. Orthod. Dentofacial Orthop.* 2004;126(5):589–603.

37 Frank CA, Nikolai RJ. A comparative study of frictional resistances between orthodontic bracket and arch wire. *Am. J. Orthod.* 1980;78(6):593–609.

38 Drescher D, Bourauel C, Schumacher HA. Frictional forces between bracket and arch wire. *Am. J. Orthod. Dentofacial Orthop.* 1989;96(5):397–404.

39 Pratten DH, Popli K, Germane N, Gunsolley JC. Frictional resistance of ceramic and stainless steel orthodontic brackets. *Am. J. Orthod. Dentofacial Orthop.* 1990;98(5):398–403.

40 Tselepis M, Brockhurst P, West VC. The dynamic frictional resistance between orthodontic brackets and arch wires. *Am. J. Orthod. Dentofacial Orthop.* 1994;106(2):131–138.

41 Loftus BP, Artun J, Nicholls JI, et al. Evaluation of friction during sliding tooth movement in various bracket–arch wire combinations. *Am. J. Orthod. Dentofacial Orthop.* 1999;116(3):336–345.

42 Burstone CJ. The biomechanical rationale of orthodontic therapy. In: Melsen B (ed.) *Current Controversies in Orthodontics*. Chicago: Quintessence, 1991.

43 Vaughan JL, Duncanson MG Jr,, Nanda RS, Currier GF. Relative kinetic frictional forces between sintered stainless steel brackets and orthodontic wires. *Am. J. Orthod. Dentofacial Orthop.* 1995;107(1):20–27.

44 Cha JY, Kim KS, Hwang CJ. Friction of conventional and silica-insert ceramic brackets in various bracket–wire combinations. *Angle Orthod.* 2007;77(1):100–107.

45 Bednar JR, Gruendeman GW, Sandrik JL. A comparative study of frictional forces between orthodontic brackets and arch wires. *Am. J. Orthod. Dentofacial Orthop.* 1991;100(6):513–522.

46 De Franco DJ, Spiller RE Jr,, von Fraunhofer JA. Frictional resistances using Teflon-coated ligatures with various bracket–archwire combinations. *Angle Orthod.* 1995;65(1):63–74.

47 Pattan SK, Peddu R, Bandaru SK, et al. Efficacy of super slick elastomeric modules in reducing friction during sliding: a comparative in vitro study. *J. Contemp. Dent. Pract.* 2014;15(5):543–551.

48 Edwards GD, Davies EH, Jones SP. The ex vivo effect of ligation technique on the static frictional resistance of stainless steel brackets and archwires. *Br. J. Orthod.* 1995;22(2):145–153.

49 Hain M, Dhopatkar A, Rock P. The effect of ligation method on friction in sliding mechanics. *Am. J. Orthod. Dentofacial Orthop.* 2003;123(4):416–422.

50 Franchi L, Baccetti T, Camporesi M, Barbato E. Forces released during sliding mechanics with passive self-ligating brackets or nonconventional elastomeric ligatures. *Am. J. Orthod. Dentofacial Orthop.* 2008;133(1):87–90.

51 Galvão MB, Camporesi M, Tortamano A, et al. Frictional resistance in monocrystalline ceramic brackets with conventional and nonconventional elastomeric ligatures. *Prog. Orthod.* 2013;14:9.

52 Sims AP, Waters NE, Birnie DJ, Pethybridge RJ. A comparison of the forces required to produce tooth movement in vitro using two self-ligating brackets and a pre-adjusted bracket employing two types of ligation. *Eur. J. Orthod.* 1993;15(5):377–385.

53 Matarese G, Nucera R, Militi A, et al. Evaluation of frictional forces during dental alignment: an experimental model with 3 nonleveled brackets. *Am. J. Orthod. Dentofacial Orthop.* 2008;133(5):708–715.

54 Budd S, Daskalogiannakis J, Tompson BD. A study of the frictional characteristics of four commercially available self-ligating bracket systems. *Eur. J. Orthod.* 2008;30(6):645–653.

55 Kusy RP, Whitley JQ, Prewitt MJ. Comparison of the frictional coefficients for selected archwire–bracket slot combinations in the dry and wet states. *Angle Orthod.* 1991;61(4):293–302. [Published correction in *Angle Orthod.* 1993;63(3):164.]

56 Braun S, Bluestein M, Moore BK, Benson G. Friction in perspective. *Am. J. Orthod. Dentofacial Orthop.* 1999;115(6):619–627.

57 Southard TE, Marshall SD, Grosland NM. Friction does not increase anchorage loading. *Am. J. Orthod. Dentofacial Orthop.* 2007;131(3):412–414.

58 Prashant PS, Nandan H, Gopalakrishnan M. Friction in orthodontics. *J. Pharm. Bioallied Sci.* 2015;7(Suppl. 2):S334–S338.

59 Kusy RP, Whitley JQ. Influence of archwire and bracket dimensions on sliding mechanics: derivations and determinations of the critical contact angles for binding. *Eur. J. Orthod.* 1999;21(2):199–208.

60 Lombardo L, Wierusz W, Toscano D, et al. Frictional resistance exerted by different lingual and labial brackets: an in vitro study. *Prog. Orthod.* 2013;14:37.

61 Nucera R, Lo Giudice A, Matarese G, et al. Analysis of the characteristics of slot design affecting resistance to sliding during active archwire configurations. *Prog. Orthod.* 2013;14(1):35.

62 Burrow SJ. Friction and resistance to sliding in orthodontics: a critical review. *Am. J. Orthod. Dentofacial Orthop.* 2009;135(4):442–447.

63 da Costa Monini A, Júnior LG, Martins RP, Vianna AP. Canine retraction and anchorage loss: self-ligating versus conventional brackets in a randomized split-mouth study. *Angle Orthod.* 2014;84(5):846–852.

64 Zhou Q, Ul Haq AA, Tian L, et al. Canine retraction and anchorage loss self-ligating versus conventional brackets: a systematic review and meta-analysis. *BMC Oral Health* 2015;15(1):136.

65 Malik DES, Fida M, Afzal E, Irfan S. Comparison of anchorage loss between conventional and self-ligating brackets during canine retraction: a systematic review and meta-analysis. *Int. Orthod.* 2020;18(1):41–53.

66 Sueri MY, Turk T. Effectiveness of laceback ligatures on maxillary canine retraction. *Angle Orthod.* 2006;76(6):1010–1014.

67 Fleming PS, Johal A, Pandis N. The effectiveness of laceback ligatures during initial orthodontic alignment: a systematic review and meta-analysis. *Eur. J. Orthod.* 2013;35(4):539–546.

68 Long H, Zhou Y, Lai W. The effectiveness of laceback ligatures during initial orthodontic alignment: a systematic review and meta-analysis. *Eur. J. Orthod.* 2013;35(4):547–548.

69 Hashish DI, Mostafa YA. Effect of lip bumpers on mandibular arch dimensions. *Am. J. Orthod. Dentofacial Orthop.* 2009;135(1):106–109.

70 Fiorelli G, Melsen B. Occlusion management in orthodontic anchorage control. *J. Clin. Orthod.* 2013;47(3):188–197.

71 Rebellato J, Lindauer SJ, Rubenstein LK, et al. Lower arch perimeter preservation using the lingual arch. *Am. J. Orthod. Dentofacial Orthop.* 1997;112(4):449–456.

72 Sullivan ZC, Harrison JE. Tissue necrosis under a Nance palatal arch: a case report. *J. Orthod.* 2017;44(4):302–306.

73 Bennett JC, McLaughlin RP. *The different uses of brackets and tubes. In: Fundamentals of Orthodontic Treatment Mechanics.* London and Dubai: Le Grande Publishing, 2014.

74 Diar-Bakirly S, Feres MF, Saltaji H, et al. Effectiveness of the transpalatal arch in controlling orthodontic anchorage in maxillary premolar extraction cases: a systematic review and meta-analysis. *Angle Orthod.* 2017;87(1):147–158.

75 Rodriguez Yanez EE. *Anchorage. In: 1,001 Tips for Orthodontics and its Secrets.* New Delhi: MedTech Publishing, 2019.

76 Fernández-González FJ, Cañigral A, Balbontín-Ayala F, et al. Experimental evidence of pharmacological management of anchorage in orthodontics: a systematic review. *Dental Press J. Orthod.* 2015; 20(5):58–65.

77 Hassan AH, Al-Fraidi AA, Al-Saeed SH. Corticotomy-assisted orthodontic treatment: review. *Open Dent. J.* 2010;4:159–164.

78 Charavet C, Lecloux G, Bruwier A, et al. Localized piezoelectric alveolar decortication for orthodontic treatment in adults: a randomized controlled trial. *J. Dent. Res.* 2016;95(9):1003–1009.

79 Fleming PS, Fedorowicz Z, Johal A, et al. Surgical adjunctive procedures for accelerating orthodontic treatment. *Cochrane Database Syst. Rev.* 2015;(6):CD010572.

80 Figueiredo DS, Houara RG, Pinto LM, et al. Effects of piezocision in orthodontic tooth movement: a systematic review of comparative studies. *J. Clin. Exp. Dent.* 2019;11(11):e1078–e1092.

81 Alfawal AMH, Hajeer MY, Ajaj MA, et al. Evaluation of piezocision and laser-assisted flapless corticotomy in the acceleration of canine retraction: a randomized controlled trial. *Head Face Med.* 2018;14(1):4.

82 Al-Imam GMF, Ajaj MA, Hajeer MY, et al. Evaluation of the effectiveness of piezocision-assisted flapless

corticotomy in the retraction of four upper incisors: a randomized controlled clinical trial. *Dent. Med. Probl.* 2019;56(4):385–394.

83 El-Angbawi A, McIntyre GT, Fleming PS, Bearn DR. Non-surgical adjunctive interventions for accelerating tooth movement in patients undergoing fixed orthodontic treatment. *Cochrane Database Syst. Rev.* 2015;(11):CD010887.

84 Jambi S, Thiruvenkatachari B, O'Brien KD, Walsh T. Orthodontic treatment for distalising upper first molars in children and adolescents. *Cochrane Database Syst. Rev.* 2013;(10):CD008375.

85 Grec RH, Janson G, Branco NC, et al. Intraoral distalizer effects with conventional and skeletal anchorage:

a meta-analysis. *Am. J. Orthod. Dentofacial Orthop.* 2013;143(5):602–615.

86 Christou P, Kiliaridis S. Vertical growth-related changes in the positions of palatal rugae and maxillary incisors. *Am. J. Orthod. Dentofacial Orthop.* 2008;133(1): 81–86.

87 Ganzer N, Feldmann I, Liv P, Bondemark L. A novel method for superimposition and measurements on maxillary digital 3D models: studies on validity and reliability. *Eur. J. Orthod.* 2018;40(1):45–51.

88 An K, Jang I, Choi DS, et al. Identification of a stable reference area for superimposing mandibular digital models. *J. Orofac. Orthop.* 2015;76(6):508–519.

4

Consent

Gavin J. Mack

CHAPTER OUTLINE

Introduction, 79
Types of Consent, 80
  Implied Consent, 80
  Verbal Consent, 80
  Written Consent, 80
Valid Consent, 80
Withdrawal of Consent, 81
Treatment Options, 81
  Avoiding Orthodontic Treatment, 81
  Orthodontics with Limited Objectives, 81
  Comprehensive Orthodontics for Occlusal Correction, 81
Key Factors to be Communicated with Patients, 82
  Treatment Duration, 82
  Expected Compliance, 82
  Retention Protocol, 82
  The Costs of Treatment, 82
Treatment Benefits, 83
  Enhanced Smile Aesthetics, 83
  Enhanced Dental Health, 83
  Enhanced Occlusal Function, 84
  Psychosocial Benefits, 84
  Unfounded Claims for the Benefits of Orthodontic Treatment, 84
Treatment Risks, 84
  Damage to Teeth, 84
  Damage to the Periodontium, 85
  Pain and Discomfort during Treatment, 86
  Rare and Unusual Injuries, 87
  Relapse, 87
Effective Communication, 88
  Patient Information Leaflets, 88
  Websites, 88
  Clinical Predictions, 89
  Involvement of Family and Friends, 89
Conclusions, 89
References, 90

Introduction

The process of gaining consent from a patient prior to undertaking an investigation or treatment is an evolving and essential aspect of medicine and dentistry. In relation to consent, the medicolegal responsibilities of health professionals practising within the UK are clearly outlined in both the General Medical Council's *Consent: Patients and Doctors Making Decisions Together*[1] and the General Dental Council's publication *Standards for the Dental Team*.[2]

The professional guidance relating to consent has evolved. Previously there was a more paternalistic approach, with a patient discussing and agreeing to a clinician's prescribed course of treatment. Increasingly, consent is now more of a more patient-centred process, with the patient being empowered to make their own decisions regarding their preferred course of treatment (see Chapter 1).

This evolution in the consent process for treatment has been clearly represented by the legal requirements that have changed regarding the amount of information patients should be provided with regarding the possible treatment options and the attendant risks and benefits.

There has been a clear transition from clinicians informing patients of the more commonly associated risks and complications associated with a type of treatment, as outlined by the Bolam Test.[3] Currently there is a professional responsibility for clinicians to outline all known possible risks and complications associated with a type of treatment, particularly if the implications of the risk and complications materialising are significant. This change in the professional standards governing the information that should be provided to patients was introduced following the court ruling in the Montgomery versus Lanarkshire Health Board case in 2015.[4]

The principles of gaining consent for treatment are evolving in relation to professional standards and can be significantly impacted through rulings of individual case law. The general trend has been for clinicians to increasingly involve patients in the decisions regarding treatment options initially and thereafter throughout the process of delivering the treatment. The benefits of this evolution are thought to be increased patient satisfaction with the result of treatment and fewer complaints and litigation should an unfavourable outcome or complication occur.

Types of Consent

Implied Consent

Implied consent is demonstrated through the actions and behaviour of the patient. A simple example would be when a patient sitting in a dental chair opens their mouth to permit an intraoral examination to take place. This type of consent is appropriate for simple and routine assessment and interventions.

Verbal Consent

Verbal consent would be expected if a more significant investigation or procedure is going to be undertaken. In advance of a pretreatment lateral cephalometric radiograph or dental panoramic radiograph, a discussion with a patient or the parents is required. The discussion would allow the clinician to outline the indications for the radiograph, and the potential clinical benefits of the radiograph would be explained in relation to the associated level of exposure to the ionising radiation.

Written Consent

Written consent represents a more comprehensive approach to confirming that a patient formally approves of proceeding with an investigation or treatment. This would be appropriate for investigations that are more intensive or invasive and for treatments that are more complex or lengthy. Written consent is obtained through the use of a form or document that is amended, read through, discussed and signed by both the patient and the clinician who is responsible for delivering the treatment. These forms can be lengthy and may include numerous sections that relate to the proposed treatment, alternative treatment options, the associated risks and benefits of treatment, and the potential use and publication of images and records that will be collected during treatment.

The documents used for obtaining written consent for a course of treatment may take a significant amount of time to complete and may require the patient to consider a significant amount of complex clinical information before confirming the decision they make regarding the treatment. For this reason, a 'two-stage' approach to obtaining consent may be appropriate for patients. This allows patients to discuss, consider and sign the consent documentation over two separate appointments. This process is thought to allow the patient an increased amount of time to consider how they would like to proceed with their treatment and, importantly, some of this time would be outside the clinical environment and away from the clinical team. This hopefully allows patients ample time to discuss their treatment options with family and friends and reflect on how they truly wish to proceed without feeling under any pressure or influence from the clinical team.

Valid Consent

The concept of valid consent is important to ensure the consent process is effective. For consent to be considered valid, patients should be fully informed about their treatment options and the associated risks and benefits of all these options. Patients should also be competent and therefore able to fully understand the information that has been provided regarding the available treatment options. And finally, it is essential that patients give their consent to treatment voluntarily, without feeling under pressure or influence from anyone else, which could potentially include members of the clinical team or the patient's family members or friends.

Withdrawal of Consent

It is extremely important to appreciate that consent is given by patients prior to starting a course of treatment, and thereafter this consent is reaffirmed and maintained throughout the treatment. For this reason, consent is more appropriately considered as an ongoing process that starts before treatment commences and is maintained during the treatment. This also means that a patient can withdraw their consent and discontinue treatment at any stage of the treatment process.

Treatment Options

For prospective orthodontic patients there can be a multitude of treatment options that relate to the agreed aims of treatment and the selection of appliances that are available. However, in relation to the possible aims of treatment the following options broadly apply to most patients.

Avoiding Orthodontic Treatment

The significant majority of orthodontic treatment undertaken is considered as elective and may not be essential to the future dental health of a patient. Even when a patient presents with an unerupted impacted tooth that is causing significant resorption to adjacent teeth, an orthodontic treatment option may be viable; however, an approach avoiding orthodontic treatment, possibly involving oral surgery and restorative treatment, may be a reasonable alternative.

This means that for some patients the option of accepting their existing alignment and occlusion or considering a different type of dental treatment to address their concerns may be a viable alternative option to orthodontic treatment.

For patients presenting with relatively mild malocclusions, the risk–benefit analysis for orthodontic treatment should also be openly discussed (see Chapter 1). This option also has the inherent benefit of avoiding the long-term burden of care that is associated with the long-term retention that is routinely indicated for most orthodontically treated patients.

Orthodontics with Limited Objectives

This approach to treatment may be appropriate for patients who present with localised dental irregularities that require some specific tooth movement. This would include a short course of treatment to upright a mesially tipped molar tooth in order to facilitate a future restorative intervention, such as the placement of a bridge or an implant.

Another example of an approach to orthodontics with limited objectives would be improving the alignment of the teeth for an adult patient presenting with an underlying skeletal discrepancy. This treatment approach may enhance the alignment of a patient's teeth but would not deliver an optimally functional occlusion.

When a course of orthodontic treatment with limited objectives is agreed between a patient and a clinician it is essential that the end result of the treatment is mutually appreciated and agreed upon. This is because when a course of treatment with limited orthodontic objectives is being proposed, there is often an element of compromise in the occlusion that has to be accepted. To ensure a patient has appropriate expectations for the treatment result, a full discussion regarding the occlusal result should be held prior to commencing the treatment. In addition, the further treatment that would be required to establish an ideal orthodontic treatment result should also be fully explored and discussed prior to the commencement of any active treatment.

Comprehensive Orthodontics for Occlusal Correction

For comprehensive orthodontic correction to be achieved on completion of treatment, static and dynamic occlusal goals should be explained to patients.

The static occlusal treatment goals are represented by the Six Keys to Normal Occlusion that were proposed by Andrews.[5] These ensure that on completion of treatment a patient's teeth are well aligned, with optimal intercuspation between the mandibular and maxillary dentition.

The dynamic occlusal goals for orthodontic treatment have also been well described by the dental profession and ensure that a balanced occlusion with anterior guidance, canine guidance or group function and an absence of non-working side interferences are established on completion of treatment.[6–8]

The ideal static occlusion is readily appreciable by patients and parents and is clearly demonstrated through the typodont study models that are very helpful in allowing potential patients an opportunity to touch and examine the braces prior to starting treatment (Figure 4.1).

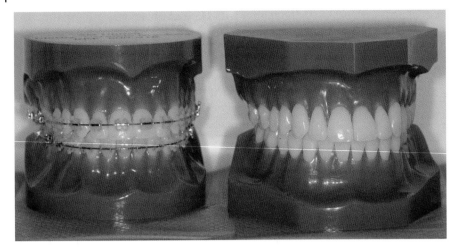

Figure 4.1 Class I typodont models.

Key Factors to be Communicated with Patients

In addition to a clear agreement on the aims of treatment, there are other key factors that should be clearly communicated by the clinician prior to confirming a treatment plan.

Treatment Duration

Studies have demonstrated that the duration of a course of treatment can vary depending on many factors. These variables include the complexity of the presenting malocclusion, the compliance of a patient, and the expertise and number of clinicians involved in delivering the treatment.[9, 10] An estimation of the duration of active treatment is extremely helpful in allowing patients to prepare for orthodontic treatment. The burden of active treatment includes attending for regular appointments and modifying oral hygiene and dietary habits. It is therefore essential for patient compliance in the short term and patient satisfaction in the long term that a reasonably accurate estimate of treatment duration is discussed as part of the consent process.

Expected Compliance

Irrespective of the orthodontic treatment that is being proposed, for successful delivery of treatment in the short term and effective retention of the corrected occlusion in the long term, a good level of patient compliance is essential to achieve successful outcomes.

The requested compliance with removable appliances will involve a discussion covering the hours of wear and appliance care. For fixed appliance treatment, cooperation with the use of inter-arch elastics may also be required to achieve a good outcome. For all orthodontic treatments, cooperation with oral hygiene routines and dietary habits is also important.

Retention Protocol

On completion of every course of orthodontic treatment a prescribed retention regime is essential. For removable retainers this will include an explanation of the type of retainer that will be provided and the suggested hours of wear. The hours of wear that is requested from the patients typically reduces over a period of time, from a 'full-time' approach to a 'night-time' only level.

When the use of fixed wire retainers is planned on completion of treatment, patients should be given very clear instructions about the specific oral hygiene techniques that are required to maintain dental health.

The long-term use of retainers is considered to be extremely important to the long-term success of orthodontic treatment.[11] It is therefore essential to carry out a full discussion regarding the type of retainers to be used and their duration of use before active treatment has commenced. This is a key aspect of the consent process.

The Costs of Treatment

A clear explanation of the costs associated with the planned orthodontic treatment is a fundamental aspect of the consent process. This should include the varying costs associated with the different orthodontic treatment options that may have been discussed. All possible additional costs that may be incurred during active treatment or during the retention regime and beyond should also be explicitly outlined. In addition, the potential costs associated with the involvement of other dental professionals for non-orthodontic components of the treatment, such as hygiene therapy, extractions and temporary or permanent restorations and prostheses, should be outlined during the pretreatment consent process. This helps to avoid patient dissatisfaction if unexpected and potentially hidden treatment costs are requested after treatment has started.

Treatment Benefits

The demand for orthodontic treatment continues to increase as patients and parents with increasing levels of dental awareness and improving standards of dental health seek to optimise their dental appearance and occlusal function. The demand for treatment has also increased as orthodontic appliances have become more easily tolerated by patients. The range of available appliances has also never been more diverse, with more aesthetically acceptable appliances available for older patients who request a more discreet orthodontic treatment approach.

As the demand for orthodontic treatment increases, it is important that a clear evidence-based explanation of the benefits of treatment is provided as part of the consent process. This ensures that patient expectations of treatment are realistic and are predictably aligned with the planned outcome. This ensures that patients are more fully aware of what the treatment will deliver and hopefully ensures future patient satisfaction.

Enhanced Smile Aesthetics

A major motivating desire for patients to undergo a course of orthodontic treatment is to improve the appearance of their smile. This often relates to the alignment of the upper and lower anterior teeth. This obvious aesthetic benefit to orthodontic treatment is easily understood by most patients.

A full discussion about the improvements to a smile that may be possible should include the benefits of achieving well-aligned anterior teeth but should also include possible limitations and compromises that may be required. Examples of this would be the pre-existing morphology of the teeth that would not be changed through orthodontic treatment. Anterior teeth that have a specific morphology, such as being tapered or barrel shaped, can still appear to have spaces present between adjacent teeth even when optimal interdental contact points have been established (Figure 4.2).

Similarly, the relief of anterior crowding and the alignment of anterior teeth may result in the establishment of spaces below the contact points of adjacent teeth. These spaces can result as a consequence of papillary eviction and the resulting 'dark triangles' between teeth at the level of the gingival margin can be a cause for concern for patients with high aesthetic expectations (Figure 4.3).

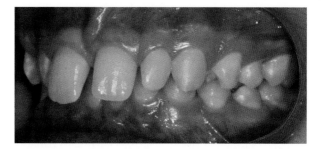

Figure 4.2 Incisors with tapered crown morphology.

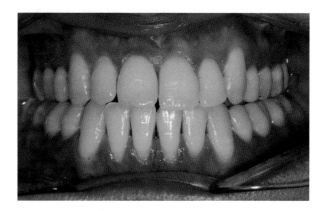

Figure 4.3 Interproximal spaces, particularly evident between the lower incisor teeth.

Enhanced Dental Health

The theoretical health benefits of orthodontic treatment can be discussed with a potential patient and these would include reduced plaque and calculus accumulation around well-aligned teeth in relation to crowded teeth. This assumption would seem logical and obvious but is not clearly supported by clinical research. Clinical studies have found that the satisfactory maintenance of ideal oral hygiene is more closely related to the dexterity and diligence of the individual patient as opposed to the alignment of the teeth.[12]

The motivation and dedication of the individual patient to maintain an optimum standard of oral hygiene has been recognised as the key factor in improving gingival health in the short term and avoiding periodontal complications in the long term. This therefore precludes clinicians from making enhanced claims regarding the potential for a course of orthodontic treatment to have a long-term benefit on periodontal health for patients in the majority of cases.

A similar rationale would apply to the potential role orthodontic treatment may confer in reducing the risk of dental caries. It would be logical to assume that well-aligned teeth are at reduced risk of developing carious lesions than crowded and impacted teeth, but this claim is also difficult to substantiate through reference to the available clinical research. Whilst plaque traps and stagnation areas may become established between crowded and impacted teeth, the development of caries in these areas can be effectively controlled through dietary and oral hygiene disciplines.[13]

A recognised and important dental health improvement that orthodontic treatment can deliver relates to the increased trauma risk that is associated with patients with increased incisor overjets. Studies have estimated that approximately 10% of 12-year-old children will have sustained some degree of trauma to their permanent incisors.[14, 15] For a patient with an overjet greater than 9 mm the associated risk of experiencing dental trauma is doubled.[16] This risk is further increased if a patient has incompetent lips.[17] The evidence to support the dental health benefits of reducing increased overjets is both logical and supported by the available clinical research. This is reflected in the weight given to increased overjets in the Index of Orthodontic Treatment Need (IOTN), where patients with overjets in excess of 9 mm are considered to have a 'very high need' for treatment.[18]

Enhanced Occlusal Function

Enhanced occlusal function may be a credible treatment benefit when patients present with severe malocclusions associated with underlying skeletal discrepancies, or anterior open bites related to digit-sucking habits. This can result in patients struggling to achieve incisal contacts that facilitate the biting and shearing components of masticatory function. Anecdotally, patients who cannot establish incisal contacts may avoid eating certain foods or adapt how they eat, particularly in social situations. For such patients, the orthodontic correction of the malocclusion would hopefully improve their ability to bite and chew food.

For less severe malocclusions, when the benefits of orthodontic treatment are related to relieving crowding or reducing a minimally increased overjet, it is unlikely that the treatment will predictably enhance a patient's experience of biting and chewing whilst eating.

Psychosocial Benefits

A major treatment benefit for orthodontic patients is the increase in confidence that can be delivered through optimising the dental appearance and smile aesthetics. This has been assessed and quantified over the years and in many countries.[19]

In addition to the internal benefit of an orthodontic patient feeling happier with their enhanced smile on completion of a course of treatment, there are also external benefits to presenting an aesthetic smile in social situations. Studies have demonstrated a more negative response from possible partners, teachers and employers when individuals present with obvious facial blemishes, including irregular or missing anterior teeth. Therefore, a possible benefit of orthodontic treatment may be that improving and normalising a patient's smile can avoid other people making negative assumptions about them, based on their dental appearance, throughout their lifetime.

Unfounded Claims for the Benefits of Orthodontic Treatment

Caution is advised when discussing the potential benefits of undergoing orthodontic treatment with prospective patients and, when applicable, their parents. The expectations of the patients should be carefully managed and guided with reference to the accepted clinical evidence and the established professional guidance.

The evidence to suggest that orthodontic correction of a malocclusion can relieve parafunction and symptoms of temporomandibular joint dysfunction is equivocal.[20] Similarly, claims to correct a speech impediment or to improve a patient's clarity of speech through a course of orthodontic treatment should be avoided as there is a similar lack of evidence to reliably support this aspiration.[21]

Treatment Risks

The majority of orthodontic treatment is generally considered to be associated with a low level of risk and harm. However, this does not mean that potentially adverse side effects and complications do not occur.

Damage to Teeth

Enamel Decalcification
This process can affect the enamel surrounding the components of a fixed appliance (Figure 4.4). Decalcification occurs during the early stages of progression of dental decay and occurs when poor standards of oral hygiene allow plaque stagnation areas to develop around the appliances. Coupled with a diet that includes cariogenic drinks and foods, this combination allows the enamel to become demineralised. At an early stage this can result in white spot lesions on the enamel surface and these have been shown to be reversible to some extent.[22] At a more severe level the lesions progress to brown spot lesions or cavitation of the enamel surface.

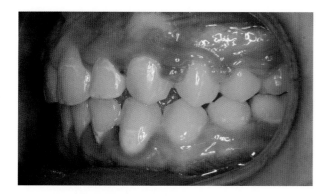

Figure 4.4 Enamel decalcification.

Enamel Fracture

This can occur when orthodontic appliances are bonded to, and then removed from, the surface enamel of the teeth. This occasional incidence of trauma to the teeth can be avoided by using the appropriate adhesives with relatively low bond strengths and careful application of force during the debonding process. Particular care should be taken when teeth are heavily restored and the enamel surfaces may be relatively unsupported and prone to fracture.

Another mechanism that can allow enamel fractures to occur is when the teeth from the opposing arch occlude on to the components of a fixed appliance. An example of this would be ceramic brackets on the lower teeth causing attritional wear to the enamel of the incisal edges of the upper teeth. This irreversible damage to the enamel of the teeth can be avoided by carefully sequencing the treatment process, appropriately positioning fixed appliances, and discluding the teeth for stages of the treatment if required. Particular care should be taken to avoid this type of attritional wear in patients who present with bruxist tendencies.

Root Resorption

Orthodontically induced inflammatory root resorption is a recognised risk of orthodontic treatment. This occurs when an orthodontic force is applied to a tooth, the periodontal ligament is both compressed and under tension, and inflammatory mediators stimulate the remodelling of the surrounding bone. This process can to some extent allow for resorption of the root surface to occur. Histological studies have reported a greater than 90% incidence of root resorption in orthodontically repositioned teeth.[23] In most cases this was minimal and of no clinical consequence to the patient in the short or long term and did not compromise the prognosis of the teeth (Figure 4.5).

However, patients may be inherently predisposed to experiencing root resorption to a more severe extent (Figure 4.6). The presenting morphology of the teeth has

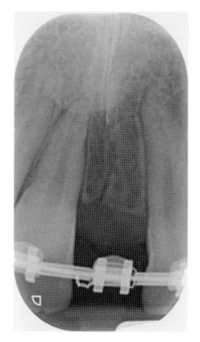

Figure 4.5 Mild root resorption.

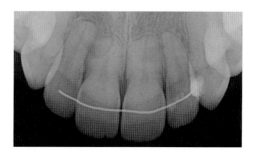

Figure 4.6 Severe root resorption.

been described as a prognostic indicator for severe resorption, with short, blunted, curved and pipette-shaped roots being considered more at risk or undergoing significant resorption (Figure 4.7).

In addition, other factors such as the duration of treatment, use of inter-arch elastics and the application of higher forces have also been considered as possible risk factors.[24]

Damage to the Periodontium

Mechanical Injury

The supporting periodontal tissues can also be damaged during a course of orthodontic treatment. This can occur through the injudicious insertion and removal of fixed appliances. An example would be over-seating a molar band around a molar tooth causing a traumatic injury to the periodontal tissues, or traumatising the gingival margin

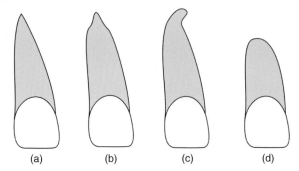

Figure 4.7 Susceptible root morphologies with a tendency towards external apical root resorption when undergoing orthodontic treatment include (a) triangular root morphologies, (b) pipette-shaped apical morphology, (c) roots with an apical bend, and (d) short blunt root apices.

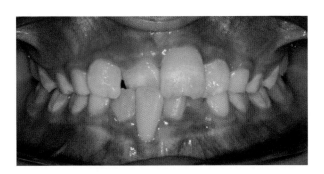

Figure 4.8 Gingival recession.

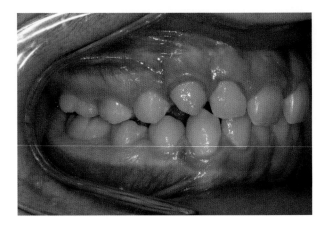

Figure 4.9 Gingivitis.

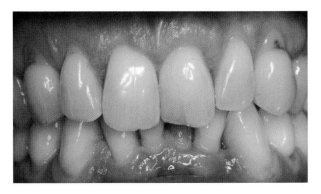

Figure 4.10 Periodontally compromised teeth.

around a molar tooth whilst applying force to the gingival margin of a band using band removing pliers.

Gingival Recession

Recession of the gingival margins and the associated attachment loss can occur as a consequence of periodontal disease and mechanical trauma. Gingival recession may also occur during the orthodontic repositioning of teeth. This may affect individual teeth that are crowded and significantly displaced from the line of the arch as the roots of these teeth may be positioned in or through the outer cortical margins of the maxilla and mandible. Recession can also occur when teeth are orthodontically repositioned and arch-form changes such as upper arch expansion and lower incisor proclination have been considered as potential causes of recession.[25] This recession can be unsightly and has the potential to be progressive unless meticulous and careful oral hygiene is maintained (Figure 4.8).

Gingivitis

The presence of orthodontic appliances can also be associated with the development of gingivitis and gingival hypertrophy. This is typically reversible and will settle on removal of the appliances but can further compromise the patient's

ability to maintain a satisfactory level of oral hygiene and compromise the fit of retainer appliances (Figure 4.9).

Periodontal Disease

For all potential orthodontic patients, a comprehensive assessment of the periodontium should be included in a pretreatment clinical examination. The progression of active periodontal disease can be accelerated through the application of orthodontic forces and the use of fixed appliances.[26] It is for this reason that orthodontic treatment is contraindicated in patients with uncontrolled periodontal disease but can be undertaken carefully when the disease process has been stabilised. For periodontally susceptible patients considering undergoing orthodontic treatment, the risks of disease recurrence and progression should be discussed prior to treatment and signs of disease carefully monitored during the active treatment (Figure 4.10).

Pain and Discomfort during Treatment

Soft Tissue Irritation

The presence of fixed appliances in the oral cavity can cause traumatic irritation to and ulceration of the proximal soft tissues. This is typically most pronounced when a fixed appliance has been recently fitted. The use of relief wax or similar products can help to prevent ulcers from developing during the time required for the local soft tissues to become more fibrous and resistant to the traumatic irritation. During the later stages of treatment, an appliance that has broken or partially debonded can also be an additional cause of trauma to the soft tissues and discomfort to the patient.

Dental Pain

During orthodontic treatment the application of forces to the teeth can lead to patients experiencing pressure and soreness in their teeth, with tenderness and discomfort when biting and chewing. This is often transient and is most commonly experienced after the braces have been initially fitted, and then subsequently adjusted and tightened. The pain experienced after the insertion of initial archwires has been reported to commence after four hours and then peak after 24 hours. This pain persists for three to four days before gradually declining.[27] This level of pain should be relatively tolerable for most patients and analgesics can be used to provide relief.[28] The use of light orthodontic forces can help to limit this type of discomfort that patients experience, and the pain threshold of individual patients can vary to the extent that very light forces may be required for certain patients (see Chapter 14).

Rare and Unusual Injuries

Whilst the majority of risks associated with orthodontic treatment can be considered to be of relatively low consequence to the long-term well-being of the patient, there are certain less commonly occurring risks that should also be considered.

Loss of Vitality of the Teeth

A tooth that is being repositioned as part of an orthodontic treatment plan can occasionally devitalise. This results in the tooth darkening in colour, developing a periapical lesion and requiring endodontic therapy (Figure 4.11). This can occur as a corollary to previous trauma or could be an iatrogenic change due to the application of excessive forces during treatment.

Allergic Reactions

Occasionally, an allergic reaction may develop as a consequence of orthodontic appliances causing hypersensitivity reactions in the adjacent tissues. This may be due to nickel-containing appliances irritating the skin or mucosa and is more likely to affect the extraoral tissues.[29]

Should an allergic reaction be experienced, a change to the treatment plan is likely to be required. Alteration of

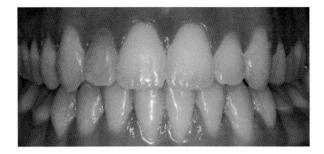

Figure 4.11 Non-vital tooth.

the prescribed appliances or the possible discontinuation of treatment may also have to be considered.

Penetrating Eye Injury

Rare and serious complications have been reported when penetrating eye injuries have occurred during treatment with headgear appliances.[30, 31] For all headgear appliances at least two safety features must be incorporated and appropriate patient selection and advice is also essential. As with all orthodontic appliances, patients should be appropriately trained in the safe and correct insertion, removal and use. All appliances must also be well fitting, correctly activated and routinely checked at every treatment appointment.

General Anaesthetic Complications

Some orthodontic patients may require surgery under sedation or general anaesthesia as part of a multidisciplinary treatment approach. It would primarily be the responsibility of the surgeon and anaesthetist to fully explain the potential risks and complications associated with the surgical procedure. The patients and parents should be fully aware of all the rare and potentially life-threatening complications associated with the surgery and the anaesthesia. Any presurgical orthodontic treatment should not be commenced if there are unresolved concerns about proceeding with the operation.[32]

Relapse

Prior to starting any course of orthodontic treatment, the risk of the teeth relapsing away from the agreed post-treatment position should be considered and planned for. Relapse can occur in the short term after completing the active orthodontic treatment, and tooth movement can also occur in the longer term as a consequence of the maturational dental changes that may take place over future decades.

Certain features of a presenting malocclusion have been identified as having a relatively high relapse tendency and these include diastemas, spacing and rotations of individual teeth. The stability of upper arch expansion is also considered to be relatively low and prone to relapse.[33]

Although there is a lack of consensus and reliable evidence regarding an optimum retention protocol, an ongoing approach to using retainers is increasingly advocated to all patients (see Chapter 17). This is because orthodontic relapse may not be associated with the potential to harm or damage a patient's teeth or compromise dental health, but it can significantly affect a patient's satisfaction with the long-term result of the treatment.

Effective Communication

The process of consenting a patient for a course of orthodontic treatment is commenced at the initial appointments when treatment options and the associated risks and benefits of delivering the treatment are discussed. This typically results in a patient signing a consent form. However, this does not signify the end of the consent process as an ongoing dialogue between the clinician and the patient continues throughout the active treatment and retention phases. This dialogue includes a discussion regarding the progress towards the planned treatment result and the potential management of risks or complications that may exist or occur.

During the initial pretreatment appointments a considerable amount of information is exchanged between the clinician and the prospective patient. This information can be provided verbally through the clinical consultations, and adjuncts to the delivery of the relevant information have been developed to aid this process. These include the following.

Patient Information Leaflets

The use of relevant patient information leaflets can allow patients to be provided with clear information regarding specific aspects of their potential treatment. These leaflets can be discussed within the clinical setting, then taken home by the patients to allow for further reflection and consideration outside of the clinical environment. Typically, these leaflets are presented in a patient-friendly style and the use of clinical terminology is avoided, allowing for a clearer understanding of the treatment by the patients (Figure 4.12).

Websites

The use of interactive websites is increasingly helpful for patients to gain access to information regarding all aspects of orthodontic treatment. The multimedia potential of

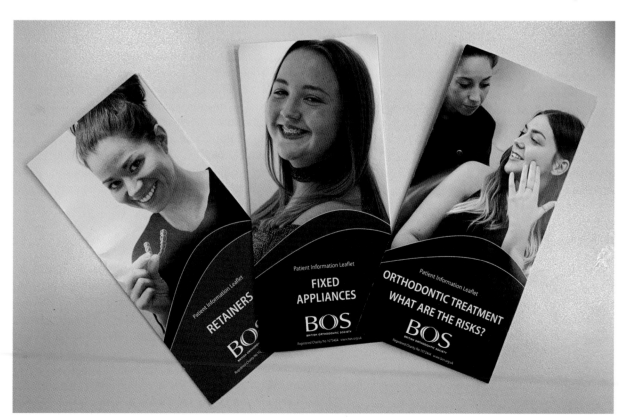

Figure 4.12 Patient information leaflets. Source: British Orthodontic Society.

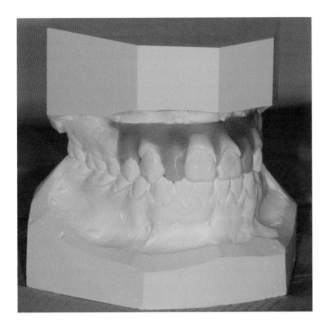

Figure 4.13 Kesling (diagnostic) set-up plaster models.

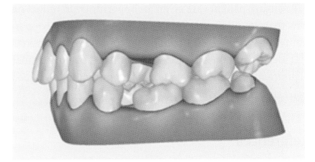

Figure 4.14 Three-dimensional images. Source: based on Barreto MS, Faber J, Vogel CJ, Araujo TM. Reliability of digital orthodontic setups. *Angle Orthod*. 2016;86(2):255–259.

websites allows for written and visual information to be presented in an interactive format. This can be further supplemented with video footage of interviews with patients and clinicians. These websites can contain links to other sites that host videos and animated films that aid patient education regarding the risks and processes involved in different treatment approaches.

Clinical Predictions

To provide more customised, individual and option-specific aids to the consent process, and to aid treatment planning, clinical predictions of the treatment outcome can powerfully support the consent process.

A Kesling (diagnostic) set-up can allow patients to visualise and appreciate how teeth can be aligned within an arch and how the teeth can approximately occlude between the arches. A conventional Kesling set-up is provided when a technician repositions teeth on plaster study models (Figure 4.13).

Photographic and digital images, along with three-dimensional scans, can also be used to produce a predicted treatment outcome that allows patients to visualise and agree to a proposed treatment plan (Figure 4.14).[34]

Involvement of Family and Friends

In addition to excellent verbal and non-verbal communication and clinical adjuncts, encouraging the involvement of parents, family members and friends in the consent process can be highly effective. The involvement of a trusted friend or family member can ensure a patient feels supported during the consent process, has an advocate who can ask additional questions on their behalf and can be a reassuring influence throughout the decision-making process of gaining effective consent.

In relation to family members supporting the consent process, it is important to consider that whilst patients over the age of 16 years are legally considered to have the capacity to give consent for their treatment, younger patients can also provide or withdraw consent for treatment if they are considered to be competent.[35] The Mental Capacity Act[36] provides the legal framework for adults who may lack the capacity to consent to treatment and this is explored in more detail in Chapter 5.

Occasionally, additional assistance may be required to facilitate the consent process and when language barriers are present the use of a professional interpreter can be invaluable. This can sometimes be preferable to relying on a patient's friend or family member to assist with the consent process and impartial assistance can be more confidently provided.

Conclusions

Clinicians should ensure that valid patient consent is provided for all treatment that is proposed and delivered. This is not just seen as good clinical practice, but is considered to be a legal requirement.

For orthodontic treatment, the range of options that may be available and the commitment to potentially lengthy treatment followed by the subsequent use of retainers means that the consent process can be complex. A considerable amount of information has to be presented by the clinician and comprehended by the patient. This process can be aided by the provision of relevant information leaflets and directing patients to other relevant sources of information and guidance.

To ensure patients are given an opportunity to reflect on how they would like to consent to treatment, ample opportunity must be given for patients to consider their options and ideally the consent process is managed over a number of pretreatment appointments and is continually reinforced as treatment is delivered.

Ensuring valid consent is given by all patients for their orthodontic treatment can be time-consuming and challenging. However, gaining valid consent from patients should be considered an essential requirement and a fundamental component of providing high-quality treatment, ensuring a high level of patient satisfaction during the active treatment and beyond.

References

1 General Medical Council. Consent: Patients and Doctors Making Decisions Together. *London: GMC*, 2008.

2 General Dental Council. Standards for the Dental Team. London: GDC, 2013. Available at https://standards.gdc-uk.org/Assets/pdf/Standards%20for%20the%20Dental%20Team.pdf

3 Bolam v. Friern Hospital Management Committee [1957] 2 All ER 118–128.

4 Montgomery v. Lanarkshire Health Board [2015] UKSC 11

5 Andrews LF. The six keys to normal occlusion. *Am. J. Orthod.* 1972;62(3):296–309.

6 Bonwill WGA. Geometric and mechanical laws of articulation: anatomical articulation. *Transactions of the Odontological Society of Pennsylvania* 1885:119.

7 D'Amico A. Functional occlusion of the natural teeth of man. *J. Prosthet. Dent.* 1961;11:899–915.

8 Beyron HL. Occlusal relations and mastication in Australian aborigines. *Acta Odontol. Scand.* 1964;22:597–678.

9 Fisher MA, Wenger RM, Hans MG. Pretreatment characteristics associated with orthodontic treatment duration. *Am. J. Orthod. Dentofacial Orthop.* 2010;137(2):178–186.

10 Mavreas D, Athanasiou AE. Factors affecting the duration of orthodontic treatment: a systematic review. *Eur. J. Orthod.* 2008;30(4):386–395.

11 Al Yami EA, Kuijpers-Jagtman AM, van't Hof MA. Stability of orthodontic treatment outcome: follow-up until 10 years postretention. *Am. J. Orthod. Dentofacial Orthop.* 1999;115(3):300–304.

12 Davies TM, Shaw WC, Worthington HV, et al. The effect of orthodontic treatment on plaque and gingivitis. *Am. J. Orthod. Dentofacial Orthop.* 1991;99(2):155–161.

13 Hafez HS, Shaarawy SM, Al-Sakiti AA, Mostafa YA. Dental crowding as a caries risk factor: a systematic review. *Am. J. Orthod. Dentofacial Orthop.* 2012;142(4):443–450.

14 Bauss O, Röhling J, Schwestka-Polly R. Prevalence of traumatic injuries to the permanent incisors in candidates for orthodontic treatment. *Dent. Traumatol.* 2004;20(2):61–66.

15 Chadwick BL, White DA, Morris AJ, et al. Non-carious tooth conditions in children in the UK, 2003. *Br. Dent. J.* 2006;200(7):379–384.

16 Nguyen QV, Bezemer PD, Habets LL, Prahl-Andersen B. A systematic review of the relationship between overjet size and traumatic dental injuries. *Eur. J. Orthod.* 1999;21(5):503–515.

17 Burden DJ. An investigation of the association between overjet size, lip coverage, and traumatic injury to maxillary incisors. *Eur. J. Orthod.* 1995;17(6):513–517.

18 Brook PH, Shaw WC. The development of an index of orthodontic treatment priority. *Eur. J. Orthod.* 1989;11(3):309–320.

19 Liu Z, McGrath C, Hägg U. The impact of malocclusion/orthodontic treatment need on the quality of life: a systematic review. *Angle Orthod.* 2009;79(3):585–591.

20 Luther F, Layton S, McDonald F. Orthodontics for treating temporomandibular joint (TMJ) disorders. *Cochrane Database Syst. Rev.* 2010;(7):CD006541.

21 Johnson NC, Sandy JR. Tooth position and speech: is there a relationship? *Angle Orthod.* 1999;69(4):306–310.

22 Bishara SE, Ostby AW. White spot lesions: formation, prevention, and treatment. *Semin. Orthod.* 2008;14:174–182.

23 Weltman B, Vig KW, Fields HW, et al. Root resorption associated with orthodontic tooth movement: a systematic review. *Am. J. Orthod. Dentofacial Orthop.* 2010;137(4):462–476.

24 Levander E, Malmgren O. Evaluation of the risk of root resorption during orthodontic treatment: a study of upper incisors. *Eur. J. Orthod.* 1988;10:30–38.

25 Morris JW, Campbell PM, Tadlock LP, et al. Prevalence of gingival recession after orthodontic tooth movements. *Am. J. Orthod. Dentofacial Orthop.* 2017;151(5):851–859.

26 Sanders NL. Evidence-based care in orthodontics and periodontics: a review of the literature. *J. Am. Dent. Asoc.* 1999;130(4):521–527.

27 Krishnan V. Orthodontic pain: from causes to management. A review. *Eur. J. Orthod.* 2007;29:170–179.

28 Ngan P, Wilson S, Shanfeld J, Amini H. The effect of ibuprofen on the level of discomfort in patients undergoing orthodontic treatment. *Am. J. Orthod. Dentofacial Orthop.* 1994;106:88–95.

29 Leite LP, Bell RA. Adverse hypersensitivity reactions in orthodontics. *Semin. Orthod.* 2004;10:240–243.

30 Holland GN, Wallace DA, Mondino BJ, et al. Severe ocular injuries from orthodontic headgear. *Arch. Ophthalmol.* 1985;103(5):649–651.

31 Booth-Mason S, Birnie D. Penetrating eye injury from orthodontic headgear: a case report. *Eur. J. Orthod.* 1998;10:111–114.

32 Yentis SM, Hartle AJ, Barker IR, et al. AAGBI: Consent for anaesthesia 2017: Association of anaesthetists of Great Britain and Ireland. *Anaesthesia* 2017;72(1):93–105.

33 Littlewood SJ, Kandasamy S, Huang G. Retention and relapse in clinical practice. *Aust. Dent. J.* 2017;62:51–57.

34 Barreto MS, Faber J, Vogel CJ, Araujo TM. Reliability of digital orthodontic setups. *Angle Orthod.* 2016;86(2):255–259.

35 Nottingham EC. Gillick v West Norfolk and Wisbech Area Health Authority [1986] AC 112: an archaeological study of a test case. Doctoral dissertation, University of Southampton, 2018.

36 Mental Capacity Act 2005. London: The Stationery Office. Available at https://www.legislation.gov.uk/ukpga/2005/9/contents

5

Dentolegal Aspects of Orthodontic Treatment

Alison Williams

CHAPTER OUTLINE

Introduction, 93
Advertising, 94
The Initial Consultation, 94
 Recording the Patient's Concerns, 94
 Pretreatment Orthodontic Examination, 95
 Dental Health Assessment, 95
 Taking Radiographs as Part of the Orthodontic Assessment, 96
Pretreatment Records, 97
 Storage of Records, 98
Dentolegal and Ethical Issues that may Arise During Treatment Planning, 99
Obtaining Consent, 100
 Who is Able to Provide Consent?, 102
Dentolegal Issues Arising During Active Orthodontic Treatment, 102
 Transfers, 105
 Non-compliance, 105
 Non-attendance, 105
 Non-payment of Fees, 106
 Supervision of Orthodontic Therapists, 106
Retention, 106
Relapse, 107
Duty of Candour, 107
Responding to a Complaint, 108
References, 109

Introduction

From the point of view of most patients, routine orthodontic treatment is usually undertaken as an elective procedure to improve dental appearance. Therefore, complaints may be generated if a patient's expectations are not met. This is particularly so for adult patients, who often expect huge psychological rewards from going through lengthy and potentially obtrusive treatment.

All registered dentists in the UK are permitted to provide orthodontic treatment. As a consequence, orthodontic treatment systems have been developed specifically for use by general dental practitioners (GDPs), with the support of a third party. However, some dentists have been tempted into providing orthodontic treatment which is beyond their knowledge and training. If the treatment does not meet the patient's expectations, the dentist is vulnerable not only to a claim for a refund from the patient, but also a complaint that they have breached the General Dental Council (GDC) Standards,[1] because they have gone beyond their clinical competence. In the worst scenario, dentists providing orthodontic treatment have damaged the teeth and supporting tissues[2] and are liable to a claim of clinical negligence.

These factors have combined to produce a steady increase in the number of complaints that were received by Dental Protection Ltd about orthodontic treatment provided by members during the period 2011–2015 (Dental Protection Ltd, personal communication, 2016) (Figure 5.1). More recently, the Dental Complaints Service, which provides

Preadjusted Edgewise Fixed Orthodontic Appliances: Principles and Practice, First Edition. Edited by Farhad B. Naini and Daljit S. Gill.
© 2022 John Wiley & Sons Ltd. Published 2022 by John Wiley & Sons Ltd.

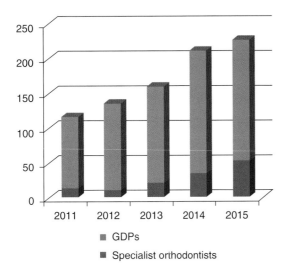

Figure 5.1 Complaints received about orthodontic treatment by members of Dental Protection. Source: Dental Protection Ltd, personal communication, 2016.

advice to patients who are dissatisfied with private dental treatment, has reported that the highest number of complaints that are discussed with them are about orthodontic treatment.[3]

This chapter discusses the dentolegal and ethical issues that may arise during orthodontic treatment and the professional standards that apply to clinicians providing orthodontic treatment. Measures that a clinician may put in place along the treatment pathway to reduce their risk of receiving a successful complaint from a patient or the GDC are suggested.

Advertising

Adult patients may self-refer for orthodontic treatment after reading an advert from the manufacturer of an orthodontic system. Advertising, including adverts that are sent electronically as a consequence of an individual's browsing history, is regulated by the Advertising Standards Authority.[4] A patient may also seek treatment after reading on a dental practice website that a particular system of orthodontics or bracket design is available at the practice. The content of dental practice websites is regulated by the GDC, which states, in Standard 1.3.3 of the GDC *Standards for the Dental Team*, 'You must make sure that any advertising, promotional material or other information that you produce is accurate and not misleading.'[1] The British Orthodontic Society (BOS) also publishes *Professional Standards for Orthodontic Practice*, which contains a section on advertising.[5]

Issues that may arise in relation to orthodontic treatment include dentists and orthodontists not making it clear, on their practice websites, that a particular orthodontic system may not be suitable for every patient and can only be provided after the patient has undergone a detailed orthodontic examination. It is also illegal, under the Dentists Act 1984,[6] to use the title 'orthodontist' or to state, in practice advertising, that you 'specialise' in providing a particular orthodontic system if you are not on the GDC's Specialist List for Orthodontics.

Another area that has been the subject of complaints by patients is the practice of offering patients 'free consultations' for orthodontic treatment, as practice-builders. The patient is examined briefly by the orthodontist who outlines, in general terms, the type of orthodontic treatment that might be appropriate for the patient. The patient then has a meeting with a treatment coordinator who outlines the costs of treatment. Patients have complained that they have been misled by the appointment being termed a 'consultation' because, without the availability of radiographs and the results of other special tests, for which a charge is then made, only generic advice can be provided about their suitability for orthodontic treatment. To avoid this type of complaint, it is important to include advice about what a 'free' consultation does, and does not, include on the practice's website.

The Initial Consultation

Recording the Patient's Concerns

For an elective treatment such as orthodontics, it is particularly important to have a detailed discussion with the patient and/or their parent regarding their concerns about their malocclusion before treatment begins, and to document these clearly in the clinical records. The old adage that 'if it isn't written down, it didn't happen' applies to all clinical practice.

It is also important to identify, at the outset, factors such as travelling time to appointments and work or school commitments, which may make it difficult for a patient to attend regularly. A discussion can then be had with the patient about the implications that this may have for their overall treatment time, rather than encountering these issues further along the treatment process.

There are some patients whose expectations of orthodontic treatment are unrealistic. It is possible that they may be suffering from undiagnosed body dysmorphic disorder (BDD)[7] and have a distorted body image. If BDD is suspected, the patient should be informed in a straightforward and polite manner, and advised to seek the help of a clinical psychologist or liaison psychiatrist with a special interest in BDD.[7] Alternatively, there may be aspects of their personality that make them crave attention or seek to control a clinician. These traits are often well hidden and dentists are not trained in the diagnosis and management of personality disorders. Unless the patient decides to seek help themselves, there may be little that a clinician can do to help the patient receive the appropriate care.

However, a clinician is not compelled to provide elective treatment for a patient. If the clinician detects, during the initial consultation, that the treatment they are able to provide will not meet a patient's expectations, then it is better to discuss this with the patient and suggest that they seek treatment elsewhere, rather than to embark on treatment in the hope that the patient will become more realistic as treatment progresses. This can be a very difficult situation to manage if the patient has already sought opinions from several other orthodontists.

Pretreatment Orthodontic Examination

'Failure to undertake and record a sufficient orthodontic examination at the beginning of treatment' is an allegation that has been made frequently by the GDC, particularly, but not exclusively, against GDPs providing orthodontic treatment with limited objectives. Some GDPs mistakenly believe that, since they are only moving the anterior teeth, a full orthodontic examination and diagnosis is not required. The GDC disagrees. Furthermore, the BOS publishes *Professional Standards for Orthodontic Practice*, which states that 'All significant findings and diagnosis must be fully documented'.[5] These Standards, which the Court is likely to use as a benchmark for a reasonable standard of clinical practice, apply to all orthodontic treatment in the UK, not just that which is provided by Specialist Orthodontists. The list of what should be assessed and recorded during an orthodontic assessment, as outlined in the paper by Roberts-Harry and Sandy,[8] has been referred to by expert witnesses in GDC investigations and so can be considered a reasonable guide for what should be recorded during the orthodontic examination.

Specialist Orthodontists have also been criticised for not recording full details of their examination of the patient in the main clinical notes. For example, if details of the examination are entered on a separate screen in an orthodontic record software package, it is also necessary to record the fact that the examination was carried out, and the location of that electronic record, in the main clinical notes. The orthodontic diagnosis should also be recorded in the main clinical records. Failure to do so makes it difficult to defend an allegation that the assessment was made from dental study models, for example, after the patient had left the surgery, and so the patient was not informed of the outcome of the examination.

Dental Health Assessment

The BOS Professional Standards also state that 'other significant dental problems (other than orthodontic problems) must be documented and communicated with the patients' primary care Dental Practitioners'.[5] However, the extent to which a Specialist Orthodontist, taking a referral from a GDP, who is responsible for the patient's overall oral health, should examine the patient for oral disease during an orthodontic assessment is unclear.

Lesions of the oral mucosa and soft tissues of the mouth may arise within the time between referral from the GDP and the orthodontic consultation. A visual inspection of the oral mucosa and soft tissues is non-invasive. It would be hard to defend an orthodontist who failed to undertake a visual inspection of the oral soft tissues and record their findings, at the first consultation and during subsequent appointments, in a patient who is subsequently found to have a neoplastic lesion which would have had a better outcome if it had been detected earlier. It is therefore good clinical practice during orthodontic treatment, which tends to focus predominantly on the position of the teeth, to establish the habit of undertaking and recording an inspection of the oral soft tissues at every patient visit.

The presence of untreated dental caries, particularly if a tooth is unrestorable, may modify an orthodontic treatment plan. 'Occult' caries may also be detected on scanning radiographs. These findings, and clear instructions for restoring the affected teeth, or requesting an opinion about the long-term prognosis for a tooth affected by significant caries, should then be communicated to the patient's GDP in writing. If the caries has been detected on a radiograph, then a copy of the radiograph should be provided to the GDP. It is also good practice to undertake a clinical examination of the dental tissues for caries at every treatment visit. Issues have arisen in which the patient assumes that the orthodontist is responsible for their general dental care as well as their orthodontic treatment, resulting in dental caries going untreated. It is therefore important to emphasise to patients, at the beginning of orthodontic treatment, that they must continue to see their GDP for regular dental care throughout their orthodontic treatment, unless of course you are also the patient's GDP.

A more difficult issue is whether a Specialist Orthodontist, seeing a patient for a consultation who is under the regular care of a GDP, should undertake a basic periodontal examination (BPE)[9] as part of the orthodontic assessment. In the past, the majority of an orthodontist's caseload was children and adolescents and BPE screening was not recommended for patients aged under 18 years. However, orthodontists would be able to detect if their patient was suffering from periodontal disease, which is a contraindication for orthodontic treatment if the disease is active, by visually inspecting periodontal bone levels in scanning radiographs taken for other clinical purposes.

The situation has now changed because not only are more adults, who may have active periodontal disease, seeking orthodontic treatment, but also because the British Periodontal Society (BPS) now recommends that a BPE screening is undertaken for adolescents from the age of 12 years,[10] the age when most orthodontic treatment begins for adolescents. As such, the BOS now recommends that 'it is good practice for a periodontal screening (BPE) to be undertaken, in particular of adult patients by the Orthodontist at new patient assessment, start of treatment visit and mid-way through treatment' (N. Atack, Chair of BOS Clinical Governance Committee, personal communication, 2016). A clinician undertaking a BPE screening would also be expected, under GDC standards,[1] to have the skills, knowledge and training to undertake the screening. Specialist orthodontists may wish to consider undertaking training in BPE screening if they have not used the index for some time.

Taking Radiographs as Part of the Orthodontic Assessment

Another area in which clinicians undertaking orthodontic treatment have been the subject of criticisms from the GDC regards the taking of pretreatment radiographs. The regulations for taking and reporting on radiographs are laid out in the recently updated Ionising Radiations Regulations 2017 (IRR17)[11] and the Ionising Radiation (Medical Exposure) Regulations 2017 (IRMER17).[12]

Under IRR17, a clinician must quality-assure or grade a radiograph that has been taken and record the grading in the clinical notes. IRMER17 states that a clinician must justify why she is exposing her patient to ionising radiation. The clinical reason for taking the radiograph and the clinical findings from that radiograph must be recorded in the clinical records, as evidence that the clinician has conformed with the regulations.

The radiographs that should be taken as part of an orthodontic assessment has been an area of disagreement. GDPs undertaking orthodontic treatment, with limited objectives, have argued that since only light tipping forces will be used, the risk of root resorption during orthodontic treatment is low. Furthermore, the Orthodontic Radiographs Guidelines, which have been produced by the BOS, advise that 'orthodontic treatment may be carried out without the need for radiographs' in patients in the 'adult dentition'.[13] It is important to appreciate, however, that

these guidelines relate to taking screening radiographs to identify unerupted or impacted teeth.

Teeth with blunt or pipette-shaped apices are more vulnerable to root resorption. This resorption has been observed within the first six months of treatment,[14] i.e. within the time-frame of short-term orthodontic treatment. In addition, many adult patients requesting orthodontic treatment with limited objectives have previously undergone orthodontic treatment which has relapsed. Most fixed appliance orthodontic treatment is associated with some minor root resorption, typically blunting of the apices. It is therefore important to identify this during the pretreatment assessment and to advise patients of their increased risk of further root resorption during the consent process. This discussion suggests that it is possible to justify clinically undertaking a radiographic review of the roots and apices of the teeth as part of the orthodontic assessment in patients in the adult dentition. This is supported, in part by the BOS recommendation, that intraoral radiographs are justified 'in patients having a repeat course of treatment'.[13]

The radiographic assessment of root morphology should include all the teeth within the fixed appliance, not just the teeth which are being moved. Newton's Third Law of Motion states that for every action there is an equal and opposite reaction. Orthodontic forces are therefore being applied to all the teeth, within the appliance, during orthodontic treatment with limited objectives. The vulnerability to root resorption of every tooth included within the orthodontic appliance should therefore be assessed before treatment begins. The Faculty of General Dental Practitioners (FGDP) Guidelines on Selection Criteria for Dental Radiography recommend that no more than one scanning radiograph should be taken for a patient within a 12-month period.[15] Referring dentists should therefore be requested to provide copies of dental pantomograms taken within the previous 12 months when referring a patient for an orthodontic assessment.

For patients in the mixed and adolescent dentition, the BOS Guidelines[13] advise that if a non-extraction treatment is planned, then it is not necessary for radiographs to be obtained as part of the orthodontic assessment or before treatment begins. Again, these Guidelines are based on the assumption that radiographs are being taken to identify unerupted or impacted teeth, rather than to assess the vulnerability of the roots to root resorption during treatment. However, the Guidelines do advise that if a tooth is identified clinically to be excessively mobile, then 'intraoral radiographs may be indicated'.[13] Nevertheless, clinical experience suggests that teeth with resorbed roots often show no clinical signs of mobility until the root resorption is quite advanced. Similarly, for adult patients there appears to be a strong argument for undertaking a radiographic assessment of the roots in adult and child patients before fixed orthodontic treatment begins to identify those at increased risk of root resorption. The BOS Guidelines[13] also recommend that if there is a long waiting list for treatment, then the scanning radiograph should be taken just before treatment begins. However, under these circumstances, it is important to advise the patient, and their parent or caregiver, that there is a possibility that when the radiograph is taken it might reveal issues that are contraindications to orthodontic treatment, thus reducing the risk of disappointment and a complaint.

The value of taking a lateral cephalometric radiograph, as part of the pre-treatment orthodontic assessment, is a contentious subject. In common law, the existence of a clinical guideline supporting their practice, can help a clinician justify the treatment that was provided. As such, the BOS[13] have provided guidance, in the form of flow charts, for when a lateral cephalometric radiograph should be taken, for a patient, as part of the orthodontic assessment. If, however, the clinician can argue why he or she did not follow the guideline for a particular patient, this may also be accepted by the Court.

When deciding whether to take a lateral cephalometric radiograph as part of the orthodontic assessment, the clinician must assess whether they are conforming to IRMER17 when prescribing the radiograph for this individual patient. Will they be able to ascertain any additional information from the radiograph to inform the treatment-planning process and thus benefit the patient? Alternatively, are they merely taking the radiograph to confirm the incisor inclination for example, which they have already assessed clinically?

To conform with IRMER17, and also to confirm that the clinician has undergone this thought process when prescribing the radiograph, the justification for taking a lateral cephalometric radiograph must be recorded in the clinical notes. The lateral cephalometric radiograph should also be traced and the measurements which have informed the treatment plan must be recorded in order to provide evidence of benefit to the patient of taking the radiograph.

Pretreatment Records

The BOS have produced advice about the records that may be collected as part of a course of orthodontic treatment.[16] However, the publication is not presented as clinical guidance. Lists of the types of records that could be collected during orthodontic treatment are provided, rather than recommendations for the records that should be collected. The lack of formal guidance about orthodontic records has led GDPs, in particular, to argue that there is no necessity to take three-dimensional (3D) records of the occlusion at the beginning of treatment.

However, a 3D record of the presenting malocclusion provides evidence of the clinical issues that were confronting the clinician at the beginning of treatment. This may help to justify the decisions that were made during treatment planning if the patient brings a claim against them. The existence of 3D records of the occlusion is also extremely helpful in the consent process (see section Obtaining Consent). They provide a means by which the clinician can explain and discuss their planned individual tooth movements with the patient.

For orthodontic treatments with limited objectives where the tooth movements may have been subtle, the existence of a 3D model of the starting occlusion provides evidence of the tooth movements that have been achieved by the operator. This provides a defence to the, not uncommon, complaint that the treatment has achieved nothing. It is important to appreciate, however, that without a wax bite or some other record of the teeth in occlusion, pretreatment 3D models have little value. Orthodontic treatment, even that with limited objectives, moves the teeth in three dimensions and so it is important that the records collected are able to provide evidence of this.

Intraoral clinical photographs of the presenting dentition and occlusion are frequently presented as an alternative to a 3D record. In my experience, however, these photographs either fail to show the buccal segments clearly or are taken with the patient posturing forward, and so are not a true record of the presenting malocclusion. Also, photographs can be manipulated after they have been taken.

The legal status of virtual models of the occlusion provided by manufacturers of aligner systems is not clear. The GDC have accepted these as records of the starting occlusion (Dental Protection Ltd, personal communication, 2016), but the clinician has no control over the production of the model and the manufacturers are usually based outside of British jurisdiction. It may be difficult, under these circumstances, to defend an accusation from a patient making a claim that the images of the occlusion at the beginning of treatment have been manipulated. Taking your own 3D records of the starting occlusion for these treatments could reduce your risk of a successful claim. Software packages are also able to provide an audit trail, and this can be provided to the Court, for example, to show that the images have not been tampered with after they have been collected. It is clearly important to check that these facilities are provided if you decide to invest in 3D imaging.

Intraoral and extraoral clinical photographs are universally taken at the beginning of treatment for patients undergoing aesthetic treatment, including orthodontics.

These photographs are often then used, with the patient's consent, in practice literature to inform other patients of what can be achieved by the treatments offered by the practice.

However, the main dentolegal value of taking intraoral clinical photographs at the beginning of orthodontic treatment is as a record of the health of the gingivae and of the structure and appearance of the dental enamel. Complaints have been received from patients that the dental enamel has been damaged during fixed orthodontic treatment. The existence of a high-quality intraoral photograph of the enamel of the teeth taken at the beginning of treatment may enable the clinician to show that the enamel defect was present before treatment began, if this was the case. Similarly, GDC case examiners have alleged that orthodontic treatment has been commenced for a patient with poor oral hygiene (Dental Protection Ltd, personal communication, 2016). A good-quality clinical photograph taken at the beginning of treatment showing that the gingivae were healthy at the beginning of treatment can be crucial in defending this type of allegation.

It is also necessary to take extraoral clinical photographs for patients who are about to undergo orthodontic treatment. This is particularly important for treatment that aims to change a patient's facial appearance, for example functional appliance and orthognathic surgical treatment. Extraoral photographs taken at the start of treatment are also very valuable for defending a claim from an adult patient that the orthodontic treatment they have received has 'ruined' their appearance. Such claims are not uncommon from adult patients with unrealistic expectations of treatment. These may be hard to defend if you have not taken a record of the patient's facial appearance at the beginning of treatment.

It is important that clinical photographs are taken with a dedicated clinical camera. You will be in breach of the Data Protection Act[17] (the UK's implementation of the European Union's General Data Protection Regulations) if you take clinical photographs using a mobile phone because the images will not be stored securely and can inadvertently be shared with your other electronic devices. GDC *Standards for the Dental Team*, Standard 4.2.7 states that 'if you want to use patient information such as photographs for any reason, you must: explain how the information will be used' and 'obtain and record the patients' consent to their use'.[1]

Storage of Records

One of the arguments against using dental study models as a 3D record of the occlusion has been the difficulties presented by storing the models. The Data Protection Act states that 'records must be stored safely and securely'.

Clinical records are confidential, except to the patient or their representative, and members of practice staff who have been instructed in the security policy. A patient's clinical records, including dental study models and radiographs, are the property of the clinician who made the record. If the practice is subsequently sold and the new owners purchase the clinical goodwill of the practice, ownership of records pertaining to previous patients passes to the new owners.

Under the Data Protection Act[17], patients are able to obtain copies of their clinical records if they provide the clinician with a written and signed request for the records. A parent, or clinical guardian who has responsibility for the patient, is able to request the records for a patient who is aged under 18 years. If the patient is aged over 18 years, even if they were under age when the treatment was provided, they must make the written request for the records themselves or provide their written permission for another person (e.g. a solicitor) to request the records on their behalf. It is important to appreciate that the clinical records include not only the written or electronic record of the treatment that has been provided but also items such as laboratory dockets, NHS forms and consent forms.

There is provision within the Data Protection Act[17] for a clinician to request that the patient covers the cost of copying their records. Unfortunately, many requests for clinical records are made by patients who are considering making a complaint against a clinician. A request from the clinician for monies to cover this cost may be the final factor which persuades the patient to pursue their complaint. It is therefore worth thinking carefully before proceeding with such a request.

The rules about how long records should be stored after the patient's treatment has ended are less clear. The Data Protection Act states that personal data should be retained 'no longer than necessary'.[17] However, the Department of Health recommends that records are retained for 11 years if an adult patient was treated in primary care, or for eight years if they were treated in secondary care. For children, it is recommended that their records are retained until the age of 25 years.[18]

A claim of negligence must be made within three years of the plaintiff becoming aware of an issue that may be a consequence of treatment they have received. However, the Court does have the discretion to extend this period, and for children this clock does not start until they reach the age of 18 years. Potentially, therefore, an issue may arise from orthodontic treatment provided during adolescence, for example, excessive tooth wear as a consequence of the teeth being left in traumatic occlusion at the end of orthodontic treatment. Therefore, ideally, clinical records should only be destroyed on the death of the clinician (it is not permitted in civil law to sue the deceased or their estate).

With the introduction of electronic patient records, it may be possible to store clinical records for the lifetime of the clinician, but clearly this is not practical for paper records and dental study models. Dental Protection advise their members to store clinical records of complex treatments for 30 years. Dental Protection also advise that you are unlikely to be criticised if 12 years have elapsed since you provided treatment for an adult patient and you have destroyed their records. Records should be destroyed in a manner that protects the patient's anonymity.[18]

Dentolegal and Ethical Issues that may Arise During Treatment Planning

GDPs undertaking short-term orthodontic treatment are particularly vulnerable to a complaint that has originated from the treatment-planning process. Specialists in orthodontics take three years to train and so it is clear that GDPs cannot be taught these skills in a short weekend course, for example. To overcome this problem, many of the orthodontic systems that have been developed for GDPs provide assistance with treatment planning. This treatment planning is often informed by artificial intelligence. Unfortunately, however, it is the GDP who provides the treatment, rather than the manufacturer of the system, who is liable if issues arise during treatment that are the consequence of an inappropriate treatment plan. It is therefore worth bearing in mind that if you are tempted to provide one of these treatments for your patient, and a problem occurs leading to a patient complaint to the GDC, you will be cross-examined about the process that you went through to plan the patient's treatment. It is worth spending time ensuring that you fully understand the biological and mechanical basis of the treatment that you are proposing before offering it to your patient.

Specialist Orthodontists may also receive a complaint or claim about their treatment planning, particularly if they have not paid attention during the examination process and have overlooked an issue, for example an impacted canine. The realisation that the surgical exposure of an impacted tooth is required is likely to result in treatment time being much longer than the patient anticipated, potentially generating a complaint. Similar issues may arise if the orthodontist has not fully appreciated the extent of a patient's skeletal discrepancy and it becomes clear, during a protracted treatment, that orthognathic surgery is ideally needed to fully correct the patient's malocclusion. The risk of these types of issues arising can be significantly reduced if the clinician adopts a systematic approach to the examination of the patient during the initial consultation.

Complaints may also occur as a consequence of poor communication between the specialist orthodontist and the referring GDP. If a patient presents with hypodontia, for example, and the orthodontist plans to create space for prosthetic replacement of teeth, this must be discussed with the clinician who will be providing the restorations before treatment begins. This is particularly important for child and adolescent patients, who may well be entitled to free orthodontic treatment under the NHS because of their hypodontia but, by the time they are of the ideal age to be fitted with a permanent restoration, are no longer routinely entitled to free dental treatment. A complaint is likely to follow if the patient or parent is informed at debond that they will have to fund the cost of a bridge or implant themselves. Furthermore, the child's GDP may not agree with your clinical suggestion for how the space should be filled or may not have the skills to provide the restoration that you discussed with the patient during treatment planning. An impasse may be reached, in which the patient is ready to have their final restoration but then has difficulty obtaining the last part of their treatment. A complaint is almost inevitable.

It is therefore important during the treatment-planning process for a hypodontia case that there is detailed consideration of the type of restorations that will be fitted at the end of treatment, when the restoration will be fitted, by whom, and how this will be funded. These points should all be recorded in the clinical notes, as part of the overall treatment plan, and then agreed with the clinician providing the restorations. Orthodontic treatment is often completed before the age when permanent restorations should be placed. Plans should therefore also be made for the temporary prosthetic replacement of the missing teeth. Again, these need to be agreed with the patient's GDP, or whoever will be managing the restorative aspects of the case, before treatment begins. As previously, the proposed arrangements should be carefully documented in the patient's clinical records.

Another area where poor communication between the specialist orthodontist and the referring GDP may lead to a complaint is in extraction cases. Many clinicians will be aware of instances when an unfortunate GDP has extracted the wrong tooth as part of an orthodontic treatment plan. Although it is ultimately the clinician who extracts the tooth who has the responsibility to identify the tooth, the orthodontist may be criticised if clear instructions have not been provided to the GDP about which tooth (teeth) are to be extracted and for what purpose. It is therefore good practice to write the notation of the tooth and also to describe the tooth (teeth) that are to be extracted in the letter that is sent to the GDP to request the extractions. It is also good clinical practice to indicate in the letter that the teeth require extraction 'to facilitate orthodontic treatment'.

If a GDP has mistakenly extracted the wrong tooth, the way in which the situation is handled by the orthodontist is likely to have a significant impact on whether the patient or parent/carer decides to make a formal complaint against the GDP or not. Clearly, the GDP has a Duty of Candour[19] (see later) to inform the patient of their error. They should also contact the orthodontist as soon as they realise their mistake, for urgent advice. However, it is up to the orthodontist to act in the patient's best interests and to modify their treatment plan, if possible, to achieve the best possible outcome for the patient. If this increases treatment time or means that not all the original treatment aims can be achieved, then this should be discussed with the patient and/or their parent or carer. A specialist orthodontist would be severely criticised if, after the wrong tooth has been extracted, they make no attempt to consider a change to their treatment mechanics, where one exists, and lay the blame for a poor outcome solely on the GDP.

Obtaining Consent

Many complaints, particularly against specialist orthodontists, arise from the consent process. For an elective treatment such as orthodontics, gaining informed consent from a patient is particularly important. A patient and their parent/carer must clearly understand the risks and benefits and what will be involved for them in proceeding with a treatment that is not clinically necessary. Standard 3 of the GDC *Standards for the Dental Team*[1] provides Professional Standards for obtaining patient consent to dental treatment. The BOS have produced specific standards[5] for obtaining consent for orthodontic treatment. It is important to appreciate that the consent process must include a discussion of the potential risks and benefits of the whole orthodontic treatment pathway, including retention and interproximal enamel reduction. Complaints have arisen because patients have been unaware that after completing a gruelling course of orthodontic treatment, they then have a lifetime of wearing retainers and the ongoing costs of maintaining these.

For consent to be valid, details of what the patient has consented to should be documented, at the time that their consent was obtained, in the patient's main clinical records. The GDC also advise that 'a signature on a form is important in verifying that a patient has given consent'.[1] However, it is important to appreciate that if it later becomes apparent that the patient did not understand the treatment that they were providing their consent for, then a signed form will not provide a defence. Unfortunately, the opposite does not usually apply. The absence of a signed consent form tends to increase the clinician's vulnerability to a successful claim that the patient did not understand the treatment. Patients should be requested to provide separate written consent to having clinical photographs taken, if there is a possibility that their photographs will be used in the future for teaching or advertising purposes.

The Supreme Court ruling in Montgomery versus Lanarkshire Health Board[20] now provides the common law on consent in the UK. This ruling puts the issues that are important to the patient at the centre of the consent process by stressing that gaining consent should involve a dialogue between the clinician and the patient, in which 'the significance of a given risk is likely to reflect … the effect which its occurrence would have upon the life of a patient and the importance to the patient of the benefits sought to be achieved by the treatment' are paramount. The ruling in Montgomery versus Lanarkshire Health Board also states that 'The doctor is therefore under a duty to take reasonable care to ensure that the patient is aware of any material risks involved in any recommended treatment, and of any reasonable or variant treatments'.[20] This potentially provides a particular challenge in orthodontics, because there is often a range of different treatment options available for treating the patient's presenting malocclusion. For GDPs offering orthodontic treatment with limited aims, the challenge is greater because they are unlikely to have the training or experience to be able to advise the patient about the full range of treatment options. To satisfy the requirements of the ruling in Montgomery versus Lanarkshire Health Board, GDPs are now expected to include a discussion about the risks and benefits of treatment involving a referral to a specialist orthodontist, when obtaining a patient's consent for orthodontic treatment. For an elective treatment, such as orthodontics, it is also important to discuss the risks and benefits to the patient of remaining as they are, i.e. the option of no treatment. The details of these discussions must be documented in the clinical notes and also included in the written consent form that the patient signs.

There is an adage which suggests that 'if you provide ten orthodontists with a malocclusion, you will generate ten different treatment plans'. The ruling in Montgomery versus Lanarkshire Health Board therefore presents specialist orthodontists with the challenge of deciding how many treatment options to discuss with the patient and in how much detail. When deciding how many options should be discussed it is important to be aware of the second part of the ruling in Montgomery versus Lanarkshire Health Board, which states that:

'The test of materiality is whether, in the circumstances of the particular case, a reasonable person in the patient's position would be likely to attach significant significance to the risk, or the doctor is or should reasonably be aware that the particular patient would be likely to attach significance to it'.[20]

A pragmatic approach would therefore be to discuss, for example, the risks and benefits of an extraction versus a non-extraction approach to treatment, if this is a concern to the patient, or the risks and benefits of a compromise treatment compared to achieving an ideal result, if the patient indicates that they are only concerned about some aspects of their malocclusion. Clearly, the circumstances will vary from patient to patient, but you are unlikely to be criticised for not discussing the risks and benefits of extracting a second premolar versus a first premolar, for example, during the consent process, unless the patient professes a particular attachment to either tooth.

This part of the ruling in Montgomery versus Lanarkshire versus Lanarkshire Health Board illustrates the importance of spending time investigating the patient's concerns with their malocclusion and what they are hoping to achieve from orthodontic treatment during the initial consultation. If, as a clinician, you feel that the patient does not understand, and also, importantly, *accept*, that the only thing that orthodontic treatment is guaranteed to do (hopefully) is to improve their dental appearance, then you should discuss your concerns with the patient. The BOS recommend that 'All patients and guardians should be given a "cooling off" period to consider their options as part of the valid consenting process'.[5] This is particularly valuable for a patient who seems to have unrealistic expectations of what orthodontic treatment can do for their life.

The BOS also state that 'consent is an on-going process'.[5] This issue may arise during the orthodontic treatment of adolescent patients, because it is often their parents or carers who engage most in the consent process when the patient first attends for treatment. As treatment progresses it may become clear, as they become more Gillick-competent (see following section), that the patient would prefer to withdraw his or her consent to the continuation of treatment. This can present the clinician with a difficult dilemma if, for example, extractions have been undertaken and there are still spaces to close. It is not appropriate for a clinician to continue to provide treatment with the knowledge that the patient has not provided their full consent. The clinician will need to have a discussion with the patient about the advantages and disadvantages of continuing with treatment and document these. Rather than debonding the patient, it may be possible to adjust the treatment plan, with the patient's consent, to aim for a compromise result if this reduces overall treatment time. Wherever possible, efforts should be made to include whoever provided consent to the original treatment plan in these discussions. Alternatively, you could write to the parent or caregiver, with the patient's consent, explaining the reasons for the proposed change to the treatment plan and offering them the opportunity to ask questions.

If after discussion of the risks and benefits of stopping treatment, an adolescent is adamant that they want to stop treatment, then, although an active intervention is required to debond the appliances, they can be considered to have withdrawn their consent. A clinician could be criticised for refusing to remove the appliances. Some clinicians invite patients who wish to have their treatment terminated to sign a disclaimer to confirm that they understand the risks. However, the legal basis of such a document has not been confirmed. Another controversial area is whether retainers should be provided for a patient who has ended their treatment prematurely. It is important to be aware that, under the current NHS contract, most practitioners will have indicated that retainers will be provided as part of the orthodontic treatment plan. Retainers are also usually included with private orthodontic treatment contracts. Therefore, by not offering to provide retainers to a patient who has requested that their appliances be removed, you could be in breach of contract. If, by contrast, you offer to provide retainers to maintain the tooth movements that have been achieved but the patient declines to be fitted with retainers, then this should be recorded in the patient's clinical records.

Many clinicians have concerns that if they discuss a possible treatment option in general terms with a patient, then they are compelled to provide this treatment. However, GDC Standard 1.4.2 states that 'if their desired outcome is not achievable or is not in the best interest of their oral health, you must explain the risks, benefits and likely outcomes to help them to make a decision'.[1] For example, if it is your clinical opinion that a non-extraction approach will lead to long-term oral health consequences for a patient, then you would not be criticised if you decline to treat the patient on this basis. Therefore, it is crucial to clearly document the rationale behind your advice in the patient's records. It would also not be appropriate, under these circumstances, for you to then refer the patient to a clinician who you are aware is a 'non-extractionist'. The patient or their parent is entitled to make whatever decision they wish about their treatment. You could be criticised, however, for referring a patient for treatment which you are aware could be potentially damaging. Similarly, GDC Standard 7.2 states that 'you must work within your knowledge, skills, professional competence and abilities'.[1] If a non-extraction approach, say, would involve the use of treatment mechanics which you do not feel confident to use –temporary anchorage devices might be an example – then, again, you are able to decline to treat the patient if you have explained and documented the reasons for your advice. In the latter example however, the GDC advises that 'you must refer the patient to an appropriately trained colleague'.[1]

Another issue that has arisen in discussions about possible treatment options for orthodontic patients regards the discussions that should be had with orthodontic patients about 'alternative' types of treatments, i.e. non-conventional treatments akin to 'alternative medicine'. These treatment modalities tend not to be accepted by the body of the orthodontic profession due to lack of evidence for their effectiveness. It has been argued, however, that these treatments should be included in the list of treatments discussed with patients as part of the consent process, although a GDC Fitness to Practice ruling did not support this view (Dental Protection Ltd, personal communication, 2016). However, in the spirit of the ruling in Montgomery versus Lanarkshire Health Board,[20] if a patient or parent raises this as a possible treatment option during the consent process, then the clinician would be expected to discuss the pros and cons of such a treatment in a measured way. Similarly, an 'alternative treatment practitioner' may be criticised for not discussing the pros and cons of conventional orthodontic treatment with the patient, if their treatment is aimed at correcting a malocclusion.

Who is Able to Provide Consent?

People over the age of 16 are entitled to provide consent for their own treatment. In cases where refusal to provide consent may lead to death or serious injury, this can be overruled by the Court of Protection, under the Mental Capacity Act 2005.[21] After the ruling in Gillick versus West Norfolk & Wisbech Area Health Authority,[22] a child aged under 16 who is considered to have enough understanding to fully appreciate what is involved in their treatment, i.e. they are **Gillick-competent**, may also provide consent for their own treatment.

A patient, or their parent or caregiver, is able to withdraw their consent to treatment at any time. For a long course of treatment, such as orthodontics, consent for each treatment visit is implied by the patient attending the appointment and sitting willingly in the dental chair. Issues may arise during treatment if the patient's parents become estranged and an irreversible procedure, for example, dental extractions, is required to which one parent does not agree. This type of scenario illustrates the importance of predicting, and incorporating, the whole

treatment pathway into the original consent process, if at all possible. However, it is not unusual for an orthodontist to have to change a treatment plan in mid-course to include extractions, for example, if a patient fails to respond to an appliance or grows unpredictably.

The Children Act[23] provides the law about who should be involved in making decisions about a child. The Act states that 'when important decisions are made about the child', including consenting to 'a child's operation or certain medical treatment', then all those with 'parental responsibility' are allowed to have a say in that decision. Under the Act, mothers and married fathers automatically have parental responsibility for their child, even if they divorce. Unmarried fathers automatically have parental responsibility if the child was born after 1 December 2003 and the father's name is on the birth certificate or they have entered into a parental responsibility agreement with the mother. Grandparents have no parental responsibility for the child unless they were appointed as guardians, and the child's parents have died or they have obtained a Child Arrangements Order from the Court and the child lives with them. Similarly, step-parents have no parental responsibility for a child, unless they have entered into a parental responsibility agreement with everyone who has responsibility for the child and they are also married to one of these individuals.[23]

The Children Act states that if parents are unable to agree on a major decision for their child, which might include extractions for orthodontic treatment, then the parents should seek family mediation. Clearly, this would extend the length of the child's orthodontic treatment if it has already started, and if you are faced with a situation where parents are unable to agree a change in the treatment plan, for example, the need for extractions, you may consider providing information to each parent separately and then invite them to discuss this together in a side room. Similarly, if you are aware that a child's parents do not live together, then it would be wise to confirm with the parent attending with the child that the child's other parent is in agreement with the proposed change to the orthodontic treatment plan. Again, all these discussions must be documented in the child's clinical records.

Dentolegal Issues Arising During Active Orthodontic Treatment

For a claim of clinical negligence to be successful, the plaintiff must prove that:

1. the clinician has a duty of care
2. the clinician has breached this duty
3. an injury has occurred as a consequence of this breach.

If these three points can be proved, then the patient is entitled to obtain compensation through the civil courts.

A **duty of care** is a legal obligation placed on an individual whilst performing an act which could foreseeably harm the other person. All clinicians therefore have a duty of care towards their patients. The common law test for the standard of care that should be provided comes from the ruling in Bolam versus Friern Hospital Management Committee.[24] The **Bolam test** states that 'a doctor is not negligent if he has acted in accordance with a practice accepted as proper by a reasonable body of men skilled in that particular art'. A second test was added to the Bolam test after the ruling in Bolitho versus City and Hackney Health Authority.[25] The **Bolitho test** is that the standard which was considered to be proper should be able to 'withstand logical analysis'. Expert witnesses who provide advice to the Court about the standard of care that should have been achieved are now expected to produce clinical guidelines that have been developed after systematic review of the evidence of the effectiveness of a recommended clinical practice, where they exist, to demonstrate that their evidence will satisfy the test in Bolitho. Bolam sets out that 'the clinician is not negligent if they have acted in accordance with a responsible body of opinion'.[24] The ruling in Bolitho narrowed the scope of the Bolam test by stating 'that the court must be satisfied that the body of opinion relied upon has a logical basis'.[25]

It is also important to appreciate that, for negligence to be proved, 'a relationship of proximity must extend between the defendant and the claimant'.[26] This is relevant to treatments, including aligner treatments, which are planned by a third party. These third parties are usually considered not to be liable because they do not have a direct relationship with the patient. The clinician will therefore bear the total costs if negligence is proved.

An important aspect of the ruling in Bolam versus Friern HMC[24] is that the standard of care that is applied is that of the clinician's peers. This may raise issues if a claim of negligence is made against a GDP providing orthodontic treatment. Should the outcome of orthodontic treatment provided by a GDP be judged against those achieved by other GDPs, which have been reported to be low,[27] or against the results that are achieved by specialists? This has not yet been tested in the courts.

However, the GDC, which includes orthodontic treatment within the scope of practice for all registered dentists, states in Standard 7.2.2 that 'you should only deliver treatment if you are confident that you have had the necessary training and are competent to do so'.[1] GDPs undertaking orthodontic treatment, with limited objectives, sometimes encounter difficulties during active treatment if the teeth do not move as predicted or there are issues such as frequent breakages. Specialist Orthodontists encounter these problems too but they have the knowledge and range of skills to correct them. GDPs, however, may be vulnerable to an allegation that they were in breach of GDC Standard 7.2.1, which states that 'You must be sure that you have undertaken training which is appropriate for you and equips you with the appropriate knowledge and skills to perform a task safely',[1] if, having identified a problem, they do not have the skills to remediate it. It may also take some time for GDPs undertaking orthodontic treatment to realise that the treatment is not proceeding as anticipated. Treatment times will then be extended, which is a frequent source of complaints from patients.

Specialist Orthodontists, who have the training to adjust their own treatment plans, are vulnerable to a different issue that may arise during active orthodontic treatment. Most adult patients are engaged in the treatment process but, for some, this engagement becomes obsessive and they become their own 'experts', requesting frequent amendments to the treatment plan, often on a tooth-by-tooth basis. In an effort to appease the patient, the orthodontist will often go along with these 'tweaks' to the treatment plan but is then at risk of losing sight of the original aims of treatment. It is often impossible to satisfy these patients and eventually a situation is reached where neither the patient nor the clinician can see treatment being completed to the patient's satisfaction. The patient may then make a complaint against the orthodontist.

Although in retrospect there may have been clues to indicate the patient's obsessive personality during the initial consultation, unfortunately these patients can be difficult to spot before treatment begins. It is therefore important, for every patient, that the clinician formulates and gains consent for a very specific treatment plan at the start of treatment. It is also prudent that if the patient requests a change to the treatment plan during active treatment, that the new aims of treatment are documented and that the risks and benefits of the revised plan, however small the changes have been, are discussed with the patient and their formal consent to the revised treatment plan obtained. This process will appear to be very tedious in the busy clinical situation, but will help you to keep control of your treatment plan.

The clinical situations discussed here are unlikely to result in injury to a patient or a claim of clinical negligence. However, the patient would be able to make a claim of breach of contract if treatment is not completed. They may also be able to make a successful complaint to the GDC if they have doubts about your ability to complete their orthodontic treatment, or if they feel that their wishes have not been taken into account during the treatment process. Fortunately, injury during orthodontic treatment, which could lead to a successful charge of negligence, is rare. Alani and Kelleher[2] have listed the dental issues which may arise during treatment. These include enamel demineralisation, gingivitis, exacerbation of periodontal disease, damage to restorations, tooth devitalisation, temporomandibular joint dysfunction, and external root resorption. Many of these conditions are either preventable or predictable. For example, a clinician providing orthodontic treatment who has not shown the patient how to care for their fixed appliances when they were fitted, not provided them with written instructions, and not documented this in the clinical notes may be vulnerable to a claim of negligence if the patient experiences significant enamel demineralisation or gingivitis during treatment. Similarly, if a patient presents with active periodontal disease and you do not take steps to ensure that this is under control before treatment begins and monitored throughout orthodontic treatment, and that these steps are documented, then you may be vulnerable to a successful claim if the patient's periodontal disease progresses. The GDC may also consider that you have not provided the expected standard of care when treating this patient.

A clinician's vulnerability to a successful claim of negligence if root resorption occurs during orthodontic treatment may be less conclusive. Blunting of the root apices is a common radiographic finding after orthodontic treatment with fixed appliances. Patients are usually warned about the risk of root resorption during the consent process for orthodontic treatment. Occasionally, however, root resorption during orthodontic treatment may be excessive, although there may be few, or no, clinical indicators that this is occurring during treatment. There is also rarely a clinical justification for taking a scanning radiograph during orthodontic treatment or at debond. The clinician may therefore be unaware that significant root resorption has occurred. The situation is further complicated because the prognosis for teeth with external root resorption is uncertain.[28]

Each case is different, but the issues which are likely to be taken into account when determining whether a clinician is negligent if external root resorption has occurred include the following. Were there radiographic signs at the beginning of treatment which indicated that the patient was particularly vulnerable to root resorption? If yes, and these were identified, was the patient warned of their increased risk? Also, did the patient report symptoms characteristic of root resorption to the clinician during treatment? If yes, did the clinician undertake the appropriate investigations? Similarly, were there any clinical signs of excessive root resorption present during treatment? If yes, did the clinician investigate these?

Another factor which may be taken into account is the time that the fixed appliances were in place and also the tooth movements that were undertaken. The risk of root resorption is correlated with treatment duration and bodily movements of the teeth, particularly those which move the root apices close to the cortical plates.[28] If it can be shown that treatment time was significantly longer than average or there were unnecessary root movements (e.g. 'round-tripping'), again the clinician may be vulnerable to a successful claim of negligence. However, it is important to appreciate that all orthodontic treatment applies forces to the periodontium that may lead to external root resorption. It is no defence to suggest that since you were only applying, say, tipping forces to the teeth in orthodontic treatment with limited objectives, there was no need to radiographically assess the vulnerability of the roots of the teeth to external resorption at the start of treatment.

Injury may also occur during orthodontic treatment, for example, if part of an orthodontic appliance is swallowed or inhaled. It is not practical to fit a rubber dam when fitting or adjusting a fixed orthodontic appliance, and so there is always a risk that a patient may swallow or, worse, inhale a piece of the appliance. The BOS have produced advice about the steps to take under these circumstances.[29] For example, if a complaint is made following the loss of a bracket down the patient's throat, the following factors may be taken into account: Did the clinician notice that part of the appliance had been lost? Was the clinician working with a trained dental surgery assistant? Was adequate suction available? Did the clinician inform the patient/parent and provide appropriate advice? Were the steps that were taken documented in the clinical notes? Was a clinical incident recorded? Did the clinician contact the patient at home to check that all was well? Accidents do happen during clinical practice but if you are able to show that you have taken steps to remediate the damage and have always put the patient's interests first, then you will reduce your risk of a successful investigation by the GDC. However, you could still be found negligent by the Court if it is found that your actions have caused injury to the patient. Most lost brackets, for example, are swallowed and pass through the gut uneventfully, i.e. no physical injury can be proven. Unfortunately, some plaintiffs are now claiming psychological injury, from worrying about the possible consequences of an untoward event during treatment. It is therefore worthwhile seeking advice from your indemnifiers if any type of untoward incident occurs during clinical practice.

Clear advice should also be provided to patients about the action they should take if their fixed appliance breaks. The main clinical concern with debonded brackets or lost archwires tends to be the impact that these may have on treatment progress. However, a case has been reported in which a patient swallowed a section of archwire that had become detached from a recently fitted fixed appliance.[30] The wire then became embedded in the wall of the gut and needed to be surgically removed. It is likely that this patient contributed to the loss of the archwire by tampering with the appliance. Patients should therefore be warned, in a non-alarmist way, about the possible consequences of interfering with their fixed appliances.

Transfers

Orthodontic treatment can be a lengthy process and sometimes it becomes necessary to transfer a patient to another clinician during active treatment. The BOS report that, on average, treatment times are six months longer in patients who transfer during treatment.[31] To avoid a complaint, it would be wise to discuss this issue with the patient and to suggest ways for them to continue under your care if possible.

If a transfer is unavoidable, then the best way to facilitate this process is to provide them with copies of their clinical records, including radiographs and study models, to inform their new clinician of their presenting malocclusion; this is not mandatory but would be considered to be in the patient's best interests. However, it is important to remember to keep the original records and archive these carefully. Unfortunately, clinicians are most vulnerable to a complaint when a patient transfers to another clinician. It is therefore very important to be able to quickly retrieve the documentation regarding the treatment you have provided.

Non-compliance

Another issue that arises during treatment is non-compliance. This may be non-compliance with oral hygiene measures or non-compliance with treatment, for example the wearing of removable appliances or elastics. It is almost always adolescent patients who fail to comply with treatment. As previously discussed, this raises the issue of consent for treatment. Non-compliance is almost always a sign that the patient has decided that orthodontic treatment is no longer for them. However, it is very important to rule out other issues, such as lack of physical dexterity, before raising your concerns with the patient about their consent to treatment. If the patient is unable to physically tolerate an appliance or elastics, for example, it may be possible to amend the treatment plan or to reduce the aims of treatment. As discussed previously, these revised aims should be documented and consent obtained from the patient and their parent/caregiver.

More difficult issues arise when the decision to stop treatment has to be made by the clinician, for example due to continued poor oral hygiene or repeated breakages. In each of these situations, if the patient or their parent/caregiver makes a complaint to the GDC, the clinician will need to be able to show that they have put the patient's best interests first when terminating treatment. The patient should be informed of your concerns immediately they arise and efforts should be made to identify why the patient is struggling and to assist the patient to care for their appliances. The GDC is likely to take a dim view if you remove the appliances without giving the patient the opportunity to improve their ways. If poor oral hygiene is the issue, then intraoral clinical photographs will not only provide evidence of the clinical situation that you as a clinician were managing, but they can also be used to inform the patient of your concerns. Start clinical photographs can also form a baseline for comparison. The only exception to removing an appliance without giving the patient a warning would be when there has been a significant loss of tooth tissue due to caries or erosion and there is a significant risk to the dentition of leaving the appliance in situ. Again, good-quality intraoral photographs should be taken to document the clinical situation. Arrangements should also be made for the patient to receive urgent restorative care.

Non-attendance

A patient may also show their lack of consent for continuing with orthodontic treatment by failing to attend for appointments. If this is an intermittent pattern, once again the clinician should show that they are acting in the best interests of the patient by discussing the impact that failed attendance will have on treatment progress and the potential for unwanted side effects to occur if the appliance is not monitored. As ever, these discussions must be documented. Efforts should also be made to identify the issues that are making it difficult for the patient to attend and, if possible, to make arrangements to assist the patient to attend. Sometimes, the situation will be impossible to correct. This highlights the value of discussing the importance of regular attendance, and also the surgery hours, with patients and their parents/caregivers during the initial consent process. Similarly, if the practice operates a policy in which patients are discharged after a minimum number of failed appointments, this must be drawn to the patient and parent/caregiver's attention during the initial consent process.

Often the patient fails to attend for any further appointments. Again, the GDC will want to see evidence that you have continued to act in the patient's best interests and that efforts were made to contact the patient to arrange an appointment to discuss treatment/debond. Clearly you cannot impose treatment on a patient who has withdrawn their consent by not attending. The BOS advises that 'efforts should be made to inform the patient that wearing an unsupervised appliance carries risks for the dentition'.[32] A non-compliant patient may be nervous of attending again for fear of rebuke; adding a line to a letter informing them that you are keen to find a solution, including possibly removing the braces, may encourage them to attend.

Non-payment of Fees

Orthodontists often arrange for private patients to spread the cost over the course of treatment. Issues may arise if treatment is continuing but patients are not keeping up with their payments. The clinician may be tempted to suspend treatment until further payments are made. Wearing an appliance that is either inactive or is not being regularly monitored is clearly not in the best interests of the patient. The clinician could be criticised for this if the patient makes a complaint to the GDC.

Non-payment of fees therefore needs to be regarded as a separate issue to the clinical treatment, which must continue as planned. It is not strictly necessary to wait until treatment has been completed to put debt recovery measures in place. Clearly, however, this has the potential to impact on the relationship with the patient and so discussions should be had, out of the surgery, with whoever is paying for the treatment to find a sensitive solution to the problem.

Supervision of Orthodontic Therapists

In the UK, orthodontic treatment is increasingly being delivered by orthodontic therapists. The clinical procedures which may be performed by orthodontic therapists are laid out in the GDC's *Scope of Practice*.[33] Orthodontic therapists are only able to undertake clinical procedures that are prescribed by a registered dentist. This includes both GDPs and specialist orthodontists. The BOS has produced Professional Standards for Orthodontic Practice which state that 'patients should not be seen and/or treated by Dental Care Professionals (DCPs) without direct supervision on at least every other appointment by a General Dental or Specialist Practitioner with adequate orthodontic competency'.[34] An expert witness will use these standards as evidence of the standard of care that should have been provided if a patient makes a complaint about an issue that has occurred during active orthodontic treatment provided by an orthodontic therapist. To reduce your risk of an allegation that you have breached this standard, it is worthwhile checking that systems are in place to record

that you have seen the patient and provided a prescription to the orthodontic therapist, if you are the supervising clinician.

Retention

Issues with retainers are a common source of complaint in orthodontics. Orthodontists now routinely recommend that patients wear their retainers for the life of their dentition. However, patients or their parents/caregivers may complain that they were not made aware of the long-term implications of wearing retainers, particularly the cost of maintaining them, before treatment began. It is therefore important that the retention which is planned for a case is included in the initial consent process.

Some patients or their parents/caregivers have preconceptions that fixed retainers are superior to removable retainers. It is not unknown for fixed retainers to be requested by parents/caregivers at the end of orthodontic treatment, because they have little confidence in their child's ability to wear their removable retainer. This raises two issues. Firstly, there are long-term oral health implications associated with fixed retainers and so the clinician could be vulnerable to criticism if there were no good clinical reasons for fitting the fixed retainers. Secondly, many clinicians now recommend that patients wear their removable retainers at night, as an adjunct to the fixed retainers. This may come as an unwelcome surprise to a parent who has paid extra to have a fixed retainer fitted. Clearly, it is better to have these discussions before treatment begins rather than to be confronted, at debond, by the patient or parent/caregiver feeling unable to provide their consent for your recommended retention regimen.

Another issue that frequently arises in orthodontic clinical practice is the long-term cost of maintaining retainers and also who will provide this. Under current NHS regulations,[35] patients are entitled to a 12-month period of supervision of retention, but there is a charge for a lost retainer. Charges for NHS treatment for children are very rare and so most parents/caregivers will be taken aback if they are suddenly presented with a bill for a lost retainer. They will also probably feel that they have no choice but to pay the charge, rather than jeopardising their child's orthodontic result. These feelings could lead to a complaint. Consequently, NHS patients, and their parents, should be informed of the possibility of additional charges before they commit to orthodontic treatment and this advice documented in the clinical notes. This advice should be repeated when the retainers are fitted. If the patient is being treated under private contract, then the fact that lost retainers will incur additional charges, and the level of those charges, should be clearly stated in the contract, if this is your practice's protocol.

For NHS patients, once the 12-month retention is over, orthodontists are entitled to charge patients for review appointments. Alternatively, the patient's GDP may review the patient's occlusion and their retainers. For specialist orthodontists who take referrals, it is worth confirming the arrangements for the ongoing maintenance of retainers with your referring dentists. Complaints have arisen when patients or parents have sought advice about a broken or lost retainer from a GDP, only to be informed that it is the orthodontist's responsibility to maintain these, and vice versa. Not all GDPs will feel confident to monitor or repair a fixed retainer. Furthermore, fixed retainers have the potential to retain plaque and calculus and so require regular review. It is ultimately the responsibility of the clinician who fits a retainer to ensure that arrangements are in place to ensure that no harm will come to the patient from wearing the retainer.

Issues may also arise when an orthodontist leaves his or her practice or retires. Many orthodontists are in the habit of making running minor repairs to a previous patient's fixed retainers, at little or no charge, if they attend with a breakage. The incoming orthodontist may not be willing to provide this type of care at low cost to the patient. Complaints have arisen because a patient has been presented with a large bill for what is often a relatively quick procedure. If the practice is being sold, it is important for an arrangement to be made for the ongoing maintenance of patients wearing fixed retainers, in particular, as part of the sale of the practice. Monies will usually need to be left by the outgoing orthodontist to cover these costs. Similarly, if an orthodontist leaves a practice, these issues should be discussed before they leave.

When removable retainers are fitted, it is important that the patient is given clear instructions about their wear and maintenance. In the UK, it is also important to be aware that if you make your own vacuum-formed retainers on site, then you must register with the Medicines and Healthcare Products Regulatory Agency (MHRA).[36] It is good practice to support the verbal advice that is given to patients with written instructions. The advice that is given to patients, particularly about when they should wear their removable retainers and how to clean them, should be documented in the clinical notes. These instructions should provide clear advice about the patient's responsibility for attending review appointments and also the action that the patient should take if they identify a problem with a retainer. If the number of hours that removable retainers should be worn is reduced during the retention period,

this advice should be clearly recorded in the clinical notes. Patients should also be provided with clear instructions about the action they should take if a retainer is lost or broken.

Relapse

Orthodontic treatment requires a significant investment of time and money from the patient or their parent or caregiver. If changes then occur in the occlusion after the appliances have been removed, the patient is likely to be extremely disappointed. If their issues are not addressed by the clinician to their satisfaction, they may make a formal complaint. A patient may also complain if their fixed retainer requires frequent repairs.

It is not uncommon for an adolescent patient in particular to fail to wear their removable retainers as directed. If clear instructions have been given to the patient and their parent about when they should wear their retainers, and these have been documented in the clinical notes, it is unlikely that the patient will be successful in their complaint about relapse if this is a consequence of lack of retention. An exception to this may be when a clinical reviewer is of the opinion that the teeth have been placed in an extremely unstable position at the end of treatment, and that the patient was not warned about this risk during the initial consent process.

Similarly, if a patient continually presents with a broken fixed retainer, rather than continually repairing it, it is worth spending time considering whether the retention that has been provided is adequate. Fixed retainers do fail due to bond failure but repeated failures should draw the clinician's attention to the possibility of relapse of individual teeth attached to the retainer. GDPs providing fixed retainers at the end of short-term treatment are particularly vulnerable to a complaint about a frequently debonding fixed retainer because they may not be able to convince the Court, or the GDC, that they have sufficient knowledge and skills to understand and remedy this type of clinical situation.

Duty of Candour

If you have identified an issue with a fixed retainer that you have fitted, or some other problem with part of the orthodontic treatment process, it is important that you inform the patient of what has occurred as soon as you become aware of it. All clinicians working within the regulated healthcare professions in the UK now have a Professional Duty of Candour.[19] The GDC states that:

this means that healthcare professionals must:

- Tell the patient (or their carer, if the patient does not have capacity) when something has gone wrong;
- Apologise to the patient;
- Offer an appropriate remedy or support to put matters right (if possible); and
- Explain fully to the patient the long and short-term effects of what has happened.[19]

It is important to appreciate that the Duty of Candour was introduced to increase transparency within the delivery of healthcare and also to increase patient engagement with the treatment process. Many clinicians are very worried about the obligation to apologise to the patient if treatment has not gone to plan, because they are under the impression that this will be taken as an admission of negligence if the patient makes a complaint or claim. However, the purpose of the apology in the Duty of Candour is to show empathy towards the patient about their feelings of disappointment and concern that something has gone wrong with their treatment. The Court will not use a record of an apology from a clinician, on its own, as evidence that he or she has been negligent. Similarly, being candid and apologising to a patient is no defence for providing clinical care that your peers would consider to be substandard.

Responding to a Complaint

Unfortunately, despite one's best efforts to avoid them, it is almost inevitable that, as a clinician, you will receive a complaint from a patient, about the orthodontic treatment that you have provided, during your practising lifetime. However, your risk of receiving a complaint can be significantly reduced by developing a good relationship with your patient and listening to them, so that issues can be discussed as soon as they arise. Nevertheless, it is not unknown for a patient who appeared to have been reassured when they left your surgery to then go home and be encouraged to make a formal complaint by a third party.

The GDC *Standards for the Dental Team*, Standard 5.1.1 states that 'It is part of your responsibility as a dental professional to deal with complaints properly and professionally'.[1] If the patient makes a complaint to the GDC, the manner in which you and your practice have handled the complaint will be examined as part of the GDC's investigation of the complaint. All the indemnifiers in the UK provide advice for their members. It is very worthwhile contacting your indemnifiers for advice as soon as you become aware that a patient is dissatisfied with the orthodontic treatment you have provided.

Circumstances vary but, in general terms, it is probable that if you have received a verbal complaint, you will be advised to arrange a meeting with the patient and their representatives to discuss their concerns. This can be a daunting prospect for the clinician but will demonstrate to the patient that you are taking their concerns seriously and wish to work with them to find a solution. As such, it is important to give sufficient time for the meeting, rather than squeezing in the complainant between other patients. Although you should never compromise your safety, it is also important to consider that a patient may feel intimidated if you are accompanied to the meeting by a third party, for example, your practice manager.

If a verbal meeting is not sufficient to resolve the complaint, then it may be necessary for you to invite the patient to put their concerns in writing. Again, it is extremely important that you seek advice immediately you receive a written complaint. It is also important to comply with GDC Standards[1], i.e. the patient is sent a written acknowledgement of their complaint within the time limits set out in your practice's complaints protocol, together with a copy of the protocol. The latter should also be displayed in the practice where patients can see it.

Some clinicians working in private practice have been tempted to simply give the patient their money back 'as a gesture of goodwill', if the patient has made a complaint about orthodontic treatment which has not gone smoothly. Although this may seem like an effective way to bring the matter to a close, it may be considered that you were not taking the patient's issues seriously and were merely paying them to go away. It is entirely possible that after reviewing your clinical records, your indemnifiers may be of the opinion that the patient has some grounds for a successful complaint or claim and that a refund is recommended to dissuade the patient from taking their complaint further. Your indemnifiers will be able to assist you to write a letter, to accompany the refund, that provides your response to the issues that the patient has raised and explains the reason for the refund. This will reduce your risk of an allegation that you have not responded to the patient's complaint professionally.

Although receiving a complaint from a patient is an extremely unpleasant experience for a clinician, it is worth keeping uppermost in your mind that the proportion of patient complaints that are taken forward by the GDC to a Fitness to Practice (FTP) Panel hearing, for example, is very small (Dental Protection Ltd, personal communication, 2016). If you are unfortunate enough to be referred to a FTP hearing, the GDC panel's main concern is about your current practice and whether you are a risk to patients. If you are able to demonstrate that you have insight into the deficiencies in your practice that have led to the patient complaint and can provide evidence that you have taken steps to remediate these, then this is likely to be considered favourably by the Panel.

The GDC are also concerned about dishonest practice and the impact of this on the reputation of the dental profession. If an allegation of dishonesty is proven against a clinician, this is likely to have consequences for their registration. However, the GDC are realistic that clinical treatment does not always go to plan and patients do not always understand the consequences of their decisions. If, as has been emphasised throughout this chapter, you have documented your discussions with your patient, and also the treatment that you have provided, carefully and **contemporaneously**, then this will demonstrate to the GDC that you have been open and honest about the care you provided even if the patient is dissatisfied.

This is not to say that providing a poor standard of care or a treatment that you do not have the knowledge, skills or experience to undertake is acceptable, even if you have made good clinical notes of what you have done. The patient may still be able to make a successful claim of negligence against you for the treatment that they themselves received, even if the GDC do not consider that your current practice is impaired. It is therefore very important to always work within your clinical competency and to maintain your continuing professional development.

References

1 General Dental Council. Standards for the Dental Team. London: GDC, 2013. Available at www.gdc-uk .org/information-standards-guidance/standards-and-guidance/standards-for-the-dental-team/ (accessed April 2020).

2 Alani A, Kelleher M. Restorative complications of orthodontic treatment. *Br. Dent. J.* 2016;221:389–400.

3 Williams M. *What the Dental Complaints Service has achieved from 2015 to 2018.* https://www.gdc-uk.org/ news-blogs/blog/detail/blogs/2019/09/09/what-the-dental-complaints-service-has-achieved-from-2015-to-2018 (accessed April 2020)

4 Advertising Standards Authority. www.asa.org.uk (accessed April 2020).

5 British Orthodontic Society. *Professional Standards for Orthodontic Practice.* London: BOS, 2014.

6 Dentists Act 1984. Available at https://www.legislation .gov.uk/ukpga/1984/24 (accessed April 2020)

7 Naini FB. A surgeon's perspective on body dysmorphic disorder and recommendations for surgeons and mental health clinicians. In: Phillips KA (ed.). *Body Dysmorphic Disorder: Advances in Research and Clinical Practice.* Oxford: Oxford University Press, 2017.

8 Roberts-Harry D, Sandy J. Orthodontics. Part 2 and Part 3: Patient assessment and examination. *Br. Dent. J.* 2003;195:489–565.

9 British Society of Periodontology. Basic Periodontal Examination (BPE). Available at https://www.bsperio .org.uk/assets/downloads/BSP_BPE_Guidelines_2019 .pdf. (accessed April 2020).

10 Clerehugh V, Kindelan S. Guidelines for Periodontal Screening and Management of Children and Adolescents Under 18 Years of Age. Available at https:// www.bsperio.org.uk/assets/downloads/executive-summary-bsp_bspd-perio-guidelines-for-the-under-18s.pdf (accessed April 2020).

11 The Ionising Radiation Regulations 2017 (IRR17). Available at https://www.legislation.gov.uk/uksi/2017/1075/ contents/made (accessed April 2020).

12 The Ionising Radiation (Medical Exposure) Regulations 2017. Available at https://www.legislation.gov.uk/uksi/ 2017/1322/contents/made (accessed April 2020)

13 Isaacson KG, Thom AR, Atack NE, et al. *Orthodontic Radiographs Guidelines*, 4th edn. London: British Orthodontic Society, 2015.

14 Smale I, Artun J, Behbehan F, et al. Apical root resorption 6 months after initiation of fixed orthodontic appliance therapy. *Am. J. Orthod. Dentofacial Orthop.* 2005;128:57–67.

15 Horner K, Eaton KA. *Selection Criteria for Dental Radiography*, 3rd edn. London: Faculty of General Dental Practice (UK), 2018.

16 British Orthodontic Society. *Orthodontic Records: Collection and Management.* London: BOS, 2015.

17 Data Protection Act 2018. Available at https://www .legislation.gov.uk/ukpga/2018/12/contents/enacted (accessed April 2020)

18 Dental Protection Ltd. Record keeping in England. https://www.dentalprotection.org/uk/articles/record-keeping-in-the-uk (accessed January 2017).

19 General Dental Council. Being open and honest with patients when something goes wrong. https://www.gdc-uk.org/information-standards-guidance/standards-and-guidance/gdc-guidance-for-dental-professionals/the-professional-duty-of-candour (accessed April 2020).

20 Montgomery v Lanarkshire Health Board [2015] UKSC 11.

21 Mental Capacity Act 2005. Available at https://www.legislation.gov.uk/ukpga/2005/9/contents (accessed April 2020)

22 Gillick v West Norfolk and Wisbeach Health Authority [1986] AC 112.

23 Children Act 1989. Available at https://www.legislation.gov.uk/ukpga/1989/41/contents (accessed April 2020)

24 Bolam v Friern Hospital Management Committee [1957] 1 WLR 582.

25 Bolitho v City & Hackney Health Authority [1997] 3 WLR 1151 House of Lords.

26 Caparo Industries plc v Dickman [1990] UKHL 2.

27 Fox N, Richmond S, Wright J, Daniels C. Factors affecting the outcome of orthodontic treatment within the general dental services. *Br. J. Orthod.* 1997;24: 217–221.

28 Lee Y, Lee T. External root resorption during orthodontic treatment in root-filled teeth and contralateral teeth with vital pulp: a clinical study of contributing factors. *Am. J. Orthod. Dentofacial Orthop.* 2016;149:84–91.

29 British Orthodontic Society. *Advice Sheet: Guidelines for the Management of Inhaled or Ingested Foreign Bodies.* London: BOS, 2011.

30 Jauhar P, Machesney M, Sharma P. Ingestion of an orthodontic archwire resulting in a perforated bowel: a case report. *J. Orthod.* 2016;43:237–240.

31 British Orthodontic Society. Moving and transferring during treatment. https://www.bos.org.uk/Information-for-Dentists/Moving-Transferring-During-Treatment (accessed April 2020).

32 British Orthodontic Society. *Advice Sheet: Ethical Management of Patient Compliance.* London: BOS, 2010.

33 General Dental Council. *Scope of Practice*, September 2013. Available at https://www.gdc-uk.org/docs/default-source/scope-of-practice/scope-of-practice.pdf (accessed April 2020).

34 British Orthodontic Society. Guidelines on Supervision of Orthodontic Therapists, April 2017. Available at www.bos.org.uk/Portals/0/Public/docs/General%20Guidance/GuidelinesonSupervisionofOrthodonticTherapistsApril2017.pdf (accessed April 2020).

35 The National Health Service (Dental Charges) Regulations 2005. Available at https://www.legislation.gov.uk/ukdsi/2005/0110736400/contents (accessed April 2020)

36 British Orthodontic Society. Vacuum Formed Retainers. www.bos.org.uk/Professionals-Members/Members-Area-Publications-General-Guidance/Information-and-Advice/General-Guidance/Vacuum-Formed-Retainers (accessed April 2020).

Section II

The Preadjusted Edgewise Appliance

6

Bracket Design

Chris D. Donaldson

CHAPTER OUTLINE

The Origins of Fixed Appliance Bracket Design, 113
  Le Bandeau, 113
  Appareil de Schangé, 114
  Edward Angle and his Appliances, 114
  Begg Appliance, 117
  Tip-Edge Appliance, 117
  Further Appliance Improvements, 117
Preadjusted Edgewise Straight-wire Appliance, 117
  Andrews Straight-wire Appliance, 118
Straight-wire Appliance: Bracket Prescriptions, 121
  Non-customised, 123
  Semi-customised, 127
  Fully Customised, 128
  Optimal Bracket Positioning, 128
Straight-wire Appliance: Bracket Modifications, 129
  Bracket Material, 129
  Slot Dimensions, 132
  Auxiliary Slots, 132
  Bracket Base, 132
  Standard, Auxiliary, Headgear and Lip Bumper Tubes, 133
  Tie-wings, 133
  Archwire Ligation, 134
Acknowledgements, 135
References, 135

The Origins of Fixed Appliance Bracket Design

The earliest records of orthodontic appliances occur in Etruscan, ancient Greek and Roman artefacts. Aulus C. Celsus (c. 25 BC to c. AD 50) in book VII of *De Medicina*,[1] initially inscribed in Latin and largely derived from Greek sources, describes the daily application of finger pressure to move newly erupted, displaced adult teeth. This is the earliest known text describing the intentional effort to apply an orthodontic force.

Le Bandeau

In 1746, Pierre Fauchard (1678–1761), a French physician, described the *Bandeau* as a device designed to align teeth (Figure 6.1).[2] The Bandeau was fixed to teeth using gold threads looped through holes in a flexible curved arch of flat silver or gold ribbon and tied under tension. He described the procedures for the alignment of teeth in chapter VIII of his book entitled *Le Chirurgien Dentiste, ou Traité des Dents*.

Preadjusted Edgewise Fixed Orthodontic Appliances: Principles and Practice, First Edition. Edited by Farhad B. Naini and Daljit S. Gill.
© 2022 John Wiley & Sons Ltd. Published 2022 by John Wiley & Sons Ltd.

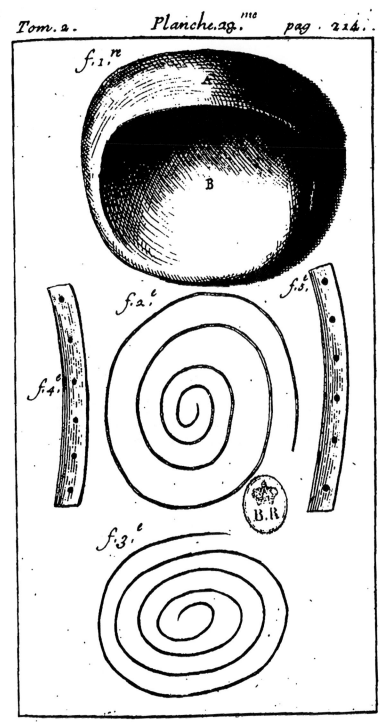

Figure 6.1 Le Bandeau (diminutive of the French word *bande*, which translates as 'small strip') designed by Pierre Fauchard, comprising of a strip of curved metal made into an arch (f.4 and f.5), through which gold thread was threaded (f.2 and f.3). Source: *Le Chiurgien Dentiste, Ou Traité Des Dents*, Vol 2.[2] Reproduced with permission of the Bibliothèque nationale de France.

Appareil de Schangé

In 1841, Jean M. Alexis Schangé, another Frenchman, published his book *Précis sur le Redressement des Dents*[3] in which he introduced a number of additional features to Fauchard's *Bandeau* in his appliance designs: an adjustable metal screw clamp to apply a pushing force to teeth from a similar flexible curved arch of flat metal ribbon as described by Fauchard and encircling metal bands on the molar teeth to secure the appliance and provide anchorage (Figure 6.2).

Edward Angle and his Appliances

Edward H. Angle (1855–1930), described as the father of orthodontics, was an educator and innovator (Figure 6.3).

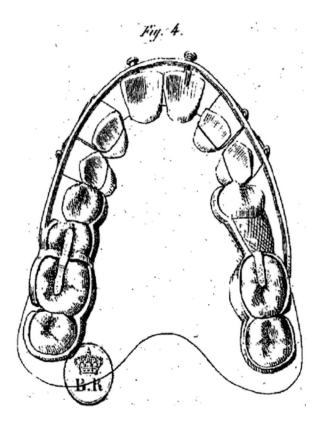

Figure 6.2 Appareil de Schangé. Jean M.A. Schangé used the features of a metal arch and threads from Le Bandeau and introduced a metal clamp screw, seen here on the upper left central incisor, to apply force and molar bands to provide anchorage. Source: *Précis Sur Le Redressement Des Dents*.[3] Reproduced with permission of the Bibliothèque nationale de France.

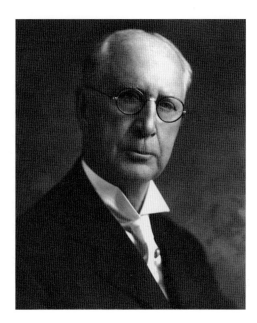

Figure 6.3 Edward H. Angle (1855–1930) known as the father of orthodontics. Source: Angle Society of Orthodontists. Reproduced with permission of Edward H. Angle Society of Orthodontists.

He was born in New York in the United States and trained as a dentist. He later restricted his practice to orthodontics and founded the Angle School of Orthodontia (1900), the American Society of Orthodontics (1901) and the journal *American Orthodontist* (1907). His philosophy for treatment was to use non-extraction treatment and aim for the 'ideal' occlusion that nature had intended, which he observed as having the following common features.[4]

1. 'The mesio-buccal cusp of the upper first molar is received in the buccal groove of the lower first molar.' He regarded the first permanent molar relationship as the 'Key to Occlusion'; as he notes, the first molars are the largest teeth and the first of the adult dentition to erupt and establish their occlusion. In support of this principle, Angle remarked that the occlusion of the primary dentition prior was 'almost always normal'.
2. The teeth of the arches are aligned along an ideal arch form which he termed 'the line of occlusion' and defined as 'the line with which, in form and position according to type, the teeth mush be in harmony if in normal occlusion'; the lower arch is slightly narrower than the upper.
3. The cusps of the upper and lower dentition should interlock, with the cusps of one arch fitting into the interspaces of two teeth of the opposing arch (except for the incisors and distobuccal cusp of the upper third molars).
4. The labial and buccal surfaces of the teeth of the upper jaw slightly overhang the lower teeth and the upper incisors overlap the lower by a third of their crown height.

This definition led to Angle's development of designs of increasing complexity that aimed to establish this ideal occlusion, aided by expansion of the arches. In seventh edition of his book *Treatment of Malocclusion of the Teeth: Angle's System* published in 1907,[4] Dr Angle acknowledged the use of a curved metal arch by Pierre Fauchard, the adjustable metal screw clamp and metal bands of Jean M.A. Schangé, and also the work of Dr Magill who had recently started to cement bands using zinc oxychloride.

E-Arch Appliance

Angle describes advancing the features of previous designs by adding horizontal welded metal tubes to the buccal surfaces of cemented molar bands and switching from using gold and platinum to using nickel silver, which had recently been introduced and could be formed from strips on reels to form bands at the chairside (Figure 6.4). The curved flat ribbons of silver or gold in the devices of Fauchard and Schangé were replaced with three sizes

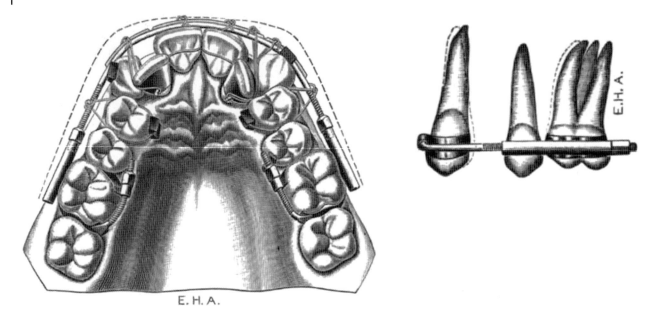

Figure 6.4 Angle's E-Arch appliance. Developing on the features of the Appareil de Schangé, Angle introduced welded metal tubes on adjustable clamp bands which anchored a round, flexible, ribbed and notched arch of metal with 'sheath-hooks' which could be slid on and soldered, and from which intermaxillary or intramaxillary elastic traction could be applied. Teeth were ligated to the expansion arches with brass wire ligatures. The use of lengths of nickel silver ribbon to construct bands meant bands for all teeth could be formed at the chairside. Traction-screws and jack-screws, secured by friction nuts, moved teeth and could expand or contract the arch forms. Source: *Treatment of Malocclusion of the Teeth: Angle's System.*[4] Reproduced with permission of Edward H. Angle Society of Orthodontists.

of notched and ribbed round gold metal arch and three diameters of braided soft brass wire used as metal ligatures, which ligated teeth to the metal arches (tightened by twisting).

This metal arch flexed when the ligatures were tied to apply traction to the teeth and when expanded developed the arch form laterally, giving the name *E-Arch* (*Expansion-Arch*).[4, 5] Angle also developed and integrated the traction-screw to apply a pulling force to teeth, the jack-screw to apply a pushing force, and 'sheath hooks' fed onto and soldered on the upper or lower metal arches, from which to apply rubber ligatures, to provide inter- and intra-arch traction or anchorage. In addition to the lateral expansion provided by activating the metal arch, jack-screws mesial to the molar tubes could also be activated to expand the arch in an anteroposterior direction. This proclined the incisors, providing further space for crowded dentitions to align.

Pin and Tube Appliance

Modifications were made by Angle to the E-Arch appliance to create the *pin and tube appliance*.[6] The diameter of the expansion arch in cross-section was reduced to 0.030 inches to increase flexibility and metal pins were soldered to it by the orthodontist and repositioned at appointments to move teeth. These pins once soldered were slotted into vertically oriented tubes soldered onto bands placed on the buccal surfaces of the premolars, canines and incisors. The tubes were to be sited at the centre of the labial surfaces of the crowns and were termed 'brackets' by Angle. These soldered archwire pins introduced root torque to appliances but meant that a high degree of operator skill was needed, and because the expansion arch was relatively inflexible frequent adjustments of the pins were necessary.

Ribbon Arch Appliance

In order to overcome these issues, Angle moved from a round to a rectangular *ribbon arch* and for this to be engaged, a generic vertical slot facing occlusally was added to the vertical tubes on the bands.[7–9] The molars were still banded and had horizontally positioned tubes buccally. The 0.022 × 0.036-inch rectangular gold archwire was smaller in dimension than that of the pin and tube appliance and therefore more flexible. It was fixed in place by a 'lock pin' placed into the vertical tube. This design reduced the operator skill required and reduced the frequency of adjustments needed. However, as the archwire was more flexible it reduced torquing ability. As control of the positioning of teeth in three dimensions increased through wire bending, so did the required operator skills.

Angle's Edgewise Appliance

To increase the torquing ability of the ribbon arch appliance, Angle made the decision to reorient the vertical slot on the band to a horizontal slot and remove the vertical tube.[10, 11] The narrow edge of the rectangular wire therefore moved from incisal to buccal to match the slot, rotating it by 90°. This horizontal slot (now 0.022 × 0.028-inch) of the bracket brazed to the band was flanked gingivally and occlusally by single overhanging wings. A round wire of 0.022-inch or a rectangular wire of 0.022 × 0.028-inch was inserted 'edgewise' as opposed to the 'flatwise' insertion of the ribbon arch appliance wire and this improved torque control. However, as the brackets were narrow mesiodistally, rotational control was poor; in order to overcome this, precious metal staples were soldered to the band mesially and distally of the bracket. When used to augment ligation of the wire into the bracket, this increased rotational control.

Begg Appliance

Percival Raymond Begg (1898–1983), an Australian who trained at the Angle School of Orthodontia, attempted to treat patients in Australia with Angle's philosophies using the ribbon arch appliance. However, Dr Begg found by using a non-extraction approach that his patients experienced an unsatisfactory degree of relapse from expansion of the arches laterally and anteroposteriorly, although Angle had advocated retention. He found that with the control of root torque from the ribbon arch appliance, he was able to control space closure after extracting teeth to resolve crowding.

He transitioned from using rectangular gold archwires to using round 0.016-inch heat-treated stainless steel and bands made from stainless steel rather than nickel silver. He also moved the direction of the vertical slot on the ribbon arch appliance from occlusally to gingivally facing. The archwires were held in place in the vertical bracket slots, which were identical for each tooth, by brass 'Begg pins' pushed into adjacent vertical tubes. As the archwire was now round, torque was applied by placing auxiliary (torquing) springs into the vertical tubes in the torquing phase. Tip was also corrected with the use of auxiliary (uprighting) springs. The appliance became known as the *Begg appliance*[12, 13] and became very popular due to its efficiency of moving teeth through free tipping and torquing movements, although achieving precision was difficult.

Tip-Edge Appliance

Co-author of the second edition of *Orthodontic Theory and Technique* with Dr Begg was Peter C. Kesling,[14, 15] who brought together design features from Angle's edgewise appliance and an earlier modification made by A. Sved[16] to create the *Tip-Edge appliance*. A sequence of round and rectangular wires is used in a modified single wing edgewise bracket, with a horizontal slot cut away mesially and distally to allow free mesiodistal tipping in smaller round wires. Once free tipping is complete, larger rectangular wires are used to upright teeth and express torque.

Further Appliance Improvements

Angle's edgewise, Begg and Tip-Edge appliances were all designed with brackets that were narrow mesiodistally and therefore were not inherently effective at rotational control, especially when closing space at extraction sites. Angle had originally used precious metal staples soldered to the band mesially and distally to the bracket to improve rotational control to help overcome this. Dr Lewis improved on this modification by developing *Lewis brackets* with 'rotation arms' that were extensions of the bracket mesially and distally, curving out to touch the wire; they acted as lever arms increasing rotational control.[17] Dr Lang subsequently modified Lewis's bracket by flattening the curved rotation arms as the curved arms tended to flatten the archwire, and these became known as *Lang brackets*.

The origins of the *Siamese* or twin bracket was a further development by Dr Brainerd Swain[18] that aimed to improve rotational control. Orthodontists had started to use two aligned single-wing brackets on the same tooth adjacent to extraction spaces in order to protect against unwanted rotations when closing space. Swain simply placed these two single-wing brackets on a single base, creating the twin-wing bracket. He termed it the 'Siamese' bracket after the conjoined twins of Siam.

Preadjusted Edgewise Straight-wire Appliance

A key development of the modern straight-wire appliance was the shift from using wire bending to deliver the majority of adjustments required during treatment to the manufacture of preadjusted brackets. This shift came from orthodontists looking to simplify treatment chairside by reducing the need for wire bending and to improve precision of tooth control.

In an important observation, in 1952 Reed A. Holdaway[19] noted that practitioners had been 'artistically positioning' brackets on the upper lateral teeth at an angle in order to avoid the need for bends in the wire. He therefore suggested that this angulation could be built into bracket design to obviate the need for the artistic bracket positioning. Observations such as this drove the shift to the preadjusted appliance concept. Dr Ivan Lee and Dr Joseph Jarabak highlighted the benefits of building torque into the edgewise bracket.

Andrews Straight-wire Appliance

In 1989, Lawrence F. Andrews published *Straight Wire: The Concept and Appliance*.[20] In this book, a culmination of 14 research projects, Dr Andrews presents justification for the *Six Keys to Optimal Occlusion*, optimal arch lines and the design of the straight-wire concept, based on the analysis of study casts of 120 naturally optimal occlusions.

An important definition by Andrews was made to help define the angulations and inclinations of individual teeth. He defined the *Andrews plane* as 'the plane on which the mid-transverse plane of every crown will fall when the teeth are optimally positioned'. He used it as a reference plane from which the angulations and inclinations of individual teeth could be assessed; these were established

by determining the relation of the crown to a 90° angle from Andrews plane (see Figures 6.5 and 6.8).

Angle's definition of an ideal static occlusion lacked key elements. For example, if there were spaces, rotations or the occlusal planes were not level, the ideal occlusion Angle referred to was not achieved. In defining the Six Keys to Optimal Occlusion,[20] Andrews refined and added to existing definitions and in doing so redefined the descriptive elements of ideal occlusion. He described existing definitions as 'individually inadequate and collectively incomplete'. The Six Keys, made from observations on the 120 naturally optimal occlusions, are as follows.

- **Key I: Inter-arch relationships**. A slight modification from Angle's definition of a Class I molar relationship: 'the mesio-buccal cusp of the permanent maxillary first molar occludes in the groove between the mesial and middle buccal cusps of the permanent mandibular first molar'.
- **Key II: Crown angulation**. The crown angulation of maxillary and mandibular teeth, relative to the Andrews plane, followed a pattern and is positive, whereby the occlusal portion of the facial axis of the clinical crown lies mesial to the gingival portion.
- **Key III: Crown inclination**. Maxillary and mandibular crown inclinations, relative to Andrews plane, like angulation also followed a pattern, whereby the occlusal portion of the labial surface of the crown lies lingual to the gingival half except for the upper incisors.
- **Key IV: Rotations**. The contact points of adjacent teeth are aligned; there are therefore no rotations.

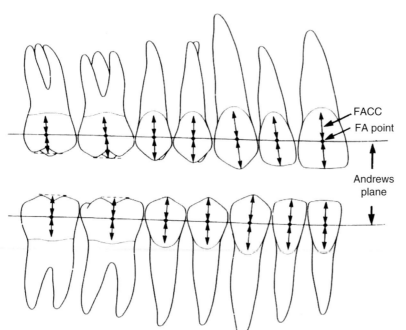

FACC
FA point
Andrews plane

Figure 6.5 Andrews defined the facial axis (FA) point as the target for bracket or tube placement; this was located halfway between the incisal edge, cusp tip or line between cusp tips and the gingival margin, along the facial axis of the clinical crown (FACC), a line following the most prominent part on the facial surface of a tooth (through the buccal groove of molars). In an optimal occlusion, all FA points of the teeth of each arch lie in order on the Andrews plane. Angulation and inclination of the teeth in relation to each other are established with the Andrews plane as a reference. Source: Andrews L. Straight Wire: The Concept and Appliance. San Diego, CA: LA Wells, 1989. Reproduced with permission of L.A. Andrews and © L.A. Andrews.

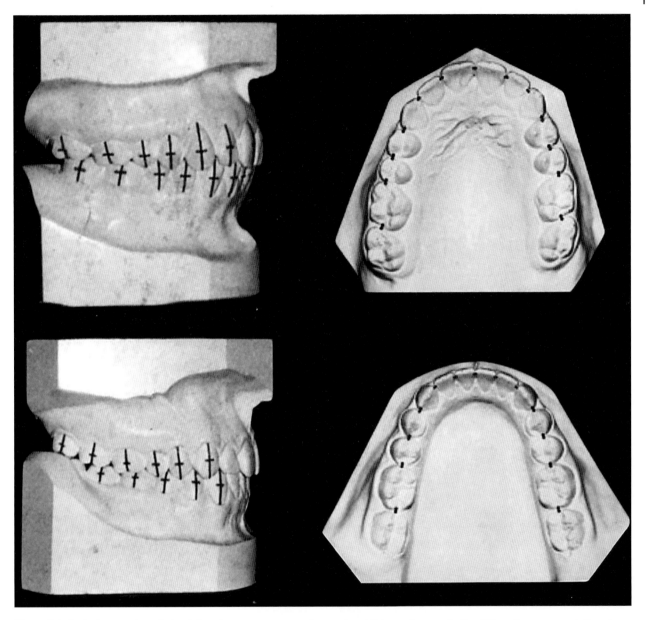

Figure 6.6 Dr Andrews acknowledged that there was a range of normal and this can be seen in the different crown angulations in these casts, both of which have an optimal occlusion. The FACC and the FA point are drawn on the teeth. He also noted that among optimal occlusions the contact points were all approximated and aligned. Source: Andrews L. *Straight Wire: The Concept and Appliance.* San Diego, CA: LA Wells, 1989. Reproduced with permission of L.A. Andrews and © L.A. Andrews.

- **Key V: Tight contacts**. The contact points of adjacent teeth are approximated, except when there is a tooth size discrepancy.
- **Key VI: Curve of Spee**. The occlusal plane is flat or slightly concave (it should be no greater than 2.5 mm in depth).

Andrews made the observation that ideal tooth positions could be established by assessing ideal occlusions and, similarly, ideal tooth positions were associated with ideal occlusions (Figure 6.6). Therefore, the 120 naturally optimal occlusions were analysed for crown angulation, crown inclination and relative facial prominence (Box 6.0). In addition, observation was made that the contact points were vertically and horizontally aligned and approximated in optimal occlusions. Measurements were also made to ensure that brackets designed would fit teeth they were placed on and therefore average measurements were collected on maxillary molar offset, facial crown height and width (to establish maximum bracket dimensions) and vertical and horizontal crown contour (to establish bracket base contour) (Figure 6.7).

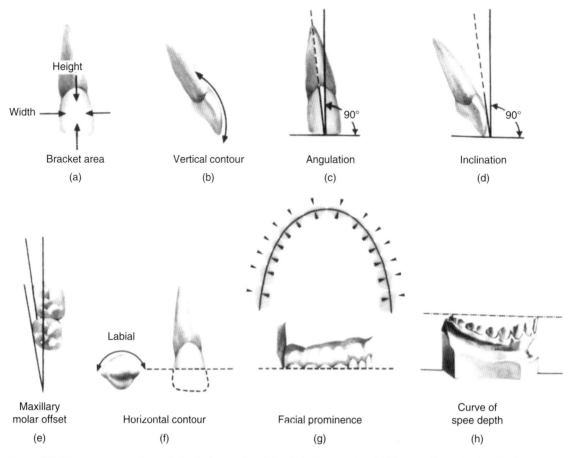

Figure 6.7 The measurements made by Andrews of each tooth in the sample of 120 naturally optimal occlusions was used to create an average prescription for each tooth. Source: Andrews L. *Straight Wire: The Concept and Appliance*. San Diego, CA: LA Wells, 1989. Reproduced with permission of L.A. Andrews and © L.A. Andrews.

Box 6.1

The collection of 120 non-orthodontic naturally optimal study casts began in 1960 and this was achieved by 1964; it is referred to as the 1960 dataset. The collection then evolved as Dr Andrews replaced the less ideal casts in the collection with those better demonstrating optimal occlusion. Measurements were taken again in 1988 from each cast included in the collection at that time; known as the 1988 dataset, these are published in the Appendix of the book *Straight Wire: The Concept and Appliance*.[20]

Andrews acknowledged that when using the straight-wire appliance, for treatment to be effective in achieving an optimal occlusion (i) teeth should have a normal shape and (ii) the jaws should be normally related. Andrews suggests that for those with a malocclusion and normal jaw relations, treatment for 10% will not be as efficient, as they will still need a significant amount of custom wire bending; these 10% represent those with 'abnormal' teeth. Those with abnormal jaw relations require treatment alongside a surgeon and those with abnormal teeth a general dentist to correct the occlusion.

Andrews introduced the following definitions as part of the straight-wire concept and also to aid bracket positioning, where precision was now more important.

- *Facial axis of the clinical crown (FACC)*: Andrews moved from using the traditional long axis of the tooth (which needed radiographs and was difficult to assess) to the more clinically relevant and easily assessed FACC to place brackets (see Figures 6.5 and 6.6). The FACC is defined as 'the most prominent portion of the central lobe on each crown's facial surface; for molars, the buccal groove that separates the two large facial cusps'. A straight line can be drawn down the most prominent part of each tooth from the incisal edge or cusp tip representing the FACC and for the molar teeth, drawn through the buccal groove.
- *Facial axis (FA) point*: a point that lies on the intersection of two lines (see Figures 6.5 and 6.6): (i) a line halfway between the gingival margin and the incisal edge, cusp tip or a line drawn connecting cusp tips in molar teeth (in late mixed dentition) and (ii) the FACC.

A 'prescription' built into the geometry of the bracket slot and customised for the bracket of each tooth was derived from the average values from Andrews' landmark study of 120 normal occlusions (Figure 6.8). This meant that the previously necessary wire bends were eliminated or greatly simplified. The prescription was essentially made up of five elements, which were controlled by the bracket geometry and by placing the bracket on the FA point.

1. Tip (angulation), which had been corrected with second-order bends, was now built into the mesiodistal angulation of the bracket slot.
2. Inclination (torque), which had been achieved through third-order bends, was achieved by customising the buccolingual angulation of the slot walls relative to the bracket base.
3. Mesiodistal contact point alignment (offset), which had been achieved using first-order bends, was now corrected by using an archwire using an Andrews arch form and differentially modifying the bracket base thickness mesiodistally.
4. Vertical contact point alignment (height) was now achieved by placing the bracket on the FA point.
5. Facial prominence (in–out), which had also been corrected with first-order bends, was built into the thickness between the bracket base and slot.

In addition to defining the Six Keys to occlusion, collecting averaged data on ideal tooth positions and building these into the bracket slot, a number of improvements to bracket design were introduced by Andrews.[22] These included eight slot-siting features designed to aid correct positioning of the bracket slot, such as 'compound curvature' whereby the bracket base is contoured vertically and horizontally; previously, bracket bases had been contoured horizontally but not vertically. Torque was built into the base of the bracket rather than in the base of the slot, which enabled all the slots to be aligned once the teeth had been aligned and torqued, thus allowing 'straight-wire' sliding mechanics for space closure and removing the need for loop mechanics to close spaces. Building torque into the base also enabled the FA point, bracket base point and bracket slot point to align on the slot axis. The slot point therefore acted as a visual reference representing the FA point, which was obscured by the bracket once sited.

Alongside slot-siting features, convenience features and auxiliary features were built into the Andrews straight-wire appliance. Convenience features were designed to increase patient comfort, such as asymmetric tie-wings that were set in occlusally, reducing the chance of interference with the opposing occlusion and set out gingivally to avoid gingival impingement. The facial surfaces of the tie-wings were curved, matching the curved base of the bracket to increase lip comfort. Convenience features included not only those that increased patient comfort but also those that made the appliance more convenient for the orthodontist, such as bracket marking to help identification and orientation, for example the distogingival tie-wing had a dot, dash or groove. Auxiliary features are non-slot-sitting features that aid mechanics and include facebow (headgear) tubes, utility tubes, bracket hooks and power arms.

Despite significant advances in design that benefited orthodontists and patients, a number of issues were commonly encountered.

- *Wagon wheel effect*: the effect of expressing torque to the upper and lower incisors from the curved archwire was to unavoidably introduce tip.
- *Rollercoaster effect*: when closing premolar extraction spaces with heavy power chain on 0.018-inch stainless steel archwires, the rollercoaster effect was encountered. The archwires were not strong enough to resist the teeth adjacent to the extraction spaces tipping into the space and this led to lateral open bites posteriorly and an increased overbite anteriorly.

The Andrews straight-wire appliance was the first 'fully programmed' appliance, with a preprogrammed prescription for tip, torque, offset and in–out values built into the bracket design. Appliances with any incomplete combination of tip, torque, offset and in–out are termed 'partly programmed'. Angle's edgewise appliance is in essence 'non-programmed'.

Bracket design has been central to the development of fixed appliances. Alongside bracket design development, it is important to acknowledge the work in defining optimal occlusion by Angle and Andrews. In doing so, this allowed significant advances in design which led to the current widespread adoption of the straight-wire appliance concept, of which there are now numerous prescriptions and design modifications.

Straight-wire Appliance: Bracket Prescriptions

Of all the features of straight-wire appliances, slot prescription has received considerable attention and modification since the non-programmed slot was introduced by Angle. There is seemingly a myriad of prescriptions available from manufacturers, many associated with individual author's philosophies and recommended mechanics. Bracket prescriptions can be defined as non-customised, semi-customised or fully customised.

Values for tip, torque and offset for a number of these prescriptions are shown Tables 6.1, 6.2 and 6.3 and recommended arch forms in Table 6.4.

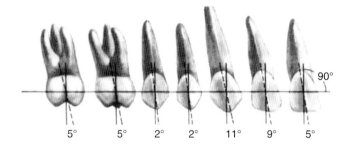

5°   5°   2°   2°   11°   9°   5°   90°

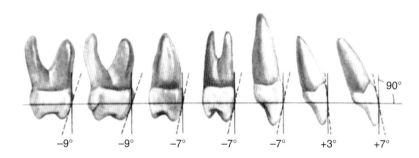

−9°   −9°   −7°   −7°   −7°   +3°   +7°   90°

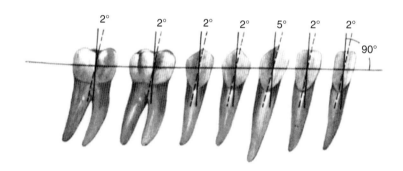

2°   2°   2°   2°   5°   2°   2°   90°

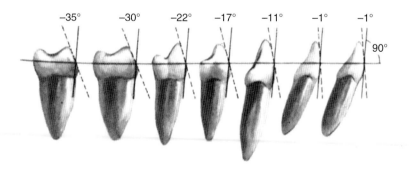

−35°   −30°   −22°   −17°   −11°   −1°   −1°   90°

Figure 6.8 The average values for angulation (tip) and inclination (torque) of the maxillary and mandibular teeth used in Andrews' prescription. (*Top to bottom*) Average maxillary crown angulations, average maxillary crown inclinations, average mandibular crown angulations, and average mandibular crown inclinations. Source: Andrews L. *Straight Wire: The Concept and Appliance*. San Diego, CA: LA Wells, 1989. Reproduced with permission of L.A. Andrews and © L.A. Andrews.

Table 6.1 Average angulation values for Andrews' 120 naturally optimal occlusions from the 1960 dataset and the positive (mesial) and negative (distal) crown tip values for the bracket prescriptions.

		Angle's Edgewise[10,11]	Andrews 120[20]	Andrews Set 'S'[20]	Andrews2	Roth[24]	Alexander Vari-simplex[25]	Ricketts' Bioprogressive[26]	MBT Versatile+[27]	Damon Q2
Maxillary	Central incisor	0	+5	+5	+4	+5	+5	0	+4	+5
	Lateral incisor	0	+9	+9	+8	+9	+8	+8	+8	+9
	Canine	0	+11	+11	+8	+13	+10	+5	+8	+5
	First premolar	0	+2	+2	+2	0	0	0	0	+2
	Second premolar	0	+2	+2	+2	0	0	0	0	+2
	First molar	0	+5	+5	+5	0	0	0	0	—
	Second molar	0	+5	+5	+5	0	0	0	0	—
Mandibular	Central incisor	0	+2	+2	+1.5	+2	+2	0	0	+2
	Lateral incisor	0	+2	+2	+1.5	+2	+3	0	0	+4
	Canine	0	+5	+5	+3	+7	+6	+5	+3	+5
	First premolar	0	+2	+2	+2	−1	0	0	+2	+4
	Second premolar	0	+2	+2	+2	−1	0	0	+2	+4
	First molar	0	+2	+2	+2	−1	−6	0	0	—
	Second molar	0	+2	+2	+2	−1	0	0	0	—

Non-customised

Andrews' Prescription

Andrews' standard prescription for non-extraction cases using the straight-wire appliance was derived from the 120 naturally optimal occlusions in the 1960 dataset and identified as 'Set S' (standard) brackets. A separate set of brackets were made for extraction cases (E1–3), which had anti-tip and anti-rotation features for teeth adjacent to premolar extraction sites. This was to counteract the unwanted tip and rotation associated with bodily movement (translation) when closing spaces in extraction cases; 2–4° of additional tip was built into the brackets along with a power arm projecting gingivally to prevent unwanted tip, whilst 2–6° of rotation was built into the brackets to prevent unwanted rotation.[22]

Incisor brackets for Class I cases were served by Set S brackets that had a normal torque prescription, whilst Class II and Class III tendencies were assigned Set A and Set C brackets, respectively, aiding camouflage of the incisor relationships using modified torque prescriptions.

Andrews also identified the need for an adjusted prescription for cases finishing with a Class II molar relationship by removing tip and molar offset in the Class II molar bracket and therefore improving the occlusal fit (the 'E4' bracket).

A number of issues with the original Andrews' prescription were noted: (i) practitioners needed to amass a large inventory of brackets and for some this led to stock control difficulties; (ii) the posterior molars tended to drift mesially due to anchorage loss; and (iii) it was found that incisor torque was not always delivered as expected.

Dr Lawrence F. Andrews and his son Dr William A. Andrews have since modified elements of bracket design and made changes to the prescription to create the Andrews2 Appliance.

Roth Prescription

The Roth prescription was developed by Dr Ronald H. Roth who was an early adopter of the Andrews straight-wire appliance in his clinical practice. In his experience of using Andrews' appliance, he aimed to 'overcome the inherent error built in' whilst applying his own orthodontic philosophies centred on gnathological concepts.[23,24]

He formed a set of treatment principles from these aims as follows: (i) overcorrection, in anticipation of a degree of relapse and settling of the alignment and occlusion after debond; (ii) achieving not only an optimal Andrews' Six Keys static occlusion, but also an optimal functional occlusion, i.e. a mutually protected occlusion and elimination of any occlusal interferences on protrusion and lateral excursion; and (iii) ensuring the condyles are in optimal positions in occlusion, in centric relation, which Stuart defined as 'the rearmost, uppermost and midmost relationship' of the condyles in the glenoid fossae. The achievement of these principles using the Roth prescription was termed the 'end of appliance therapy goal'.

Roth assessed many of his cases at the end of treatment using panoramic tomograms and by mounting casts on the Stuart articulator and found that Andrews' Six Keys to Optimal Occlusion appeared to be concordant with the treatment principles he had set out. Roth therefore concluded that achieving optimal static occlusion

Table 6.2 Average inclination values for Andrews' 120 naturally optimal occlusions from the 1960 dataset and the positive (palatal) and negative (buccal) root torque values for the bracket prescriptions.

		Angle's Edgewise [10, 11]	Andrews 120 [20]	Andrews Set 'S' [20]	Andrews Set 'A' and Set 'C' [22]	Andrews2	Roth [24]	Alexander Vari-simplex [25]	Ricketts' Bioprogressive [26]	MBT Versatile+ [27]	Damon Q2, standard torque	Damon Q2, High ▲, Std/Low ▽, Low ▼
Maxillary	Central incisor	0	+7	+7	+2 (A) +12 (C)	+7	+12	+14	+22	+17	+12	+22 ▲ +2 ▼
	Lateral incisor	0	+3	+3	−2 (A) +8 (C)	+4	+8	+7	+14	+10	+8	+13 ▲ −5 ▼
	Canine	0	−7	−7		−7	−2	−3	+7	+7 / 0 / −7	+7	+11 ▲ −9 ▼
	First premolar	0	−7	−7		−7	−7	−7	0	−7	−11	
	Second premolar	0	−7	−7		−7	−7	−7	0	−7	−11	
	First molar	0	−9	−9		−10	−14	−10	0	−14	—	
	Second molar	0	−9	−9		−10	−14	−10	0	−14	—	
Mandibular	Central incisor	0	−1	−1	+4 (A) −6 (C)	−6	−1	−5	0	−6	−3	−6 ▽ −11 ▼
	Lateral incisor	0	−1	−1	+4 (A) −6 (C)	−6	−1	−5	0	−6	−3	−6 ▽ −11 ▼
	Canine	0	−11	−11		−11	−11	−7	+7	+6 / 0 / −6	+7	+13 ▲ 0 ▼
	First premolar	0	−17	−17		−17	−17	−11	0	−12	−12	−5 ▲
	Second premolar	0	−22	−22		−22	−22	−17	0	−17	−17	
	First molar	0	−30	−30		−30	−30	−22	0	−20	—	
	Second molar	0	−35	−35		−35	−30	0 or −27	0	−10	—	

was harmonious with optimal functional occlusion and optimal condyle positioning.

Roth also felt the need for a reduced, simplified inventory of brackets, so the *Roth prescription* consisted of a single set of modified Andrews' prescription brackets. To aid over-correction, Roth advocated for the anterior brackets to be placed 'slightly more incisally' to the FA point in order to help level the arches and for a Tru-Arch form to be used, which is widest at the mesiobuccal cusp of the first molars.

Upper incisor torque prescriptions were increased to compensate for the brackets being placed more incisally, the torque being the same as Andrews' Set C brackets. Anti-tip and anti-rotation were built into the buccal brackets as standard, as extraction treatment was common at that time. Super-torque upper incisor brackets were

available, acknowledging the expected high demands on delivering incisor torque for Class II/2 patients.

Roth had also noted posterior anchorage issues in both arches with the Andrews' prescription which he felt led to mesial drift due to the prescribed mesial tip. He therefore removed the mesial tip of the upper and lower premolars and molars.

Alexander Vari-simplex Prescription

Dr R.G. 'Wick' Alexander introduced the Alexander Discipline, which comprises an appliance that uses a variety of different bracket types programmed with the Alexander Vari-simplex prescription, alongside a set of 20 published treatment principles.[25] The term 'vari-simplex' refers to two key elements: bracket variety and the principle of keeping treatment simple. *Lang brackets* are used on the

Table 6.3 Average mesiodistal rotation values for Andrews' 120 naturally optimal occlusions from the 1960 dataset and the distal (positive) and mesial (negative) offset values for the bracket prescriptions.

		Angle's Edgewise[10, 11]	Andrews 120[20]	Andrews Set 'S'[20]	Andrews2	Roth[24]	Alexander Vari-simplex[25]	Ricketts' Bioprogressive[26]	MBT Versatile+[27]	Damon Q2
Maxillary	Central incisor	0	—	0	0	0	0	0	0	0
	Lateral incisor	0	—	0	0	0	0	0	0	0
	Canine	0	—	0	0	−2	0	0	0	0
	First premolar	0	—	0	0	−2	0	0	0	0
	Second premolar	0	—	0	0	−2	0	0	0	0
	First molar	0	+10	+10	+10	+14	+15	0	+10	—
	Second molar	0	+10	+10	+10	+14	–	0	+10	—
Mandibular	Central incisor	0	—	0	0	0	0	0	0	0
	Lateral incisor	0	—	0	0	0	0	0	0	0
	Canine	0	—	0	0	+2	0	0	0	0
	First premolar	0	—	0	0	+4	0	0	0	0
	Second premolar	0	—	0	0	+4	0	0	0	0
	First molar	0	—	0	0	+4	+5	0	0	—
	Second molar	0	—	0	0	+4	+6	0	0	—

Table 6.4 Straight-wire appliance arch forms for the bracket prescriptions.

Bracket prescription	Arch form
Andrews	Andrews
Roth	Tru-Arch
Alexander Vari-simplex	Vari-simplex arches
Ricketts' Bioprogressive	Pentamorphic arches
MBT Versatile+	Tapered, ovoid or square
Damon	Damon

canines, *Lewis brackets* on the premolars and lower incisors and twin-wing brackets on the upper incisors, using an 0.018-inch slot.

Alexander was influenced by the philosophies of Dr Charles Tweed, who had felt that for stability it was important to keep the lower incisors over basal bone, at an angle of 90 ± 5° from the mandibular plane (i.e. incisor mandibular plane angle or IMPA), and for the intercanine distance not to be significantly altered.

The benefit of using single-wing Lewis brackets on the premolars and lower incisors is in achieving greater rotational control through their unique rotation wings. A −6° tip was used in the lower first molar prescription, as this was felt to increase the arch length. This, combined with the negative root torque in the lower incisors designed to counter proclination when levelling the arch, constitute significant elements in the prescription.

The treatment principles include the following recommendations: (i) brackets are not placed routinely on the FA point and are instead placed at prescribed distances from incisal edges or cusp tips; (ii) placing anterior maxillary incisor brackets 0.5 mm more incisal and maxillary posterior brackets 0.5 mm more gingivally to help correct low angle cases; (iii) avoiding extractions where possible; (iv) aiming to consolidate arches early in treatment and using orthopaedic correction if the patient is growing, using headgear, facemasks and inter-arch elastics where this is appropriate; (v) applying torque early in the lower arch; and (vi) using 'driftodontics' where possible in extraction cases. The Vari-simplex arch forms were developed to be used with the Alexander Discipline; the mandibular arch form is available in two different forms.

The Vari-simplex bracket system was introduced in 1978 and has since been developed into the Mini-Wick and Long Term Stability (LTS) systems.

Ricketts' Bioprogressive Prescription

Dr Robert M. Ricketts developed a set of treatment principles along with Drs Bench, Gugino, Hilger and Schulhof which became the Bioprogressive Philosophy and which were published in 1979 in the book entitled *Bioprogressive Therapy*.[26] A key element was the use of the visualised treatment objective (VTO), a cephalometric tracing technique to plan treatment by predicting growth and forecasting the effects of treatment mechanics.

In addition to the VTO, a number of mechanical concepts were put forward. In treating patients with existing preadjusted appliances unwanted anchorage loss in extraction cases had been noted, and this was attributed to excessive use of force leading to hyalinisation of bone. Controlled light forces were therefore recommended, facilitated by (i) the use of 'root ratings' indicating approximate forces required for each tooth movement; (ii) using an 0.018-inch slot rather than a 0.022-inch slot; and (iii) sectional (segmental) archwires, for example, for retracting canines and intruding incisors. It was also recommended that the occlusion should be unlocked progressively and in a biologically logical way, for example reducing the overbite before the overjet.

Anchorage control was augmented with the use of lip bumpers and by moving the roots of the mandibular teeth into the dense buccal cortical bone of the external oblique ridge. Five arch forms were developed – the pentamorphic arches, for use with Ricketts' Bioprogressive prescription – and overtreatment of cases was recommended in anticipation of some degree of relapse. Ricketts' Bioprogressive prescription was developed to help deliver these aims.

Ricketts' Bioprogressive prescription is perhaps the simplest of the preadjusted prescriptions and of the few prescribed values the upper and lower canine torque of +7°, designed to maintain the canine root in trabecular bone, is of note. Initially, the advocated progressive lower molar buccal root torque, to move roots into cortical bone, was bent into the wire; this was later added to the prescription.

MBT Versatile+ Prescription

Dr Richard McLaughlin, Dr John Bennett and Dr Hugo Trevisi (MBT) developed the MBT Versatile+ Appliance System, which comprises of a series of brackets that employ the MBT Versatile+ prescription using a 0.022-inch slot and a set of archwires, along with a set of recommended treatment mechanics. The authors felt that a number of commonly encountered issues with the straight-wire appliance could be overcome. A textbook was published illustrating recommended treatment mechanics entitled *Systemized Orthodontic Treatment Mechanics*.[27]

It had been noted that the preadjusted appliance did not consistently deliver the torque that was prescribed in the bracket,[28] and therefore palatal root torque was added to the upper incisors and labial root torque was increased for the lower incisors. Labial root torque was added to the lower incisors to help avoid excessive proclination when levelling the lower arch. It had also been observed that the lower cuspids and bicuspids were prone to gingival recession using Andrews' prescription, so buccal root torque was reduced. To avoid occlusal interferences from hanging palatal cusps, upper molar buccal root torque was increased.

Versatility is a key element of the MBT Versatile+ prescription in that (i) three canine torque prescriptions are available to use with three recommended arch forms (tapered, ovoid and square); (ii) the lower second molar tubes can be used on the contralateral upper first and

Table 6.5 Recommended vertical bracket positions for MBT Versatile+ prescription.[27] Examples are given for average size teeth, measured from the incisal edge, cusp tip or line between cusp tips.

		MBT Versatile+, non-extraction	MBT Versatile+, premolar extraction
Maxillary	Central incisor	5.0 mm	5.0 mm
	Lateral incisor	4.5 mm	4.5 mm
	Canine	5.0 mm	5.0 mm
	First premolar	4.5 mm	4.5 mm
	Second premolar	4.0 mm	
	First molar	3.0 mm	3.5 mm
	Second molar	2.0 mm	2.0 mm
Mandibular	Central incisor	4.0 mm	4.0 mm
	Lateral incisor	4.0 mm	4.0 mm
	Canine	4.5 mm	4.5 mm
	First premolar	4.0 mm	4.0 mm
	Second premolar	3.5 mm	
	First molar	2.5 mm	3.0 mm
	Second molar	2.5 mm	2.5 mm

second molars in cases finishing to a Class II molar relationship; (iii) the upper lateral bracket may be inverted when the crown is palatally positioned to increase buccal root torque; and (iv) two second premolar brackets are available with different in–out values to accommodate small second premolars.

The rollercoaster effect when using 0.018-inch stainless steel wires and heavy power chain had been commonly encountered, leading to lateral open bites. Therefore, extraction site space closure using light elastic forces on 0.019 × 0.025-inch hooked stainless steel wires en masse is recommended, whilst managing anchorage demands appropriately.

Bracket placement charts and bracket positioners are also recommended, highlighting the importance of accurate vertical bracket placement (Table 6.5). In addition, to help control anchorage, the use of lacebacks, bendbacks and tiebacks is advised.

The latest version of the system is McLaughlin Bennett 5.0.

Damon Prescription

Damon brackets have undergone significant development since their introduction in 1996 as Damon SL; the latest, eighth iteration is the Damon Q2. The Damon Q2 bracket is a passive self-ligating bracket with a sliding gate closure, which has a built-in vertical slot for a drop-in hook.

The Damon bracket and prescription are part of the Damon System, developed by Dr Dwight H. Damon, and encompass a number of distinctive treatment philosophies,[29] including the use of (i) light 'biologically sensible' forces; (ii) multiple bracket torque options to help overcome the lack of control torque using a 0.019 × 0.025-inch stainless steel wire in the 0.022-inch slot; (iii) the smile arc to determine vertical placement of the brackets; (iv) Damon arch form copper NiTi archwires; (v) temporary anchorage devices (TADs) where required; (vi) the Herbst appliance for skeletal II correction; (vii) very light, early inter-arch elastics; (viii) Damon splints to retain anteroposterior and transverse corrections; and (ix) permanent lower 3-3 retention.

Dr Damon also discusses the benefits of non-extraction treatment and the potential effects on aesthetics of the mid-face and facial profile from developing the arches and on the airway, due to the potential of orthodontic treatment to alter tongue position.

ProTorque Latin/Hispanic and Sugiyama Evidence-based Asian (SEBA) Prescriptions

The development of the ProTorque Latin/Hispanic and SEBA prescriptions came from differences noted in comparisons between the average inter-incisal angles of Caucasian, Hispanic and Asian cephalometric analyses. It was noted that the average Hispanic inter-incisal angle is approximately 12° less than Caucasian averages and the average Asian inter-incisal angle is approximately 10° less.[30] The prescribed torques of the anterior teeth in the ProTorque and SEBA prescriptions have therefore been increased accordingly to help achieve these inter-incisal angles in Hispanic and Asian patients.

Semi-customised

Appliances can be semi-customised by using high, standard or low torque bracket options, inverting, reversing or swapping brackets from the same prescription, or by swapping brackets between different prescriptions. These customisations can be useful where tooth or skeletal base morphology is not within normal ranges and to help mitigate the effect of play between the wire and bracket slot. Achieving optimal tooth positioning often needs customisation and can significantly improve the final aesthetic and occlusal result.

Understanding torque play is important in understanding fixed appliance mechanics. Torque play (see third-order clearance and Figure 19c in Introduction), measured in degrees, is a result of slop between the wire and the bracket slot and the flex of the wire and bracket.

A 0.019 × 0.025-inch wire engaged in a 0.022-inch slot will have approximately 10° of slop between the wire and the slot walls due to the differences in their physical dimensions. However, slop also exists as a result of the rounding of wire edges and the dimensional tolerances set by the manufacturers of bracket wires and slots.[28] Standard dimensional tolerances are set by bracket and wire manufacturers so that, on average, wires are undersized and bracket slots are oversized to reduce the chance of a wire not fitting into a slot at the chairside. Torque play can create a significant issue with the delivery of torque using the straight-wire appliance and this has long been noted by orthodontists. More recent non-customised prescriptions have aimed to improve the delivery of torque, but customisation is often also required to deliver the torque desired.

Bracket Torque Options

Some prescriptions, such as the Damon prescription, offer high, standard and low torque bracket options. For example, high-torque brackets are useful if the upper or lower incisors are retroclined at the start of treatment. Conversely, if the upper or lower incisors are proclined, then low-torque brackets are helpful. Similarly, high- and low-torque incisor and canine brackets are helpful when canines are disimpacted from buccal or palatal positions respectively. High- and low-torque brackets on upper and lower incisors can also help to reduce the unwanted effects from inter-arch Class II and III elastics.

Inverting Brackets

When brackets are turned 180°, the prescribed torque is reversed and tip remains unchanged. This technique can be useful when a lateral incisor crown is palatally displaced at the start of treatment. If the bracket is not inverted, play between the wire and the bracket slot will result in this tooth being under-torqued and will therefore not achieve its intended inclination. The 10° of palatal root torque built into the MBT Versatile+ prescription, when inverted, provides 10° of buccal root torque, helping to correct the inclination given what is lost through play.

'Reversing' Brackets

The tip is reversed and the torque remains the same when a bracket is reversed. To reverse a bracket, it is placed on its contralateral counterpart tooth in the same arch. When camouflaging Class III skeletal bases, reversing the lower canine brackets can be useful. Using the MBT Versatile+ prescription this converts 3° of mesial crown tip into 3° of distal crown tip.

Swapping Brackets

Brackets from the same prescription can be swapped between teeth, and brackets from different prescriptions can be mixed. Care needs to be taken when swapping brackets, as the in–out value within the same prescription and among different prescriptions is often not the same.

Using a lower second molar tube of the MBT Versatile+ prescription inverted on the contralateral upper molar when finishing cases to a Class II molar relationship can be used to remove the molar offset. In doing so, this can help improve cuspal interdigitation when finishing to a Class II molar relationship.

Fully Customised

There has been progression in bracket design from being based on average values towards individualised custom appliances. For an appliance to be fully customised, a detailed history should be taken alongside a comprehensive clinical and radiographic examination. Examination should include identifying the physiology, morphology and any pathology of an individual's maxillary dentition, mandibular dentition, skeletal bases and orofacial soft tissues. Once these have been identified, a comprehensive management plan made in the light of the best available evidence can be established, allowing for full customisation of appliances and bracket prescription. Fully customised appliances are established by clinicians trained to an appropriate level after a full clinical assessment and this impacts the quality of the result achieved. The use of algorithms in assisting bracket and wire customisation will no doubt be of benefit in achieving fully customised appliances and a number of systems are now available, one of which is Ormco's *Insignia*.

Insignia (Ormco Corporation, Brea, California, USA) software produces its version of fully customised brackets and wires that are reverse engineered from an algorithmically determined virtual optimal occlusion. A Standard Tessellation Language (.stl) file obtained from a structured light optical scanner of the crowns of the teeth and supporting periodontium, or impressions of these, are uploaded to *Insignia* online. Semi-automated segmentation of the virtual crowns of the teeth and landmarking means their ideal positions in three dimensions can be derived once tooth size discrepancies and optimal occlusion have been established. Cortical limits are derived from the scanned form of the supporting mandibular periodontium. A virtual straight wire is then constructed, and Boolean operations determine bracket base, stem and slot dimensions that enable custom reverse engineering of the bracket design.

Optimal Bracket Positioning

A key determinant of the prescription of a bracket or tube slot of the preadjusted straight-wire appliance being expressed is its correct siting (Figure 6.9). Andrews advocated using the FA point to site brackets and this is still the default convention for bracket placement. Brackets can be placed under direct or indirect vision and a number of features have been built into brackets to aid this, along with the use of bracket positioning devices.

Bracket Positioning Technique

Direct Visualisation Direct visualisation of the labial and occlusal surfaces and their landmarks is the recommended method for determining the FA point. Optimal patient and operator positioning improve direct visualisation of the labial surface. The operator should align themselves facing perpendicular to the labial or occlusal surface of each tooth. When this is not possible the bracket position should be viewed indirectly.

Indirect Visualisation A dental mirror allows indirect visualisation of labial, lingual and occlusal surfaces. The operator should align themselves with the FACC and position the mirror at 45° to the observed surface. Indirect vision can also be achieved by using intraoral or extraoral clinical photographs or by viewing bracket positions on study models or on a virtual dentition constructed from intraoral scans.

Bracket Positioning Features

In order to aid direct and indirect bracket placement, a number of bracket positioning features are incorporated into bracket design, including visual aids and base locating contours (Figure 6.10).

Rhomboid Shape Conventional bracket design for teeth where tip prescriptions are greater or less than 0° leads to a bracket shape with incongruent visual cues. Offsetting rectangular brackets to the same degree as the tip in the bracket prescription produces rhomboid brackets which resolves this. These brackets have mesial and distal edges that are parallel to the FACC and these edges, together with a centred vertical scribe line, enhance visual cues to align the bracket correctly to the FACC.

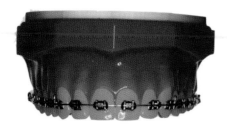
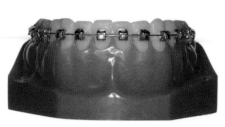

Figure 6.9 Upper typodont with conventional ligation brackets ligated with black elastomeric modules, and lower typodont with self-ligating brackets bonded on the FA point (note the minor vertical bracket positioning error on the lower right central incisor).

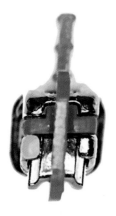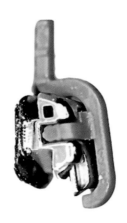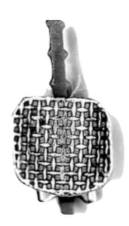

Figure 6.10 Damon Q self-ligating lower right canine bracket showing sliding gate mechanism, compound contoured rhomboid base, distogingivally placed, colour-coded identification and orientation mark, auxiliary horizontal and vertical slots, removable plastic positioning jig and an 80-gauge mesh base.

Torque-in-base Using brackets or tubes with torque-in-base, as described by Andrews, where the FA point, bracket base point and bracket slot point are all aligned on the slot axis, means the slot point represents the bracket base point. This alignment of slot base and bracket base helps prevent minor vertical positioning errors when bracket siting.

Compound Contoured Bases Contoured bracket bases, designed using data from average tooth surface contours, help guide the centre of the base of the brackets onto the FA point in averagely contoured teeth. Bondable molar tube designs are also available with a vertical ridge in the base of the tube that aids correct siting into the mid-buccal groove.

Bracket Positioning Devices

Bracket positioning devices principally aid correct vertical siting. When a bracket is positioned incorrectly in the vertical dimension, not only will there be a vertical error but also a torque error. This will be greater for teeth which are more convex occlusogingivally. A variety of bracket positioning devices are available, including positioning jigs and bracket height gauges.

Positioning Jigs Positioning jigs are either plain or have half millimetre or millimetre markings or ridges that align with the incisal edge or cusp tip (Figure 6.10). The jigs are supplied pre-engaged into the bracket slot and are removed once the brackets are bonded in position with forceps or tweezers.

Bracket Height Gauges These instruments typically have a forked metal design, with one tine engaging into the bracket slot and the other tine gauged to the occlusal reference point. These gauges can be used alongside bracket placement charts and they enable the bracket slot to be placed a prescribed distance from the incisal edge or cusp tip.

Straight-wire Appliance: Bracket Modifications

Bracket Material

The materials used for bracket manufacture can be divided into metal, ceramic and plastic.

Metal

Orthodontic brackets made from various metals have been the mainstay of orthodontic bracket design since their early introduction. Metal brackets are principally made from stainless steel or titanium; however, they are also available in cobalt-chromium or stainless steel plated with gold or platinum.

Stainless Steel This is the standard material for orthodontic brackets, most commonly AISI (American Iron and Steel Institute) Type 316L 'marine grade' stainless steel. Type 316L stainless steel is an austenitic chromium-nickel steel containing approximately 63–70% iron, 16–18% chromium, 10–14% nickel and 2–3% molybdenum, and has good deformation and corrosion resistance. A wide variety of bracket designs in stainless steel are available (Figure 6.11) and a number of methods are used to construct these en masse.

Milled The Andrews straight-wire appliance brackets were originally cold (room temperature) drawn and manually milled, although this was liable to manufacturing errors and proved not to be cost-effective.[24] More recently, computer numerical controlled (CNC) milling of the

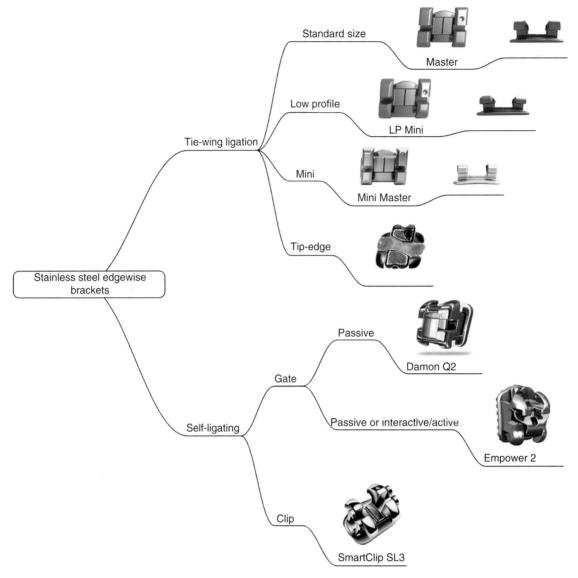

Figure 6.11 Examples of stainless steel brackets. Note that images are not to scale; please refer to the manufacturer for product specifications. Sources: Master, LP Mini, Mini Master and Empower 2: American Orthodontics, reproduced with permission of American Orthodontics and © American Orthodontics. Tip-Edge: C.D. Donaldson. Damon Q2: Ormco, reproduced with permission of Ormco and © Ormco. SmartClip: 3M, reproduced with permission of 3M and © 3M.

bracket slot has become available that uses computer-aided design (CAD) and computer-aided manufacture (CAM) to deliver high milling accuracy and improved manufacturing efficiency.

Metal Casting In the process of metal casting, typically liquid metal is poured through a spruce (channel) into a reusable hollow mould. Once the metal has solidified it is removed from the mould in the form of a cast. Orthodontic brackets made using metal casting produces brackets that are less hard than cold drawn and milled stainless steel brackets.

Metal Injection Moulding The process of metal injection moulding (MIM) involves combining metal powder with a polymer binder that is then heated and injected into a mould. The binder is then removed through the use of solvents and/or low heat in a process known as debinding. Subsequently, sintering uniformly removes the porosities created through high temperature heating.

Notably, significant shrinkage occurs during the sintering process as the porosities are removed and this is accommodated for by oversizing the mould. MIM produces resultant metal parts with 98% metal density. MIM became widely adopted in the 1980s and significantly reduced the cost of manufacture of complex small metal parts produced in large volumes and became the standard manufacturing process for metal orthodontic brackets.

Titanium Titanium brackets manufactured using commercially pure titanium or titanium alloy (Ti-6Al-4V)[31] can be used in patients with a nickel allergy;[32] they also have greater resistance to corrosion than stainless steel brackets.

Ceramic

Ceramic brackets have a significant advantage over stainless steel brackets in being a more aesthetic option for patients and are also available in a variety of designs (Figure 6.12). However, ceramic has a number of inherent disadvantages compared to stainless steel when used to manufacture brackets.

Ceramic brackets have the ability to cause rapid abrasive wear of the opposing dentition, as they have greater hardness than enamel. As a result, ceramic brackets should not be used where there is a risk of occlusal interference. Ceramic slots encounter increased resistance to friction compared to stainless steel slots and ceramic brackets have

since become available with metal slots. Because ceramic bracket bases have low ductility when traditional debond pliers are applied, an engineered 'line of weakness' is built into some ceramic bases and are often supplied alongside specific debonding pliers. Stainless steel bracket bases are more ductile and flex when debonding pliers are applied, leading to bond failure at the base–composite interface rather than the base–enamel interface, lowering the risk of enamel loss. As ceramic bracket designs have developed, the risk of enamel fracture has reduced.

Ceramic brackets are available as polycrystalline or monocrystalline, with differing manufacturing processes and physical properties.

Polycrystalline Alumina Polycrystalline brackets are opaque and manufactured by ceramic injection moulding. In this process, aluminium oxide particles are injected along with a binder into a mould. Pressure and heat of over 1800°C removes the binder and condenses the aluminium oxide particles into a polycrystalline structure.

Monocrystalline Alumina Monocrystalline (sapphire) brackets are translucent and are formed by milling a single block

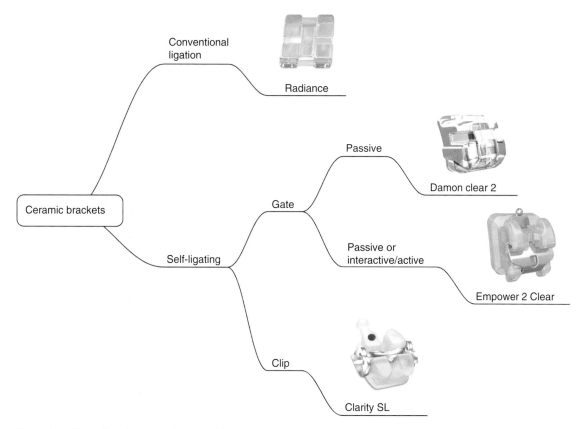

Figure 6.12 Examples of ceramic brackets. Note that images are not to scale; please refer to the manufacturer for product specifications. Sources: Radiance and Empower 2 Clear: American Orthodontics, reproduced with permission of American Orthodontics and © American Orthodontics. Damon Clear 2: Ormco, reproduced with permission of Ormco and © Ormco. Clarity SL: 3M, reproduced with permission of 3M and © 3M.

of synthetic sapphire crystal. This sapphire crystal is produced by fusing aluminium oxide particles at 2100°C and then cooled slowly to allow control of crystallisation to form a monocrystalline structure.

Plastic

Plastic brackets are an alternative aesthetic option and are made from polycarbonate or polyurethane. However, polycarbonate brackets are susceptible to elastic deformation and permanent (creep) deformation, secondary to exposure to mechanical stress below the material's yield threshold. This has led to the manufacture of reinforced brackets with ceramic fillers and the use of engineered metal slots.

Both polycarbonate and polyurethane brackets are at risk of discoloration, although polyurethane brackets are less likely to discolour.

Slot Dimensions

The two standard sizes used in modern fixed straight-wire appliances are 0.018 × 0.028-inch and 0.022 × 0.028-inch slots. As the slot depth is the same in both slots, they are typically referred to as the 0.018-inch slot and the 0.022-inch slot. Different working and finishing archwire dimensions are used in 0.018-inch and 0.022-inch systems.

The 0.018-inch Slot

The typical finishing archwire dimensions for an 0.018-inch slot is 0.017 × 0.025-inch, whilst round wire sliding mechanics are typically completed on a 0.016-inch round stainless steel wire.

The 0.022-inch Slot

The working archwire for an 0.022-inch slot is a 0.019 × 0.025-inch wire; however, a 0.021 × 0.025-inch archwire is also available in cases where more complete torque expression is useful at the end of treatment. Round wire sliding mechanics can be completed on a 0.018-inch or 0.020-inch round stainless steel.

The principal difference between the 0.018-inch and 0.022-inch systems is that the 0.022-inch slot allows for a greater maximum prescribed force to be expressed due to the final wire having greater maximum dimensions and therefore has (i) greater ability to expand arches through lateral force application delivery and (ii) greater arch levelling ability. The 0.022-inch slot also has greater resistance to unwanted tip and rotations during sliding mechanics. The 0.018-inch slot brackets can achieve lateral expansion and arch levelling but may require the use of auxiliary archwires.

Auxiliary Slots

Auxiliary slots are found in a number of brackets (see Figure 6.10) and they can be oriented vertically or horizontally. Horizontal slots are typically used for narrow-gauge piggyback wires, alongside a rigid base archwire ligated in the main bracket slot. Vertical slots can be used for drop-in hooks or alternatively in Tip-Edge appliances for auxiliary (uprighting and torquing) springs.

Bracket Base

Base Surface

Bracket base surfaces can be divided into those that have retentive features built in and those that do not, and this division is related to whether the base is to be welded or bonded.

Retentive Bases The surface of bondable bracket bases is designed to prevent unintentional bond failure via macro-mechanically retentive and/or micro-mechanically retentive features whilst allowing for planned bond failure at debond.

Macro-mechanical The main type of macro-mechanical feature used on bracket bases is mesh (see Figure 6.10). Mesh bases are typically 80 gauge and can be single, double or triple layered. Comparing debond rates at 24 hours between single and double mesh bases has found similar shear bond strengths.[33] Grooves and undercuts can also be used, and these can be milled, cast or laser cut.

Micro-mechanical These features create microscopic porosities and voids, and methods include the use of acids, lasers or by coating the base with microporous metal or ceramic particles. These techniques are termed micro-etching, laser-microstructuring and particulate coating, respectively. Bracket bases can also be sand-blasted.

Non-retentive Bases Weldable metal brackets and tubes have bases that are smooth and can be welded to metal bands.

Base Contour

Originally, bracket bases were contoured horizontally but not vertically, which meant that the brackets were not stable when fully seated. The design of the compound contoured base was derived for individual teeth using the average vertical and horizontal curvature measurements by Andrews. The compound contoured base design has become a common feature of modern bracket design and aids bracket base siting on the FA point (see Figure 6.10).

Rhomboid Shape

Andrews straight-wire appliance had tip built into the slot; however, this led to unhelpful visual cues when placed on a tooth, even though compound contour bases helped locate brackets onto the FA point. To help create congruent visual cues, rhomboid brackets were introduced which mirrored the tip of the prescription and further aid placement (see Figure 6.10).

Torque-in-base

Moving bracket design from torque-in-face to torque-in-base meant moving the torque prescription from the slot base to the bracket base. In torque-in-base brackets the slot point, base point and FA point are aligned, and this feature helps vertical bracket positioning (see Figure 6.10).

Pre-coated

3M have developed brackets pre-coated with composite and these are known as APC (adhesive pre-coated) brackets (Figure 6.13). APC Plus pre-coated bracket bases are coated with a pink composite; when excess is extruded from under the bracket base, the colour aids identification and therefore removal. Once the composite is cured it loses its colour. APC Flash-Free pre-coated brackets use a non-woven mat of entangled polypropylene fibres soaked with an amount of composite resin. When compressed against a tooth surface, the resin is designed to spread evenly to the edges and corners of the bracket base avoiding excess.

Standard, Auxiliary, Headgear and Lip Bumper Tubes

Molar tubes are available in single, double or triple tube configurations, including a prescription tube with or without auxiliary prescription, headgear or lip bumper tubes.

Molar tubes are available pre-welded to molar bands, separately for in-surgery or in-laboratory welding to bands, or with a bondable base for direct or indirect bonding.

Non-convertible, convertible and reconvertible molar tubes are available (Figure 6.14). Convertible tubes have a removable buccal wall and tie-wings that essentially enables the slot to be 'converted' to a bracket. Reconvertible tubes incorporate a self-ligating mechanism that enables them to be 'converted' to a bracket when opened and then 'reconverted' to a tube again when closed. Tubes are also available which have a widened and chamfered mesial entrance to aid wire insertion.

Auxiliary prescription tubes can be included on upper molar bands or bondable tubes and can be offset gingivally or occlusally. Auxiliary tubes are designed for auxiliary archwires, such as a jockey arch for arch expansion, and can be round or rectangular in cross-section depending on whether torque is desired.

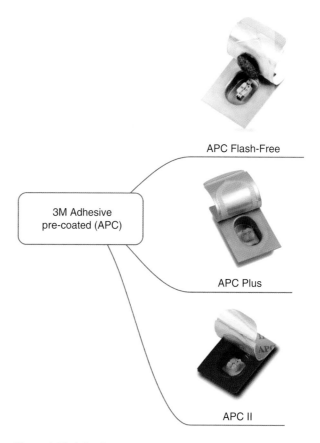

Figure 6.13 Adhesive pre-coated APC bracket options from 3M. Note that images are not to scale; please refer to the manufacturer for product specifications. Source: APC Flash-Free, APC Plus and APC II: 3M, reproduced with permission of 3M and © 3M.

Headgear tubes are designed to receive the inner bow of a facebow and can be gingivally or occlusally offset relative to the prescription slot, providing occlusal or gingival relief and changing the force vector. Headgear tubes are typically 0.045-inch or 0.051-inch in diameter to receive corresponding diameter inner bow terminal ends.

On lower molars, lip bumper tubes can be used to engage and anchor lip bumpers.

Tie-wings

Single Versus Double Wing

Angle's edgewise appliance had a single tie-wing. Standard bracket design quickly adopted the double wing design as this gave better rotational control and also more options for ligation. The double-wing bracket design has also been called the twin, double and Siamese bracket and was developed by Dr Swain.[18] Single-wing bracket designs are still available, alongside the modified single-wing designs by Lang and Lewis.

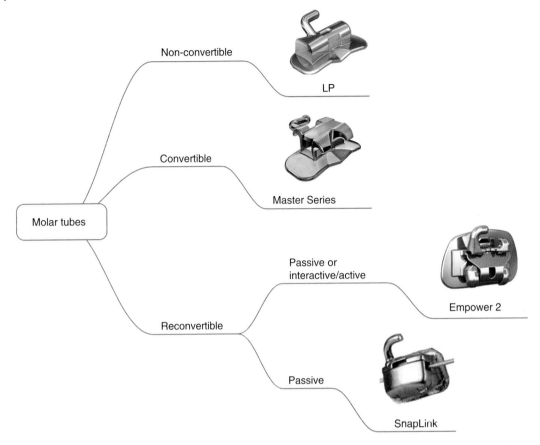

Figure 6.14 Examples of molar tubes. Note that images are not to scale; please refer to the manufacturer for product specifications. Sources: LP, Master Series and Empower 2: American Orthodontics, reproduced with permission of American Orthodontics and © American Orthodontics. SnapLink: Ormco, reproduced with permission of Ormco and © Ormco.

Low Profile

Low-profile bracket wings aid patient comfort, although this reduces tie-wing undercut depth and may limit the use of multiple tie-wing ligatures (see Figure 6.11).

Chamfered Corners

Chamfering wing corners occlusally and gingivally allows for greater patient comfort, whilst chamfering the slot side of the wings mesially and distally facilitates the cutting of wire ligatures with a wire cutter, as is found in the Andrews2 bracket.

Archwire Ligation

Tie-wing Ligation

The buccal wall of conventional bracket slots is open to allow the archwire to be inserted and then ligated into the slot with elastomeric or stainless steel ligatures secured around the bracket tie-wings. The degree of friction and force applied can be controlled by varying the method of ligation, for example using single-wing, double-wing or figure-of-eight ligation.

Elastomeric Ligatures Elastomeric or 'Ormolast' ligatures are easy to use, available in a wide range of colours and are easy to secure. However, elastomeric ligatures are known to accumulate plaque and have the potential to increase bleeding on probing scores when oral hygiene is suboptimal.[34] Elastomeric ligatures can be lost between appointments, allowing unwanted tooth movements.

Stainless Steel Ligatures Stainless steel ligatures provide a more secure method of ligation but are more time-consuming to place and remove. Ligature wire is available in various gauges on the spool or preformed in short and long lengths. Preformed short lengths are available as short or Kobayashi ligatures (Figure 6.15) and preformed long lengths as long ligatures.

Short 'Quick lig' Ligatures This is the most common form of wire ligation. Ordinarily they are preformed for convenience and are manufactured using 0.010-inch gauge wire.

Kobayashi Ligatures These ligatures are typically made from 0.012-inch or 0.014-inch gauge wire. Once ligated to

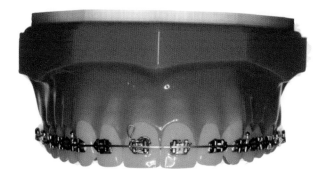

Figure 6.15 Typodont with Quick ligature on the upper left central incisor and Kobayashi ligature ligation of the upper right central incisor tooth, providing a hook which can be orientated mesially or distally.

a bracket they form a hook that can be used, for example, to secure elastic auxiliaries.

Long Ligatures Long length ligatures are used for lacebacks or tiebacks, to secure any group of teeth together or to simply reinforce the archwire and can be tied under the wire (under-tied) or over the wire (over-tied).

Self-ligating

The development of self-ligating appliances has been driven by the aim of creating a low friction environment for the archwire to slide that is simple and quick to ligate. The gate or clip mechanism to ligate the wire to a self-ligating bracket slot is typically opened or closed with an instrument or digitally. Self-ligating mechanisms can be divided into active/interactive or passive depending on whether the mechanism actively engages the wire with a potential active force or passively (see Figures 6.11 and 6.12).

The self-ligating bracket was commercially introduced in 1935 as the Russell Lock bracket[35] and since then there have been significant developments in manufacture and design. Development has focused on producing a self-ligating mechanism that is reliable and exerts minimal or no tooth displacement when opening and closing, whilst retaining other convenient and mechanical features of conventional brackets.

'Quick ligs' provide reliable full engagement of the wire into the slot but are something of a misnomer as they are slower to ligate than when using elastomeric ligation or a self-ligation mechanism.[36] Increased speed of ligation has been reported by a number of authors using a number of different self-ligating appliances.[36, 37]. In addition, reduced chairside assistance is required using self-ligating brackets.

However, the clinical benefit of engaging the wire with reduced friction – a key difference between conventional and self-ligating brackets[38] – has been widely debated. It has been suggested that the increased friction and resistance to sliding of conventionally ligated bracket–wire interfaces is overcome by the forces produced by the orofacial musculature during mastication, speaking and swallowing.[39] The *in vivo* benefits of self-ligating brackets continue to be debated.

Acknowledgements

I would like to thank the Edward H. Angle Society of Orthodontists and Dr Lawrence F. Andrews for their kind agreement to the use of a number of images in this chapter. Dr Angle's and Dr Andrews' work significantly advanced bracket and appliance design and set together their necessary elements.

References

1 Celsus AC. *De Medicina*. Florence: Nicolaus [Laurentii], 1478.

2 Fauchard P. Le *Chirurgien Dentiste, Ou Traité Des Dents, Vol 2, 2nd edn*. Paris, 1746.

3 Schangé JMA. *Précis Sur Le Redressement Des Dents, Ou Exposé Des Moyens Rationnels de Prévenir Ent de Corriger Les Déviations Des Dents*. Paris, 1842.

4 Angle HE. *Treatment of Malocclusion of the Teeth: Angle's System*. Philadelphia: The S.S. White Dental Manufacturing Company, 1907.

5 Angle EH. Orthodontia: new combinations of well-known forms of appliances. *The Dental Cosmos* 1899;41:836–841.

6 Angle EH. Further steps in the progress of orthodontia. *The Dental Cosmos* 1913;55(1):1–13.

7 Angle EH. Some new forms of orthodontic mechanisms and the reasons for their introduction. *The Dental Cosmos* 1916;58:969–994.

8 Angle EH. Orthodontia: the ribbon-arch mechanism and some new auxiliary instruments. *The Dental Cosmos* 1920;62(10):1157–1176.

9 Angle EH. Orthodontia: the ribbon-arch mechanism and some new auxiliary instruments (continued). *The Dental Cosmos* 1920;62(11):1279–1294.

10 Angle EH. The latest and best in orthodontic mechanism. *The Dental Cosmos* 1928;70(12):1143–1158.

11 Angle EH. The latest and best in orthodontic mechanism. *The Dental Cosmos* 1929;71(2):164–174.

12 Begg PR, Kesling PC. *Orthodontic Theory and Technique*, 2nd edn. Philadelphia, London: Saunders, 1971.

13 Begg PR. Differential force in orthodontic treatment. *Am. J. Orthod.* 1956;42(7):481–510.

14 Kesling PC. Dynamics of the tip-edge bracket. *Am. J. Orthod. Dentofacial Orthop.* 1989;96(1):16–25.

15 Kesling PC. Expanding the horizons of the edgewise arch wire slot. *Am. J. Orthod. Dentofacial Orthop.* 1988;94(1):26–37.

16 Sved A. Principles and technique of modified edgewise arch mechanism. *Am. J. Orthod. Oral Surg.* 1938;24(7):635–654.

17 Lewis PD. Canine retraction. *Am. J. Orthod.* 1970;57(6):543–560.

18 Swain BF. Dr. Brainerd F. Swain on current appliance therapy. Interview by Sidney Bradt. *J. Clin. Orthod.* 1980;14(4):250–264.

19 Holdaway RA. Bracket angulation as applied to the edgewise appliance. *Angle Orthod.* 1952;22(4): 227–236.

20 Andrews L. *Straight Wire: The Concept and Appliance.* San Diego, CA: LA Wells, 1989.

21 Andrews LF. The six keys to normal occlusion. *Am. J. Orthod.* 1972;62(3):296–309.

22 Andrews LF. The straight-wire appliance. *Br. J. Orthod.* 1979;6:125–143.

23 Roth RH. Five year clinical evaluation of the Andrews straight-wire appliance. *J. Clin. Orthod.* 1976;10(11):836–850.

24 Roth RH. The straight-wire appliance 17 years later. *J. Clin. Orthod.* 1987;21(9):632–642.

25 Alexander RG 'Wick'. *The Alexander Discipline: Contemporary Concepts and Philosophies.* Glendora, CA: Ormco Corp., 1986.

26 Ricketts RM, Bench RW, Gugino CF, et al. *Bioprogressive Therapy.* Denver, CO: Rocky Mountain Orthodontics, 1979.

27 McLaughlin RP, Bennett JC, Trevisi HJ. *Systemized Orthodontic Treatment Mechanics.* Edinburgh: Mosby, 2002.

28 Cash A, Curtis R, McDonald F, Good S. An evaluation of slot size in orthodontic brackets: are standards as expected? *Angle Orthod.* 2004;74(4):450–453.

29 Damon D, Keim RG. Dwight Damon, DDS, MSD. *J. Clin. Orthod.* 2012;46(11):667–678.

30 Fastlicht J. Tetragon: a visual cephalometric analysis. *J. Clin. Orthod.* 2000;33(6):353–360.

31 Gioka C, Bourauel C, Zinelis S, et al. Titanium orthodontic brackets: structure, composition, *hardness and ionic release. Dent. Mater.* 2004;20(7):693–700.

32 Bass JK, Fine H, Cisneros GJ. Nickel hypersensitivity in the orthodontic patient. *Am. J. Orthod. Dentofacial Orthop.* 1993;103(3):280–285.

33 Bishara SE, Soliman MMA, Oonsombat C, et al. The effect of variation in mesh-base design on the shear bond strength of orthodontic brackets. *Angle Orthod.* 2004;74(3):400–404.

34 Türkkahraman H, Sayin MÖ, Bozkurt FY, et al. Archwire ligation techniques, microbial colonization, and periodontal status in orthodontically treated patients. *Angle Orthod.* 2005;75(2):231–236.

35 Stolzenberg J. The Russell attachment and its improved advantages. *Int. J. Orthod. Dent. Children* 1935;21(9):837–840.

36 Shivapuja PK, Berger J. A comparative study of conventional ligation and self-ligation bracket systems. *Am. J. Orthod. Dentofacial Orthop.* 1994;106(5):472–480.

37 Maijer R, Smith DC. Time savings with self-ligating brackets. *J. Clin. Orthod.* 1990;24(1):29–31.

38 Thomas S, Sherriff M, Birnie D. A comparative in vitro study of the frictional characteristics of two types of self-ligating brackets and two types of pre-adjusted edgewise brackets tied with elastomeric ligatures. *Eur. J. Orthod.* 1998;20(5):589–596.

39 Braun S, Bluestein M, Moore BK, Benson G. Friction in perspective. *Am. J. Orthod. Dentofacial Orthop.* 1999;115(6):619–627.

7

Bracket Placement

Hemendranath V. Shah, Daljit S. Gill, and Farhad B. Naini

CHAPTER OUTLINE

Introduction, 137
Design Features of Preadjusted Edgewise Appliance Brackets, 137
  Primary Design Features, 138
  Slot Siting Features, 138
  Auxiliary Features, 139
  Convenience Features, 140
Direct versus Indirect Bonding, 140
  Advantages of Direct Bonding, 141
  Disadvantages of Direct Bonding, 141
  Advantages of Indirect Bonding, 141
  Disadvantages of Indirect Bonding, 141
Direct Bonding Technique, 141
  Localising the FA Point, 141
  Measuring the Distance from the Incisal Edge, 141
Indirect Bonding Technique, 142
  Stages of Indirect Bonding, 142
Banding Molars and Premolars, 143
  Separators, 143
  Banding Technique, 145
Tips for Bracket Selection in Certain Situations, 145
References, 146

Introduction

Orthodontic mechanotherapy with labial fixed appliances allows precise three-dimensional tooth movement in all planes of space. For predictable treatment results, correct diagnosis and treatment planning are of primary importance, followed by execution of treatment with an appropriate appliance that is correctly placed. The accurate placement of fixed orthodontic brackets is especially important in achieving the desired outcome and a detailed understanding of the technology is vital for the orthodontist in treatment delivery. For an outline of the history of the preadjusted appliance and a description of the anatomy of an orthodontic bracket, please refer to the Introduction of the book.

Design Features of Preadjusted Edgewise Appliance Brackets

During the design of the original straight-wire appliance, Andrews described four sets of features that were essential to their design:

1. Primary design features
2. Slot siting features
3. Auxiliary features
4. Convenience features.

Andrews[1] defined different parts of a bracket that were integral to the design of the appliance and important in the direct placement of a bracket onto the correct part of the tooth surface.

Preadjusted Edgewise Fixed Orthodontic Appliances: Principles and Practice, First Edition. Edited by Farhad B. Naini and Daljit S. Gill.
© 2022 John Wiley & Sons Ltd. Published 2022 by John Wiley & Sons Ltd.

Primary Design Features

This is the prescription of the bracket.

1. Prominence (in–out or first order): this is built into the bracket base to account for the differing buccolingual thicknesses of individual teeth.
2. Angulation (tip or second order): in the original Andrews brackets, the slot was cut at an angle to the vertical axis of the bracket to ensure the correct mesiodistal angulation of the specific tooth upon completion of treatment.
3. Inclination (torque or third order): in the preadjusted edgewise appliance, torque is placed in the base of the bracket. The slot point, base point and facial axis point all lie along the slot axis (see Introduction, Figure 15).

Slot Siting Features

A key factor in achieving successful treatment with the preadjusted edgewise appliance is the accuracy of bracket placement. There are several key components in the design of a bracket for the purpose of accurate placement as shown in Figure 7.1.

- Bracket base: the most lingual portion of the bracket stem, which holds the stem on to the enamel surface.
- Bracket stem: the portion of a bracket between the bracket base and the most lingual portion of the slot.
- Slot base: the lingual wall of the slot.
- Base point: on the bracket base, the point that would fall on a lingual extension of the slot axis.
- Slot axis: the labiolingual/buccolingual centreline of the slot. It is equidistant from the gingival and occlusal slot walls and is centred mesiodistally.

Slot siting features were designed into the original standard edgewise appliance brackets. These are features which site the bracket slot when placed in the correct position. Andrews defined a specific siting location on the labial enamel surface of the clinical crown to reliably place the bracket, known as the **facial axis (FA) point**, which is found midway between the incisal edge or cusp tip and the cementoenamel junction, along a line described as the **long axis of the clinical crown (LACC)** (Figure 7.2); this is the case for all teeth except the molars. The LACC is located on the long axis of the crown, midway between the mesial and distal surfaces. The location point for molars is the buccal grove, which separates the mesiobuccal and distobuccal cusps (Figure 7.3). For the preadjusted appliance to function as designed, the centre of the bracket must be placed on the FA point.

There are eight slot siting features considered in all three planes of space of a tooth.

In the mid-transverse plane (Figure 7.4)

1. The bracket slot, bracket stem and crown must be in the same plane.
2. The base of the bracket for each tooth type must have the same inclination as the facial plane of the crown at the FA point.
3. Each bracket's base must be contoured occlusogingivally to match the curvature of the crown.

In the mid-sagittal plane

4. The bracket slot, bracket stem and crown must be coincident.
5. The plane of the bracket base at its base point must be the same as the facial plane of the crown at the FA point. In all crowns this is 90° to the mid-sagittal

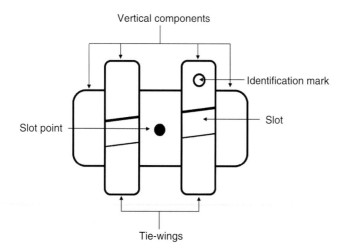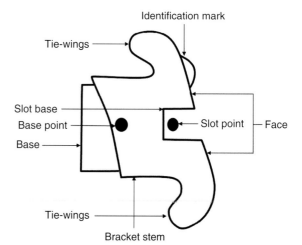

Figure 7.1 Key components of an orthodontic bracket. Source: Andrews LF. The straight-wire appliance. *Br. J. Orthod.* 1979;6(3):125–143. © 1979, SAGE Publications.

Figure 7.2 (a) Upper right central incisor demonstrating the long axis of the clinical crown (LACC) (blue line) and the facial axis (FA) point (red). (b) Labial view of a bracket placed in the correct position on the upper right central incisor.
(c) Lateral view of a bracket placed in the correct position on the upper right central incisor.

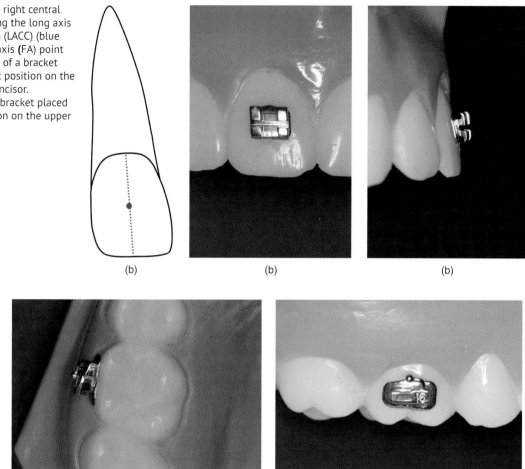

(b) (b) (b)

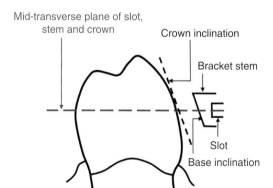

(a) (b) (c)

Figure 7.3 (a) Upper right first permanent molar demonstrating the LACC (blue line) and the FA point (red). (b) Occlusal view of molar tube in the correct position on the upper right first permanent molar. (c) Buccal view of molar tube in the correct position on the upper right first permanent molar.

Mid-transverse plane of slot, stem and crown

Crown inclination

Bracket stem

Slot

Base inclination

Figure 7.4 Slot siting features in mid-transverse plane.

plane (Figure 7.5), but in maxillary molars this is 100° (Figure 7.6).

6. Each bracket's base must be contoured mesiodistally to match the curvature of the crown.

In the mid-frontal plane

7. The vertical components of the bracket should be parallel to one another and to the LACC. The horizontal components of the bracket should be sited equidistant from the gingival margin and the cusp tip/incisal edge (Figure 7.7).

8. Within an arch, all slot points must have the same distance between them and the crown's embrasure line. This eliminates the need for first-order wire bends that allow for varying crown prominence.

Auxiliary Features

These contribute to the biological aspects of treatment, for the attachment of auxiliaries to apply force to teeth for movement, but are not involved in the slot siting, e.g. parallel tie-wings, integral hooks, power arms, facebow and auxiliary tubes.

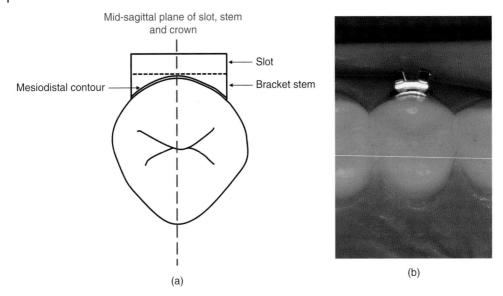

(a)   (b)

Figure 7.5 (a) Slot siting features in the mid-sagittal plane of a premolar. (b) A premolar bracket in the correct mesiodistal position on the upper right first premolar.

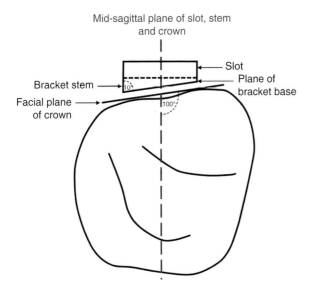

Figure 7.6 Slot siting features in the mid-sagittal plane of a molar.

Convenience Features

These are features of the bracket which are not either involved in siting the slot or the biological aspects of treatment but facilitate use by the orthodontist or make the appliance more comfortable for the patient.

- Bracket identification: orientation marker placed on the distogingival tie-wing.
- Facial contouring of brackets: improves soft tissue comfort.

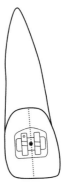

Figure 7.7 Bracket positioning of the right maxillary central incisor in the mid-frontal plane with the slot point directly on the FA point of the tooth.

- Extended gingival tie-wings: designed to extend laterally so there will not be any gingival impingement.
- Bracket material.

Accurately placed brackets result in better control of the three-dimensional position of the teeth with the correct expression of the prescription built into the bracket. This also reduces the requirement for wire bending or bracket repositioning during treatment, reducing overall treatment time.

Direct versus Indirect Bonding

Bracket placement can be either direct, or indirect using a transfer tray. The direct bonding technique is the more commonly used technique by most orthodontists. The principles for determining the position of a bracket either directly onto a prepared tooth surface or on a model remain the same.

Advantages of Direct Bonding

- No laboratory costs
- Excess adhesive can be removed immediately
- Positioning of brackets is directly visible
- Useful for single bracket placement.

Disadvantages of Direct Bonding

- Field of vision can be obscured due to soft tissues, limited mouth opening, instruments
- Possibly greater chairside time.

Advantages of Indirect Bonding

- Accurate bracket placement
- Less chairside time
- No manipulation of bracket position in the mouth
- Improved ability to bond to posterior teeth eliminating the need for separators and band placement on posterior teeth
- Improved patient comfort and hygiene.

Disadvantages of Indirect Bonding

- Technique sensitive
- Need for an extra set of impressions
- Increased laboratory time and costs
- Removal of set excess adhesive is time-consuming.

Direct Bonding Technique

Direct bracket placement can most commonly be undertaken onto a prepared enamel surface either using the acid etch technique or with the use of self-etch primer.[2] There are two methods for determining the position of the bracket or bonded tube for direct placement on the prepared enamel surface.

Localising the FA Point

The bracket can be located directly onto the surface of the tooth so that the slot point overlies the FA point, with the mesial and distal sides of the bracket parallel to the LACC, and equidistant from the mesial and distal surfaces of the tooth. This does not require any special measuring device.

Measuring the Distance from the Incisal Edge

Some clinicians advocate the positioning of brackets a measured distance from the incisal edge to account for differences in the FA points caused by their not being in the same plane between teeth.[3]

It is recommended that the tooth size for each patient is measured either directly in the mouth or on study models. Fully erupted teeth are chosen. By dividing the measurements by two, the distance from the occlusal surface to the vertical centre of the clinical crown is calculated.[4]

An additional technique is to use a bracket positioning chart (Table 7.1).[4] This involves identifying the row with the greatest number of recorded measurements. This will be the row which is used for bracket placement for that patient. This creates an individualised bracket positioning chart for the patient that can be recorded in their clinical notes. This can be used for both direct and indirect bonding.

The bracket is placed along the LACC and a bracket placement gauge (e.g. Boone gauge/Dougherty gauge) is used to confirm the vertical height of the bracket (Figure 7.8). Instead of using gauges, some bracket manufacturers supply jigs for placement of brackets, e.g. Damon brackets and Tip-edge brackets (Figure 7.9).

There is no overall evidence to suggest that using the FA point or measuring from the incisal edge is a more accurate method of bracket positioning.[5]

Incorrect positioning of horizontal brackets can lead to the introduction of rotations, especially in canines and premolars, which have rounded buccal surfaces (Figure 7.10). Incisors and molars, which have flat labial and buccal surfaces, are less likely to be affected by small errors in the horizontal placement of an attachment. However, there is an increased chance of horizontal and vertical placement

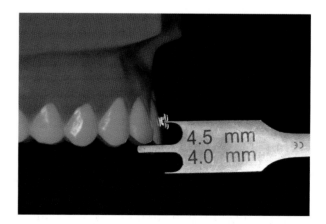

Figure 7.8 Bracket height gauge to determine the vertical position of the bracket on the upper right central incisor.

Table 7.1 Bracket positioning chart.

7	6	5	4	3	2	1	Upper
2.0	4.0	5.0	5.5	6.0	5.5	6.0	+1.0 mm
2.0	3.5	4.5	5.0	5.5	5.0	5.5	+0.5 mm
2.0	3.0	4.0	4.5	5.0	4.5	5.0	**Average**
2.0	2.5	3.5	4.0	4.5	4.0	4.5	−0.5 mm
2.0	2.0	3.0	3.5	4.0	3.5	4.0	−1.0 mm
7	6	5	4	3	2	1	Lower
3.5	3.5	4.5	5.0	5.5	5.0	5.0	+1.0 mm
3.0	3.0	4.0	4.5	5.0	4.5	4.5	+0.5 mm
2.5	2.5	3.5	4.0	4.5	4.0	4.0	**Average**
2.0	2.0	3.0	3.5	4.0	3.5	3.5	−0.5 mm
2.0	2.0	2.5	3.0	3.5	3.0	3.0	−1.0 mm

Source: McLaughlin RP, Bennet JC, Trevisi HJ. *Systemized Orthodontic Treatment Mechanics*. London: Mosby, 2001. © 2001, Elsevier.

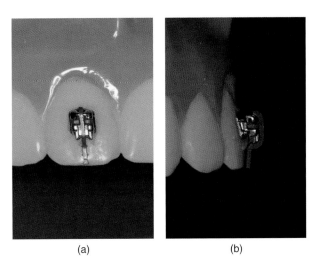

(a)　　　　　　　　(b)

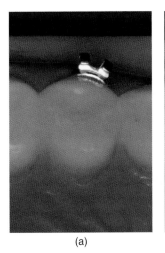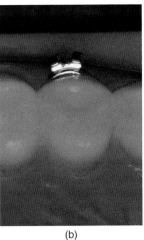

(a)　　　　　　　　(b)

Figure 7.9 Upper right central incisor Damon bracket with a jig to determine the vertical position of the bracket: (a) labial view; (b) lateral view.

Figure 7.10 (a) A premolar bracket placed too far mesially on the upper right first premolar tooth; this will lead to a mesiopalatal rotation of the crown. (b) A premolar bracket placed too far distally on the upper right first premolar tooth; this will lead to a distopalatal rotation of the crown.

errors when using brackets with reduced mesiodistal and occlusogingival dimensions.

Indirect Bonding Technique

Indirect bonding requires the initial positioning of brackets on a working model, either by locating the FA point or measuring from the incisal edge. These are transferred using a transfer tray from the dental model to the patient's mouth for bonding.

Stages of Indirect Bonding

1. Working models are cast in orthodontic stone from accurate alginate impressions.
2. Placement of separating medium.
3. Bonding resin applied to bracket base.
4. Brackets placed in correct position on plaster model and excess bonding resin removed (Figure 7.11a).
5. Bracket position checked.
6. Bonding resin cured with light curing unit (Figure 7.11b).

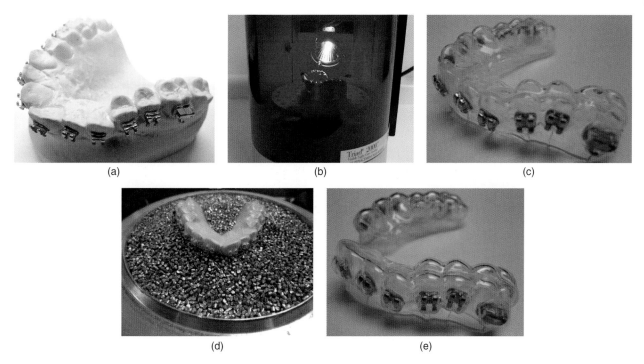

Figure 7.11 (a) Brackets placed in ideal positions using bonding resin. (b) The resin is light cured. (c) Soft transparent silicone is used to fabricate the inner flexible tray. The flexibility allows the tray to be peeled away from the brackets. (d) Rigid outer tray made over inner tray. The rigidity prevents distortion of the inner tray. (e) The final indirect bonding trays.

7. Undercuts blocked out on working model.
8. Inner tray fabricated using a soft silicone material which is transparent (Figure 7.11c).
9. Rigid outer tray is fabricated over the soft inner tray (Figure 7.11d).
10. Trays are trimmed (Figure 7.11e).
11. Brackets are inspected and any plaster is removed.
12. Composite surface is roughened.
13. Enamel surface is cleaned.
14. The maxillary and mandibular dentitions are isolated and etched.
15. Resin A applied to teeth.
16. Resin B applied to roughened composite surface on bracket.
17. Trays inserted separately over maxillary then mandibular dentitions.
18. Adhesive allowed to set or light cure.
19. Rigid outer tray removed.
20. Soft inner tray carefully removed.
21. Any excess composite removed.

Advancements in digital technologies, such as intraoral scanning, three-dimensional printing and computer simulation of bracket placement, are leading to the development of indirect bonding digital workflows.[6]

A clinical study using a split-mouth design concluded that bracket placement errors with direct or indirect bonding to the labial segments appear to be similar with both techniques.[7] Similarly, investigation of bond failure rates showed no difference in the failure rates between direct and indirect bonding.[8] Furthermore, this study found that the total number of appointments and overall treatment times did not differ between the two techniques. A systematic review and meta-analysis found weak evidence for any significant difference in bracket placement accuracy, oral hygiene status and bond failure rate when comparing direct and indirect bonding of orthodontic brackets.[9]

Banding Molars and Premolars

Molar bands are routinely used for the distal attachments on the posterior teeth of a fixed appliance. However, some practitioners favour molar tubes. Premolar bands are infrequently used, but do have a use in certain situations, for example when using a rapid maxillary expansion appliance.

Separators

Separators are placed for one week between the mesial and distal contact points of the teeth to be banded to create space for the placement of bands (Figure 7.12).

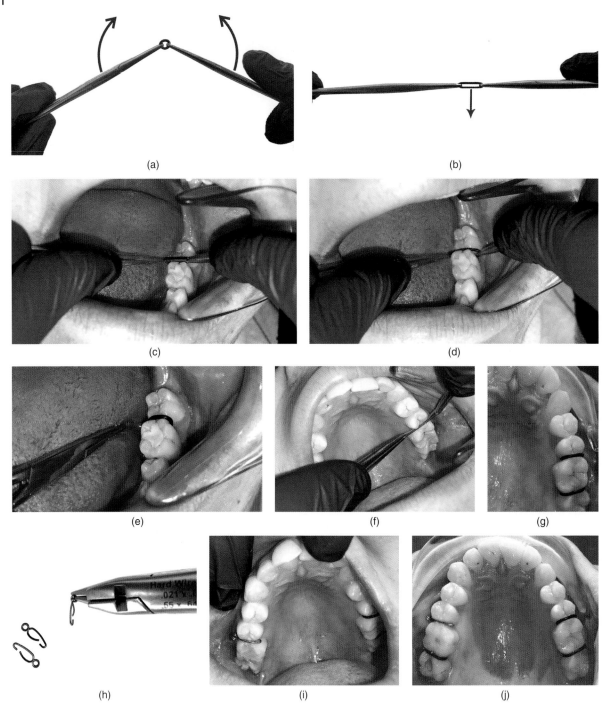

Figure 7.12 Elastomeric separators may be placed with separating pliers (see Appendix I). They may also be placed using two mosquito pliers. (a) The mosquito pliers should hold the elastomeric separator at an oblique angle, as shown, rather than from diametrically opposing sides. The benefit is that when the mosquito pliers are pulled, the part of the separator to be placed interdentally becomes taught, as shown in (b). (c–e) The taut part of the separator is gently squeezed in the interdental space, taking great care that should the separator tear or a mosquito clip inadvertently open, the patient is not injured by rebound of the clinician's hands and instruments. The taut part of the separator is placed interdentally and the opposing part remains visible. (f) The same procedure is carried out in each arch on the teeth to be subsequently banded. A left-to-right gentle sawing motion usually permits placement of the separators on the mesial and distal aspects of the teeth to be banded, as shown in (g). (h,i) In cases with very tight contact points, where an elastomeric separator cannot be placed, a stainless steel spring-clip separator may be used. These are held with the tips of light wire pliers at the base of the shorter leg, next to the helix (the image shows the separator being held in the helix for demonstration purposes). The tip of the longer leg is placed in the lingual/palatal embrasure between the teeth to be separated and the spring is pulled open so the shorter leg can slip beneath the interdental contact on the buccal side. (j) Separators *in situ* for the maxillary molar teeth. These are usually kept *in situ* for one week. The patient is advised to maintain a soft diet and particularly to avoid sticky foods. The following week, the separators are removed, providing space for the bands to be fitted.

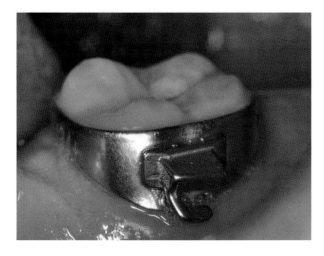

Figure 7.13 Buccal view of a molar band in the correct vertical position with equal amounts of enamel visible on the mesiobuccal and distobuccal cusps.

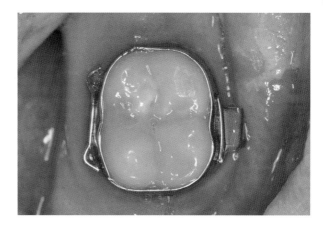

Figure 7.14 Occlusal view of a well-adapted molar band with the buccal tube in the correct mesiodistal position to ensure that rotation of the tooth is not created.

Banding Technique

The size of the band can be estimated from the patient's study models prior to their arrival if these are available. Once the separators are removed, the bands are tried for fit until the correct fitting band size is selected, which is closely adapted to the surface of the tooth. Bands are usually fabricated with an occlusogingival taper towards the cervical margin in order to better fit molar teeth. The selected bands should fit closely round the selected teeth, providing some mechanical retention before cementation, usually with glass ionomer cement. A band pusher and a band seater/biter (see Appendix I) may be used to help seat each band into position, both during initial trying in of the bands to check for fit and during cementation. The inner surface of bands may be conditioned, e.g. using sandblasting or laser-etching, to increase retention.

The maxillary and mandibular molar bands, when placed in the correct position, should demonstrate equal amounts of mesiobuccal and distobuccal cusp enamel when viewed from the buccal aspect and the occlusal edge of the band parallel to the cusps (Figure 7.13). If the band is placed with the molar tube either too mesial or distal, this will introduce an undesired rotation of the tooth (Figure 7.14). Premolar bands should be positioned so that the occlusal edge of the band is parallel to the buccal, with equal amounts of enamel visible on both the mesial and distal aspects of the buccal cusp.

When a band is selected, it is important that it is adequately adapted to the tooth surface and not too large, which risks the incorrect positioning of the band during cementation into a gingival position and increases the likelihood of failure and loosening mid-treatment.

Tips for Bracket Selection in Certain Situations

- Missing maxillary lateral incisor: when closing the lateral incisor space with substitution of the maxillary canine for the absent lateral incisor, it is advisable to invert a canine bracket with –7° torque to deliver +7° if using the MBT prescription to reduce the canine prominence in the labial alveolus. The bracket can be placed further gingivally to give the correct gingival contour and allow for reshaping of the canine tip. The bracket placement for the maxillary first premolar may be further distal and occlusal. This will help to position the premolar gingival margin more gingivally, resembling the canine gingival margin. The intrusion of the premolar also allows space for composite addition to the buccal cusp of the premolar, although such intrusion is rarely required. The distal placement of the premolar bracket allows some mesiopalatal rotation of the buccal cusp, again to appear more like a canine. These manoeuvres may be required to improve the position of the gingival margin in a patient who is concerned and has a high smile line. It should be noted, however, that intrusion and rotation are susceptible to relapse and may require long-term retention.
- Class III camouflage treatment: using contralateral mandibular canine brackets to minimise mesial movement of the canine crown with resultant incisor proclination. With the MBT prescription which has 8° of mesial tip in the mandibular canine prescription, use of contralateral brackets will provide a 16° difference and aid the retroclination of the lower labial segment by minimising mesial tipping of the canine during the alignment phase.

- Palatally placed maxillary lateral incisors: inverting the brackets (placing upside down) to deliver −10° of torque instead of +10° when using MBT prescription brackets. This will express greater labial root torque when the treatment progresses into a full dimension rectangular stainless steel wire.

Further information on local bracket variations may be found in Chapter 14.

References

1 Andrews LF. The straight-wire appliance. *Br. J. Orthod.* 1979;6:125–143.

2 Ireland AJ, Knight H, Sherriff M. An in vivo investigation into bond failure rates with a new self-etching primer system *Am. J. Orthod. Dentofacial Orthop.* 2003;124:323–326.

3 McLaughlin RP, Bennett JC. Bracket placement with the preadjusted appliance. *J. Clin. Orthod.* 1995;29:302–311.

4 McLaughlin RP, Bennet JC, Trevisi HJ. *Systemized Orthodontic Treatment Mechanics.* London: Mosby, 2001.

5 Armstrong D, Shen G, Petocz P, Darendeliler MA. A comparison of accuracy in bracket positioning between two techniques: localizing the centre of the clinical crown and measuring the distance from the incisal edge. *Eur. J. Orthod.* 2007;29:430–436.

6 Christensen LR, Cope JB. Digital technology for indirect bonding. *Semin. Orthod.* 2018;24:451–460.

7 Hodge TM, Dhopatkar AA, Rock WP, Spary DJ. A randomized clinical trial comparing the accuracy of direct versus indirect bracket placement. *J. Orthod.* 2004;31:132–137.

8 Deahl ST, Salome N, Hatch JP, Rugh JD. Practice-based comparison of direct and indirect bonding. *Am. J. Orthod. Dentofacial Orthop.* 2007;132:738–742.

9 Li Y, Mei L, Wei J, et al. Effectiveness, efficiency and adverse effects of using direct or indirect bonding technique in orthodontic patients: a systematic review and meta-analysis. *BMC Oral Health* 2019;19:137.

8

Bonding in Orthodontics
Declan Millett

CHAPTER OUTLINE

History, 147
Bonding Procedure, 148
  Bracket Types and Bonding, 148
  Enamel Preparation, 148
  Bonding Process after Enamel Etching, 150
Bonding to Artificial Substrates, 151
Indirect Bonding, 151
Bonding Adhesives, 152
Health Risks Associated with Bonding, 154
  Blue Lights, 154
  Cytotoxicity of Adhesives, 154
Effectiveness of Adhesives, 154
  Factors Affecting Clinical Bond Failure, 154
  Bonding of Orthodontic Brackets, 154
  Rebonding a Debonded Attachment, 154
  Bonding of Molar Tubes, 154
  Effectiveness of the Light-curing Units, 155
Debonding, 156
  Patient Appraisal, 156
  Procedure and Enamel Damage, 156
  Risks, 156
  Tooth Colour Change, 156
  Management of Demineralisation Lesions Post Debond, 156
Bonded Retainers, 157
  Types and Bonding, 157
  Adhesives for Bonding of Fixed Retainers, 157
Additional Uses of Bonding in Orthodontics, 158
Future Possibilities of Orthodontic Bonding, 158
Summary, 158
Acknowledgements, 159
Further Reading, 159
References, 159

History

Bonding was introduced to orthodontics in 1968 by Newman et al.[1] following acid etching of enamel[2] and the initiation of dental bonding.[3] It has since become routine.[4]

Previously, circumferential stainless steel bands with welded attachments cemented to individual teeth were the norm. Although banding of first permanent molars has been preferred by 60% of UK clinicians,[5] banding of upper first permanent molars has been adopted by less than one-third of US orthodontists.[6] As the focus of this chapter is on bonding in orthodontics, it is not the intention to discuss band cements other than to inform the reader of those currently used, their types and basic properties (Table 8.1 and Figure 8.1).

Preadjusted Edgewise Fixed Orthodontic Appliances: Principles and Practice, First Edition. Edited by Farhad B. Naini and Daljit S. Gill.
© 2022 John Wiley & Sons Ltd. Published 2022 by John Wiley & Sons Ltd.

Table 8.1 Currently used band cements and their properties.

Cement	Means of setting	Properties
Glass ionomer (GIC)	Acid–base reaction (ABR)	Brittle, low solubility, bond to enamel and metal, 24 hours to develop maximum compressive and tensile strength, release fluoride
Resin-modified GIC	ABR and photochemical	Low solubility, high tensile and polymerisation compressive strength
Poly-acid modified composite resins	light-cured	Low solubility, higher compressive and tensile strength than zinc phosphate, high fracture resistance

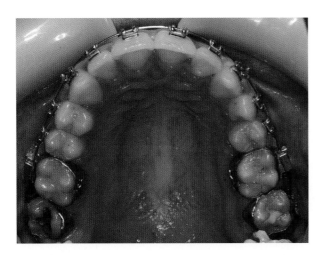

Figure 8.1 Bands cemented to upper first and second permanent molars with GIC.

Bonding has evolved in orthodontics from two-paste chemically cured to visible light-cured adhesives, and then to adhesive pre-coating, self-etching primers (SEPs), light-cured colour change adhesives, all-surface hydrophilic primers and flash-free adhesives (Figure 8.2).[7] The advantages of bonding over banding are listed in Table 8.2.

Although *in vitro* bond strength tests have been conducted as an initial assessment of new bonding adhesives to potentially guide clinical practice, well-designed and -conducted randomised clinical trials provide the ultimate assessment.[8] However, bond strength of no less than 6–8 MPa has been suggested for effective clinical practice.[4] Provision of analysis that predicts bond survival at different stresses may be a useful adjunct.[9]

Bonding Procedure

Bracket Types and Bonding

The most common types are metal and ceramic (Figure 8.3a). Stainless steel, titanium and gold variants exist. The bond to stainless steel relies on mechanical means, usually by a mesh base (Figure 8.3b), although micro-etched, laser-structured or integral bases exist.[10]

Table 8.2 Advantages and disadvantages of bonding over banding.

Advantages

Better aesthetics

No separation of teeth required

Improved patient comfort

Improved gingival/periodontal health

Precise placement possible

Removes enamel demineralisation risk under loose band (but see below)

Possible to bond partially erupted teeth

Mesiodistal enamel reduction possible

No interdental spaces post debond

Reduced inventory

Disadvantages

Enamel loss with etching and debonding clean-up

Possible enamel fracture during debonding

Greater likelihood of bracket debond than debanding

More preparation required to rebond a loose bracket than to re-cement a loose band

More time required for debonding than debanding

Enamel demineralisation around bonded attachment

Ceramic brackets, composed of either monocrystalline or polycrystalline aluminium oxide, are bonded chemically by a silane-coupling agent or mechanically by undercuts and grooves in the base (Figure 8.3c).

Attachments may be bonded directly or indirectly. While overtly simple, bonding by either means relies on (i) appropriate preparation of the bonding surfaces through *cleaning and conditioning*, (ii) possibly *sealing and priming*, and (iii) bonding of the attachment to the tooth surface via an *adhesive*, which has adequate bond strength and appropriate polymerisation.[11]

Enamel Preparation

Cleaning and Conditioning

Pumice prophylaxis prior to acid etching does not influence bond failure rate significantly.[12] As pumicing of clean

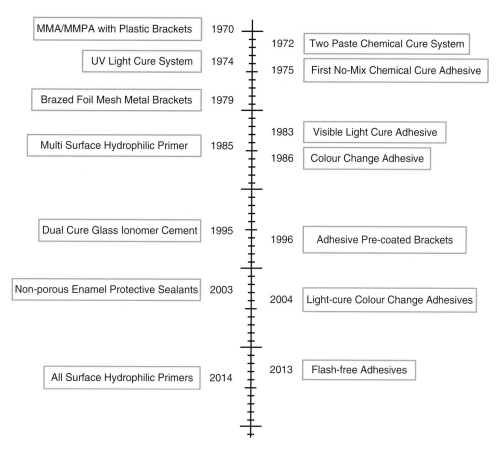

Figure 8.2 Chronological evolution in orthodontic bonding (1970 to present). Source: Gange P. The evolution of bonding in orthodontics. *Am. J. Orthod. Dentofacial Orthop.* 2015;147(4):S56–S63. © 2015, Elsevier.

enamel before bonding does not alter the etch pattern or bond strength significantly,[13] removal of any pellicle by this means seems advisable. Pumice prophylaxis, however, is essential prior to bonding with a self-etching primer.[14, 15]

Maintenance of a Dry Field

Antisialogogues are unnecessary.[16, 17] Saliva ejectors and Dri-Aids (Patterson Dental, St. Paul, MN, USA; Figure 8.4) placed over the parotid ducts are effective for full arch bonding.

Enamel Etching

Etching with 37% phosphoric acid for 15 seconds is sufficient for all teeth[12, 18, 19] (Figure 8.5), except molars where a 30-second etch is advisable.[20] The relationship of etch pattern to bond strength is complex and not completely understood.[21] For enamel more resistant to etching, longer than 15–30 seconds is required.[22] Gels (Figure 8.6a) give better control of the area to etch than liquid but enamel porosity does not appear to differ significantly between either;[23] localising the etch reduces susceptibility to development of white spot lesions.[24]

Special considerations (recommendations) with regard to bonding to primary teeth, acquired or developmental demineralisation, bleached teeth or those pre-exposed to fluoride are as follows.

- Primary teeth: sandblast with 50 μm alumina for three seconds, and then etch for 30 seconds with phosphoric acid gel.
- Acquired or developmental demineralisation: avoid or minimise etch, apply a sealant and bond directly.
- Bleached teeth: bond one to four weeks after bleaching,[25] as high post-bleaching enamel surface oxygen hinders free radical polymerisation.
- Teeth pre-exposed to fluoride: extra etching time[18] and micro-etching confer no benefit when using an adhesion promoter.[26, 27] With conventional etching, bond strength appears unchanged by fluoridation.[28]

Conventional etching removes 3–10 μm of enamel but deeper dissolution may reach beyond 100 μm;[29] however, etching is not damaging to enamel in the long term.

Crystal growth,[30] etching with maleic acid,[31] and laser etching[32] have been explored as alternatives but have not

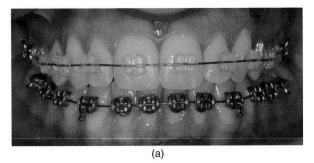

(a)

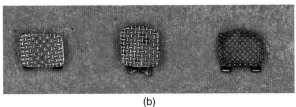

(b)

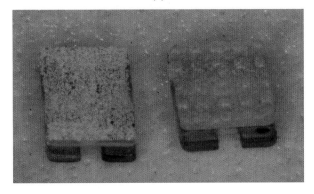

Figure 8.3 (a) Brackets: lower arch, stainless steel; upper arch, ceramic. (b) Roth, MBT and Damon Q brackets with mesh base. (c) Roth and MBT ceramic bracket bases.

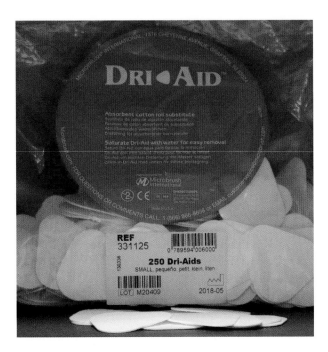

Figure 8.4 Dri-Aids used to control saliva flow from the parotid duct.

gained widespread acceptance. With lasers, enamel roughness depends on type and wavelength.[32]

Bonding Process after Enamel Etching

Use of an adhesive resin (resin primer) after etching and prior to bracket placement with a light-cured adhesive has attracted much attention in recent years;[33-35] without primer, less adhesive remains after debond but the effect on demineralisation is undetermined.[36]

Until further studies provide confirmation, once etched (Figure 8.6b) a thin layer of sealant (Figure 8.6c) is applied with a brush and light cured where moisture contamination is likely but is otherwise unnecessary; should this happen, air drying is only required prior to bracket placement. Brackets are bonded (Figure 8.6d), usually directly using a no-mix light-cured system.[5, 6] The bracket base should not be contaminated with oil from bare hands or by moisture.[28] Other than with adhesive pre-coated brackets (Figure 8.7a), adhesive resin is then applied to the bracket

base, ensuring undercuts and voids are filled, transferred to the tooth, positioned firmly to the labial or buccal surface before removal of excess resin prior to light curing.[37] The operating light should be turned away from the mouth and the adhesive during bracket transfer and prior to final positioning (Figure 8.6e).[28] Height measuring guides (Figure 8.8) assist placement.[38] Colour additive reduces excess adhesive,[39] but for a flash-free adhesive pre-coated system (Figure 8.7b) there is equivocal evidence regarding the adhesive remnant index despite operator preference for the latter.[40]

For light curing, the light source should be positioned as close as possible to the bracket base (Figure 8.9), then started for two seconds to maximise light energy. Bringing the light source into contact with the bracket is best to reduce divergent photon release. For metallic brackets, 10 seconds light curing (mesial and distal) is required, whereas for ceramic brackets only five seconds is necessary. With plasma-emulating light-emitting diodes (LEDs),[41] the rise in pulpal temperature is less profound than with longer exposure times.[42] For best results, the right combination of light source and resin is required.[43]

The occlusion must be checked prior to bonding the lower arch to avoid the risk of debonding. Occlusal build-up with either composite or glass ionomer cement may be required temporarily (Figure 8.10). Once bonding is complete, it is recommended that the patient rinse twice to reduce levels of bisphenol A that have leaked from

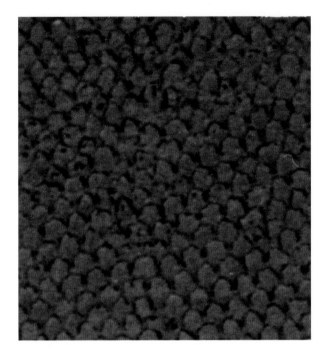

Figure 8.5 Scanning electron microsopy image of typical etch surface with 37% phosphoric acid etch. Source: courtesy of Dr R. Mattick.

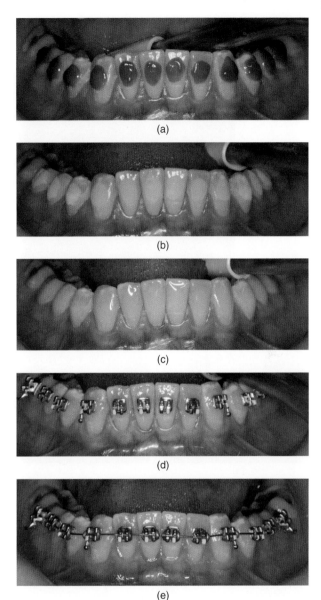

(a)

(b)

(c)

(d)

(e)

Figure 8.6 Bonding sequence: (a) enamel etching with 37% phosphoric acid gel; (b) frosted enamel surfaces after etching, washing and air drying; (c) primer applied to prepared enamel surfaces; (d) stainless steel brackets bonded; (e) initial aligning archwire placed and ligated with elastomeric ties.

the adhesive.[28] Aftercare instructions are then issued, including provision of wax to cushion against mucosal trauma and a 0.05% sodium fluoride mouthrinse for daily use (Figure 8.11).

Bonding to Artificial Substrates

The increase in adult orthodontics worldwide has brought a concomitant need for the ability to bond metal attachments reliably to artificial substrates such as large composite restorations, amalgam, gold and porcelain. Recommendations regarding bonding to these surfaces are summarised in Table 8.3.

Indirect Bonding

Described in 1972 by Silverman and Cohen[48] and presented in 1979 by Thomas,[49] this involves initially the creation of a stone model from an impression or digital scan of the dental arch, to which a separating medium is applied, a bracket is then attached to each tooth with resin adhesive;[50–52] these are conveyed to the mouth via a transfer tray (Figure 8.12), silicone being more accurate than double vacuum forms.[53] Brackets are bonded with a chemically

cured or light-cured adhesive. Differing composite/sealant combinations have been used, such as a thermally cured base composite with a chemically cured sealant or light-cured base composite with a chemically cured sealant.[54]

Advantages of indirect over direct bonding include improved bracket height positioning[55, 56] and savings in time.[57] Similar rates of bracket failure have been reported.[58, 59]

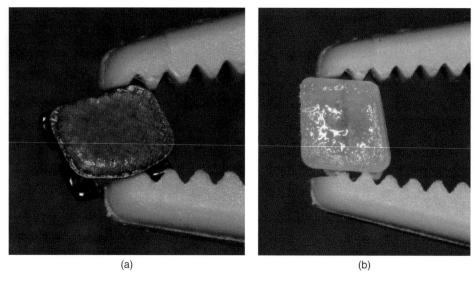

(a) (b)

Figure 8.7 Adhesive pre-coated (a) stainless steel bracket base (MBT prescription); (b) flash-free ceramic bracket base (MBT prescription).

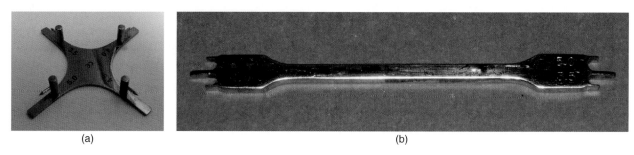

(a) (b)

Figure 8.8 Bracket height measuring gauges: (a) Boone; (b) 3M.

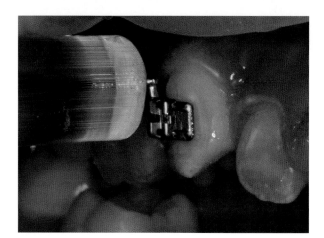

Figure 8.9 Light source positioned close to bracket for curing of adhesive.

Bonding Adhesives

These can be broadly subdivided into composite and glass ionomer, each of which may be either chemically or

light-cured. The majority of composite resins are founded on bisphenol A glycidyl methacrylate (bis-GMA).

- *Chemically cured no-mix composite* (Figure 8.13a): contains a benzoyl peroxide initiator that reacts with a tertiary amine and sets when primer on the etched surface is brought into contact with composite on the already primed bracket base and maintained in position through application of light pressure.

- *Light-cured composite* (Figure 8.13b): now the most popular bonding agent, comprising a matrix co-monomer system of bis-GMA/TEGDMA, curing starts on activation of a photoinitiator (mostly a camphoroquinone, 0.2–1% in the resin) by visible blue light of 470 nm wavelength.[60] 1-Phenyl-1,2-propanedione (PPD) has replaced camphoroquinone in some light-cured composites due to the yellowish tint of the latter.[61]

- *Primer*: usually an unfilled resin, this may be applied to the etched enamel surface and used with chemically cured or light-cured composite. Polymerisation occurs by chemical or light activation. The need for primer application after etching has been questioned;[33]

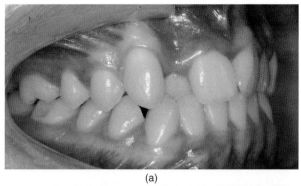

(a)

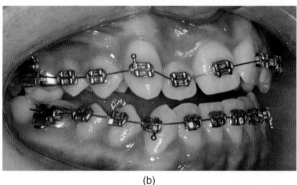

(b)

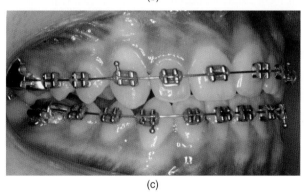

(c)

Figure 8.10 (a) Maxillary right lateral incisor in crossbite. (b) Temporary occlusal build-up of maxillary first molars with GIC to facilitate anterior crossbite correction. (c) Crossbite corrected.

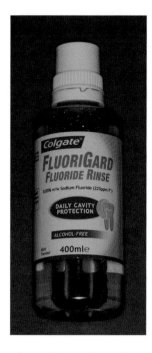

Figure 8.11 Fluoride mouthrinse. Source: Colgate-Palmolive.

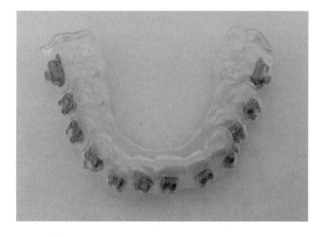

Figure 8.12 Brackets and molar tubes positioned in thermoplastic tray prior to indirect bonding.

however, primer application decreases the need for an absolute dry operating field while also filling in deficiencies at the enamel–adhesive interface. The addition of silver nanoparticles in pursuit of prevention of demineralisation has not compromised bond strength.[62]

- Moisture-insensitive primer (MIP): a light-cured hydrophilic unfilled resin capable of successful bonding in the presence of some moisture;[63] application after enamel preparation but prior to any saliva contamination and use with the relevant bonding adhesive is necessary for bonding to be effective.[64] Bond failure rate with (3.1%) and without (5.5%) Transbond™ MIP (3M Unitek) was similar over 18 months.[35]

- *Chemically cured glass ionomer (polyalkenoate)* (Figure 8.14a): composed of three elements (ion-leachable glass, polymeric water-soluble acid and water), setting takes two to three minutes via an acid–base reaction.[65] Poor bond strength makes these cements unsuitable for routine orthodontic bonding.[66]

- *Light-cured (resin-modified) glass ionomer* (Figure 8.14b): composed of both glass ionomer and composite components, setting is by chemical reaction and light activation of HEMA groups which induces free radical polymerisation. Despite superior bond strength

Table 8.3 Recommended methodology of bonding to composite, amalgam, gold and porcelain.

Substrate	Bonding procedure
Composite	Air dry, roughen with a fine diamond bur, consider intermediate primer, conventional bonding agent
Amalgam [45]	*Amalgam only:* sandblast[(a)] use 4-META intermediate resin (Reliance Metal[(b)] primer sealant, conventional bonding agent
	Amalgam with intact surrounding enamel: sandblast[(a)] amalgam, etch enamel with 37% phosphoric acid, sealant, conventional bonding agent
Gold[45, 46]	Sandblast[(a)] apply All-bond primers A and B (Bisco Inc., Schaumburg, IL, USA) or 4-META primer[(b)] conventional bonding agent or Panavia Ex and Panavia 21 (Kuray America Inc., New York, NY, USA)
Porcelain[45]	Sandblast[(a)] 9.6% HF acid gel or 37% phosphoric acid gel,[47] silane coupling agent (optional), conventional bonding agent

(a) With 50 μm alumina oxide for two to four seconds,
(b) Bisco-Z Prime Plus may be used universally as a primer to enhance adhesion with porcelain or metal and resin adhesives;
Source: Zachrisson BU, Buyukyilmaz T. Bonding in orthodontics. In: Graber TM, Vanarsdall R, Vig K (eds). *Orthodontics: Current Principles and Techniques*, 6th edn. St Louis, MO: Mosby, 2016: 812–867. © 2016, Elsevier.

to conventional glass ionomers, these adhesives have gained limited use.[5, 6]

- *Self-etching primer (SEP)* (Figure 8.15): the bond to enamel appears to be primarily chemical to calcium ions,[64] which complex with the primer on polymerisation with no obvious tag indentation of either core or prism (see Figure 8.5).[44] Compared to conventional acid etch and excluding time for pumice prophylaxis, SEP results in an eight-minute time saving for full-mouth bond-up but over 12 months there is a slightly higher odds of bond failure.[67, 68] Evidence regarding demineralisation is conflicting.[69, 70]

Health Risks Associated with Bonding

Blue Lights

It appears that any biological effects are restricted to the long term. Owing to the range of effects, vigilance is advised with use of high-energy plasma lamps when bonding molar tubes due to closeness to the mucosa.[61]

Cytotoxicity of Adhesives

Evidence is inconclusive for adhesives presently available, with no undue cause for alarm.[71] Concern has focused on the potential cytotoxicity of unreacted residual monomer in orthodontic composites and resin-modified glass ionomer cements.[72, 73] No elution of bisphenol A or any oestrogenic effect has been recorded.[74, 75] Advice is to rinse thoroughly with water twice after bracket bonding, since this returned bisphenol A levels to those before bonding.[71] Grinding adhesive at debond may hasten the production of bisphenol A.[61] Evidence-based measures are commended to keep exposure to bisphenol A to a minimum in the patient and orthodontic team members.[76]

Effectiveness of Adhesives

Factors Affecting Clinical Bond Failure

Bond failure rate is affected by factors related to the operator, patient, tooth and adhesive. Conflicting findings exist regarding the influence of each but greater bond failure was recorded with customised than non-customised labial appliances.[77]

Bonding of Orthodontic Brackets

Mandall et al.[78] found insufficient evidence to support the use of one type of adhesive over another with regard to failure rate or prevention of demineralisation around the bonded brackets. Demineralisation data did not support superiority of resin-modified glass-ionomer cement (RMGIC) over light-cured composite.[79] However, RMGIC had a rougher surface and may cause greater bacterial adhesion than composite or compomer.[80]

Rebonding a Debonded Attachment

Following removal of residual adhesive and enamel clean-up with a tungsten carbide bur (Figure 8.16), the enamel should be re-etched with 37% phosphoric acid and bonding undertaken as originally with a replacement bracket. The same topographical changes with etching will not occur due to resin remnants obstructing the prism cores. If the bracket slot is not distorted, some operators may opt to sandblast the debonded bracket base to remove adhesive remnants and then rebond with conventional adhesives.

Bonding of Molar Tubes

Over the full course of treatment, failure of molar tubes bonded with a chemically cured or a light-cured adhesive

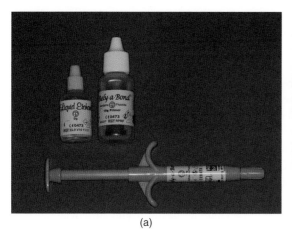 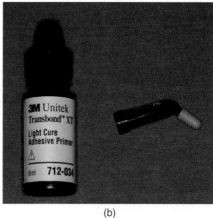

Figure 8.13 Examples of (a) chemical-cured (Rely-a-bond) and (b) light-cured (Transbond) composites.

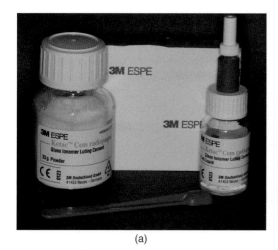 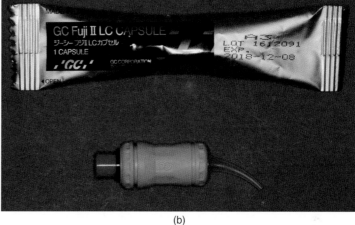

Figure 8.14 (a) Conventional and (b) resin-modified glass ionomer cements.

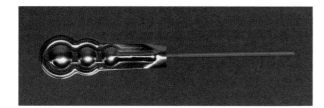

Figure 8.15 Self-etching primer.

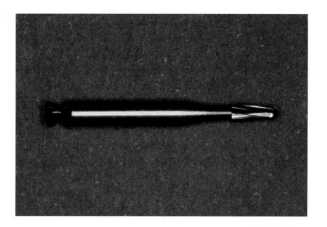

Figure 8.16 Tungsten carbide bur.

was greater than that of first molar bands cemented with glass ionomer cement.[81] However, over 12 months, failure of molar tubes bonded with a light-cured adhesive was similar to first molar bands with a conventional glass ionomer cement.[82] Assessed over 15 months, first and second molar tubes (Figure 8.17) bonded with SEP and a light cured adhesive had a similar failure rate to those bonded with a conventional acid etch technique.[83]

Effectiveness of the Light-curing Units

Following bond failure over at least six months of treatment, evidence does not favour one particular light

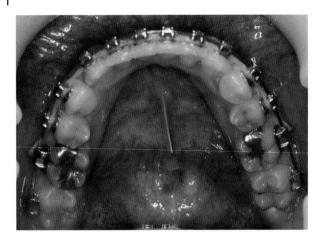

Figure 8.17 Tubes bonded to lower first and second permanent molars.

source.[67] LEDs are most commonly used with a narrow wavelength of about 460 nm and power ranging between 1 and 3200 mW/cm^2; their functioning over a long working life requires little power.[84]

Debonding

Patient Appraisal

Prior to bonding, enamel fracture lines should be identified to the patient, who should then be re-appraised of their presence prior to debond. Debonding increases tooth sensitivity for the following seven days and is greater for teeth with visible enamel microcracks.[85] Teeth with large composite or amalgam restorations, and those with a porcelain laminate or full coronal restoration are at risk of restoration fracture and may require replacement.

Procedure and Enamel Damage

Stainless steel brackets can be easily and gently removed by first applying a compressing force in a mesiodistal direction and then peeling the bracket from the tooth surface while maintaining the bracket ligated to the archwire throughout;[44] a lift-off instrument produced the least discomfort but the archwire was removed prior to debonding.[86] Alternatively a bracket-removal pliers may be used (Figure 8.18).

Mechanically, rather than chemically, retained ceramic brackets run a lesser risk of enamel fracture[87] and likelihood of enamel tear-outs.[88] Those retained mechanically and designed with a vertical slot can 'crumple' when gripped mesiodistally. A single pulse Er:YAG laser has proved effective and safe for debonding ceramic brackets.[89]

The adhesive remaining on the enamel (Figure 8.18c) must be removed. Careful light strokes with a tapered tungsten carbide bur (Figure 8.18d) nonetheless removes some enamel and leaves the enamel scratched;[90, 91] however, the latter is reduced by using a proprietary kit.[92] Ultraviolet light facilitates greater adhesive removal.[91] Sof-Lex discs and a pumice slurry or an enamel polishing kit[93] are recommended[91] but 0.1–0.2 mm^3 of adhesive remains (Figure 8.18c).[94] Removal of these resin remnants is facilitated by use of Stainbuster burs (Figure 8.19). The teeth should then be polished using either a prophylaxis paste or pumice slurry (Figure 8.18e,f). Enamel loss during debonding, clean-up and prophylaxis varies according to the method used, but can be kept to a minimum.[95, 96]

Risks

Debonding presents risks to the eyes and airway. Eye protection must be worn by both operator and patient during debonding especially of ceramic brackets in order to avoid ceramic shards. Keeping the bracket tied to the archwire during debonding is preferable for all bracket types to avoid the risk of ingestion or inhalation. Aerosol generated during adhesive removal runs an attendant risk of inhalation of small particles such as silica.[97]

Tooth Colour Change

Very low quality evidence shows that tooth colour alteration, while not reliably obvious clinically, might be linked to orthodontic treatment. This was greater with chemically cured than with light-cured composite and most common on the maxillary lateral incisor.[98]

Management of Demineralisation Lesions Post Debond

The appearance of the lesions (Figure 8.20) is likely to halve in size in the first six months post debond,[99] with improved access for oral hygiene. High-concentration fluoride varnish (Figure 8.21) is contraindicated; this hypermineralises the lesion, reduces enamel porosity and arrests natural healing from saliva, making the lesion more noticeable.[100] The application of Tooth Mousse (Recaldent, comprising casein phosphopeptide and amorphous calcium phosphate; Figure 8.22) did not improve lesion healing one-year post debond.[101]

Recalcitrant white-spot lesions may be treated by microabrasion and resin infiltration with a low-viscosity resin that is based on triethylene glycol dimethacrylate (TEGDMA). This produces more sustained colour change than microabrasion.[102, 103]

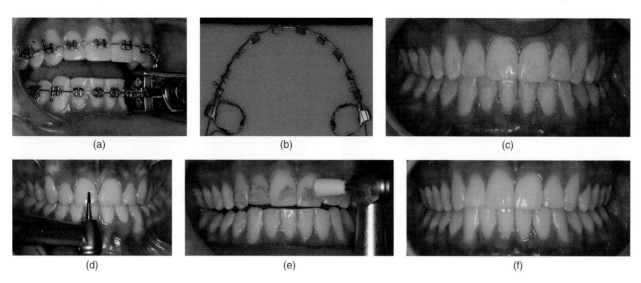

Figure 8.18 Debonding sequence: (a) debonding pliers applied to bracket; (b) brackets debonded ligated to the archwire; (c) adhesive remaining on enamel following bracket removal; (d) tungsten carbide bur in contra-angle handpiece for adhesive removal (another patient); (e) enamel polishing; (f) final appearance.

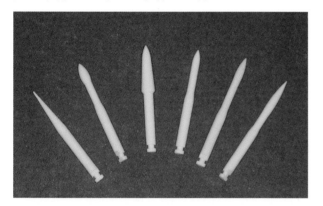

Figure 8.19 Stainbuster burs.

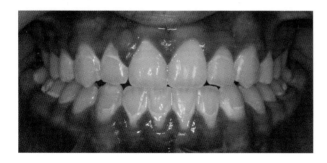

Figure 8.20 Enamel demineralisation visible on several teeth following bracket debonding.

Bonded Retainers

Types and Bonding

While plain orthodontic wire, either round or rectangular, has been used as a fixed retainer, multistrand wire (Figure 8.23) custom-made or commercially available

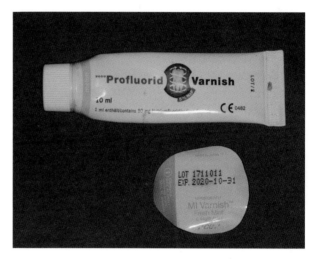

Figure 8.21 Fluoride varnish. Source: GC America Inc.

is now most commonly adopted;[104, 105] fibre-reinforced composite[106] and polyethylene ribbon[107] have also been utilised but the failure rate of the former means it is not recommended.

A fixed retainer may be bonded directly or indirectly with no significant difference in risk of failure at six months[108] or over 24 months between either technique.[109] However, indirect bonding is quicker.[106] The mean failure risk of retainers bonded to canines only versus those bonded to incisors and canines was similar (0.25 vs. 0.29, respectively).[110]

Adhesives for Bonding of Fixed Retainers

Chemically cured or light-cured adhesives perform equally well.[111] Adhesives used to bond fixed retainers must withstand long-term exposure to the oral environment

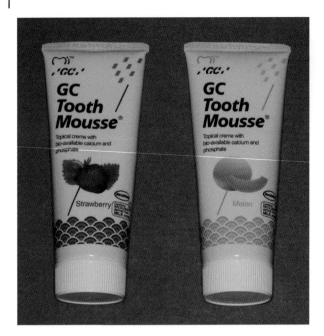

Figure 8.22 Tooth Mousse. Source: GC America Inc.

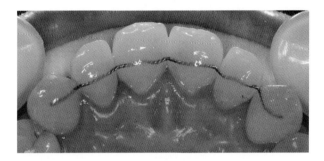

Figure 8.23 Upper bonded retainer.

as well as satisfying patient comfort and possessing abrasion resistance. Light-cured adhesives may achieve this (Figure 8.24).[112] Minimal polymerisation shrinkage, high bond strength and hardness are essential to minimise microleakage and elution of unreacted monomers.[61]

Additional Uses of Bonding in Orthodontics

Resin-modified glass ionomer may be bonded temporarily to posterior teeth to prop the occlusion for crossbite (anterior or posterior) correction during fixed appliance therapy (see Figure 8.10) or to retain a removable appliance for rapid maxillary expansion with Class III protraction. To

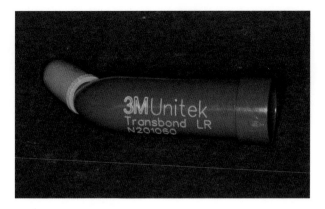

Figure 8.24 Light-cured adhesive for bonded retainer. Source: 3M.

facilitate removal, it is advisable to confine etch to the cuspal areas.

Future Possibilities of Orthodontic Bonding

Smart bonding agents, capable of detecting plaque and which change colour when oral hygiene levels fall, are an exciting prospect. The development of biometric bonding adhesives which are 'enamel-friendly', ideally capable of self-repair and self-cleaning, are similarly of great interest.[113]

Smart brackets with microsensors[114, 115] exist but whether their base could detect inadequacies or microleakage in the bonding layer is yet to be explored.

Composites containing nano-amorphous calcium phosphate[116] and the addition of niobium pentoxide phosphate invert glass[117] also offer exciting possibilities regarding prevention of demineralisation. Novel bisphenol A-free adhesives may also be an area for further exploration with orthodontic retainers.

Summary

Unsurprisingly, over the past five decades, bonding in orthodontics has advanced at a pace in line with developments in restorative dentistry, dental materials science and technology in general. As these continue to evolve with input from other disciplines, further efforts will be made in the challenge towards the optimal bonding adhesive that removes the need for enamel conditioning, retains adequate bond strength in wet and dry conditions while on debond does not affect enamel colour, as well as being self-cleaning or alerting and preventing demineralisation during treatment. A tall order indeed.

Acknowledgements

Dr Siobhan McMorrow, Dr Paul Dowling, Dr Jackie Clune, Dr Raphy Paul, Dr Rye Mattick, Dr Michael Ormond and Dr J. Donovan are thanked for their assistance with the illustrations. Particular thanks are due to Ms Niamh Kelly for her expertise with the bibliography and editing of the text/photographic material.

Further Reading

Eliades T, Sifakakis L. Clinically relevant aspects of dental materials science in orthodontics. In: Eliades T, Brantley WA (eds). *Orthodontic Applications of Biomaterials: A Clinical Guide*. Duxford, UK: Woodhead Publishing, 2016: 187–199.

Gange P. The evolution of bonding in orthodontics. *Am. J. Orthod. Dentofac Orthop.* 2015;147:S56–S63.

Miles PG, Eliades T, Pandis N. Bonding and adhesives in orthodontics. In: Miles PG, Rinchuse DJ, Rinchuse DJ (eds). *Evidence-based Clinical Orthodontics. Hanover Park, IL: Quintessence Publishing Company Inc.*, 2012: 17–29.

Zachrisson BU, Usumez S, Buyukyilmaz T. Bonding in orthodontics. In: Graber LW, Vanarsdall RV, Vig KWL, Huang GJ (eds). *Orthodontics: Current Principles and Techniques*, 6th edn. St. Louis, MO: Elsevier, 2016: 812–867.

References

1 Newman GV, Snyder WH, Wilson CE Jr. Acrylic adhesives for bonding attachments to tooth surfaces. *Angle Orthod.* 1968;38:12–18.

2 Buonocore MG, Matsui A, Gwinnett AJ. Penetration of resin dental materials into enamel surfaces with reference to bonding. *Arch. Oral Biol.* 1968;13:61–70.

3 Bowen RL. Use of epoxy resins in restorative materials. *J. Dent. Res.* 1956;35:360–369.

4 Reynolds IR. A review of direct orthodontic bonding. *Br. J. Orthod.* 1975 ;2:171–178.

5 Banks P, Elton V, Jones Y, et al. The use of fixed appliances in the UK: a survey of specialist orthodontists. *J. Orthod.* 2010;37:43–55.

6 Keim RG, Gottlieb EL, Vogels DS. JCO study of orthodontic diagnosis and treatment procedures, part 1: results and trends. *J. Clin. Orthod.* 2014;48:607–630.

7 Gange P. The evolution of bonding in orthodontics. *Am. J. Orthod. Dentofacial Orthop.* 2015;147: S56–S63.

8 Eliades T, Brantley WA. The inappropriateness of conventional orthodontic bond strength assessment protocols. *Eur. J. Orthod.* 2000;22:13–23.

9 Miles PG. Does microetching enamel reduce bracket failure when indirect bonding mandibular posterior teeth? *Aust. Orthod. J.* 2008;24:1–4.

10 Sharma-Sayal SK, Rossouw PE, Kulkarni GV, Titley KC. The influence of orthodontic bracket base design on shear bond strength. *Am. J. Orthod. Dentofacial Orthop.* 2003;124:74–82.

11 Lopes GC, Greenhaugh D, Klauss P, et al. Enamel acid etching: a review. *Compend. Contin. Educ. Dent.* 2007;28:18–24.

12 Barry GR. A clinical investigation of the effects of omission of pumice prophylaxis on band and bond failure. *Br. J. Orthod.* 1995;22:245–248.

13 Ireland AJ, Sherriff M. The effect of pumicing on the in vivo use of a resin modified glass poly (alkenoate) cement and a conventional composite for bonding orthodontic brackets. *J. Orthod.* 2002;29:217–220.

14 Burgess AM, Sherriff M, Ireland AJ. Self-etching primers: is prophylactic pumicing necessary? *Angle Orthod.* 2006;76:114–118.

15 Grover S, Sidhu MS, Prabhakar M. Evaluation of fluoride varnish and its comparison with pumice prophylaxis using self-etching primer in orthodontic bonding: an in vivo study. *Eur. J. Orthod.* 2012;34:198–201.

16 Ponduri S, Turnbull N, Birnie D, et al. Does atropine sulfate improve orthodontic bond survival? A randomized clinical trial. *Am. J. Orthod. Dentofacial Orthop.* 2007;132:663–670.

17 Roelofs T, Merkens N, Roelofs J, et al. A retrospective survey of the causes of bracket and tube bonding failures. *Angle Orthod.* 2017;87:111–117.

18 Brannstrom M, Nordenvall KJ, Malmgren O. The effect of various pre-treatment methods of the enamel in bonding procedures. *Am. J. Orthod.* 1978;74:522–530.

19 Kinch AP, Taylor H, Warltier R, et al. A clinical trial comparing the failure rates of directly bonded brackets using etch times of 15 or 60 seconds. *Am. J. Orthod. Dentofacial Orthop.* 1988;94:476–483.

20 Johnston CD, Burden DJ, Hussey DL, Mitchell CA. Bonding to molars: the effect of etch time (an in vitro study). *Eur. J. Orthod.* 1998;20:195–199.

21 Hobson RS, McCabe JF. Relationship between enamel etch characteristics and resin–enamel bond strength. *Br. Dent. J.* 2002;192:463–468.

22 Nordenvall KJ, Brannstrom M, Malmgren O. Etching of deciduous teeth and young and old permanent teeth. A comparison between 15 and 60 seconds of etching. *Am. J. Orthod.* 1980;78:99–108.

23 Brannstrom M, Malmgren O, Nordenvall KJ. Etching of young permanent teeth with an acid gel. *Am. J. Orthod.* 1982;82:379–383.

24 Knosel M, Bojes M, Jung K, Ziebolz D. Increased susceptibility for white spot lesions by surplus orthodontic etching exceeding bracket base area. *Am. J. Orthod. Dentofacial Orthop.* 2012;141:574–582.

25 de Rego MV, dos Santos RM, Leal LMP, Braga CGS. Evaluation of the influence of dental bleaching with 35% hydrogen peroxide in orthodontic bracket shear bond strength. *Dental Press J. Orthod.* 2013;18:95–100.

26 Noble J, Karaiskos NE, Wiltshire WA. In vivo bonding of orthodontic brackets to fluorosed teeth using an adhesion promoter. *Angle Orthod.* 2008;78:357–360.

27 Endo T, Ishida R, Komatsuzaki A, et al. Effects of long-term repeated topical fluoride applications and adhesions promoter on shear bond strengths of orthodontic brackets. *Eur. J. Dent.* 2014;8:431–436.

28 Cai Z, Iijima M, Eliades T, Brantley WA. Frequent handling mistakes during bonding. In: Eliades T, Brantley WA (eds). *Orthodontic Applications of Biomaterials: A Clinical Guide.* Duxford, UK: Woodhead Publishing, 2016: 171–177.

29 Burapavong V, Marshall GW, Apfel DA. Enamel surface characteristics on removal of bonded orthodontic brackets. *Am. J. Orthod.* 1978;74:176–187.

30 Read MJ, Ferguson JW, Watts DC. Direct bonding: crystal growth as an alternative to acid etching. *Eur. J. Orthod.* 1986;8:118–122.

31 Bas-kalkan A, Orhan M, Usumez S. The effects of enamel etching with different acids on the bond strength of metallic acids. *Turkish J. Orthod.* 2007;20:35–42.

32 Sağır S, Usumez A, Ademci E, Usumez S. Effect of enamel laser irradiation at different pulse settings on shear bond strength of orthodontic brackets. *Angle Orthod.* 2013;83(6):973–980.

33 Nandhra S, Littlewood S, Houghton H, et al. Do we need a primer for orthodontic bonding? A randomized controlled trial. *Eur. J. Orthod.* 2014;37:147–155.

34 Altmann AS, Degrazia FW, Celeste RK, et al. Orthodontic bracket bonding without previous adhesive priming: a meta-regression analysis. *Angle Orthod.* 2016;86:391–398.

35 Bazargani F, Magnuson A, Löthgren H, Kowalczyk A. Orthodontic bonding with and without primer: a randomized controlled trial. *Eur. J. Orthod.* 2016;38:503–507.

36 Eliades T. Do we need a randomized controlled trial to assess trivial, albeit standard used, clinical steps in bonding? The answer is yes, but there are some interpretation issues. *Eur. J. Orthod.* 2014;37:156–157.

37 Usumez S, Erverdi N. Adhesives and bonding in orthodontics. In: Nanda R, Kapila S (eds). *Current Therapy in Orthodontics.* St Louis, MO: Mosby, 2009: 45–67.

38 Armstrong D, Shen G, Petocz P, Darendellier MA. A comparison of accuracy in bracket placement positioning between two techniques: localizing the centre of the clinical crown and measuring the distance from the incisal edge. *Eur. J. Orthod.* 2007;29:430–436.

39 Armstrong D, Shen G, Petrocz P, Darendellier MA. Excess adhesive flash upon bracket placement. A typodont study comparing APC PLUS and Transbond XT. *Angle Orthod.* 2007;77:1101–1108.

40 Grunheld T, Sudit GN, Larson BE. Debonding and adhesive remnant clean up: an in vitro comparison of bond quality, adhesive remnant clean up and orthodontic acceptance of a flash-free product. *Eur. J. Orthod.* 2015;35:497–502.

41 Corekci B, Irgin C, Halicioglu K, et al. Effects of plasma-emulating light-emitting diode (LED) versus conventional LED on cytotoxic effects and polymerization capacity of orthodontic composites. *Hum. Exp. Toxicol.* 2014;33:1000–1007.

42 Ramoglu SI, Karamehmetoglu H, Sari T, Usumez S. Temperature rise caused in the pulp chamber under simulated intrapulpal microcirculation with different light-curing modes. *Angle Orthod.* 2015;85:381–385.

43 Roulet J-F, Price R. Light curing guidelines for practitioners: a consensus statement from the 2014 symposium on light curing in dentistry, Dalhousie University, Halifax, *Canada. J. Adhes. Dent.* 2014;16:303–304.

44 Zachrisson BU, Buyukyilmaz T. Bonding in orthodontics. In: Graber TM, Vanarsdall R, Vig K (eds). *Orthodontics: Current Principles and Techniques*, 6th edn. St Louis, MO: Mosby, 2016: 812–867.

45 Zachrisson BU, Buyukilmaz T. Recent advances in bonding to gold, amalgam and porcelain. *J. Clin. Orthod.* 1993;27:661–665.

46 Büyükyilmaz T, Zachrisson YO, Zachrisson BU. Improving orthodontic bonding to gold alloy. *Am. J. Orthod. Dentofacial Orthop.* 1995;108:510–518.

47 Bourke BM, Rock WP. Factors affecting the shear bond strength of orthodontic brackets to porcelain. *J. Orthod.* 1999;26:285–290.

48 Silverman E, Cohen M. A report on a major improvement in the indirect bonding technique. *J. Clin. Orthod.* 1975;9:270–276.

49 Thomas RG. Indirect bonding: simplicity in action. *J. Clin. Orthod.* 1979;13:93–106.

50 Klocke A, Shi J, Kahl-Nieke B, Bismayer U. In vitro investigation of indirect boding with a hydrophilic primer. *Angle Orthod.* 2003;73:445–450.

51 Polat O, Karaman AI, Buyukyilmaz T. In vitro evaluation of shear bond strengths and in vivo analysis of bond survival of indirect-bonding resins. *Angle Orthod.* 2004;74:405–409.

52 Cozzani M, Menini A, Bertelli A. Etching masks for precise indirect bonding. *J. Clin. Orthod.* 2010;44:326–330.

53 Schmid J, Brenner D, Recheis W, et al. Transfer accuracy of two indirect bonding techniques: an in vitro study with 3D scanned models. *Eur. J. Orthod.* 2018;40:549–555.

54 Aksakalli S, Demir A. Indirect bonding: a literature review. *Eur. J. Gen. Dent.* 2012;1:6–9.

55 Koo BC, Chung CH, Vanarsdall RL. Comparison of the accuracy of the bracket placement between direct and indirect bonding techniques. *Am. J. Orthod. Dentofacial Orthop.* 1999;116:346–351.

56 Kalange JT, Thomas RH. Indirect bonding: a comprehensive review of the literature. *Semin. Orthod.* 2007;13:3–10.

57 Aguirre MJ, King GJ, Waldron JM. Assessment of bracket placement and bond strength when comparing direct bonding to indirect bonding techniques. *Am. J. Orthod.* 1982;82:269–276.

58 Bozelli JV, Bigliazzi R, Barbosa HA, et al. Comparative study on direct and indirect bracket bonding techniques regarding time length and bracket detachment. *Dental Press J. Orthod.* 2013;18:51–57.

59 Menini A, Cozzani M, Sfondrini MF, et al. A 15-month evaluation of bond failures of orthodontic brackets bonded with direct and indirect bonding technique: a clinical trial. *Prog. Orthod.* 2014;15:67.

60 Mitchell L. Orthodontic bonding adhesives. *J. Orthod.* 1994;21:79–82.

61 Eliades T, Sifakakis L. Clinically relevant aspects of dental materials science in orthodontics. In: Graber LW, Vanarsdall RV, Vig KWL, Huang GJ (eds). *Orthodontics: Current Principles and Techniques*, 6th edn. St. Louis, MO: Elsevier, 2016: 187–199.

62 Blöcher S, Frankenberger R, Hellak A, et al. Effect on enamel shear bond strength of adding microsilver and nanosilver particles to the primer of an orthodontic adhesive. *BMC Oral Health* 2015;15:42.

63 Shukla C, Maurya R, Jain U, et al. Moisture-insensitive primer: a myth or truth. *J. Orthod. Sci.* 2014;3:132–136.

64 Swartz ML. Orthodontic bonding. *Orthod. Select* 2004;16:1–4.

65 Sidhu SK, Nicholson JW. A review of glass-ionomer cements for clinical dentistry. *J. Funct. Biomater.* 2016;7:1–15.

66 Millett DT, McCabe JF. Orthodontic bonding with glass ionomer cements: a review. *Eur. J. Orthod.* 1996;18:385–399.

67 Fleming PS, Johal A, Pandis N. Self-etching primers and conventional acid-etch technique for orthodontic bonding: a systematic review and meta-analysis. *Am. J. Orthod. Dentofacial Orthop.* 2014;142:83–94.

68 Hu H, Li C, Li F, et al. Enamel etching for bonding fixed orthodontic braces. *Cochrane Database Syst. Rev.* 2013;(11):CD005516.

69 Ghiz MA, Ngan P, Kao E, et al. Effects of sealant and self-etching primer on enamel decalcification. Part II. An in-vivo study. *Am. J. Orthod. Dentofacial Orthop.* 2009;135:199–205.

70 Visel D, Jacker T, Jost-Brinkmann PG, Präger TM. Demineralization adjacent to orthodontic brackets after application of conventional and self-etching primer systems. *J. Orofac. Orthop.* 2014;75:358–373.

71 Kloukos D, Pandis N, Eliades T. Bisphenol -A and residual monomer leaching from orthodontic adhesive resins and polycarbonate brackets: a systematic review. *Am. J. Orthod. Dentofacial Orthop.* 2013;143:S104–S112.e1-e2.

72 Goldberg M. In vitro and in vivo studies on the toxicity of dental resin components: a review. *Clin. Oral Investig.* 2008;12:1–8.

73 Tsitrou E, Kelogrigoris S, Koulaouzidou E, et al. Effect of extraction media and storage time on the elution of monomers from four contemporary resin composite materials. *Toxicol. Int.* 2014;21:89–95.

74 Eliades T, Hiskia A, Eliades G, Athanasiou AE. Assessment of bisphenol A release from orthodontic adhesives. *Am. J. Orthod. Dentofacial Orthop.* 2007;131:72–75.

75 Eliades T, Gioni V, Kletas D, et al. Oestrogenicity of orthodontic adhesive resins. *Eur. J. Orthod.* 2007;29:404–417.

76 Eliades T. Bisphenol A and orthodontics: an update of evidence-based measures to minimize exposure for the orthodontic team and patients. *Am. J. Orthod. Dentofac Orthop.* 2017;152:435–441.

77 Penning EW, Peerlings RHJ, Govers JDM, et al. Orthodontics with customized versus non customized appliances: a randomized controlled clinical trial. *J. Dent. Res.* 2017;96:1498–1504.

78 Mandall NA, Hickman J, Macfarlane TV, et al. Adhesives for fixed orthodontic brackets. *Cochrane Database Syst. Rev.* 2018;(4):CD002282.

79 Benson PE, Alexander-Abt J, Cotter S, et al. Resin-modified glass ionomer cement versus composite for orthodontic bonding: a multi-centre single blind randomized controlled trial. *Am. J. Orthod. Dentofacial Orthop.* 2019;155:10–18.

80 Jung-Sub An, Kyungsun K, Soha Cho, et al. Compositional differences in multi-species biofilms formed on various orthodontic adhesives. *Eur. J. Orthod.* 2017;39:528–533.

81 Millett DT, Mandall NA, Mattick RCR, et al. Adhesives for bonded molar tubes during fixed brace treatment. *Cochrane Database Syst. Rev.* 2017;(2):CD008236.

82 Oeiras VJ, Almeida e Silva VA, Azevedo LA, et al. Survival analysis of banding and bonding molar tubes in adult patients over a 12-month period: a split-mouth randomized clinical trial. *Braz. Oral Res.* 2016;30:e136.

83 Pandis N, Polychronopoulou A, Eliades T. A comparative assessment of the failure rate of molar tubes bonded with a self-etching primer and conventional acid-etching. *World J. Orthod.* 2006;7:41–44.

84 Mills RW, Jandt KD, Ashworth SH. Dental composite depth of cure with halogen and blue light emitting diode technology. *Br. Dent. J.* 1999;186:388–391.

85 Dumbryte I, Linkeviciene L, Linkevicius T, Malinauskas M. Does orthodontic debonding lead to tooth sensitivity? Comparison of teeth with and without enamel microcracks. *Am. J. Orthod. Dentofacial Orthop.* 2017;151:284–291.

86 Pithon MM, Figueiredo DSF, Oliveira DDM, Coqueiro R da S. What is the best method for debonding metallic brackets from the patient's perspective? *Prog. Orthod.* 2015;16:17.

87 Winchester LJ. Bond strengths of five different ceramic brackets: an in vitro study. *Br. J. Orthod.* 1991;13:293–305.

88 Suliman SN, Trojan TM, Tantbiroijn D, Versluis A. Enamel loss following ceramic bracket debonding: a quantitative analysis analysis in vitro. *Angle Orthod.* 2015;85:651–656.

89 Mundethu AR, Gutknecht N, Franzen R. Rapid debonding of polycrystalline ceramic orthodontic brackets with an Er:YAG laser: an in vitro study. *Lasers Med. Sci.* 2014;29:1551–1556.

90 Zachrisson BU, Artun J. Enamel surface appearance after various debonding techniques. *Am. J. Orthod.* 1979;75:121–137.

91 Janiszewska-Olszowska J, Szatkiewicz T, Tomkowski R, et al. Effect of orthodontic debonding and adhesive removal on the enamel: current knowledge and future perspectives. A systematic review. *Med. Sci. Monit.* 2014;20:1991–2001.

92 Janiszewska-Olszowska J, Tandecka K, Szatkiewicz T, et al. Three-dimensional analysis of enamel surface alteration resulting from orthodontic clean-up: comparison of three different tools. *BMC Oral Health* 2015;15:146.

93 Ribeiro AA, Almeida LF, Martins LP, Martins RP. Assessing adhesive remnant removal and enamel damage with ultraviolet light: an in vitro study. *Am. J. Orthod. Dentofacial Orthop.* 2017;151:292–296.

94 Boncuk Y, Cehreli ZC, Polat-Ozsoy O. Effects of different orthodontic adhesives and resin removal techniques on enamel color alteration. *Angle Orthod.* 2014;84:634–641.

95 Ferreira FG, Nouer DF, Silva NP, et al. Qualitative and quantitative evaluation of human dental enamel after bracket debonding: a noncontact three-dimensional optical profilometry analysis. *Clin. Oral Investig.* 2014;18:1853–1864.

96 Ryf S, Fluy S, Palaniaappan S, et al. Enamel loss and adhesive remnants following bracket removal and various clean-up procedures in vitro. *Eur. J. Orthod.* 2012;34:25–32.

97 Day CJ, Price R, Sandy JR, et al. Inhalation of aerosols produced during the removal of fixed orthodontic appliances: a comparison of 4 enamel clean-up methods. *Am. J. Orthod. Dentofacial Orthop.* 2008;113:1853–1864.

98 Kamber R, Papageorgiou SN, Eliades T. Does orthodontic treatment have a permanent effect on tooth colour? A systematic review and meta-analysis. *J. Orofac. Orthop.* 2018;79:73–82.

99 Willmot DR. White lesions after orthodontic treatment: does low fluoride make a difference? *J. Orthod.* 2004;31:235–242.

100 Bergstrand F, Twetman S. A review on prevention and treatment of post-orthodontic white spot lesions: evidence -based methods and emerging technologies. *Open Dent. J.* 2011;5:158–167.

101 Beerens MW, ten Cate JM, Buijs MJ, van der Veen MH. Long-term remineralizing effect of MI Paste Plus on regression of early caries after orthodontic fixed appliance treatment: a 12-month follow-up randomized controlled trial. *Eur. J. Orthod.* 2018;40:457–464.

102 Knosel M, Eckstein A, Helma HJ. Durability of esthetic improvement following Icon resin infiltration of multibracket-induced white spot lesions compared with no therapy over 6 months: a single-center, split-mouth randomized clinical trial. *Am. J. Orthod. Dentofacial Orthop.* 2013;144:86–96.

103 Yetkiner E, Wegehaupt F, Weigand A, et al. Colour improvement and stability of white spot lesions

following infiltration, micro-abrasion, or fluoride treatments in vitro. *Eur. J. Orthod.* 2014;36:595–602.

104 Bearn DR. Bonded orthodontic retainers: a review. *Am. J. Orthod. Dentofacial Orthop.* 1995;108:207–213.

105 Zachrisson BU. Multistranded wire retainers. From start to success. *Am. J. Orthod. Dentofacial Orthop.* 2015;148:724–727.

106 Tacken MPE, Cosyn J, De Wilde P, Aerts J. Glass fibre reinforced versus multistranded bonded orthodontic retainers: a 2 year prospective multi-centre study. *Eur. J. Orthod.* 2010;32:117–123.

107 Salehi P, Najafi HZ, Roeinpeikar SM. Comparison of survival time between two types of orthodontic fixed retainer: a prospective randomized clinical trial. *Prog. Orthod.* 2013;14:25.

108 Bovali E, Kiliaridis S, Cornelis MA. Indirect vs direct bonding of mandibular fixed retainers in orthodontic patients: a single-center randomized controlled trial comparing placement time and failure over a 6-month period. *Am. J. Orthod. Dentofacial Orthop.* 2014;146:701–708.

109 Egli F, Bovali E, Kiliaridis S, Cornelis MA. Indirect vs direct bonding of mandibular fixed retainers in orthodontic patients: comparison of retainer failures and posttreatment stability. A 2-year follow-up of a single-center randomized controlled trial. *Am. J. Orthod. Dentofacial Orthop.* 2017;151:15–27.

110 Al-Moghrabi D, Pandis N, Fleming PS. The effects of fixed and removable orthodontic retainers: a systematic review. *Prog. Orthod.* 2016;17:24.

111 Pandis N, Fleming PS, Kloukos D, et al. Survival of bonded lingual retainers with chemical or photo polymerization over a two-year period: a single-center, randomized controlled clinical trial. *Am. J. Orthod. Dentofacial Orthop.* 2013;144:169–175.

112 Elaut J, Asscherickx K, Vande Vannet B, Wehrbein H. Flowable composites for bonding lingual retainers. *J. Clin. Orthod.* 2002;36:597–598.

113 Eliades T. Orthodontic material applications over the past century: evolution of research methods to address clinical queries. *Am. J. Orthod. Dentofacial Orthop.* 2015;147:S224–S231.

114 Lapatki BG, Bartholomeyczik J, Ruther P, et al. Smart bracket for multi-dimensional force and moment measurement. *J. Dent. Res.* 2007;86:73–78.

115 Rues S, Panchaphongsaphak B, Gieschke P, et al. An analysis of the measurement principle of smart brackets for 3D force and moment monitoring in orthodontics. *J. Biomech.* 2011;44:1892–1900.

116 Jahanbin A, Farzanegan F, Atai M, et al. A comparative assessment of enamel mineral content and *Streptococcus mutans* population between conventional composites and composites containing nano amorphous calcium phosphate in fixed orthodontic patients: a split-mouth randomized clinical trial. *Eur. J. Orthod.* 2017;39:43–51.

117 Altmann ASP, Collares FM, Balbinot G de S, et al. Niobium pentoxide phosphate invert glass as a mineralizing agent in an experimental orthodontic adhesive. *Angle Orthod.* 2017;87:759–765.

9

Debonding

Lucy Davenport-Jones

CHAPTER OUTLINE
Introduction, 165
Preparation, 166
Stainless Steel Brackets, 166
Ceramic Brackets, 166
Polycrystalline Alumina Brackets, 167
Monocrystalline Alumina Brackets, 167
Bracket Fracture, 167
Self-ligating Brackets, 168
Lingual Appliances and Bite Turbos, 168
Solvent Use, 168
Organic Solvents, 168
Peppermint Oil, 168
Electrothermal Debonding, 168
Laser Debonding, 168
Band Removal, 169
Composite Resin Removal, 169
Multifluted Tungsten Carbide Bur, 169
Diamond Finishing Bur, 169
Scalers, 169
Lasers, 169
Finishing Techniques, 169
Enamel, 169
Composite, 170
Porcelain, 171
Iatrogenic Damage, 171
Burns, 171
Enamel Fractures and Tear-out Injuries, 171
Pulpal Injury, 171
Debanding Injuries, 171
Particulates, 171
Conclusions, 172
References, 172

Introduction

The decision to debond is made once all the aims of treatment have been achieved, and early debond may be required if the oral hygiene is not of an acceptable level to support treatment with fixed appliances and the teeth are at risk of decalcification or caries. Efficient and safe debonding is dependent upon the bracket system used and the adhesive protocol. The aim is to remove all the components of the fixed appliance along with the composite adhesive remnants, without causing damage to the tooth surface, whilst minimising any risks to the patient and

Preadjusted Edgewise Fixed Orthodontic Appliances: Principles and Practice, First Edition. Edited by Farhad B. Naini and Daljit S. Gill.
© 2022 John Wiley & Sons Ltd. Published 2022 by John Wiley & Sons Ltd.

operator. How the appliance components are adhered to and removed from the tooth surface influences the risk and degree of enamel damage.[1]

Unlike bonding in other areas of dentistry, the bonding of orthodontic brackets is limited to the duration of treatment and whilst robust and predictable bond strength is required for successful treatment, the ability to predictably debond the brackets without causing harm is vital. The inception of acid etch bonding[2] made it possible to bond orthodontic brackets to enamel with composite resin systems. With more sophisticated bonding systems, the bond strength has increased and with ceramic brackets has the potential to be higher than is clinically necessary. The ideal site of bond failure is at the bracket–composite interface as this minimises the chance of enamel loss during bracket removal but results in more composite to remove following the debond.

Preparation

Coordination with the orthodontic laboratory to plan the availability of fixed retainers and the turn-around time for removable retainers is helpful. Personal protective equipment (PPE) must be worn as with any clinical procedure. Facemasks prevent inhalation of particulates produced during debond and visors are especially important when debonding ceramic brackets as they have the potential to shatter when force is placed on them. If the debond is an aerosol-generating procedure, then a high-volume aspirator for adequate suction is mandatory in order to reduce aerosols.

Stainless Steel Brackets

With conventional stainless steel bracket systems, the archwire can be left *in situ* and fully ligated for debonding; this makes the process quicker and also keeps the components of the appliance together, preventing possible ingestion or inhalation of a foreign body. A metal bracket will deform significantly before the debond is achieved, resulting in a predictable debond.

There are many instruments available for debonding orthodontic brackets. Different techniques use ligature cutters, debracketing instruments, Howe pliers and conventional bracket-removing pliers. The instrument of choice is positioned over the bracket with the beaks in an occlusal–gingival position.

The beaks engage the tie-wings around 1 mm from the enamel surface and are squeezed together. The clinician should squeeze the debonding pliers gently using finger

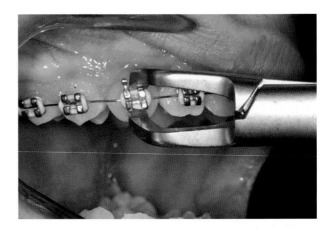

Figure 9.1 Debonding pliers being used to remove metal brackets with the beaks placed under the occlusal–gingival tie-wings.

pressure whilst avoiding rocking motions with their wrist. The bracket base should distort or collapse in on itself and the bond should fail predominantly at the bracket–adhesive interface (Figure 9.1). The brackets will remain ligated to the archwire and the process is repeated until all brackets are debonded. It is important to keep the beaks as far away from the enamel surface as possible as this will reduce stress on the enamel surface.[3]

Another method is to use an instrument called the lift-off bracket remover. This has a loop that engages the tie-wings of the brackets and when the loop is activated a peel force is applied to the bracket.

Some authors discuss using a blunt pair of ligature cutters in the same way as debonding pliers are used. However, there is an increased risk of enamel damage along with higher reported pain during the debond process.[4] In addition, if the blades are still sharp and care is not taken, the tips could damage the enamel surface directly during debond.

Care should be taken that no loose brackets slide off the archwire into the patient's mouth (Figure 9.2). This can be ensured by cinching the archwire distal to the terminal molar tube prior to commencing debonding, checking that all brackets are securely ligated, or by sliding the molar tubes off the archwire whilst they are still in the beaks of the debonding pliers.

Ceramic Brackets

The market has an abundance of different types of ceramic brackets. With each system the manufacturer's instructions should always be followed and the appropriate debonding tool used. Most systems have a specific debonding tool that

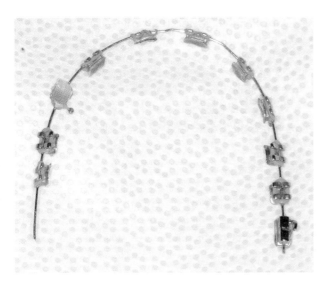

Figure 9.2 The entire archwire and brackets can be removed in one piece. Note here that one of the molar tubes has slipped off the archwire; care must be taken to secure the components in place to prevent inhalation or ingestion.

is calibrated to the specific dimensions of the profile and base design of the bracket to be debonded.

Historically, the bond strengths with ceramic brackets have been very high. However, advances in bracket design have moved from ceramic brackets with a predominantly chemical bond to those that are mechanically retained, in a bid to reduce bond strengths and prevent enamel fractures or tear-out injuries. Prior to debonding, it is important to remove any composite flash with a finishing bur as this allows the tie-wings to be fully engaged and minimises the risk of fracture. Rather than describe the individual debonding techniques for all available bracket systems, an example of each is described.

Polycrystalline Alumina Brackets

The base of the 3M Clarity™ bracket, an example of a polycrystalline alumina bracket, incorporates a *stress concentrator* for more dependable debonding and this allows the bracket to collapse under a gentle squeezing pressure. The Clarity brackets can be debonded on or off the archwire. The adhesive first breaks at the edge of the bracket, initiating a crack that continues through the adhesive layer to the bracket base. The stress concentrator collapses the bracket vertically in half, allowing the bracket to be entirely removed and peeled from the tooth. Specific debonding pliers are available but Weingart or Howe pliers can be used. However, there is some evidence that conventional Weingart or Howe pliers may result in a higher risk of bracket fracture.[5]

The debonding tool is placed in a mesiodistal direction against the sides of the bracket with the ledges of the debonding instrument symmetrically positioned against the labial surface of the bracket, and the bracket is squeezed and rocked to debond.

Monocrystalline Alumina Brackets

The base of the AO Radiance™ bracket, an example of a monocrystalline alumina bracket, has a strong mechanical retention in the centre of the base with a weaker chemical retention on the outside of the base.

Sushi pliers can be used or specific ceramic debonding pliers. The debonding beaks should be parallel when placed along the side of the bracket. The beaks are placed on the enamel–adhesive interface, and the handles squeezed together gently until the bracket debonds from the tooth. It is recommended to place the beaks in an occlusogingival position for the upper central incisor brackets and in a mesiodistal position on all other teeth. Each bracket should be squeezed gently until the operator feels it collapse. It is important not to squeeze too hard or the bracket may fracture prematurely. The brackets may be gently rocked in a mesiodistal direction to completely separate from the enamel. After debonding, the surfaces of the instrument should be wiped to remove any remnants of adhesive or ceramic material. Monocrystalline brackets are less likely to fracture during debond.[6]

Bracket Fracture

A recent study compared enamel loss when debonding modern polycrystalline and monocrystalline brackets (Clarity 3M Unitek and Inspire-ICE, Ormco, Orange, CA, USA) and found the enamel loss to be 20–30 μm for both systems. This is comparable to metal bracket systems with enamel loss of 20–50 μm. The polycrystalline bracket was more likely to fracture during debonding, resulting in a lengthier clean-up process.[6, 7]

If a ceramic bracket does fracture during removal, a high-speed handpiece with a diamond bur and water coolant can be used to remove the remainder of the bracket. However, it can be difficult to differentiate between the ceramic bracket, the composite layer and the enamel. This must be carried out with high-volume suction as the fractured bracket could potentially be at risk of inhalation or ingestion. Once the composite layer has been identified and all fragments of the ceramic bracket have been eliminated, the routine composite removal technique can resume.

Self-ligating Brackets

With the Damon™ metal brackets the debonding protocol is similar to that of conventional brackets and can occur with or without the archwire *in situ*. The standard debonding pliers can be used. The only difference is that only two tie-wings are engaged to allow for deformation and subsequent debond.

Damon Clear brackets have a specific debonding tool, which means that removal of the flash is not necessary. The instrument is placed over the occlusal and gingival tie-wings and the handles of the debonding tool are squeezed together to close the beaks; on continued squeezing a wedge is advanced towards the tooth surface, which peels the bracket away from the enamel. It is important to keep the instrument at 90° to the tooth surface as any twisting action will increase the chance of tie-wing fracture and is likely to result in an increase in patient discomfort.

Lingual Appliances and Bite Turbos

There are specific debonding instruments for the removal of lingual appliances and these vary from system to system. In most systems there are separate anterior and posterior debonding tools. The archwire can be left *in situ* but is sectioned between the canine and first premolar to divide the archwire into three sections. The anterior section is debonded with anterior lingual bracket-removing pliers. One beak of the pliers is placed on the base and the other rests on the incisal edge of the bracket; the handles are squeezed to release the bracket from the tooth surface.

Debonding posterior teeth can be more challenging. One beak of the posterior debonding tool is rested on the occlusal edge of the bracket and the other beak on any edge of the bracket to get a grip. The bracket is squeezed to deform the base and allow for debond. It may be necessary to use a fine diamond bur in a fast handpiece with water coolant to remove any composite that may block access to the incisal/occlusal edge of the bracket.

Solvent Use

There is some discussion in the literature regarding the use of solvents to reduce the bond strength prior to debonding.

Organic Solvents

A solution of 50% ethanol has been shown to have a significant effect on the bond strength of two bonding systems by degradation of the bisphenol A glycidyl methacrylate (bis-GMA) present in the composite resin. It has been postulated that use of an alcohol-containing mouthrinse may aid bracket removal.[8] The use of acetone as a gel solvent has been shown to be ineffective in reducing shear bond strength.[9]

Peppermint Oil

There is some evidence that the application of peppermint oil will reduce bond strength and it has been marketed as a debonding agent. However, the duration of application would need to be in the region of one hour[10] for it to have a significant effect on plasticising the composite resin. In addition, allergy to menthol is well documented,[11] along with its potential toxicity to the mucosa.

Electrothermal Debonding

An electrothermal device may be used to transfer heat through the bracket structure to soften the composite layer, encouraging bond failure between the bracket base and the adhesive. Whilst this method has been shown to be quick and efficient, the thermal changes generated at the tip could lead to pulpal damage and, if poorly handled, mucosal trauma.

Whilst some evidence exists that an electrothermal debonding tool may be useful in improving the ease of debonding of ceramic brackets, the electrothermal unit can be bulky.[12]

Laser Debonding

In 1917, Albert Einstein put forward the theory of *stimulated emission*, the basis for modern lasers. Laser stands for 'light amplification by stimulated emission of radiation'. Laser debonding has been shown to degrade composite resins by directing a focused source of light energy to result in thermal softening, thermal ablation or photoablation.

The labial surfaces of the brackets are exposed to the laser at a wavelength ranging from 248 to 1060 nm. Whilst the mode of action is similar to that of the electrothermal debonding system, the application of the laser is possibly more precise in the targeting and the duration of exposure and may provide better control of the intensity of heat to which the tooth is subjected.[13, 14]

Both carbon dioxide (CO_2) lasers and the erbium-doped yttrium aluminium garnet (Er:YAG) laser have been used as a method of reducing the bond strength of ceramic brackets. However, the reduction in possible iatrogenic damage to the enamel must be weighed against the thermal changes within the enamel, which can increase the temperature of the enamel by 200°C.[15]

Band Removal

Orthodontic bands are commonly cemented with a glass ionomer cement or a compomer cement and the bond strength is considerably lower than that of the composite resin system used for the bonding of brackets. The band is retained in position during treatment by the adhesive bond and the tight mechanical fit of the selected band. Band removing pliers are used to loosen the band and break the bond. The band removing pliers consist of a plastic support that sits on the occlusal surface of the molar tooth and a beak that engages the gingival part of the band (Figure 9.3). When the handles are squeezed together the beak engaging the band pulls it in an occlusal direction.

The weaker bond is generally easy to break and the band will come away from the tooth easily. If the tooth is heavily restored, then the risk of cuspal fracture is increased and additional care may need to be taken. The occlusal surface can be supported during the debanding process with a cotton wool roll. It is sensible to place the plastic support on the palatal surface of the molar rather than the buccal surface, as there is often a larger mass of enamel to support the force being applied to the band. It is important to inspect the instrument prior to use, as the plastic pads can become worn, and replacement pads can be ordered as needed.

If the tooth is compromised and the operator feels that there is a high chance of fracture or loss of a restoration during debanding, or the band will not easily move, then a vertical cut can be made through the band to reveal the cement layer beneath; this will significantly decrease the retention from the mechanical fit and the band can be peeled away from the tooth. This can be carried out with a tungsten carbide bur in a slow or fast handpiece or with crown slitting pliers.

Composite Resin Removal

Despite extensive published research, there is no agreement on which technique is most effective at removing the remaining resin whilst maintaining the integrity of the enamel surface. Some techniques will take considerably less time than others, especially when using a slow-speed handpiece. However, it is important to choose the technique that best preserves the enamel, rather than that which takes up less chair time. The use of disclosing solution to differentiate visually between the enamel and composite has been described.[16]

Multifluted Tungsten Carbide Bur

The conventional technique for composite removal is the use of a multifluted [8, 16] tungsten carbide bur in a slow-speed handpiece (Figure 9.4). This has been shown to result in very little enamel loss and because water coolant is not needed, it is possible to differentiate between the enamel surface and the composite remnants.[17] The tungsten carbide burs can be used in a high-speed handpiece, but whilst it has been shown to produce a smoother surface finish,[16] it results in higher levels of enamel loss. It is important that the long axis of the bur is kept parallel to the tooth surface as the tip of the bur has the potential to scratch or gouge the enamel surface.

Diamond Finishing Bur

The use of a diamond bur in a high-speed handpiece for composite removal has been shown to take half the time in comparison to a tungsten carbide bur in a slow-speed handpiece.[18] However, there is some evidence demonstrating both an increase in enamel loss with this system,[19, 20] and unwanted thermal changes within the tooth structure. This technique is not recommended for post-debond composite removal.

Scalers

The use of an ultrasonic scaler to remove composite has been shown to be more damaging to the surface enamel than removal with a slow-speed handpiece and a 16-fluted tungsten carbide bur or an aluminium oxide polishing disc (Sof-Lex™) in a slow-speed handpiece.[21] The use of hand scalers can also lead to gouging of the enamel surface.[19]

Lasers

Whilst the application of CO_2 and Er:YAG lasers to reduce the force needed to debond ceramic brackets has been widely reported in the literature, their use in composite removal is less evident.[22] Currently this method may not be suitable for removing resin remnants following debonding.

Finishing Techniques

Enamel

Following composite removal, the enamel may demonstrate surface scratches or irregularities that could harbour bacteria and plaque (Figure 9.5).[23] However, polishing will lead to further enamel loss. A decision must be made regarding the best technique depending on the post-debond

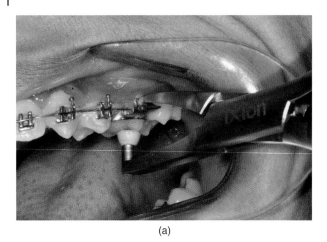

(a)

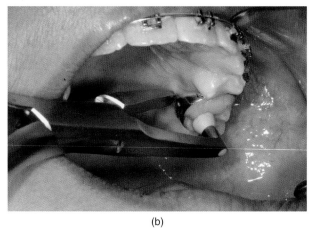

(b)

Figure 9.3 (a) Band-removing pliers can be placed on the buccal aspect to break the bond and remove the molar band, or (b) they can be used on the palatal aspect to prevent injury to the buccal cusps if vulnerable. Lower molar bands are removed with pressure applied primarily to their buccal surface, due to the usual lingual inclination of the crowns of lower molar teeth. Upper molar bands are removed with the initial pressure applied primarily to their palatal surface, which is easier if the bands have integrated palatal cleats.

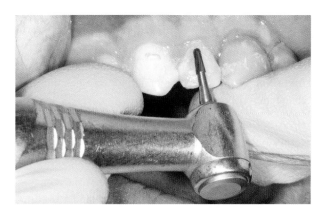

Figure 9.4 A slow-speed handpiece with a tungsten carbide bur is used parallel to the enamel surface to prevent gouging and to create a smooth enamel surface.

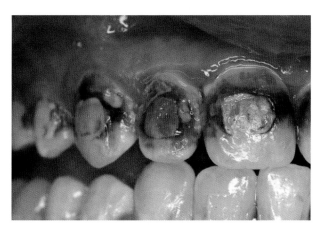

Figure 9.5 This patient had been lost to follow-up and attended requesting debond five years after bond-up. Excessive staining and dental caries can be seen.

enamel surface and the risk of further enamel loss. White spot lesions, where the enamel layer has become demineralised, have been shown to be particularly susceptible to further enamel loss during debond.

Composite removal with a tungsten carbide bur in a slow-speed handpiece removes approximately 10 μm of enamel, whereas an average of 14.2 μm of enamel is lost when prophylaxis with zirconium silicate was performed with a rotating bristle brush.[24] For the majority of debond procedures carried out with a multifluted tungsten carbide bur, no further polishing procedures are necessary.[18]

Enamel finishing techniques include the use of a rubber cup with pumice slurry, abrasive discs, and composite polishing burs. Further damage to the enamel during polishing procedures is more dependent on the choice of polishing brush or rubber cup rather than the choice of pumice.[1]

Increasingly, orthodontic treatment is carried out on adult patients and with this comes the challenge of not only bonding but also debonding brackets from restored teeth. Returning composite restorations or ceramic veneers and crowns to their pretreatment condition uses different techniques to those used on enamel (see following section). In addition, there is a risk of fracture of the restorations.

Composite

Composite polishing techniques, such as using polishing discs (e.g. Sof-Lex™) to smooth the labial surface and adjust incisal edges, can be carried out with a composite polishing kit to restore the anatomy, characterisation and surface gloss.

Porcelain

Bracket and composite removal alters the surface of the porcelain that post-debond polishing does not restore. Inevitably, there will be some change in the glaze integrity and also the shade, value and hue of the porcelain.[25] Porcelain polishing and glazing kits can be used to improve the surface using rubber points with 30–60 micron fine grit.

Iatrogenic Damage

Burns

Thermal burns can occur during debonding. Defective handpieces, motors or ultrasonic scalers can cause the temperature of the instrument to increase during use. If the handpiece or motor is noticeably hot to the operator, the procedure should be stopped immediately and steps taken to ensure that the equipment is safe for use. Electrothermal and laser debonding also has the potential to result in mucosal burns. Chemical burns can occur with use of acid etchant during the placement of bonded retainers.

Enamel Fractures and Tear-out Injuries

It is important to fully assess the condition of the teeth prior to bond-up and to have excellent photographs and study models. Once an appliance is removed, imperfections in the enamel may be noticed that were pre-existing (Figure 9.6). The pattern and location of a fracture has an impact on long-term prognosis, so it is important to accurately assess and categorise the fracture. The fracture type can be described as follows:[26]

- craze lines (i.e. minute surface cracks)
- fractured cusp
- cracked tooth
- split tooth
- vertical root fracture.

Transillumination can be used to differentiate between different patterns of cracks. If the tooth only has craze lines, then the light will travel through the entire tooth structure, whereas a true fracture line will block the light, allowing only a fragment of the tooth to light up.

The bond failure of ceramic brackets is more likely to occur at the enamel–adhesive junction, as opposed to metal brackets where bond failure more commonly occurs at the bracket–adhesive interface.[27] Enamel fracture and tear-out injuries are primarily a problem when debonding chemically retained ceramic bracket systems.[28] Some of the

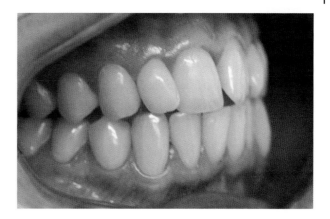

Figure 9.6 Pre-existing enamel defects prior to bond-up.

early ceramic bracket systems resulted in a 63.3% chance of enamel damage.[29]

As the force required to debond a bracket increases so does the frequency of enamel crack propagation and bracket fracture.[30] The enamel in adult patients has a higher modulus of elasticity than that of younger patients and may therefore have the potential to be more brittle.[31] It has been demonstrated that where microcracks exist prior to bonding, there is a significant increase in the width, but not the length, of these cracks post debond. This increase in width is likely to be greatest in the cervical third of the tooth, rather than the middle or incisal third.[32]

Microcracks can absorb staining and act as a harbour for plaque accumulation. What is not evident is the long-term effect on the vitality and integrity of the tooth following the instigation of enamel craze lines.

Pulpal Injury

Thermal debonding and adhesive removal can generate heat that can result in irreversible trauma to the pulp. A temperature rise of more than 5.5°C will result in pulpal inflammatory change, and more than 11°C can result in pulpal necrosis.[33] Care must be taken to minimise any thermal changes.

Debanding Injuries

The debanding instrument should be used with caution; any unsupported enamel could fracture during band removal.[34]

Particulates

The size and aerodynamic behaviour of the particulates released during debond can affect their infiltration into the lungs, possibly transmitting pathogens and resulting in inflammation and reduced lung function. In addition, remnants of ceramic brackets and microscopic amounts of tungsten and iron may be generated. There is some evidence that more particulates are produced during the removal of ceramic brackets than metal brackets. Particulate spread can be reduced by the use of high-volume suction and the use of a slow-speed handpiece rather than a high-speed handpiece with water coolant.

The aerosol produced during the clean-up stage of debonding contains polymer matrix, filler degradation by-products and particulates from the wear of the debonding bur.[35] As well as the potential risk of the generated aerosols containing sufficiently small-diameter particles capable of reaching the respiratory system,[36] there is also a potential hormone-disrupting action of particles derived from the presence of the double benzoic ring in the bis-GMA monomer. This may, under certain conditions,[37] particularly the introduction of heat into the material that occurs with grinding during clean-up with burs, lead to the formation of bisphenol A, which may have xeno-oestrogenic properties.[38] This is an additional reason to avoid a high-speed handpiece, due to the heat generated and aerosol produced. However, using a slow-speed handpiece will result in heat production in the material being removed from the enamel surface, whether water coolant is used or not. Using a water coolant may increase the aerosol production. Therefore, currently it is not known whether it is better to use or avoid water coolant with a slow-speed handpiece during debond. This requires further investigation. As such, access to adequate ventilation in the treatment room or clinic is important.

Appropriate PPE must be worn by the clinician and assistants. A standard type IIR surgical facemask has been shown to reduce particulate inhalation by 96%.[39, 40] The FFP3 respirator mask has demonstrated a higher filtration efficacy for composite dust, although some penetration of small particulates is inevitable.[41]

Conclusions

The main risks of debonding orthodontic appliances relate to enamel loss during either bracket or band removal or composite clean-up. These risks are significantly increased with the use of ceramic brackets. These can be minimised by careful selection of an appropriate orthodontic bonding technique along with a bracket system that has an in-built mechanism for a straightforward debond. Significant iatrogenic damage is thankfully rare, but patients should be assessed for risk factors and a thorough consent must be taken.

References

1 Reynolds IR. A review of direct orthodontic bonding. *Br. J. Orthod.* 1975;2:171–178.

2 Buonocore MG. A simple method of increasing the adhesion of acrylic filling materials to enamel surfaces. *J. Dent. Res.* 1955;34:849–853.

3 Pithon MM, Santos Fonseca Figueiredo D, Oliveira DD, Coqueiro R da S. What is the best method for debonding metallic brackets from the patient's perspective? *Prog. Orthod.* 2015;16:17.

4 Oliver RG, Knapman YM. Attitudes to orthodontic treatment. *Br. J. Orthod.* 1985;12(4):179–188.

5 Bishara SE, Truelove TS. Comparisons of different debonding techniques for ceramic brackets: an in vitro study. *Am. J. Orthod. Dentofacial Orthop.* 1990;98(2):145–153.

6 Suliman SN, Trojan TM, Tantbirojn D, Versluis A. Enamel loss following ceramic bracket debonding: a quantitative analysis in vitro. *Angle Orthod.* 2015;85:651–656.

7 Al Shamsi AH, Cunningham JL, Lamey PJ, Lynch E. Three-dimensional measurement of residual adhesive and enamel loss on teeth after debonding of orthodontic brackets: an in-vitro study. *Am. J. Orthod. Dentofacial Orthop.* 2007;131(3):301.e9–15.

8 Hobson RS, McCabe JF, Hogg SD. The effect of food stimulants on enamel–composite bond strength. *J. Orthod.* 2000;27(1):55–59.

9 Santana RM, Rached RN, Souza EM, et al. Effect of organic solvents and ultrasound on the removal of orthodontic brackets. *Orthod. Craniofac. Res.* 2016;19(3):137–144.

10 Larmour CJ, McCabe JF, Gordon PH. An ex-vivo investigation into the effects of chemical solvents on the debond behavior of ceramic orthodontic brackets. *Br. J. Orthod.* 1998;25(1):35–39.

11 Tran A, Pratt M, DeKoven J. Acute allergic contact dermatitis of the lips from peppermint oil in a lip balm. *Dermatitis* 2010;21(2):111–115.

12 Sheridan JJ, Brawley G, Hastings J. Electrothermal debracketing. Part 1. An in vitro study. *Am. J. Orthod.* 1986;89(1):21–27.

13 Hayakawa K. Nd:YAG laser for debonding ceramic orthodontic brackets. *Am. J. Orthod. Dentofacial Orthop.* 2005;128(5):638–647.

14 Feldon PJ, Murray PE, Burch JG, et al. Diode laser debonding of ceramic brackets. *Am. J. Orthod. Dentofacial Orthop.* 2010;138(4):458–462.

15 Lijima M, Yasuda Y, Muguruma T, Mizoguchi I. Effects of CO_2 laser debonding of a ceramic bracket on the mechanical properties of enamel. *Angle Orthod.* 2010;80:1029–1035.

16 Campbell PM. Enamel surfaces after orthodontic bracket debonding. *Angle Orthod.* 1995;2:103–110.

17 Hosein I, Sherriff M, Ireland AJ. Enamel loss during bonding, debonding and cleanup with use of a self-etching primer. *Am. J. Orthod. Dentofacial Orthop.* 2004;126:717–724.

18 Eliades T, Gloka C, Eliades G, Makou M. Enamel surface roughness following debonding using two resin grinding methods. *Eur. J. Orthod.* 2004;26(3):333–338.

19 Zachrisson B, Arthun J. Enamel surface appearance after various debonding techniques. *Am. J. Orthod. Dentofacial Orthop.* 1979;75(2):121–137.

20 Hong YH, Lew KK. Quantitative and qualitative assessment of enamel surface following five composite removal methods after bracket debonding. *Eur. J. Orthod.* 1995;17(2):121–128.

21 Cochrane N, Ratneser S, Reynolds EC. Effect of different orthodontic adhesive removal techniques on sound, demineralized and remineralised enamel. *Aust. Dent. J.* 2012;57:365–372.

22 Ahrari F, Akbari M, Akbari J, Dabiri G. Enamel surface roughness after debonding of orthodontic brackets and various clean-up techniques. *J. Dent. (Tehran)* 2013;10:82–93.

23 Ryf S, Flury S, Palaniappan S, et al. Enamel loss and adhesive remnants following bracket removal and various clean-up procedures in vitro. *Eur. J. Orthod.* 2012;34:25–32.

24 Pus MD, Way D. Enamel loss due to orthodontic bonding with filled and unfilled resins using various clean-up techniques. *Am. J. Orthod.* 1980;77:269–283.

25 Jarvis J, Zinelis S, Eliades T, Bradley TG. Porcelain surface roughness, color and gloss changes after orthodontic bonding. *Angle Orthod.* 2006;76(2):274–277.

26 American Association of Endodontists. Cracking the cracked tooth code: detection and treatment of various longitudinal tooth fractures. Summer 2008. Available at https://www.aae.org/uploadedfiles/publications_and_research/endodontics_colleagues_for_excellence_newsletter/ecfesum08.pdf

27 Odegaard J, Segner D. Shear bond strength of metal brackets compared with a new ceramic bracket. *Am. J. Orthod. Dentofacial Orthop.* 1988;94(3):201–206.

28 Kitahara-Ceia FM, Much JN, Marques dos Santos PA. Assessment of enamel damage after removal of ceramic brackets. *Am. J. Orthod. Dentofacial Orthop.* 2008;134(4):548–555.

29 Redd TB, Shivapuja PS. Debonding ceramic brackets: effects on enamel. *J. Clin. Orthod.* 1991;25(8):475–481.

30 Diaz C, Swartz M. Debonding a new ceramic bracket: a clinical study. *J. Clin. Orthod.* 2004;38(8):442.

31 Park S, Quinn JB, Romberg E, Arola D. On the brittleness of enamel and selected dental materials. *Dent. Mater.* 2008;24:1477–1485.

32 Dumbryte I, Linkeviciene L, Malinauskas M, et al. Evaluation of enamel micro-cracks characteristics after removal of metal brackets in adult patients. *Eur. J. Orthod.* 2011;35(3):317–322.

33 Zach L, Cohen G. Pulp response to externally applied heat. *Oral Surg. Oral Med. Oral Pathol.* 1965;19:515–530.

34 McGuinness N. Prevention in orthodontics: a review. *Dent. Update* 1992;19:168–175.

35 Eliades T. Orthodontic materials research and applications: part 1. Current status and projected future developments in bonding and adhesives. *Am. J. Orthod. Dentofacial Orthop.* 2006;130:445–451.

36 Ireland AJ, Moreno T, Price R. Airborne particles produced during enamel cleanup after removal of orthodontic appliances. *Am. J. Orthod. Dentofacial Orthop.* 2003;124:683–686.

37 Eliades T, Hiskia A, Eliades G, Athanasiou AE. Assessment of bisphenol-A release from orthodontic adhesives. *Am. J. Orthod. Dentofacial Orthop.* 2007;131:72–75.

38 Eliades T, Gioni V, Kletsas D, et al. Oestrogenicity of orthodontic adhesive resins. *Eur. J. Orthod.* 2007;29:404–407.

39 Johnson NJ, Price R, Day C, et al. Quantitative and qualitative analysis of particulate production using simulated clinical orthodontic debonding. *Dent. Mater.* 2009;25:1155–1162.

40 Brooke Stewart A, Chambers C, Sandy JR, et al. Orthodontic debonding: methods, risks and future developments. *Orthodontic Update* 2014;7:6–13.

41 Brel S, Van Landuyt K, Reichl F, et al. Filtration efficiency of surgical and FFP3 masks against composite dust. *Eur. J. Oral Sci.* 2020;128(3):233–240.

10

Archwires
Leila Khamashta-Ledezma

CHAPTER OUTLINE

Introduction, 175
Properties of Archwires, 176
  Stress–Strain Curves and Physical Properties, 176
  Cantilever and Three-point Bending Tests, 178
  Effects of Changing the Diameter or Length of Archwires, 178
  Other Laboratory Tests and Physical Properties, 179
Archwire Shape and Arch Form, 179
Archwire Materials, 180
  Precious Metal Alloys, 180
  Stainless Steel, 180
  Cobalt Chromium, 181
  Nickel Titanium, 181
  Beta-Titanium, 184
Aesthetic Archwires, 185
  Coated Metal Archwires, 185
  Fibre-reinforced Composite Archwires, 186
Fatigue, 187
Corrosion of Metal Alloys, 188
  Types of Corrosion, 188
  Clinical Significance of Corrosion, 190
  Methods to Reduce Corrosion, 190
Which is the Best Aligning Archwire or Archwire Sequence?, 191
Pain from Initial Archwires, 192
  Pharmacological Management, 192
  Non-pharmacological Management, 193
Root Resorption from Different Archwires, 194
  Is there Evidence that Different Archwires Cause Different Amounts of Root Resorption?, 194
Allergy to Nickel, 195
  Pathological Process, 195
  Signs and Symptoms and Management, 195
  When and How Much Nickel is Released from Appliances?, 196
  Allergies to Other Metals, 197
Acknowledgements, 197
References, 197

Introduction

There are many archwires available on the market and it is the clinician's decision which material, shape and diameter archwire to use in a determined clinical situation. During the different stages of treatment different physical proper-ties of an archwire are required and there is no ideal arch-wire that can deliver on all aspects.[1] Therefore an under-standing of the physical properties of the different archwire materials available and their clinical application is crucial. An appreciation for the effect of a change in length or diam-eter of an archwire used during treatment in relation to the

Preadjusted Edgewise Fixed Orthodontic Appliances: Principles and Practice, First Edition. Edited by Farhad B. Naini and Daljit S. Gill.
© 2022 John Wiley & Sons Ltd. Published 2022 by John Wiley & Sons Ltd.

force it will exert on the teeth is also required.

The oral environment presents a challenge for the materials used in orthodontics, as it is a moist environment with a changing pH, materials are under masticatory cyclic loading and in a medium rich in microorganisms, all of which can lead to changes in the surfaces and properties of the materials used. Therefore, the processes of intraoral ageing and fatigue and the different types of corrosion are important considerations in orthodontics, as these may change the physical properties of archwires. Furthermore, nickel ions may be released from nickel-containing materials following intraoral placement, during use, and as a result of corrosion. For sensitised patients this may lead to allergic reactions. Hence orthodontists are required to identify the signs and symptoms and manage patients with the use of alternative materials. It is also important for orthodontists to be aware of other potential side effects (e.g. pain, root resorption) and know how to minimise or avoid these.

Finally, for an evidence-based approach, clinician experience and judgement together with patient preferences and the relevant scientific evidence are taken into account when making a clinical decision. The available research in this field is discussed and future studies will no doubt help improve our understanding of the clinical effectiveness of different archwires and their effects on oral structures and guide the development/improvement of future archwire materials.

Properties of Archwires

In general, all archwires share some ideal properties (Table 10.1). The definitions of their physical properties and at what stages of treatment specific ones are more advantageous will be discussed. However, all materials placed intraorally should be **biocompatible**, i.e. there is a biological tolerance to the material and it does not produce toxic or harmful effects, including resistance to corrosion and not causing immunological reactions. Furthermore, it should have poor **biohostability**, i.e. it should not actively or passively act as a substrate for microorganisms, which will smell foul, cause colour changes, or build up and lead to changes in mechanical properties of the archwire.[1]

Table 10.1 General ideal properties of orthodontic archwires.

Ideal properties of archwires		
Strong	Good Range	Aesthetic
Resilient	Good Springback	Low friction
Formable	Biocompatible	Poor biohostability
Joinability (able to solder or weld auxiliaries)		

Archwire materials should be strong enough to withstand masticatory forces and have low friction to reduce resistance to sliding and aid tooth movement (single or by sliding mechanics). Formability, joinability, resilience and good springback are desired in order to bend wires (e.g. loops or finishing bends), join parts via soldering or welding and during their use maximise their stored elastic energy and yet still return to their initial shape.

Stress–Strain Curves and Physical Properties

The elastic behaviour of any material is defined in terms of its stress–strain response to an external load, which can be plotted on a stress–strain curve (Figure 10.1). Stress is the internal distribution of the load (force per unit area). It is commonly measured in units of pounds per square inch (psi) or megapascals (MPa), where 1 pascal is the stress resulting from a force of 1 newton (N) acting upon 1 square metre of surface, and is equal to 0.000145 psi. Strain is the internal distortion produced by the load, i.e. the change in length per unit length when stress is applied (deflection per unit length). It is expressed in the common unit inch per inch or centimetre per centimetre. As an archwire is loaded under tension the external force applied and the deflection (bending) produced by the force are external measurements that can be plotted on a force–deflection curve (Figure 10.1).

The following physical properties can be defined from a stress–strain curve.

- *Stiffness*: the flexural rigidity of a material and is represented by the gradient of the linear (elastic) portion of the curve in a stress–strain curve or by Young's modulus of elasticity (E = stress/strain). Young's modulus of elasticity is usually expressed in units of psi or MPa. Therefore, the steeper the slope, the stiffer the wire and the more force is required to bend it.
- *Springiness*: is inversely proportional to Young's modulus of elasticity (1/E). The more horizontal the linear portion of the curve in a stress–strain curve, the springier the wire.
- *Proportional limit*: the point at which permanent deformation commences. It is the maximum stress at which the straight line relationship between stress and strain is valid (Hooke's law).
- *Yield strength*: the point at which a deformation of 0.1% can be measured.
- *Ultimate tensile strength*: the maximum load carrying capacity of the wire before the material will fracture.
- *Range*: the distance the wire will bend elastically before permanent or plastic deformation occurs and the wire still returns to its original dimension when the load is removed. However, this is measured to the yield point, where 0.1% permanent deformation has occurred upon removal of the load.

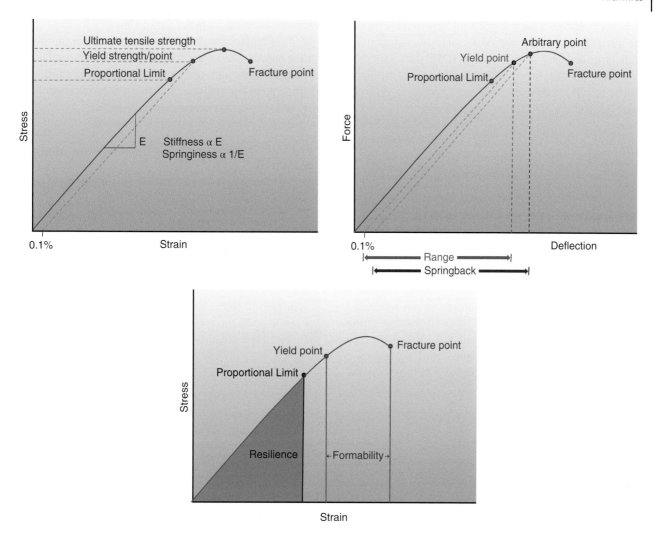

Figure 10.1 Stress–strain curves, force-deflection curve and the physical properties of wires determined from these. Within the elastic range, the material deforms directly proportional to the stress applied so that stress = modulus of elasticity × strain (Hooke's law). With further stress applied, the material response moves to a plastic range, where there is no longer a linear relationship until it fails at fracture point. Strength is a measure of the maximum possible load the wire can sustain or deliver. Considering the graphic representation of the stress–strain curve, three points can be taken as representative of the strength of a material: proportional (elastic) limit, yield strength and ultimate tensile strength.

- *Springback*: the distance the wire can bend before it is permanently deformed and still returns to its original shape, hence its elastic recovery. Clinically useful springback still occurs when the wire is deflected past its yield strength, where some permanent deformation occurs and it will not return to its original shape. Hence it is measured as the distance to a point of arbitrary loading between the elastic limit and ultimate strength.
- *Strength*: the maximum force a material can sustain. On a stress–strain graph, strength can be measured by multiplying the stiffness of a material by its range (strength = stiffness × range). It is also a measure of the force-storing capacity of a wire.
- *Resilience*: the energy storage capacity of a wire, represented by the area under the stress–strain curve up to the proportional limit. The energy absorbed by a wire whilst undergoing elastic deformation, up to the elastic limit,

is then released when the wire springs back towards its original shape after removal of an applied stress.
- *Formability*: the amount of permanent deformation (bending into a desired shape) that a wire can withstand before it fractures, represented by the area under the curve between the yield and fracture points.
- *Ductility*: the ability of a material to withstand permanent deformation under tensile load without failure.

Different properties are beneficial at different stages of orthodontic treatment. During initial alignment and levelling, a wire with low stiffness, large springback, and ideally pseudoelasticity and shape memory (described later under nickel titanium) will allow it to be engaged to crowded teeth without it being permanently deformed and to deliver a constant low force to align the teeth and in doing so return to its original shape. Instead, for working archwires a high stiffness and low surface friction are preferable, as they should be able to maintain the arch form and provide a stable arch that can withstand deformation when, for example, space closure with sliding mechanics or mechanics such as piggyback arches are used. A low friction is ideal for space closure as it is a factor leading to resistance to sliding. At the finishing stages of treatment, a high stiffness archwire with good formability is required to allow for small finishing bends to be applied in all three orders (first, second and third order).

Cantilever and Three-point Bending Tests

In the laboratory, wires are tested for their physical properties with either cantilever-type tests or three-point bending tests (Figure 10.2). In a cantilever set-up the wire is supported at one end only and a force is applied to the unsupported end, which clinically would relate to a spring on a removable appliance or an uprighting spring. In contrast, in a three-point bending test, the tested wire is supported at both ends a set distance apart and a force is applied at the midpoint of the wire span between the two

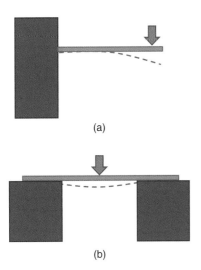

(a)

(b)

Figure 10.2 (a) Cantilever test: this is the simplest beam test and involves applying force to a piece of wire of known size and length attached firmly at one end to a block. When a force (F) is applied at a certain point on the wire (L), a bending moment is generated (force × length). This type of set-up relates well to a cantilever spring on a removable appliance or an uprighting spring, but it does not simulate accurately a multibracket system. (b) Three-point bending test: a known length of wire supported at both ends is deflected at a known rate (certain amount of deflection in a determined time) by a metal pole applying force at the midpoint of the wire span between the two attachments. This test provides a better simulation of a multibracket system, the attachments being the brackets and the span of wire between the two attachments being the interbracket distance. It is commonly used when assessing the physical properties of archwire materials in laboratory studies.

supports, providing a better simulation of a multi-bracket system.[2] From the results of these tests, stress–strain curves for the tested material are produced. Different formulas are applicable to the different types of beam tests (cantilever or three-point bending test) and different geometries of the wire tested (round or rectangular) (Box 10.0a).

Box 10.1 Formulas applicable to the different types of beam tests

(a)
Round cross-section

$$\delta = FL/\pi R^3$$

Rectangular cross-section

$$\delta = 3FL/2bd^2$$

where δ represents flexural stress (MPa), F the load at a given point on the load deflection curve (N), L the support span (mm), R the radius of the beam (mm), b the width of the test beam (mm) and d the depth or thickness of the test beam (mm).

(b)

$$F \infty dr^4/l^3$$

where F represents force, d the distance the archwire is deflected, r the radius and l the length.

Effects of Changing the Diameter or Length of Archwires

Clinically, a change in the diameter or length (interbracket span length) of an archwire will have a great impact on the force it exerts on the teeth. The aforementioned formulas are complicated and a simpler relationship between radius (r), length (l), deflection of an archwire (d) and the force it will exert (F) is helpful for an appreciation of the effect of a change in these parameters (Box 10.0b):

$$F \infty dr^4/l^3$$

It can be seen that by increasing the diameter of the archwire the force exerted by it is significantly increased and by increasing the length (or the span of wire between brackets, e.g. with loops or narrower brackets) the force is significantly reduced. These changes also impact on the physical properties, as the stiffness, strength and range of a material is determined by the length, size and shape of the wire and the material hardness. By increasing the diameter of the wire, the springiness decreases to the fourth power, strength increases as a cubic function, and range decreases proportionally.[3] When increasing the length of the wire, the effects depend on the set-up, i.e. whether a cantilever or a supported beam situation is present. In a cantilever set-up, an increase in wire length will lead to a proportional reduction in the material's strength, an increase in its springiness as a cubic function of the ratio of the length, and the range will increase as the square of the ratio of the length.[3] Thus, doubling the length would halve the bending strength and increase the springiness eight times and the range four times. In a supported beam scenario, the mathematical equations become more complicated but the general principle remains that as the length increases a proportional decrease in strength will occur, but springiness and range are exponentially increased.[3]

Other Laboratory Tests and Physical Properties

When materials are tested in the laboratory, different types of stress can be induced and tested.

- Tension or tensile stress is when the material is pulled apart, so it has the tendency to stretch or elongate a material.
- Compression or compressive stress refers to when a body is placed under a force that tends to compress or shorten the material.
- Shear stress is applied by two forces acting in opposite directions but not in the same plane, with the tendency to slide one part of the material past another along planes parallel to the applied force.

Other laboratory tests relevant to orthodontic archwire materials include measures of surface roughness and coefficient of friction in dry and wet (saliva) conditions. Stainless steel is known to have the smoothest surface, followed by beta-titanium, and nickel titanium has the roughest.[4] A smooth surface is preferred as it is thought to harbour less microorganisms and may lead to less corrosion and friction. Friction is the resistive force between surfaces that opposes motion (due to contact between asperities on the surfaces). However, it has been shown that there is little or no correlation between surface roughness and the coefficient of friction of archwires. The coefficient of friction is highest for beta-titanium, followed by nickel titanium, with least friction shown by stainless steel.[4] The reason for beta-titanium having a smoother surface but a higher coefficient of friction than nickel titanium is the higher content of titanium in beta-titanium, which affects its surface reactivity. Ion implantation methods are available to reduce this (see section Beta-Titanium).

The coefficient of friction affects how easily an archwire slides through a bracket, and hence impacts on tooth movement with sliding mechanics. Though clinically friction is a factor in the resistance to sliding, it is not the only factor. In sliding mechanics teeth move by 'tipping and uprighting' along the archwire rather than moving freely along the archwire with no contact between the archwire and the edges of brackets. Kusy and Whitley were instrumental in highlighting the lack of validity for the clinical situation of laboratory testing with the latter set-up and introduced the use of different contact angles between the archwire and the edges of the brackets to test resistance to sliding.[5, 6] They showed that there are three stages to resistance to sliding and during these the following factors contribute more or less to it: friction, elastic binding and physical notching.[5, 6] Binding occurs when the tooth tips or the wire flexes and the archwire contacts the corners of the bracket. Notching is the permanent deformation of the archwire, bracket or both at the wire–bracket corner interface, which causes tooth movement to stop. Tooth movement resumes when masticatory forces displace teeth and the notch is released. The critical contact angle (θc), at which binding increasingly prevents sliding mechanics from occurring, should not be more than 4° and this varies depending on the bracket–archwire combination. The θc angle increases as the diameter of the wire decreases, the width of the bracket decreases, and a larger bracket slot is used.[6] Therefore, some discrepancies seen between laboratory and clinical studies investigating friction of materials and its effect on tooth movement may be due to binding and notching not being taken into account in the laboratory set-up.

Archwire Shape and Arch Form

Archwires can be classified by shape or material. The shapes available can be classified as round, rectangular, hybrid (a combination such as Wonder wire, which is round in the buccal segments and rectangular in the labial segment) or by arch form type. There are several arch forms available on the market. However, no one arch form shape applies to all and although prefabricated arch forms are useful in achieving a closest fit, individual adjustments are necessary.[7] The overriding principle is to maintain as much as possible the original arch form in order to increase the chances of stability following treatment. The teeth are in a 'neutral zone', which is the position of balance between the different forces from the soft tissues around them: lips, tongue, cheeks and periodontal ligament.[8] The most stable position is to maintain them within this zone after treatment. Long-term retention studies have shown that there is more relapse observed when the pretreatment (original) arch form is altered, especially when the intercanine width is altered.[7, 9] In specific cases, where the lower incisors were 'trapped' for example by a lower lip trap or a digit sucking habit, it may be possible to allow for some stable lower incisor proclination and so a change in the arch form, when the factors that caused the retroclination of the lower incisors are corrected.[10] Lee has provided a good summary of the current thoughts on stable arch expansion.[11] The lower intercanine width should be maintained, as expansion at this site has been shown to have the highest risk of relapse. Some expansion at the premolar and, to a lesser extent, the molar sites can be stable.

Historically, the Bonwill–Hawley arch form, based around an equilateral triangle, was used.[12] The lower canine to canine formed the arch of the circle and the patient's original arch form was not considered. The catenary curve provides a more fitting description of a natural arch form. This is the shape formed by a length of chain when held at each end and allowed to drop. This shape tends to fit relatively well the arch form up to the first permanent molars but tends to miss the narrowing that exists at the level of the second molars.[13] Many prefabricated archwires are based on this curve, with some modifications for tapered or squared arch forms. The Brader arch form, based on a trifocal ellipse, has the same anterior segment as the catenary curve but is wider at the premolar region and tapers in posteriorly, giving a narrower width at the second molar region.[14] The latter is also used as a basis for prefabricated archwires. There have been numerous other mathematical models proposed for dental arch forms and there is a myriad of different prefabricated archwire shapes and sizes available to the orthodontist. After years of debating this is still a topic of discussion between orthodontists: what is the ideal arch form, to which arch form should one treat and in which archwires is this introduced? A questionnaire-based study found no consistency between clinicians in how the arch form should be measured and methods were used differently between clinicians.[15] Most of the clinicians found it important to maintain the pretreatment arch form, especially the intercanine width, at the later stages of treatment (e.g. working archwires) but it was not perceived as important at the initial stages with alignment nickel titanium archwires.[15]

In summary, although there are several prefabricated arch forms and these are quicker and more practical to use, there is still a need for the orthodontist to make a conscious selection of the arch form to be used for the individual patient's dental arch and make adjustments to the prefabricated archwire as necessary. This is especially crucial in the later stages of treatment, when rectangular stiffer archwires are used. For further discussion of arch form see Chapter 14.

Archwire Materials

Several materials are available and it is important to have an understanding of the physical properties of the different materials when selecting archwires for the different stages of treatment.

Precious Metal Alloys

Before the development of stainless steel, precious alloys were used for archwires, as they were one of the few materials that would withstand oral conditions. These often included platinum, palladium, gold and copper. The gold materials used in orthodontic archwires correspond to the type IV gold casting alloys and are subjected to softening and hardening heat treatments in the archwire manufacture process. Nowadays, these have been superseded by the materials detailed in the following sections.

Stainless Steel

Stainless steel exists in three forms: ferritic, martensitic and austenitic. Martensitic stainless steel exhibits a higher strength and hardness and is therefore often used for surgical and cutting instruments. The austenitic type is the most corrosion resistant of the stainless steels. Typically for orthodontic materials an austenitic stainless steel is used that contains approximately 71% iron, 18% chromium and 8% nickel, giving it the name '18-8 stainless steel'. AISI 302 is the basic type containing 0.15% carbon. Type AISI 304 stainless steel has a similar composition, the main difference being the reduced carbon content of 0.08%. Both types AISI 302 and 304 are referred to as '18-8 stainless steel' and are the types generally used in orthodontics for bands and archwires. Chromium provides the corrosion resistance, as when exposed to air a chromium oxide layer is formed on the surface. The nickel helps to increase ductility. A small of amount of carbon (<0.2%) helps to achieve a high yield strength and high modulus of elasticity. The properties of steel can be controlled during manufacture; **annealing** (the process of heating and cooling of the wire) softens the wire whilst **cold working** (repeated deformation of a wire whilst cold) hardens it. Heat treatment to temperatures of between 750 and 820°C removes residual stresses. Ligature wires, which are soft and highly formable, are made of nearly fully annealed stainless steel wire. The more the wire is hardened, the higher the yield strength but the lower its formability. Arthur J. Wilcock of Victoria, Australia, produced ultra-high tensile austenitic stainless steel wires for its use in the Begg technique. These are available in different diameters and in spools or cut lengths of wire. They are generally hard and brittle. The highest yield strength wires, 'super' grades or Wilcox 'special' and 'special plus', will break easily when bent, especially if bent sharply. The 'regular' grades of orthodontic steel wire provide sufficient strength and still allow bends to be introduced without fracture and are therefore the most common grade used for archwires.

The high modulus of elasticity of stainless steels makes the archwire stiff and so able to resist deformation. For this reason, it is commonly used as a working archwire, as it will maintain the arch form created in it whilst allowing for tooth movement to occur such as in space closure. Its low surface friction (lower than titanium molybdenum alloy [TMA] and nickel titanium) is an additional advantage for this purpose. During the finishing stages, bends may be required for torque and other corrections. In comparison to TMA, the number of bends and their size need to be smaller when using stainless steel, otherwise too much force would be elicited on the teeth, it may be difficult to engage the archwire in the slot (due to the low springiness) and the fracture point of the wire may be reached quicker. The high stiffness, low springiness, low springback and low range make stainless steel a poor alignment archwire. To increase spingback in order to use it during initial alignment, the length of wire between brackets used to be increased by bending loops in the archwire (see Chapter 14, Figure 14.7). However, this is time-consuming, technically difficult and has been superseded by the introduction of alternative options.

Multistranded Stainless Steel

Multistranded stainless steel archwires provide increased flexibility and lower stiffness.[16] The principle is the use of multiple thin stainless steel archwires wound together to make an archwire. The reason for the increased flexibility is that when the wire is deflected there are contact slips between adjacent wrap wires. There are three types of multistrand stainless steel wires.

- Coaxial: smaller wires wrapped around a larger central wire (e.g. a core wire of 0.0065 inch and six 0.0055-inch wrap wires produce an overall diameter of approximately 0.0165 inch).
- Twisted: three strands twisted together (e.g. three strands of 0.008 inch wound together to make an overall diameter wire of 0.0175 inch).
- Braided: eight strands of a smaller wire producing an overall rectangular archwire.

They are available in round and rectangular archwire cross-sections. Because of their increased flexibility the round wires can be used during initial alignment. Kusy and Dilley reported that 0.0175-inch multistranded stainless steel has a similar stiffness to 0.010-inch single-stranded stainless steel and is 25% stronger than it.[17] The stiffness was found to be similar to that of 0.016-inch nitinol, although nitinol tolerated 50% greater activation than the multistranded stainless steel.[17] The rectangular braided wires are helpful to allow settling whilst maintaining torque control and arch form during post-surgical or finishing stages of treatment.

Cobalt Chromium

Cobalt chromium alloy was initially manufactured for watch springs by Elgin Watch Company and later introduced in the market by Rocky Mountain Orthodontics as Elgiloy in the 1950s. It consists of 40% cobalt, 20% chromium, 15% nickel, 16% iron, 7% molybdenum and 2% manganese. It has a similar stiffness to stainless steel but is more formable and has a higher surface friction. The advantage it provides is that it can be supplied in a softer and more formable state and once shaped to the desired form it can be hardened by heat treatment in a dental furnace, which increases its resilience and strength but not its stiffness. With the availability of preformed archwires and reduced need for complex wire bends, this material is used less as an archwire nowadays but is still used for the construction of some auxiliaries or sometimes appliances such as a quadhelix. It is supplied in four tempers, which vary in formability: blue (soft), yellow (ductile), green (semi-resilient) and red (resilient, hard and not recommended for heat treatment).

Nickel Titanium

The introduction of nickel titanium (NiTi) archwires could be considered as one of the great advances in orthodontics. During the initial alignment phase of treatment, the archwire needs to be deflected to reach the malaligned teeth without permanently deforming and ideally produce low forces over a long range to align the teeth. NiTi alloy archwires are exceptionally flexible, exhibit high springiness, low modulus of elasticity, shape memory, and superelasticity and deliver low forces over a long range, making them the ideal archwire and the most commonly used for the alignment stages of treatment. Although NiTi wires are exceptional alignment wires, they are not suitable as working or finishing archwires due to their low stiffness and poor formability. There are three forms of NiTi archwires available:

- martensitic stable (e.g. nitinol, Titanal and Orthonol)
- superelastic austenitic active (e.g. Sentalloy 3)
- thermodynamic martensitic active (e.g. copper-NiTi and NeoSentalloy).

Martensitic Stable

The Naval Ordinance Laboratory in the USA first discovered nickel titanium in 1962 for their space programme and noted its shape memory effect potential. It was then brought into orthodontic use by Andreasen and Hilleman[18] through the University of Iowa as a 50% nickel and 50% titanium alloy archwire and later patented and marketed as Nitinol. The original Nitinol is a martensitic stable alloy produced by cold working. Ironically, the latter process suppresses the shape memory effect.[19] It has a low modulus of elasticity, great springiness and large springback, making it very flexible and useful for the alignment phase of treatment. The friction on this wire is higher than that with stainless steel but less than that with TMA. Nitinol, in the martensitic stable state, exhibits no shape memory or superelastic effect.

Superelastic Austenitic Active

These two unique physical properties were introduced later in orthodontics with NiTi alloys in the austenitic and martensitic active states and occur due to phase transformations in the crystalline structure of the alloy. **Superelasticity** is the ability to deliver the same force over a large range of deformation. The force deflection curve for austenitic active NiTi alloy shows its superelasticity property when compared to stainless steel and nitinol (martensitic stable state) (Figure 10.3). Burstone et al.[20] and Miura et al.[2] reported similar force deflection curves when they tested, respectively, Chinese NiTi and Japanese NiTi austenitic active nickel titanium archwires. The austenitic active nickel titanium archwire has a considerably flatter load deflection curve, lower modulus of elasticity and greater springback than nitinol and stainless steel. Nitinol exhibits greater springback than stainless steel but shows no superelasticity.

In Figure 10.4, a stress–strain curve for austenitic active nickel titanium alloy shows in more detail how the stress-induced crystalline phase transformation brings about this superelastic effect, sometimes also referred to as **pseudoelastic** behaviour. As the archwire is ligated into a displaced tooth, a stress-induced phase transformation from austenitic (stiffer crystal structure) to martensitic (lower stiffness crystal structure) phase occurs. Initially, from points A to B on the graph, the wire will behave elastically. The stress must reach a certain level, B, on the graph (i.e. the wire must be deflected clinically enough, at least 2 mm)[21] for a stress-induced **phase transformation** to be induced from austenitic to martensitic, which is represented by the loading plateau (B–C). As the tooth moves and the stress is released, elastic unloading of the martensitic phase takes place. At a certain point the reverse phase transformation is induced, represented by the unloading plateau D–E, which returns the crystal structure to its original austenitic active phase by E. E–F represents the elastic unloading of the austenitic phase. As the reverse phase transformation takes place, the wire returns to its original shape, showing its shape memory effect. It is important to note that the loading and unloading plateaus extend over a large range of deformation, meaning the wire delivers the same force over a large range, hence the term 'superelasticity'. The unloading plateau is lower than the loading plateau, showing less force is delivered by the

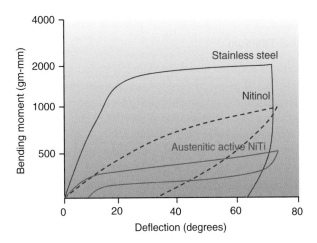

Figure 10.3 Force deflection curve comparing stainless steel, nitinol (martensitic stable) and austenitic active nickel titanium archwires. The high stiffness of stainless steel is represented by the steep slope of the elastic portion of the curve in comparison to nitinol and the austenitic active NiTi wires, which have lower stiffness respectively. The austenitic active NiTi is almost twice as elastic as nitinol and the springback is also much higher than stainless steel and nitinol. Source: adapted from Burstone CJ, Qin B, Morton JY. Chinese NiTi wire: a new orthodontic alloy. *Am. J. Orthod. Dentofacial Orthop.* 1985;87:445–452.

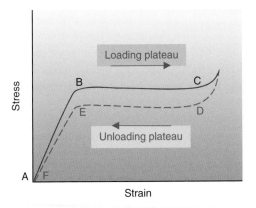

Figure 10.4 Stress–strain curve showing superelasticity due to a stress-induced transformation of an austenitic active nickel titanium archwire. Source: adapted from Burstone CJ, Qin B, Morton JY. Chinese NiTi wire: a new orthodontic alloy. *Am. J. Orthod. Dentofacial Orthop.* 1985;87:445–452.

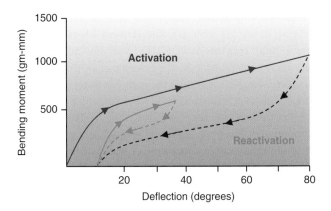

Figure 10.5 Loading and unloading curves of austenitic active nickel titanium when released and retied. Source: adapted from Burstone CJ, Qin B, Morton JY. Chinese NiTi wire: a new orthodontic alloy. *Am. J. Orthod. Dentofacial Orthop.* 1985;87:445–452.

archwire as it unloads than the force that is required to activate the wire. This loss of energy in the reversal process is termed **hysteresis**. In addition, the force produced by the archwire remains the same over a considerable range of deflection. Clinically, this would mean that even if the wire is deflected more (e.g. to ligate it to a very displaced tooth), the force exerted on the tooth will be the same as if it were deflected less, a definite advantage in the initial alignment phase of treatment. Because of irreversible changes during loading or unloading, the total strain may not be fully recovered, as shown on the graph by the position of F, which is not necessarily the same as A.

A final interesting point about this unique archwire is the finding by Burstone et al.[20] that the force delivered by an austenitic active nickel titanium wire can be changed clinically by simply releasing the wire and tying it again (Figure 10.5). In clinical orthodontics, this process is termed **reactivation** of the archwire. As can be seen on the graph, after the wire is deflected, for example by 80°, once it is released and retied (deflected again), the force delivered to the teeth (unloading plateau) is higher when retied than the first time it was activated.

Thermodynamic Martensitic Active

A phase transformation between martensitic and austenitic phases can also be induced by a temperature change, termed **thermoelasticity**. At higher temperatures the alloy is in its austenitic phase where plastic deformation can be induced and a predetermined shape, which is 'memorised', is set. As the wire is cooled, it changes to a more flexible martensitic phase (where no plastic deformation is possible), only to return again to its predetermined austenitic phase when warmed again. **Shape memory effect** is the ability of a wire to 'remember' its original

shape and return to it when triggered by stress or thermal stimulus. Since only austenite memorises the shape, NiTi exhibits a **one-way** shape memory effect. For most other alloys the temperature range at which the phase transformation occurs, named **transition temperature range** (TTR), is very high, but for nickel titanium alloys the TTR is relatively low, around body temperature. Nevertheless, it was difficult to control sufficiently precisely the transition temperature uniformly in the wire product, which led to the delay in thermally active wires being available in orthodontics.

Manufacturers managed to make **thermally active NiTi archwires** (martensitic active) with different TTRs by replacing some of the nickel with copper, which allows greater precision in the setting of the austenitic transformation temperature. Copper tends to raise the transformation temperature above body temperature and this is counteracted by the addition of 0.2–0.5% chromium, hence the term **nickel titanium copper chromium alloys**, often referred to as **copper NiTi** (CuNiTi) wires. These generate a lower and more constant force over long activation spans and exhibit better springback characteristics and lower hysteresis as compared to other NiTi alloys. The austenitic finish (Af) phase is reached at different temperatures, called the austenitic finish temperature. There are four types of copper NiTi wires available with the following Af temperatures and potential clinical applications.

- Type I, Af at 15°C: not commercially available.
- Type II, Af at 27°C: the loading force is less than that of other superelastic wires because of the low hysteresis unique to the CuNiTi alloy, while the unloading forces are comparable to traditional superelastic nickel titanium wires. Clinically, these would be used for patients with normal periodontal health and average pain threshold.
- Type III, Af at 35°C: undergoes the phase transformation (activated) once it is ligated and it heats to body temperature. Allows for easier engagement of full-size archwires and provides relatively lower and sustained unloading forces at body temperature. Clinically, suitable for patients with low to normal pain threshold and/or normal to compromised periodontal health.
- Type IV, Af at 40°C: only activated with hot food and beverages and so generates intermittent light forces and would be useful as an initial wire in patients with a low pain threshold, with periodontally compromised dentitions or with severely malaligned teeth.

These wires are produced in a martensitic active phase (low stiffness phase). In this state the wire is very flexible, allowing easy ligation into displaced teeth. As the wire is placed in the mouth and the temperature changes to that of body temperature/TTR (e.g. for types III and IV), a phase transformation is induced to its austenitic state (high stiffness state), returning the wire to its original shape (shape memory effect). Cooling these wires (e.g. in the fridge or with cooling sprays) before intraoral placement is thought to allow for easier insertion, ensuring the more flexible martensitic state. Within the TTR there is coexistence of austenitic and martensitic phases, which leads to the improved mechanical properties of low nearly constant deactivation forces.[22] In addition, local stress-induced transformation to martensite will occur where the wire is ligated to displaced teeth (pseudoelasticity) (see Figure 10.4). When the tooth has aligned and the stress on the wire is reduced, the reverse phase transformation to austenitic active state is induced (see Figure 10.4). Therefore, in these wires a combination of superelasticity and thermoelasticity is occurring, and the ideal would be a TTR corresponding to the temperature variations of the oral environment.[22] It has been shown that the application of stress usually raises the Af of the alloys. For example, CuNiti 35°C, though its unloaded Af is 35°C, with minimum loading it is 37°C and maximum loading 41°C.[22] Hence the amount of deflection expected (e.g. severe crowding) may need to be taken into account when selecting the wire.

The principle of manufacturing NiTi archwires with clinically useful TTR temperatures has been developed further to produce variable transition temperatures within the same archwire, known as **Bioforce** archwires. These are aesthetic graded thermodynamic NiTi archwires manufactured so that they provide differential force anteriorly and posteriorly, aiming to provide biologically ideal forces. In this way gentle forces can be exerted to the anterior teeth (which have a small root surface area and are therefore at higher risk of root resorption with higher forces), with progressively increasing forces applied to the posterior teeth until plateauing at the molars. This may be clinically helpful; for example, if during the initial stages of treatment torque is required, a Bioforce rectangular archwire may be engaged earlier than otherwise, as the forces delivered to the anterior teeth are lower in this wire.

Finally, there are a number of special preformed NiTi archwires available, with bends that would be difficult to achieve chairside. NiTi archwires with an exaggerated preformed reverse curve of Spee ('rocking horse wires') may be used in the lower arch to help in deep bite cases. It is important to closely monitor their effect clinically, since when left for prolonged periods they can lead to undesirable changes in the arch form. In addition, NiTi archwires can be pre-torqued, in combination or not with the reverse curve of Spee.

Different superelastic properties set within the same NiTi archwire are also possible. **Direct electric resistance heat treatment** (DERHT) was the new type of heat treatment that made this possible.[23] In this process, an electric current is passed through the wire, generating enough heat to bend it as well as imparting a change in the superelastic property of the wire. The heat-treated segments demonstrate better superelastic properties and the amount of heat is controlled by the heating time and amperage. Therefore, it is possible to produce different loading/unloading curve force levels in the anterior and posterior segments of an archwire by heat-treating the different segments for different lengths of time, the aim being for lower unloading forces anteriorly.

The latest development in the field of nickel titanium archwires is the higher performance of a seven-stranded superelastic NiTi coaxial wire called Supercable (Strite Industries Ltd, Cambridge, Ontario, Canada) compared with a single-stranded NiTi archwire. It is claimed to exert one-third of the force of an equivalent diameter single-stranded superelastic NiTi, hence delivering very low forces in the initial alignment stages.[24] A study undertaken by Sebastian compared 0.016-inch single-stranded superelastic NiTi wire (Rematitan Lite Wire) to 0.016-inch coaxial superelastic NiTi wire (Regular 7 Stranded Supercable Wire) and reported alignment rate per month for the lower labial segment.[25] Measurements were made on dental casts taken at 4, 8 and 12 weeks after initial archwire placement, using a coordinate measuring machine that calculated mean tooth movement at each time point. Coaxial superelastic NiTi archwires produced greater tooth movement over 12 weeks than the single-stranded NiTi wires.[25] This study was rated of moderate quality by a systematic review of randomised controlled trials, which also found that, other than this finding, there was insufficient evidence to determine whether any of the particular archwire materials is superior to another in terms of alignment rate, time to alignment, pain and root resorption.[26]

Beta-Titanium

Beta-titanium alloy was introduced in the early 1980s by Charles Burstone and developed primarily for use in orthodontics to provide an archwire that would produce lower biomechanical forces than stainless steel or cobalt chromium. It consists of 79% titanium, 11% molybdenum, 6% zirconium and 4% tin and because of its composition is often marketed as TMA (titanium molybdenum alloy). It offers better formability and greater springback than stainless steel, has about one-third of the stiffness of stainless steel and is twice as stiff as martensitic stabilised nickel titanium alloy. It is a useful archwire in the intermediate and finishing stages of treatment, where bends may be required. It contains no nickel and therefore is useful in patients with a nickel allergy. This wire can be welded but not soldered and its corrosion resistance is similar to that of stainless steel and cobalt chromium alloys.

When the initial patent for the alloy expired, several variations of the alloy with slight differences in their stiffness and yield strength were introduced and are described by Verstrynge et al.[27] **Titanium niobium** is one of the variations of TMA and offers 60% of the stiffness of TMA, and hence is easier to bend and marketed as a finishing archwire.

Ion Implantation

Kusy and Whitley found these wires to have a rough surface and the highest surface friction coefficients when compared with all other archwire materials.[5] The technique of **ion implantation** has been used with TMA archwires in an attempt to reduce their friction. Nitrogen ions are produced from a heated filament in a source chamber and thereafter accelerated and sent into an evacuated implantation specimen.[28] The results of *in vitro* studies seem to support this concept. Ryan et al.[29] found stainless steel produced the least frictional force, followed by ion-implanted nickel titanium, ion-implanted beta-titanium, untreated nickel titanium and untreated beta-titanium. However, to what extent this has an impact clinically is questionable. A split-mouth design study found no difference in the rate of space closure between ion-implanted beta-titanium archwires and untreated beta-titanium archwires.[30]

Aesthetic Archwires

The increased acceptability and demand for orthodontic treatment, especially in the adult population, and the wish for more aesthetic options has driven the development of aesthetic orthodontic material alternatives. Initially, ceramic and composite brackets were introduced, although the archwires were still metallic. Extensive research and development over the last few years has led to several commercially available aesthetic archwire options, which we can classify as coated metal archwires or fibre-reinforced composite archwires. The latter arise from aerospace technology, where composite plastics are readily in use in the manufacture of high-performance aircraft.

Coated Metal Archwires

Coated NiTi archwires are readily available and are the most frequently used aligning archwires. Stainless steel archwires are also available in a coated version.

The coatings are generally either an epoxy resin or polytetrafluoroethylene (Teflon), which provides a tooth-coloured coating, and this may be applied to the whole surface of the wire or only partially to the labial surface. Rhodium-coated stainless steel or NiTi wires are produced by ion implantation and provide a whiter appearance to the metal alloy, and are therefore more aesthetic than the uncoated equivalents. The surface roughness of rhodium-coated archwires seems to be not significantly different from the uncoated controls, yet most of the tooth-coloured coated archwires were found to have a higher surface roughness.[31] Although no correlation was detected between surface roughness and frictional resistance, it may still have an impact on corrosion potential and plaque accumulation.[31] The epoxy coating is manufactured by a depository process that plates the base wire with an epoxy resin approximately 0.002 inches thick, achieving a strong adhesion between the epoxy coating and the wire. The Teflon coating is achieved by using clean compressed air as a transport medium of the atomised Teflon particles, and this is further heat treated in a chamber furnace.[32] The layer has a typical thickness of 20–25 μm and is tooth coloured. Teflon has a low coefficient of friction and is a stable anti-adherent material.

The main change to consider in terms of coated archwire characteristics in comparison to their uncoated metal alloy equivalents is that the surface of the metal alloy has been modified and the diameter of the metal alloy reduced to compensate for the coating thickness, which can affect force delivery, friction, corrosive properties, and the mechanical durability of the wires. In addition, the coating must provide a durable aesthetic solution for patients, with acceptable colour stability and durability (not peeling off from the underlying metal alloy). It is also worth noting that manufacturers differ in their abilities to produce wires accurately and in general the tendency is for most inner alloy core dimensions for coated archwires to be smaller than the nominal sizes given by manufacturers.[33] Of the archwires included in the study by Da Silva et al.,[33] only the coated archwires from TP Orthodontics maintained the nominal sizes.

The reduction of the inner alloy dimension to compensate for the coating thickness seems to be the variable responsible for the changes in the mechanical properties of aesthetic coated archwires.[34] It has been shown with three-point bending tests that aesthetic coated archwires produce lower loading and unloading forces, lower modulus of elasticity and lower modulus of resilience as compared to control uncoated archwires of the same dimensions, even when from the same manufacturer.[34–36] The exception to this finding was provided by archwires that were only coated labially, as these practically maintained the inner alloy core dimension with reference to the control uncoated archwire and were able to show comparable mechanical properties and force delivery.[34, 36] The thickness of the epoxy coating was found to be almost similar between coated wires and ranged between 0.00055 and 0.0006 inches.[36] The only labially coated archwires had a 0.0014-inch coating on one side.[36] The analysis of the end values of aesthetic wires showed almost complete recovery after 2- and 3-mm deflections for all coated archwires, except Plastic-Coated NiTi (Ortho Organizer), which showed significantly higher end values at 2- and 3-mm deflections suggestive of force degradation.[36] Though a low force delivery is desirable in orthodontics, it may not be effective if it is below the required optimum orthodontic range for tooth movement. If larger-diameter archwires are used to achieve the greater force delivery, friction may be increased. Nevertheless, the efficiency of alignment by different coated archwires seems to be within an acceptable range and comparable to one another. A multicentre randomised controlled trial found that following an average clinical use of 63.65 days, there was no difference in efficiency of alignment between the four coated NiTi archwires tested: BioCosmetic, Titanol, TP Aesthetics and Tooth Tone. However, BioCosmetic performed statistically significantly better than did the other types for both colour change and coating loss.[37]

The problem seems to be more the considerable aesthetic variation in colour stability and coating loss between commercially available archwires.[38] Fifty patients undergoing upper fixed appliance treatment with ceramic brackets were allocated to have one of three coated archwires (American Orthodontics Ever White™, Forestadent Biocosmetic™ and GAC High Aesthetic™), which were retrieved following six weeks *in situ*.[38] The greatest mean coating loss of 50.7% was by the Ever White archwires, whereas the High Aesthetic archwires underwent a minimal loss of 0.07% ($P < 0.001$). The coating loss was mainly anteriorly for the Ever White archwires, but posterior for the other two groups, which would impact on the perceived aesthetics as less visible if posteriorly lost. The participants reported on the perceived aesthetics and a negative correlation was found between coating loss and final visual analogue scale scores.[38]

A rough archwire surface (for example if partial loss of the coating or changes to the coating surface occur) encourages greater plaque accumulation, colour instability and increased corrosion, all of which may influence the clinical performance mechanically and aesthetically of the archwire.[39] Coated archwires become rougher clinically and undergo delamination, with crack propagation and debris observed along the coating scratches, which could influence its durability in the oral environment.[34]

Coated wires are also found to be routinely damaged from mastication and activation of enzymes.[1] A recent study found a statistically significant increase in surface roughness after four weeks of clinical use of all archwire types tested (rhodium-coated NiTi, NiTi partially coated with Teflon, uncoated stainless steel and uncoated NiTi) and microorganism adhesion was present in all archwires, but there was no correlation between surface roughness and bacterial adhesion.[40] The increase in surface roughness was probably related to abrasion during toothbrushing, mastication and interactions between the archwires, brackets and ligatures. The authors suggest the absence of a correlation may be related to surface free energy and superficial chemical changes. The fully coated NiTi group demonstrated a statistically significant higher bacterial biofilm count while the partially coated NiTi had the lowest count.[40] These results, together with the improved mechanical performance of partially coated archwires, seems to suggest these may provide overall a better alternative than fully coated archwires. Further *in vivo* studies are needed to assess the clinical efficacy of the different coatings available and whether partial coating of archwires imparts any benefit over fully coating the archwires.

Fibre-reinforced Composite Archwires

These archwires consist of a composite polymer matrix reinforced with glass fibre. By varying the reinforcing fibre content of the composite matrix, the elastic modulus of these wires can be adjusted to the preferred range. Work by Zufall and Kusy[41] characterised the fundamental properties of the experimental material such as water absorption and concluded that the experimental product at that stage was promising. The coefficient of friction was shown to be within the limits outlined by conventional archwire–bracket couples, and they highlighted that notching would need to be reduced in order to minimise frictional resistance. Clinically, it was suggested for low ligation forces to be used with composite archwires, as notching occurred less frequently with lower normal forces. The selection of orthodontic brackets designed with well-rounded slot edges was also suggested in order to help reduce notching and consequently improve clinical sliding mechanics.[41]

The introduction of commercially available composite archwires has been slow. One example available is BioMers Products (Jacksonville, FL, USA), which is available both as a round wire (Align A, B, and C with diameters of 0.018, 0.019 and 0.021 inches, respectively) or rectangular wire (TorQ A and TorQ B with dimensions of 0.019 × 0.025 inches and 0.021 × 0.025 inches, respectively). These wires are manufactured by incorporating glass fibres into a resin contained within a shrinkable and flexible die that reacts to heat. As the die shrinks, the composite is compressed to form its predetermined transverse cross-sectional shape.

The need for orthodontic archwires to remain in the oral cavity for prolonged periods presents a challenge for fibre-reinforced composite materials, as their strength reduces when stored in water.[42] Water molecules diffuse into the resin matrix and act as a plasticiser, increasing the fluidity of resin polymer chains and making their movement under stress easier and decreasing the strength of the composite. Chang et al.[42] studied the effect of water storage on the bending properties of fibre-reinforced composite archwires (BioMers) and compared it to NiTi, stainless steel and TMA archwires. Water immersion for 30 days was damaging to the larger fibre-reinforced composite archwires, because they were more likely to craze during bending, resulting in decreased amounts of force applied at a given deflection. On the other hand, alloy wires were not significantly affected by water storage. The authors suggested that hydrolytic degradation of resin may explain the lower force level delivery by the wires in the water-stored group, but another mechanism is likely at play since the drop in force is largely tied to the higher crazing rate.

Overall, the alloy wires showed more consistent force values compared to the composite wires. All fibre-reinforced composite wires had lower stiffness and force delivery levels than the manufacturer-specified comparison except for TorQ A. For instance, Align C had the greatest deviation from the comparison, and the force delivery during activation would probably be more comparable to that of 0.020-inch martensitic stabilised NiTi, instead of 0.016-inch stainless steel. The stiffness of the rectangular fibre-reinforced composite wires was less than a TMA of the same size but slightly higher than an equivalent size martensitic-stabilised NiTi wire. For round wires, composite wires had a lower stiffness than stainless steel and martensitic-stabilised NiTi wires of comparable size.

Overall, the dimensions of the alloy wires were consistent among the same group and along a segment, but the dimensions of the fibre-reinforced composite wires were not. For rectangular fibre-reinforced composite wires the dimensions varied by 7–21% of that expected. This inconsistent variation from the specified dimension could also cause the composite wires to not fit in the slot of the brackets and could increase friction, if the sizes are greater than expected. In view of the latter finding and the reduced stiffness of composite wires relative to the stainless steel or TMA equivalents, it may make composite wires less suitable for certain types of mechanics that require rigid archwires, such as closing spaces using sliding mechanics, correcting anteroposterior relationships using inter-arch elastics, or maintaining transverse dimension.[42]

The commercially available composite wire's ability to maintain continuous forces without undergoing force decay when deflected continuously was tested by Spendlove et al.[43] Quasi force decay was evaluated by comparing three-point bending profiles of NiTi and fibre-reinforced composite archwires (BioMers) prior to and after 30 days of continuous deflection of either 1 or 2 mm. The composite 1-mm deflection group demonstrated that fibre-reinforced composite archwires are able to deliver a consistent force after 30 days of deflection. However, the clinical applicability of composite archwires may be limited, as they are unable to sustain deflections of 2 mm without experiencing crazing and loss of force delivery. The clinical efficacy of aesthetic fibre-reinforced composite orthodontic archwires remains to be observed.

Fibre-reinforced composite archwires seem promising however, so further clinical research to ascertain their efficacy compared to coated archwires and their metal alloy counterparts is needed. This may also help highlight aspects for improvement in their manufacture, such as more accurate dimensions and stable force deliveries. Future research in this field may also focus on shape-memory plastics. The first plastics that can be reformed into temporary preprogrammed shapes by illumination with ultraviolet light were developed in a joint project between German and US researchers. When exposed to ultraviolet light of a different wavelength, the bent plastic wires return to their original shapes. The mechanism involved relates to the grafting of photosensitive groups into the polymer network; this acts as a molecular switch.[44]

Fatigue

Fatigue is the weakening of a material due to repeated stress and can lead to fatigue failure (fracture) of the material. The stresses applied to a material tend to concentrate in the weaker areas, such as where the material has a change in size, there is a joint (e.g. where two materials are welded together), or where there are defects such as notches or cracks (e.g. where the wire was previously bent or crushed with pliers). These are the most common points where the weakening effect of fatigue takes place and the wire may eventually fracture. Clinically, fatigue failure is often seen where multiple bends were undertaken or where there are sharp bends in the archwire. In addition, due to repeated occlusal loading of the archwire, it may also occur when long interbracket distances exist, such as in a 2 × 4 archwire set-up or when there are multiple missing or erupting teeth and the archwire is not engaged into brackets at these sites.

A study that characterised retrieved intraorally fractured NiTi archwires found that the preferential site for fracture was posteriorly at the midpoint between the premolar and molar, probably due to high masticatory forces. All retrieved archwires (11 superelastic NiTi and 19 copper NiTi) had the distinct features of brittle fracture without plastic deformation or crack propagation and showed no increased hardness.[45] It had been previously suggested by an *in vitro* study that **hydrogen absorption**, an effect known to increase hardness and induce brittle fracture of titanium alloys, could be a mechanism of NiTi archwire failure.[46] However, the results of this retrieval study contradict this theory and suggest that hydrogen embrittlement is not the cause of fracture.[45] Archwires seem to fracture clinically more than would be expected from the results of *in vitro* studies. The reason could be that intraoral ageing of archwires is complex and cannot be replicated *in vitro*. Intraorally, archwires are under complex masticatory loading, stress during ligation, are in a changing salivary pH and may be affected by the activity of microorganisms, biofilm formation and precipitations on their surface, which may affect their surface morphology and mechanical properties, hence also the fracture characteristics.[45]

Corrosion of Metal Alloys

Corrosion refers to the change in mechanical properties and the loss of weight under the effect of various chemical agents. It occurs from either the loss of metal ions directly into a solution or the progressive dissolution of a surface film. Though some metals are noble and essentially inert, such as gold and platinum, many of the metals used in orthodontics (stainless steel, cobalt chromium and titanium alloys) rely on a passive oxide surface layer to render them corrosion resistant. These protective oxide films are susceptible to mechanical and chemical disruption. Even if not disrupted, they often undergo a process whereby they slowly dissolve (passivation), exposing and permitting corrosive attack of the underlying alloy. As the metal is exposed to oxygen from the air or the surrounding medium, the passive oxide layer is reformed (repassivation). Acidic conditions and chlorine ions can accelerate the passivation process. A study found that chlorine ions and sulphuric compounds in the presence of microorganisms can lead to corrosion of stainless steel.[47, 48] Furthermore, fluoridated acidic conditions (pH of 3.5 and below) have been found to increase the susceptibility to corrosion of some metals *in vitro*, especially stainless steel and titanium alloys, by dissolving the passive oxide film on the surface of the alloys and thus eliminating the protective layer against corrosion.[49]

Based on this research, a diet rich in sodium chloride and acidic carbonated drinks and regular use of acidulated fluoridated preparations should be avoided in patients undergoing orthodontic treatment with metal alloys susceptible to corrosion, especially titanium-containing alloys (e.g. NiTi or TMA archwires and titanium brackets). However, an *in vivo* study concluded that the changes clinically seen were so minor that titanium brackets can be safely used for up to 18 months.[50] Of 18 patients bonded with titanium brackets on the left quadrants and stainless steel brackets on the right quadrants of upper and lower arches, 15 used Gel Kam-containing soluble tin fluoride (pH 3.2) and three used a fluoride-free toothpaste three times a day. The brackets were removed for evaluation by light and scanning microscopy 5.5–7.0 months and 7.5–17 months after bonding. Regardless of the toothpaste used, plaque accumulation on titanium brackets was greater than on stainless steel brackets, due to titanium's rougher surface. Deeper pitting and wider crevices were observed in only three of the 165 titanium brackets tested (2%), which revealed no fluoride with analysis of the elements. In contrast to the results of the *in vitro* investigations, only a few brackets were affected by corrosion. The authors suggested the reason for this difference could be the short reaction time of fluoride ions (as brackets were exposed to the fluoridated toothpaste only during toothbrushing) and the rinsing effect of saliva, water and food that dilutes the fluoride ion concentration. Therefore, the use of titanium brackets in combination with acidic fluoride dentifrice and fluoridated foods was suggested to be harmless.[50]

Types of Corrosion

The different types of corrosion can be classified as follows: uniform, pitting, crevice, intergranular, galvanic, fretting, stress, fatigue and microbiologically influenced corrosion.[39, 47, 48]

- **Uniform attack**: this is the most common type of corrosion. It occurs with all metals, though at different rates, due to an oxidation and reduction (redox) reaction of the metal with the surrounding environment. Uniform attack may be undetectable until a large amount of the metal is affected.
- **Pitting corrosion**: this form has been identified on the surfaces of brackets and archwires and can be already present on as-received brackets and archwires, as they are not perfectly smooth. The microscopic surface pits and crevices increase the susceptibility to corrosion of the alloy. They may harbour plaque-forming microorganisms, which in turn cause localised pH reduction

and oxygen depletion, enhancing the passivation process. However, the interplay between surface roughness and corrosion resistance is not as simple, and at least for nickel titanium archwires, surface residual stress produced during the manufacturing process has been suggested to also affect corrosion resistance.[51]

- **Crevice corrosion**: this is a common defect found on orthodontic attachments and may also occur in removable appliances. In the latter case, a brown discoloration may appear beneath the acrylic surface in contact with the metal. It occurs especially at sites where the metal is in contact with materials such as adhesives, acrylic and elastics. It is thought to be due to a surface biofilm at these sites, where bacteria lead to a lack of oxygen and the by-products of microbial flora also deplete the oxygen, disturbing the regeneration of the passive oxide layer.

- **Intergranular corrosion**: this type of corrosion affects particularly stainless steel. Exposing stainless steel to a sensitising temperature, such as that when heated during brazing and welding, leads to sensitisation. This refers to the reaction of chromium and carbon in the steel to form chromium carbide, which precipitates at grain boundaries. This in turn makes the alloy more brittle, due to slip interferences, and decreases the resistance to corrosion as there is less remaining chromium available to form the chromium oxide layer, leading to intergranular corrosion.[47] In contrast to the other types of corrosion involving dissolution of a part of a metal, in this type of corrosion there is a localised attack at the grain boundaries with relatively little corrosion of the grains themselves. The appearance of the metal and its weight may not change, but there is a loss of the metal's mechanical properties, and it may lead to failure. Methods used to control or minimise this type of corrosion in stainless steel include quench-annealing (the heated metal is quenched in water to dissolve the chromium carbide and avoid it from precipitating at the boundaries), reducing the carbon content (but lower strengths are exhibited at high temperatures) and incorporating strong carbide formers such as niobium or titanium in the stainless steels. Such elements have a much greater affinity for carbon than does chromium, hence carbide formation with these elements reduces the carbon available in the alloy for formation of chromium carbides.

- **Galvanic corrosion**: this occurs when different metals (or even the same alloy, subjected to different treatments) are joined together and placed in a conductive solution or an electrolyte. The less noble metal is oxidised and becomes anodic, producing soluble ions in the process. The nobler metal becomes cathodic and so a galvanic cell is created because of the differences in electrochemical potential of the two metals. In orthodontics, this may occur when two metals are joined by soldering, for example posted archwires, tubes on bands or during bracket construction. It was already noted in the 1980s that the brazing alloy used in the construction of brackets appeared to be a significant factor in the initiation of corrosion, as did the mesh base, especially in cases in which spot welds were present.[48] With soldered wires, the greatest problem is the release of ions such as iron, zinc, copper and cadmium ions from the cadmium-containing silver solder. In an *in vitro* cytotoxicity study of new and used orthodontic components, only the used stainless steel molar bands with a soldered tube demonstrated potential cytotoxicity.[52]

- **Fretting corrosion**: this occurs in areas of metal contact under sustained loads. In orthodontics, this would be at the archwire–bracket slot interface. The two metals under load undergo a process of cold welding, and continued force application can cause the welded junction to shear, disrupting the passive oxide layer and leaving the metal susceptible to corrosion. This type of ageing is not seen on archwires aged using *in vitro* models, which employ electrolyte or artificial saliva solutions.[39]

- **Stress corrosion**: this occurs when the reactivity status of the alloy increases at sites of stress due to loading, such as when an archwire is ligated to brackets bonded to crowded teeth. The increased reactivity results from the generation of tensile and compressive stresses developed locally because of the multiaxial three-dimensional loading of the wire. This leads to the establishment of an electrochemical potential difference along the archwire, with specific sites acting as anodes and others as cathodes, hence facilitating corrosion.

- **Corrosion fatigue**: metals have an increased tendency to fracture when under repeated cyclic stressing (termed fatigue). Corrosion fatigue refers to the accelerated process of fatigue when metal alloys are also exposed to a corrosive medium, such as saliva, as this reduces the fatigue resistance. It occurs frequently in archwires left in the intraoral environment for extended periods of time under load. It is characterised by the smoothness of the fractured areas, which also include a site of increased roughness and crystalline appearance.[39]

- **Microbiologically influenced corrosion**: this type of corrosion is pertinent in orthodontics, as microorganisms in oral biofilms and their by-products can lead to corrosion of metal alloys. Certain species are able to directly absorb and metabolise metal from alloys (e.g. iron-consuming microorganisms include *Sphaerotilus*, *Hyphomicrobium* and *Gallionella*) leading to corrosion of the metal. Also, the normal metabolic by-products of many species and/or the interplay between the metabolic processes of different species in the biofilm may lead to an environmental condition that is more conducive to corrosion, for example by increasing acidity levels. It is thought microbial corrosion under a biofilm occurs as a cathode–anode reaction. *Streptococcus mutans* uses oxygen, so a non-uniform distribution of the microorganism in the biofilm causes differences in the oxygenation of particular areas: under the thicker layer of the biofilm the surface will behave anodically whilst under the thinner layer the surface will behave cathodically, and so a local corrosion cell is created on the metal surface.[53] Similarly, these corrosion cells can also be produced with more developed biofilms containing a mixture of aerobic and anaerobic bacteria.[53] It is known that sulphate-reducing and nitrate-reducing bacteria are aggressive and inflammatory to the hosting tissues, and that these bacteria also affect the corrosion processes of various alloys.[39, 53] Evidence of microbial attack on adhesives used in orthodontics has also been shown, together with the result of formation of craters in the bracket bases.[47]

Interestingly, certain salivary proteins, amylase and gammaglobulin in the oral environment form a biofilm that acts as a corrosion inhibitor. It has been observed *in vitro* that proteins and glycoproteins in phosphate buffered saline solution act as corrosion inhibitors and thus limit the electrochemical degradation of titanium alloys.[54] Eliades et al.[55] demonstrated the presence of a proteinaceous biofilm on retrieved NiTi archwires that had been in use for one to six months. The composition and thickness of the film depended on the individual patient's oral conditions and the intraoral exposure time, rather than archwire brand or size. The organic components of the biofilm were found to be mainly amides, alcohols and carbonates with crystalline precipitates of sodium chloride, potassium chloride and calcium phosphate. It was suggested that this mineralised layer could act as a protective layer against corrosion, especially in acidic conditions. Furthermore, this study found that the topography of the intraorally exposed NiTi wires and the structure of the alloy surface were altered. There was evidence of alloy delamination, pitting and crevice corrosion, as well as a reduction in the alloy grain size at compression sites where the archwire was tied to the brackets. The type of ageing that wires undergo intraorally, as shown by this study, is not yet possible to replicate *in vitro*.

Clinical Significance of Corrosion

The clinical significance of corrosion includes the following.

- Corrosion may increase orthodontic friction at the archwire–bracket interface due to increase in surface roughness.
- Corrosion products have been implicated in causing local pain or swelling in the region of orthodontic appliances in the absence of infection, which can lead to secondary infection.
- Corrosion products have been reported to cause staining on enamel following bracket removal.[39, 47]
- Cytotoxic and biological responses may take place (e.g. nickel allergy).
- Weakening of appliance and potential failure of the metal alloy (i.e. fracture).

Methods to Reduce Corrosion

Manufacturers are aware of the various types of corrosion orthodontic alloys are exposed to and try to minimise this in different ways. One method already discussed is the **addition or substitution of an alloy**. This principle is used in the production of orthodontic stainless steel and NiTi materials. The corrosion resistance for NiTi is provided by the large titanium content (48–54%), which can form several oxide configurations (titanium dioxide being the most common and stable) and provides the surface oxide layer.[51] In stainless steel, chromium is added to provide a chromium oxide surface layer. The nickel in stainless steel also helps, by competing with chromium to form salts, hence more chromium is available for the passive oxide layer formation. The chromium oxide layer in stainless steel is not as stable as the titanium oxide counterpart in NiTi, so stainless steel has inferior corrosion resistance compared to NiTi alloys.[39] **Coatings** have also been used but provide corrosion resistance to varied extents. Titanium nitride has been used as a coating for brackets and archwires to provide improved hardness and reduced friction. Epoxy resin coatings of archwires provide a tooth-coloured archwire, and therefore also have an aesthetic benefit. Kim and Johnson[56] compared these coated wires to stainless steel, uncoated NiTi and titanium and found that corrosion occurred readily in stainless steel, while in NiTi uncoated wires there was variation depending on the manufacturer. The nitride coating provided no protection against corrosion and the titanium and epoxy-coated NiTi archwires experienced the least corrosion.[56] Finally, **modifications to manufacturing and post-manufacturing** finishing and polishing can help in reducing the corrosive potential. During bracket production, galvanic corrosion can be reduced by laser welding the body of the bracket to its base instead of brazing and avoiding the use of different grades of stainless steel between these two components of the brackets. During manufacture of brackets and arch-wires, several of the processes used, such as alloying, heat treatment, cold working and polishing, affect the microstructure and surface of the alloy, which in turn may affect the alloy's corrosion resistance. An increased surface roughness has been often linked to an increased corrosion potential. However, an *in vitro* study assessing surface characterisation and corrosion resistance of as-received commercial NiTi archwires from different manufacturers casts some doubt on this.[57] The surface structure of the passive film on the tested NiTi wires were identical (mainly TiO_2, with small amounts of NiO), but the surface topographies varied between manufacturers. The corrosion tests showed that both the wire manufacturer and solution pH had a statistically significant influence on the corrosion potential, corrosion rate and crevice-corrosion susceptibility. However, the difference in corrosion resistance among the different NiTi archwires did not correspond with the surface roughness and pre-existing defects.[57]

In conclusion, the oral environment provides a challenge to the materials used in orthodontics in terms of their corrosion resistance, as it is a moist environment with a changing pH depending on the food and beverage ingested, with microorganisms and masticatory forces that may also have an effect. All these parameters lead to a unique ageing of materials that affects their structure and corrosion resistance. Studies assessing corrosion of alloys are generally undertaken *in vitro*, from retrieved material (which had been used intraorally) or *in vivo*. Eliades and Athanasiou[39] described very eloquently the reasons why *in vitro* studies in this field are unfortunately not as helpful in understanding what really happens *in vivo*, as it is not possible to replicate *in vitro* the effects of the oral conditions on corrosion. Therefore, *in vivo* studies in the future will help clarify the effects of intraoral ageing on corrosion resistance and the effect *in vivo* of some agents that *in vitro* lead to reduced corrosion resistance, and will therefore provide some guidance as to their clinical significance for orthodontic materials and the tailored advice, if required, for orthodontic patients.

Which is the Best Aligning Archwire or Archwire Sequence?

Generally, it is thought that continuous light forces are the most efficient and desirable for orthodontic tooth movement, making superelastic NiTi archwires the most popular choice nowadays over multistranded stainless steel archwires in the alignment phase of treatment. Stainless steel wires deliver an initially higher but rapidly declining force, meaning the force needs to be re-established and patients potentially seen more often than with superelastic NiTi archwires, which provide a continuous light force for a longer time.

Several studies have been undertaken comparing these two materials as aligning archwires and results are varied. One study found the 0.014-inch superelastic NiTi wire produced a statistically significant improvement in alignment in the mandibular anterior segment in comparison to the 0.0155-inch multistrand stainless steel wire (Dentaflex), but there was no difference in the labial segment of the maxilla.[58] However, others have found no statistically significant difference in rate of alignment between these materials.[59] Furthermore, no difference was found in rate of alignment between multistrand stainless steel and thermoelastic NiTi archwires.[59] Also, studies comparing conventional and thermoelastic NiTi archwires found no significant difference in rate of alignment between these two archwire types.[60, 61]

The Cochrane review by Wang et al.[26] which included 12 randomised controlled trials with a total of 799 participants undertook several comparisons between different materials (multistranded stainless steel, conventional NiTi, superelastic NiTi, thermoelastic NiTi and coaxial NiTi) and found insufficient evidence to determine whether any particular archwire material was better in terms of alignment rate, time to alignment, pain or root resorption. The authors commented on the general poor quality of the included trials and suggested that the results should be viewed with caution. One included study, graded as providing moderate-quality evidence, found that a 0.016-inch coaxial superelastic wire (regular 7 stranded Supercable Wire, Speed System Orthodontics, Cambridge, Ontario, Canada) produced greater tooth movement over 4, 8 and 12 weeks than a 0.016-inch single stranded superelastic wire (Rematitan Lite Wire, Dentauram GmbH & Co. KG, Ispringen, Germany). The mean difference was 6.7 mm over 12 weeks, although this was a small trial including 24 patients.[25] The authors suggested the difference may be due to the Supercable wire having greater springback, increased resistance to deformation and low force delivery due to it being multistranded.[25] In addition, although the diameter of the wires are the same, the Supercable wire will deliver a lower force (has a lower elastic modulus) and will allow the orthodontist to reach the malaligned tooth and ligate it, whereas with an equivalent diameter superelastic single-stranded archwire it would need to have been partially ligated. Therefore, superelastic coaxial wires offer the advantage of being able to engage a relatively larger archwire at the start of treatment, achieving a greater degree of uprighting, levelling and rotational control, yet still delivering a low force.

Pain from Initial Archwires

Pain experienced following initial archwire placement has been found to start approximately two hours after placement, with the mean pain intensity peaking at 24 hours and thereafter gradually declining over seven days.[62] In the latter study, 90% of patients experienced pain in the first week after initial archwire placement. Whether different archwire materials produce more or less pain has been investigated in a number of studies. A Cochrane group concluded that there is moderate-quality evidence to suggest there may be no difference in pain at day 1 between multistranded stainless steel and superelastic NiTi archwires.[26] These results were based on studies that compared 0.015-inch multistrand stainless steel (Twistflex) with 0.014-inch superelastic NiTi wire (heavy Japanese NiTi)[63] and 0.0175-inch multistrand stainless steel (six-stranded) with 0.016-inch superelastic NiTi (austenitic active).[64] Other comparisons between materials have also been undertaken, but it was deemed there was insufficient evidence to decide whether any particular initial archwire material is better or worse than another, with regard to speed of straightening, pain or root resorption.[26] One study evaluated 0.014-inch nitinol compared to 0.014-inch superelastic NiTi wire (Sentalloy) and found no difference in pain intensity or analgesic consumption between groups on day 1 or 7.[65] Another group compared 0.016-inch superelastic NiTi to a 0.016-inch thermoelastic heat-activated NiTi archwire and also found no difference in mean reported pain between the groups on day 1 or 7.[66] More high-quality studies are required with a standardised approach to measuring reported pain.[26]

There are increasing number of studies assessing the effectiveness of different pharmacological and non-pharmacological methods for managing orthodontic-induced pain.

Pharmacological Management

A study comparing the effectiveness of a single dose of a placebo, aspirin (650 mg) or ibuprofen (400 mg) following placement of separators or an initial archwire found that ibuprofen is significantly more effective than aspirin in reducing discomfort, though both reduced it.[67] Another randomised controlled trial compared ibuprofen (400 mg) and paracetamol (1 g) given one hour before and six hours after separator placement.[68] Taken in this way (preoperative and postoperative), ibuprofen was found to be clinically significantly more effective than paracetamol from two hours to bedtime on the day of treatment.[68] Interestingly, from day 1 to 3 there was also a trend for those who had taken ibuprofen to experience lower pain levels compared with the paracetamol group. The authors suggest it is possible that ibuprofen could therefore have more beneficial long-term effects in the relief of orthodontic pain than paracetamol, even when blood levels of the drug are undetectable or below the therapeutic window of efficacy.[68]

It has been suggested that non-steroidal anti-inflammatory drugs (NSAIDs) such as ibuprofen may be a more effective analgesic compared to paracetamol in orthodontic-induced pain due to their different mode of action. NSAIDs inhibit the synthesis of prostaglandins peripherally at the site of the tissue injury, via inhibition of the cyclooxygenase enzymes COX-1 and COX-2 and have an anti-inflammatory effect. Hence the concentration of prostaglandins, which are important pain mediators, is reduced. Paracetamol has its effect centrally by inhibition of COX-3 in the brain and spinal cord. On the other hand, prostaglandins are important promoters of bone resorption in orthodontic tooth movement. Therefore, the disadvantage of local prostaglandin inhibition by NSAIDs is reduced bone resorption and hence reduced orthodontic tooth movement.[69] Currently the effect and clinical significance of NSAIDs on human orthodontic tooth movement is unclear, especially when they are only taken for a short period of time at the beginning of treatment. Long-term intake of NSAIDs would probably be better avoided if possible. However, more high-quality research is needed to investigate these comparisons, and to evaluate pre-emptive versus post-treatment administration of analgesics.[70] Currently, the meta-analysis of studies (rated as low quality) gave no clear evidence of a difference between the effect of ibuprofen and paracetamol for reducing pain intensity at two hours, six hours or 24 hours following either the placement of separators or an initial aligning archwire.[70] The benefit of taking ibuprofen preoperatively versus only postoperatively could also not be confirmed.[70] What is certain is that analgesics are more effective at reducing orthodontic pain than a placebo or no treatment.[70] Numerous analgesics have been shown to help relieve orthodontic pain (ibuprofen, paracetamol, naproxen sodium, aspirin, etoricoxib, meloxicam, piroxicam and tenoxicam), but there is still no consensus on the most effective analgesic, effective dose and protocol to be used.[71]

Non-pharmacological Management

Interestingly, there is an increasing number of non-pharmacological methods available that would avoid the negative side effects of drugs and help those who may have allergies or who are unable to take certain drugs. However, the low quality of the studies in this field and the need for more high-quality studies has been highlighted and so the results should be viewed with caution.[72] Some examples of the non-pharmacological methods studied include:

- chewing gum
- bite wafers
- vibratory stimulation
- low-level laser therapy
- transcutaneous electrical nerve stimulation (TENS)
- acupuncture/acupressure
- psychological interventions (e.g. structured telephone call or text message).

A number of these methods (vibratory stimulation devices such as AcceleDent®, chewing gum and bite wafers) are based on the belief that vibratory/masticatory stimulation may lead to loosening of the periodontal ligament, increase of vascularity and limiting of ischaemia following orthodontic appliance placement and hence force application on the teeth. This in turn would reduce inflammation, ischaemia and so the pain response.

Chewing gum was found to significantly reduce reported pain following initial archwire engagement.[73] Although this contradicts the normal advice given to patients of avoiding chewing gum, no evidence was found that chewing gum increases the incidence of appliance breakages.[73] The effectiveness of biting wafers is unclear. One study undertaken in the USA reported that 40% of 82 patients included in the study found that the wafers alleviated pain.[74] However, this study had no control group or robust methodology, and the results could be interpreted as a placebo effect instead of actual pain reduction. This led another research group to test a similar wafer in the UK. Contrary to the previous research results, this group found more pain was reported by those using bite wafers than by those who avoided masticatory activity after placement of fixed appliances.[75] There is also contradictory evidence on the effect of vibratory devices on orthodontic pain control, with some studies reporting some pain reduction,[76, 77] and another reporting no difference between patients using an AcceleDent device and the control group (who used a placebo device) during initial orthodontic alignment.[78]

Low-level laser therapy (LLLT) is defined as laser treatment in which the energy produced by the laser is low enough not to cause an increase in body temperature. The laser produces a pure light with a single wavelength that stimulates the biological processes within the tissue being treated. LLLT has anti-inflammatory effects that can result in pain relief.[79] A meta-analysis involving a total of 118 participants provided low-quality evidence that LLLT reduced pain at 24 hours and seemed to also reduce pain at six hours, three days and seven days.[72] Although most studies report favourable results in terms of pain reduction,[80–82] there is variation in how LLLT is applied and there is a need for more evidence on its effectiveness and the ideal clinical protocol.[71]

Finally, there is some evidence to show there is a relationship between anxiety and reported pain,[83] and therefore that psychological support, involving communication with patients and reassurance, could also help in reducing anxiety and reported pain. An interesting study found that a telephone call from the orthodontic practice within 24 hours of bonding of orthodontic brackets and initial archwire placement reduced patient's reported pain and anxiety scores, the content of the call being irrelevant.[84] In this study two groups received a call; one group received a structured call where patients were asked about their well-being and were reminded of what to expect and how to care for the braces, whereas the other group's call was only to thank them for their participation. Both groups reported lower pain and anxiety scores compared to the control group who received no call.[84] The effectiveness of a telephone call has been supported by another randomised controlled study, which found that a structured telephone call was a more effective and consistent method than a structured text message in reducing reported pain, both forms of communication reducing reported pain more than no post-procedure communication (control group).[85]

There are only a few studies comparing the efficacy of pharmacological and non-pharmacological pain control methods in relation to orthodontic-related pain. The results of these seem to suggest that the use of non-pharmacological methods may help reduce the need for drug intake. For instance, Ireland et al.[86] conducted a multicentre randomised controlled trial involving 1000 patients and found that following bonding of fixed appliances and placement of initial archwires, chewing sugar-free gum reduced the consumption of ibuprofen. Over 80% of patients in the chewing gum group did so on the day of appliance placement and over 50% used it at some time over the next three days. Despite this high rate of chewing gum, there was no clinical or statistically significant difference in appliance breakages between the two groups.[86] The authors also found a weak positive correlation between anxiety reported and pain experienced following both the initial fitting of the fixed appliances and at the subsequent archwire change.[83] Patients who were more anxious tended to take more ibuprofen for their pain relief.[83] Another study in this field, though with a small sample size of only 10 female patients per group, compared the use of a placebo, ibuprofen (400 mg), chewing gum, soft viscoelastic wafers and hard viscoelastic wafers following fixed appliance and initial archwire placement.[87] The authors concluded that ibuprofen might be replaced by either chewing gum or the use of wafers. However, in view of the small sample size, the results should be viewed with caution. Future studies are needed to ascertain the effectiveness of non-pharmacological pain control methods and determine to what extent they reduce the need for analgesic intake by orthodontic patients. It would be helpful to include patient anxiety assessments, as it may be that certain patient cohorts may benefit more than others from the use of non-pharmacological pain control methods.

Root Resorption from Different Archwires

Orthodontically induced external root resorption (OIERR) is a common side effect of orthodontic treatment. When orthodontic forces exceed capillary pressure in the periodontal ligament, it leads to hyalinised zones and undermining resorption takes place. During active removal of the hyalinised necrotic tissue, root resorption occurs when the reparative capacity of the cementum is exceeded, leaving dentine exposed to activated odontoclasts, which cause the irreversible loss of root structure.[88] It is reported that 80% of patients will experience this, although it is usually not clinically significant. A recent systematic review and meta-analysis of studies assessing root resorption with the use of cone beam computed tomography found an average amount of OIERR of 0.79–0.86 mm.[89] Severe apical root resorption (loss of more than one-third of the root length or more than 4 mm) has been reported to occur in less than 3% of orthodontic patients.[90–92] Risk factors for OIERR are patient and treatment related.[90–93] Patient-related factors include genetics, ethnicity, gender, age, tooth type (maxillary incisors most commonly affected; lateral incisors more than central incisors), systemic factors, root morphology (blunt or pipette-shaped roots having a higher risk), and history of trauma or previous root resorption. Treatment-related factors include appliance type, treatment duration (longer treatment having a higher risk), type of tooth movement (intrusion and movement of roots against the cortical bone having a higher risk), use of Class II elastics, applied force magnitude, duration of force application, and extraction treatment.

Is there Evidence that Different Archwires Cause Different Amounts of Root Resorption?

The little research available assessing the effect of aligning archwires on root resorption and pain was highlighted in the Cochrane review by Wang et al.[26] Weiland[94] showed that the increased amount of tooth movement that occurred in the 12-week period with the superelastic wires (which delivered a continuous force of 0.8–1 N) compared to that of the stainless steel archwire group (which delivered an initially higher but rapidly declining force) came at a price. Although the depth of the resorption lacunae noted on the teeth that were moved did not significantly differ between the two groups, the perimeter, area and volume of the resorption lacunae on the superelastic teeth group were 140% greater and the amount of resorption in the superelastic group was significantly greater.[94]

A prospective study of 82 patients compared the alignment archwire sequences of superelastic NiTi archwires (0.014-inch and 0.016-inch Sentalloy, and 0.018 × 0.025-inch Bioforce) versus stainless steel archwires (0.0175-inch Penta-one multistranded, 0.016-inch Australian regular and 0.016 × 0.022-inch resilient 3M Unitek).[95] Root resorption was assessed on intraoral periapical radiographs. All evaluated teeth except one did not have a statistically significant difference in OIERR. The exception was the mandibular left central incisor tooth in the superelastic group, which showed a statistically significant increased amount of OIERR by 1.00 mm (SD 0.71, range 0.00–2.70) compared to the stainless steel group (0.47 mm, SD 0.58, range −0.30 to 1.90). In this sample, levelling was accomplished sooner by the superelastic archwires (mean 6.17 months, SD 0.77) compared with the stainless steel archwires (mean 6.98 months, SD 1.42) and treatment duration was longer for the stainless steel group.[95]

Another randomised controlled trial compared three different archwire sequences including all archwires required until a 0.019 × 0.025-inch stainless steel working archwire was placed and assessed root resorption by means of a periapical radiograph of only the maxillary left central incisor.[96] The archwire sequences compared were as follows: Group A: 0.016-inch NiTi, 0.018 × 0.025-inch NiTi and 0.019 × 0.025-inch SS; Group B: 0.016-inch NiTi, 0.016-inch stainless steel, 0.020-inch stainless steel and 0.019 × 0.025-inch stainless steel; Group C: 0.016 × 0.022-inch copper (Cu)NiTi, 0.019 × 0.025-inch CuNiTi and 0.019 × 0.025-inch stainless steel. There were no statistically significant differences between archwire sequences A, B or C for patient discomfort or root resorption.[96] The authors suggest that all archwire sequences were comparable and when making a clinical choice other factors such as cost, number of visits and clinical factors (e.g. severely rotated teeth may align more efficiently when fully tied by a thinner diameter archwire) would play a factor in the clinician's decision-making process.

It is known that teeth which experience severe root resorption already show signs of it (even if minor root irregularity or minor resorption) within the first six to nine months of orthodontic treatment.[91] Therefore, when there are known factors (e.g. blunt or pipette-shaped roots with higher risk of OIERR), a radiograph is advised approximately six months into treatment.[91] When root resorption is noted clinically it is generally advised to pause treatment for a few months to allow for some root surface repair and healing.[93, 97] In a study of 40 patients who were shown to be experiencing OIERR within the first six months of orthodontic treatment, half were assigned to continuing with treatment and half to a pause. The overall loss of root length was statistically significantly greater in patients treated continuously compared with those who were treated with a pause of two to three months.[97]

Allergy to Nickel

Nickel allergy is a type IV delayed cell-mediated hypersensitivity reaction that was first recognised as an allergic response in 1925. Questions about a potential allergy to nickel should figure in the health questionnaire given in a dental practice and should be something the orthodontist bears in mind and is able to recognise and manage if symptoms occur. It has been estimated that approximately 11% of all women and 20% of women between the ages of 16 and 35 years have an allergy to nickel. In contrast, only 2% of males are affected.[98, 99] The difference in gender is thought to be due to ear piercing being a major cause of sensitisation to nickel. On one study the prevalence in subjects with pierced ears was found to be 31% compared to 2% in those without pierced ears.[100] Interestingly, patients who are allergic to nickel and have allergic reactions on the skin often do not present intraoral reactions in response to orthodontic appliances. The occurrence of an intraoral harmful response to nickel is estimated to be 0.1–0.2%.[101] This reduced response is thought to be due to saliva diluting potential antigens and digesting them before they enter the oral mucosa, the extensive vascularity of the oral mucosa removing the potential allergens quickly before an allergic reaction takes place, and a greater concentration of nickel being required to elicit a response in the oral mucosa than in the skin.

Pathological Process

The pathological process for this reaction has two phases. The first phase, sensitisation, occurs when nickel initially enters the body. Antigen-presenting cells (Langerhans cell) phagocytose the antigens and present parts of it to CD4⁺

T-cell or T-helper cells in lymph nodes. If these recognise the substance as dangerous, they multiply and send out more of itself to the site of exposure. There is often no reaction, but the body is sensitised and when re-exposure to the antigen occurs (second/elicitation phase) a full clinical reaction takes place. Upon re-exposure, memory T-cells in the skin recognise the antigen and release cytokines, which cause more T-cells to migrate from blood vessels. A complex immune cascade starts leading to contact dermatitis (skin inflammation with itching and a rash), which develops over a period of days or, rarely, up to three weeks.

Signs and Symptoms and Management

The signs and symptoms of a nickel allergy reaction could include the following.

- *Extraoral*: generalised urticaria, widespread eczema, allergic dermatitis and/or exacerbation of pre-existing eczema.
- *Intraoral*: burning sensation or soreness at the site of contact, oral ulcers, swelling of lips and gingivae, stomatitis, gingival hyperplasia, mild erythema of gingivae and buccal mucosa, labial desquamation, loss of taste or metallic taste, numbness and/or erythema multiforme.

When a nickel allergy is suspected, a dermatologist can confirm a diagnosis by undertaking a patch test. For the latter, a disc with 5% nickel sulphate in petroleum jelly is placed on the skin and the intensity of the skin's reaction is assessed by the dermatologist after 48 and 72 hours.

If a patient has a known allergy to nickel, the orthodontist will need to think carefully about what materials to use during the orthodontic treatment, as many contain nickel.

The most commonly used aligning archwire is nickel titanium, which contains 47–50% nickel and NiTi is also found in some auxiliaries, such as closing coils. Stainless steel, which contains 8% nickel, is also used extensively as a material for brackets, archwires, auxiliaries, headgear bows and removable appliances. There have been reports of extraoral nickel allergy caused by the outer stainless bow of a headgear.[102] It is interesting to note that patients who have reactions extraorally may not have reactions intraorally or may not react to materials such as stainless steel intraorally. Bass et al.[103] assessed 29 patients with skin patch tests. Of these, five had an allergy to nickel, although none experienced a reaction or discomfort with orthodontic treatment. The nickel content in stainless steel is low (8%) and it is thought to be more tightly bound to the alloy's crystal lattice, making it difficult for it to leach out. If stainless steel is tolerated, multistrand stainless steel

Table 10.2 Table of nickel free alternatives to commonly used components during orthodontic treatment.

Component	Nickel-free alternatives
Brackets (metallic brackets are often made of stainless steel and the gates of some active self-ligating ceramic brackets contain nickel titanium)	• ceramic brackets (produced using polycrystalline alumina, single-crystal sapphire or zirconia) • pure titanium brackets • polycarbonate brackets • gold-plated brackets • low nickel SS brackets (nickel content ≤0.2%) • or consider the use of aligners
Bands (often made of stainless steel)	• gold-plated bands are available
Archwires	• TMA (available from round alignment archwires through to working and finishing archwires) • fibre-reinforced composite • pure titanium • gold plated
Auxiliaries (closing coils tend to be made of SS or NiTi, and SS is used for ligatures, Kobayashi hooks, crimpable hooks, etc)	• elastomeric modules can be used instead of SS ligatures to tie in archwires in conventional brackets • elastomeric chain can be used for closing spaces and also as ligatures (when spaces are already closed) • closing loops may be bend on TMA archwires for space closure, avoiding the need for closing coils and crimpable hooks • the hooks on canine nickel-free brackets can be used for inter-maxillary elastics instead of crimpable hooks on archwires • Teflon coated ligatures and Kobayashi hooks are available and could be tried clinically to assess on an individual basis if they cause reactions or not (as the Teflon coat may rub away with use)
Other fixed appliances (Quad-helix, transpalatal arches, lingual arches, rapid maxillary expansion screws)	• TMA or low nickel SS (nickel content ≤ 0.2%) wires may be used for Quad-helices and transpalatal or lingual arches • rapid maxillary expansion screws made of titanium are available
Fixed retainers	• Titanium retainer wire is available
Removable appliance wirework (wirework for removable appliances and Hawley retainers is made of stainless steel)	• Plastic retainers (e.g. Polyvinylsiloxane) can be used instead of Hawley retainers • Aligners may be used, if appropriate, instead of removable appliances
Headgear	• Teflon coated stainless steel facebow

archwires could be used for alignment. Furthermore, a low-nickel stainless steel (≤0.2% nickel) is available and could be useful for patients with nickel allergy. Stainless steel materials could be tested with caution and if reactions occur, then nickel-free alternatives are an option (Table 10.2).

When and How Much Nickel is Released from Appliances?

The leaching of nickel from bands, brackets and stainless steel or NiTi archwires *in vitro* has been shown to maximally occur within the first week and then decline thereafter.[104] The nickel in the alloys can also be released intraorally throughout the use of the appliances due to corrosion. NiTi archwires have been shown *in vitro* to release significantly more nickel ions in artificial saliva when in a fluoride media.[105] An *in vitro* study assessing the corrosion characteristics of nickel-containing archwires (stainless steel, NiTi, nitride-coated NiTi, epoxy-coated NiTi and titanium archwires) found that only the epoxy coating of NiTi archwires provided some corrosion resistance and these together with titanium archwires exhibited the least corrosion potential.[56] However, clinically the epoxy coating is often disrupted, which would still leave the underlying NiTi alloy exposed to corrosion with potential nickel ions being released, so these are best avoided in a true nickel allergy patient.

How much nickel is released during orthodontic treatment is difficult to estimate as it is dependent on multiple factors: intraoral temperature, pH, salivary composition, wear of the materials due to friction, leaking of ions through corrosion, presence of soldered joints and fluoride, amongst other variables. Daily nickel and chromium dietary intakes are estimated to be on average 200–300 μg and 280 μg, respectively. An *in vitro* study showed that a full-mouth orthodontic appliance exposed to 0.05% saline released on average 40 μg nickel and 36 μg chromium per day, levels far below the normal daily intake of nickel in diet.[106] Kerosuo et al.[107] assessed nickel and chromium levels in saliva following fixed appliance insertion for a period of up to a month and found no significant difference in the salivary levels relative to the levels present before insertion. Another study involving the assessment of nickel in retrieved stainless steel and NiTi archwires with a mean clinical use of four months (range 1.5–12 months) found no significant difference between the retrieved and the as-received archwires with respect to nickel-content ratios.[108] Therefore, although it is known there may be some nickel released from orthodontic appliances, at the moment it seems the amount is low and the use of orthodontic materials containing nickel may continue in patients who are not allergic to it. In addition, it is currently believed the risk is extremely low for orthodontic-derived nickel to act as a sensitising agent for patients who are not already nickel hypersensitive at the start of orthodontic treatment. However, for patients who already have a history of nickel hypersensitivity, the recommendation is for nickel-free alternatives to be used instead.[39]

Allergies to Other Metals

Although rare, allergy to other metal alloys such as mercury, gold, platinum, palladium, silver and cobalt are also possible. Therefore, orthodontists should be alert to symptoms and take careful histories, including any previous allergic responses after wearing metal items or after having dental restorations undertaken, as well as the timing of the symptoms (if the onset coincides with the insertion of an orthodontic appliance). If in doubt it is best for the patient to see a specialist dermatologist for testing, and samples of the orthodontic materials used in the patient can be given to the patient for the dermatologist to have as a reference.

Acknowledgements

I would like to thank Dr Daljit Gill and Dr Farhad B. Naini for inviting me to write this chapter. My special thanks to Dr Farhad B. Naini for his support and expert guidance over the years and his patience and excellent suggestions when reading and editing this chapter. To my parents, who gave me everything with their hard work, love, and effort and are my strength, example to follow and support me always, I am forever grateful. To my husband, for his patience during the process of writing this chapter and his love and support, which mean everything to me; words cannot express my gratitude to you.

References

1 Kusy RP. A review of contemporary archwires: their properties and characteristics. *Angle Orthod.* 1997;67:197–207.

2 Miura F, Mogi M, Ohura Y, Hamanaka H. The super-elastic property of the Japanese NiTi alloy wire for use in orthodontics. *Am. J. Orthod. Dentofacial Orthop.* 1986;90:1–10.

3 Proffit WR, Fields HW, Sarver DM. *Contemporary Orthodontics*, 4th edn. St Louis, MO: Mosby Elsevier, 2007.

4 Kusy RP, Whitley JQ. Effects of surface roughness on the coefficients of friction in model orthodontic systems. *J. Biomech.* 1990;23:913–925.

5 Kusy RP, Whitley JQ. Friction between different wire–bracket configurations and materials. *Semin. Orthod.* 1997;3:166–177.

6 Kusy RP, Whitley JQ. Influence of archwire and bracket dimensions on sliding mechanics: derivations and determinations of the critical contact angles for binding. *Eur. J. Orthod.* 1999;21:199–208.

7 De la Cruz A, Sampson P, Little RM, et al. Longterm changes in arch form after orthodontic treatment and retention. *Am. J. Orthod. Dentofacial Orthop.* 1995;107:518–530.

8 Proffit WR. Equilibrium theory revisited. Factors influencing position of teeth. *Angle Orthod.* 1978;48:175–186.

9 Little RM. Stability and relapse of dental arch alignment. *Br. J. Orthod.* 1990;17:235–241.

10 Mills JRE. The stability of the lower labial segment. A cephalometric survey. *Dent. Pract.* 1968;18:293–306.

11 Lee RT. Arch width and form: a review. *Am. J. Orthod. Dentofacial Orthop.* 1999;115:305–313.

12 Hawley CA. Determination of the normal arch and its application to orthodontics. *Dent. Cosmos* 1905;47:541–557.

13 McConnail MA, Scher EA. The ideal arch form of the human dental arcade with some prosthetic application. *Dent. Rec.* 1949;69:285–302.

14 Brader AC. Dental arch form related with intraoral forces: PR = C. *Am. J. Orthod.* 1972;61:541–561.

15 McNamara C, Drage KJ, Sandy JR, Ireland AJ. An evaluation of clinician's choices when selecting arch-wires. *Eur. J. Orthod.* 2009;32:54–59.

16 Kusy RP, Stevens LE. Triple stranded stainless steel wires: evaluation of mechanical properties and comparison with titanium alloy alternatives. *Angle Orthod.* 1987;57:18–32.

17 Kusy RP, Dilley GJ. Elastic property ratios of a triple-stranded stainless steel archwire. *Am. J. Orthod.* 1984;86:177–188.

18 Andreasen GF, Hilleman TB. An evaluation of 55 cobalt substituted Nitinol wire for use in orthodontics. *J. Am. Dent. Assoc.* 1971;82:1373–1375.

19 Kusy RP. Orthodontic biomaterials: from the past to the present. *Angle Orthod.* 2002;72:501–512.

20 Burstone CJ, Qin B, Morton JY. Chinese NiTi wire: a new orthodontic alloy. *Am. J. Orthod. Dentofacial Orthop.* 1985;87:445–452.

21 Santoro M, Nicolay OF, Cangialosi TJ. Pseudoelasticity and thermoelasticity of nickel–titanium alloys: a clinically oriented review. Part II: Deactivation forces. *Am. J. Orthod. Dentofacial Orthop.* 2001;119:594–603.

22 Santoro M, Beshers DN. Nickel–titanium alloys: stress-related temperature transitional range. *Am. J. Orthod. Dentofacial Orthop.* 2000;118:685–692.

23 Miura F, Mogi M, Ohura Y. Japanese NiTi alloy wire: use of the direct electric resistance heat treatment method. *Eur. J. Orthod.* 1988;10:187–191.

24 Berger JL. The speed system: an overview of the appliance and clinical performance. *Semin. Orthod.* 2008;14:54–63.

25 Sebastian B. Alignment efficiency of superelastic coaxial nickel–titanium vs superelastic single stranded nickel–titanium in relieving mandibular anterior crowding. A randomized controlled prospective study. *Angle Orthod.* 2012;82:703–708.

26 Wang Y, Liu C, Jian F, et al. Initial arch wires used in orthodontic treatment with fixed appliances. *Cochrane Database Syst. Rev.* 2018;(7):CD007859.

27 Verstrynge A, Van Humbeeck J, Willems G. In-vitro evaluation of the material characteristics of stainless steel and beta-titanium orthodontic wires. *Am. J. Orthod. Dentofacial Orthop.* 2006;130:460–470.

28 Mizhari E, Cleaton Jones PE, Luyckx S, Fatti LP. The effect of ion implantation on the beaks of orthodontic pliers. *Am. J. Orthod. Dentofacial Orthop.* 1991;99:513–519.

29 Ryan R, Walker G, Freeman K, Cisneros GJ. The effects of ion implantation on rate of tooth movement: an in vitro model. *Am. J. Orthod. Dentofacial Orthop.* 1997;112:64–68.

30 Kula K, Phillips C, Gibilaro A, Proffit WR. Effect of ion implantation of TMA archwires on the rate of orthodontic sliding space closure. *Am. J. Orthod. Dentofacial Orthop.* 1998;114:577–580.

31 Rudge P, Sherriff M, Bister D. A comparison of roughness parameters and friction coefficients of aesthetic archwires. *Eur. J. Orthod.* 2015;37:49–55.

32 Husmann P, Bourauel C, Wessinger M, Jager A. The frictional behavior of coated guiding archwires. *J. Orofac. Orthop.* 2002;63:199–211.

33 da Silva DL, Mattos CT, Sant' Anna EF, et al. *Cross-section dimensions and mechanical properties of esthetic orthodontic coated archwires. Am. J. Orthod. Dentofacial Orthop.* 2013;143:S85–S91.

34 da Silva DL, Santos E Jr,, Camargo S de S Jr, Ruellas AC. Infrared spectroscopy, nano-mechanical properties, and scratch resistance of esthetic orthodontic coated archwires. *Angle Orthod.* 2015;85:777–783.

35 Elayyan F, Silikas N, Bearn D. Mechanical properties of coated superelastic archwires in conventional and self-ligating orthodontic brackets. *Am. J. Orthod. Dentofacial Orthop.* 2010;137:213–217.

36 Kaphoor AA, Sundareswaran S. Aesthetic nickel titanium wires: how much do they deliver? *Eur. J. Orthod.* 2012;34:603–609.

37 Ulhaq A, Esmail Z, Kamaruddin A, et al. Alignment efficiency and esthetic performance of 4 coated nickel–titanium archwires in orthodontic patients over 8 weeks: a multicenter randomized clinical trial. *Am. J. Orthod. Dentofacial Orthop.* 2017;152:744–752.

38 Collier S, Pandis N, Johal A, et al. A prospective cohort study assessing the appearance of retrieved aesthetic orthodontic archwires. *Orthod. Craniofac. Res.* 2018;21:27–32.

39 Eliades T, Athanasiou AE. In vivo aging of orthodontic alloys: implications for corrosion potential, nickel release, and biocompatibility. *Angle Orthod.* 2002;72:222–237.

40 Costa Lima KC, Benini Paschoal MA, de Araujo Gurgel J, et al. Comparative analysis of microorganism adhesion on coated, partially coated, and uncoated orthodontic archwires: a prospective clinical study. *Am. J. Orthod. Dentofacial Orthop.* 2019;156:611–616.

41 Zufall SW, Kusy RP. Sliding mechanics of coated composite wires and the development of an engineering model for binding. *Angle Orthod.* 2000;70:34–47.

42 Chang JH, Berzins DW, Pruszynski JE, Ballard RW. The effect of water storage on the bending properties of esthetic, fiber-reinforced composite orthodontic archwires. *Angle Orthod.* 2014;84:417–423.

43 Spendlove J, Berzins DW, Pruszynski JE, Ballard RW. Investigation of force decay in aesthetic, fibre-reinforced composite orthodontic archwires. *Eur. J. Orthod.* 2015;37:43–48.

44 Eliades T. Orthodontic materials research and applications: Part 2. Current status and projected future developments in materials and biocompatibility. *Am. J. Orthod. Dentofacial Orthop.* 2007;131:253–262.

45 Zinelis S, Eliades T, Pandis N, et al. Why do nickel–titanium archwires fracture intraorally? Fractographic analysis and failure mechanism of in-vivo fractured wires. *Am. J. Orthod. Dentofacial Orthop.* 2007;132:84–89.

46 Birnbaum HK, Sofronis P. Hydrogen-enhanced localized plasticity: a mechanism for hydrogen-related fracture. *Mater. Sci. Eng. A* 1994;176:191–202.

47 Matasa CG. Attachment corrosion and its testing. *J. Clin. Orthod.* 1995;29:16–23.

48 Maijer R, Smith DC. Biodegration of the orthodontic bracket system. *Am. J. Orthod. Dentofacial Orthop.* 1986;90:195–198.

49 Schiff N, Dalard F, Lissac M, et al. Corrosion resistance on three orthodontic brackets: a comparative study of three fluoride mouthwashes. *Eur. J. Orthod.* 2005;27:541–549.

50 Harzer W, Schroter A, Gedrange T, Muschter F. Sensitivity of titanium brackets to the corrosive influence of fluoride-containing toothpaste and tea. *Angle Orthod.* 2001;71:318–323.

51 Huang H. Variation in corrosion resistance of nickel titanium wires from different manufacturers. *Angle Orthod.* 2005;75:661–665.

52 Mockers O, Deroze D, Camps J. Cytotoxicity of orthodontic bands, brackets and archwires in vitro. *Dent. Mater.* 2002;18:311–317.

53 Mystkowska J, Niemirowicz-Laskowska K, Łysik D, et al. The role of oral cavity biofilm on metallic biomaterial surface destruction: corrosion and friction aspects. *Int. J. Mol. Sci.* 2018;19:743–761.

54 Khan MA, Williams RL, Williams DF. The corrosion behavior of Ti-6Al-4V, Ti-6Al-7Nb and Ti-13Nb-13Zr in protein solutions. *Biomaterials* 1999;20:631–637.

55 Eliades T, Eliades G, Athanasiou AE, Bradley TG. Surface characterization of retrieved NiTi orthodontic archwires. *Eur. J. Orthod.* 2000;22:317–326.

56 Kim H, Johnson JW. Corrosion of stainless steel, nickel–titanium, coated nickel–titanium, and titanium orthodontic wires. *Angle Orthod.* 1999;69:39–44.

57 Huang HH. Surface characterizations and corrosion resistance of nickel–titanium orthodontic archwires in artificial saliva of various degrees of acidity. *J. Biomed. Mater. Res.* 2005;74:629–639.

58 West AE, Jones ML, Newcombe RG. Multiflex versus superelastic: a randomized clinical trial of the tooth alignment ability of initial arch wires. *Am. J. Orthod. Dentofacial Orthop.* 1995;108:464–471.

59 Quintão CCA, Jones ML, Menezes LM, et al. A prospective clinical trial to compare the performance of four initial orthodontic archwires. *Korean J. Orthod.* 2005;35:381–387.

60 Abdelrahman RSh, Al-Nimri KS, Al Maaitah EF. A clinical comparison of three aligning archwires in terms of alignment efficiency: a prospective clinical trial. *Angle Orthod.* 2015;85:434–439.

61 Pandis N, Polychronopoulou A, Eliades T. Alleviation of mandibular anterior crowding with copper–nickel–titanium vs nickel–titanium wires: a double-blind randomized control trial. *Am. J. Orthod. Dentofacial Orthop.* 2009;136:152–153.

62 Erdinç AM, Dincer B. Perception of pain during orthodontic treatment with fixed appliances. *Eur. J. Orthod.* 2004;26:79–85.

63 Jones M, Chan C. The pain and discomfort experienced during orthodontic treatment: a randomized controlled clinical trial of two initial aligning arch wires. *Am. J. Orthod. Dentofacial Orthop.* 1992;102:373–381.

64 Sandhu SS, Sandhu J. A randomized clinical trial investigating pain associated with superelastic nickel–titanium and multistranded stainless steel archwires during the initial leveling and aligning phase of orthodontic treatment. *J. Orthod.* 2013;40:276–285.

65 Fernandes LM, Øgaard B, Skoglund L. Pain and discomfort experienced after placement of a conventional or a superelastic NiTi aligning archwire. A randomized clinical trial. *J. Orofac. Orthop.* 1998;59:331–339.

66 Cioffi I, Piccolo A, Tagliaferri R, et al. Pain perception following first orthodontic archwire placement: thermoelastic vs superelastic alloys. A randomized controlled trial. *Quintessence Int.* 2012;43:61–69.

67 Ngan P, Wilson S, Shanfield J, Amini H. The effect of ibuprofen on the level of discomfort in patients undergoing orthodontic treatment. *Am. J. Orthod. Dentofacial Orthop.* 1994;106:88–95.

68 Bradley RL, Ellis PE, Thomas P, et al. A randomized clinical trial comparing the efficacy of ibuprofen and

paracetamol in the control of orthodontic pain. *Am. J. Orthod. Dentofacial Orthop.* 2007;132:511–517.

69 Walker JB, Buring SM. NSAID impairment of orthodontic tooth movement. *Ann. Pharmacother.* 2001;35:113–115.

70 Monk AB, Harrison JE, Worthington HV, Teague A. Pharmacological interventions for pain relief during orthodontic treatment. *Cochrane Database Syst. Rev.* 2017;(11):CD003976.

71 Topolski F, Moro A, Correr GM, Schimim SC. Optimal management of orthodontic pain. *J. Pain Res.* 2018;11:589–598.

72 Fleming PS, Strydom H, Katsaros C, et al. Non-pharmacological interventions for alleviating pain during orthodontic treatment. *Cochrane Database Syst. Rev.* 2016;(12):CD010263.

73 Benson PE, Razi RM, Al-Bloushi RJ. The effect of chewing gum on the impact, pain and breakages associated with fixed orthodontic appliances: a randomized clinical trial. *Orthod. Craniofac. Res.* 2012;15:178–187.

74 Hwang J, Tee C, Huang A, Taft L. Effectiveness of thera-bite wafers in reducing pain. *J. Clin. Orthod.* 1994;5:291–292.

75 Otasevic M, Naini FB, Gill DS, Lee RT. Prospective randomized clinical trial comparing the effects of a masticatory bite wafer and avoidance of hard food on pain associated with initial orthodontic tooth movement. *Am. J. Orthod. Dentofacial Orthop.* 2006;130:6.e9–e15.

76 Lobre WD, Callegari BJ, Gardner G, et al. Pain control in orthodontics using a micropulse vibration device: a randomized clinical trial. *Angle Orthod.* 2016;86:625–630.

77 Miles P, Smith H, Weyant R, Rinchuse DJ. The effects of a vibrational appliance on tooth movement and patient discomfort: a prospective randomized clinical trial. *Aust. Orthod. J.* 2012;28:213–218.

78 Woodhouse NR, DiBiase AT, Johnson N, et al. Supplemental vibrational force during orthodontic alignment: a randomized trial. *J. Dent. Res.* 2015;94:682–689.

79 Hashmi JT, Huang YY, Osmani BZ, et al. Role of low-level laser therapy in neurorehabilitation. *PM R* 2010;2(12 Suppl 2):S292–S305.

80 Doshi-Mehta G, Bhad-Patil WA. Efficacy of low-intensity laser therapy in reducing treatment time and orthodontic pain: a clinical investigation. *Am. J. Orthod. Dentofacial Orthop.* 2012;141:289–297.

81 Tortamano A, Lenzi DC, Haddad ACSS, et al. Low-level laser therapy for pain caused by placement of the first orthodontic archwire: a randomized clinical trial. *Am. J. Orthod. Dentofacial Orthop.* 2009;136:662–667.

82 Deshpande P, Patil K, Mahima V, et al. Low-level laser therapy for alleviation of pain from fixed orthodontic appliance therapy: a randomized controlled trial. *J. Adv. Clin. Res. Insights* 2016;3:43–46.

83 Ireland AJ, Ellis P, Jordan A, et al. Chewing gum vs. ibuprofen in the management of orthodontic pain: a multi-centre randomised controlled trial. The effect of anxiety. *J. Orthod.* 2017;44:3–7.

84 Bartlett BW, Firestone AR, Vig KWL, et al. The influence of a structured telephone call on orthodontic pain and anxiety. *Am. J. Orthod. Dentofacial Orthop.* 2005;128:435–441.

85 Cozzani M, Ragazzini G, Delucchi A, et al. Self-reported pain after orthodontic treatments: a randomized controlled study on the effects of two follow-up procedures. *Eur. J. Orthod.* 2016;38:266–271.

86 Ireland AJ, Ellis P, Jordan A, et al. Comparative assessment of chewing gum and ibuprofen in the management of orthodontic pain with fixed appliances: a pragmatic multicenter randomized controlled trial. *Am. J. Orthod. Dentofacial Orthop.* 2016;150:220–227.

87 Farzanegan F, Zebarjad SM, Alizadeh S, Ahrari F. Pain reduction after initial archwire placement in orthodontic patients: a randomized clinical trial. *Am. J. Orthod. Dentofacial Orthop.* 2012;141:169–173.

88 Jung YH, Cho BH. External root resorption after orthodontic treatment: a study of contributing factors. *Imaging Sci. Dent.* 2011;41:17–21.

89 Samandara A, Papageorgiou SN, Ioannidou-Marathiotou I, et al. Evaluation of orthodontically induced external root resorption following orthodontic treatment using cone beam computed tomography (CBCT): a systematic review and meta-analysis. *Eur. J. Orthod.* 2019;41:67–79.

90 Linge L, Linge BO. Patient characteristics and treatment variables associated with apical root resorption during orthodontic treatment. *Am. J. Orthod. Dentofacial Orthop.* 1991;99:35–43.

91 Levander E, Malmgren O. Evaluation of the risk of root resorption during orthodontic treatment: a study of upper incisors. *Eur. J. Orthod.* 1988;10:30–38.

92 Sameshima GT, Sinclair PM. Characteristics of patients with severe root resorption. *Orthod. Craniofac. Res.* 2004;7:108–114.

93 Currell SD, Liaw A, Blackmore Grant PD, et al. Orthodontic mechanotherapies and their influence on external root resorption: a systematic review. *Am. J. Orthod. Dentofacial Orthop.* 2019;155:313–329.

94 Weiland F. Constant versus dissipating forces in orthodontics: the effect on initial tooth movement and root resorption. *Eur. J. Orthod.* 2003;25:335–342.

95 Alzahawi K, Færøvig E, Brudvik P, et al. Root resorption after leveling with super-elastic and conventional steel arch wires: a prospective study. *Prog. Orthod.* 2014;15:35.

96 Mandall NA, Lowe C, Worthington HV, et al. Which orthodontic archwire sequence? A randomized clinical trial. *Eur. J. Orthod.* 2006;28:561–566.

97 Levander E, Malmgren O, Eliasson S. Evaluation of root resorption in relation to two orthodontic treatment regimes. A clinical experimental study. *Eur. J. Orthod.* 1994;16:223–228.

98 Nielsen NH, Menné T. Allergic contact sensitization in an unselected Danish population. The Glostrup Allergy Study, *Denmark. Acta Derm. Venereol.* 1992;72: 456–460.

99 Nielsen NH, Menné T. Nickel sensitization and ear piercing in an unselected Danish population. *Glostrup Allergy Study. Contact Dermatitis* 1993;29:16–21.

100 Kerosuo H, Kullaa A, Kerosuo E, et al. Nickel allergy in adolescents in relation to orthodontic treatment and piercing of ears. *Am. J. Orthod. Dentofacial Orthop* 1996;109:148–154.

101 Menre T. Quantitative aspects of nickel dermatitis: sensitization and eliciting threshold concentrations. *Sci. Total Environ.* 1994;148:275–281.

102 Lowey MN. Allergic contact dermatitis associated with the use of Interlandi headgear in a patient with a history of atopy. *Br. Dent. J.* 1993;17:67–72.

103 Bass JK, Fine H, Cisneros GJ. Nickel hypersensitivity in the orthodontic patient. *Am. J. Orthod. Dentofacial Orthop.* 1993;103:280–285.

104 Barrett RD, Bishara SE, Quinn JK. Biodegration of orthodontic appliances. Part I. Biodegradation of nickel and chromium in vitro. *Am. J. Orthod. Dentofacial Orthop.* 1993;103:8–14.

105 Schiff N, Grosgogeat B, Lissac M, Dalard F. Influence of fluoride content and pH on the corrosion resistance of titanium and its alloys. *Biomaterials* 2002;23:1995–2002.

106 Park HY, Shearer TR. In vitro release of nickel and chromium from simulated orthodontic appliances. *Am. J. Orthod. Dentofacial Orthop.* 1983;84:156–159.

107 Kerosuo M, Moe G, Hensten-Pettersen A. Salivary nickel and chromium in subjects with different types of fixed appliances. *Am. J. Orthod. Dentofacial Orthop.* 1997;111:595–598.

108 Eliades T, Zinelis S, Papadopoulos MA, et al. Stainless steel archwires: assessing the nickel release hypothesis. *Angle Orthod.* 2004;74:151–154.

11

The Use of Auxiliaries in Orthodontics

Andrew T. DiBiase and Jonathan Sandler

CHAPTER OUTLINE

Introduction, 203
Anchorage and Space Management, 203
   Intermaxillary Traction and the Use of Elastics, 203
   Palatal Arches, 204
   Lingual Arches and Space Maintainers, 205
   Headgear and Extraoral Traction, 207
Class II Correction, 208
   Herbst Appliance, 209
   Fixed Class II Correctors, 211
Tooth Movement, 211
   Nickel Titanium Coil Springs, 211
   Closing Loops, 212
   Utility and Intrusion Archwires, 212
   Sectional Archwires, 214
   Torquing Spurs, 214
   Hooks, 216
   Piggyback Archwires, 216
   Ballista Spring, 217
Conclusion, 217
References, 218

Introduction

While the use of preadjusted and customised labial and lingual fixed appliances systems had made most of our orthodontic treatments very predictable, there are many circumstances when the use of auxiliaries is necessary in order to achieve acceptable treatment aims and to optimise the occlusal result. In this chapter we explore some of these scenarios.

Anchorage and Space Management

Orthodontics is based around the planned movement of teeth. Anchorage, simply put, is the resistance to unwanted tooth movement. One of the criticisms of straight-wire appliances is, because of the angulation built into the brackets and the resulting bodily movement of teeth, they are more anchorage demanding than other appliance systems that move teeth initially by tipping, i.e. Begg and Tip-Edge. Anchorage therefore often needs careful management, particularly at the beginning of treatment so the planned treatment aims can be achieved.

Intermaxillary Traction and the Use of Elastics

Elastics have been used for as long as fixed appliances have been around. Indeed, the use of heavy elastics was how Angle achieved anteroposterior correction in the absence of tooth extraction. They are also an integral part of the Begg and Tip-Edge appliances systems, again to achieve anteroposterior movement.

Elastics can be worn in many different formulations. The commonest are Class II elastics and this is closely followed

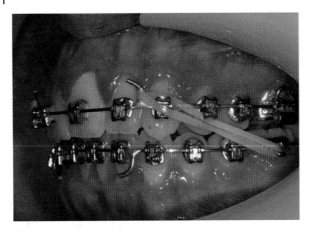
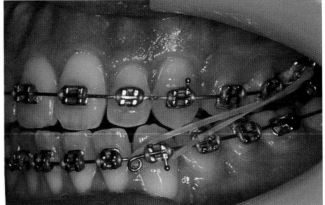

Figure 11.1 Class II (*left*) and Class III (*right*) elastics.

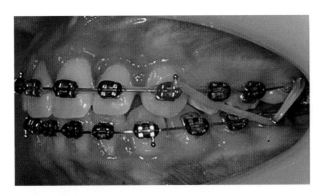
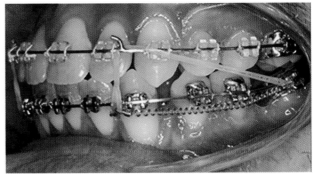

Figure 11.2 Class II elastics with vertical component to extrude molars (*left*) and with vertical component to close an open bite (*right*).

by Class III (Figure 11.1). Vertical components can be added to these configurations either to help in overbite reduction in deep bite cases by encouraging extrusion of the molars or to close an anterior open bite by extrusion of the incisors (Figure 11.2).

Elastics can be worn full or part time and different levels of force can be used. The strength of an elastic is defined as the force delivered when it is stretched to three times its diameter and is usually measured in either ounces or grams. The following gives a range of forces often used:

- 2–5 ounces (60–150 g) – light
- 6–10 ounces (150–300 g) – medium
- 11 ounces plus (300 g plus) – heavy.

Elastics can also be used for a number of other purposes, such as crossbite and centreline correction (Figure 11.3) and for occlusal setting at the end of treatment during finishing (Figure 11.4).

When using elastics, they are usually changed twice a day due to force degradation as they absorb moisture in the oral cavity and a successful outcome, like many things in orthodontics, depends on excellent compliance. They can also have unwanted side effects. For example, prolonged

use of Class II intermaxillary traction can result in excessive proclination of the lower incisors, which in most cases is inherently unstable and was one of the criticisms of Angle's modality of treatment. However, their use remains an important part of orthodontic treatment with fixed appliances.

Palatal Arches

Palatal arches can be used for both anteroposterior and vertical anchorage control. The simplest is the transpalatal or Goshgarian arch. This is constructed of 0.9 or 1.0 mm stainless steel and attached either with soldering or use of a lingual sheath spot welded to bands cemented on the first or second molars (Figure 11.5). There is a U loop facing either mesially or distally which can allow activation to rotate the molars and to achieve a small degree of expansion. The effectiveness of the palatal arch to do this can be improved by increasing the size of the U loop and hence the amount of the wire and the range of action (Figure 11.5).[1] Theoretically, the arch provides anteroposterior anchorage by fixing the intermolar width, preventing the molars coming forward when force is applied to them. They can

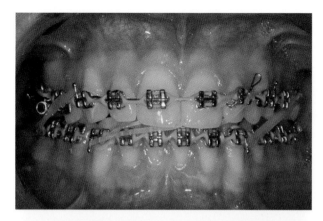

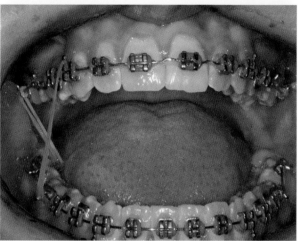

Figure 11.3 Asymmetrical elastics including anterior cross elastic for correction of centrelines (*top*) and cross elastic to correct posterior crossbite (*bottom*).

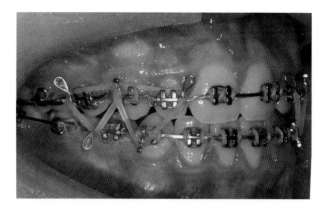

Figure 11.4 Vertical elastics for finishing and detailing occlusion.

still tip, however, and the anchorage provided by a simple transpalatal arch appears to be minimal.[2] Vertically a transpalatal arch can be useful in stabilising the molars and providing a point of application when mechanically extruding a canine or applying headgear.

To increase the anchorage value the palatal arch wirework can be extended forward into the anterior vault of the palatal, which is engaged by addition of an acrylic pad into which the palatal arch is embedded. The acrylic that ideally rests against the vertical part of the hard palate is called a Nance button after its inventor, Hays Nance (Figure 11.6). This uses the anterior hard palate to prevent the molars coming forward, providing greater anchorage than a simple transpalatal arch alone, during the initial stages of tooth alignment. Care must be taken to have a sufficiently large and well-designed Nance button otherwise the acrylic button will become embedded in the palate.

Another scenario in which palatal arches are very useful is for discouraging a digit-sucking habit and resolution of an anterior open bite. A patient presented in the early permanent dentition with a 5-mm anterior open bite on the upper central incisors, largely due to an enthusiastic thumb-sucking habit (Figure 11.7). Non-invasive techniques to discourage the digit-sucking habit had failed and therefore a 'hay-rake' appliance was fitted with four vertical metal loops extending well beyond the incisor tips. The hay-rake was supported by a Nance button palatal arch which, if the patient persists in the active thumb-sucking habit, will prevent the metal loops embedding in the anterior part of the hard palate. The extraoral photograph demonstrates how the tongue is prevented from sitting immediately behind the upper incisors because of the hay-rake. The appliance removes all the pleasurable sensations of thumb sucking, and dissuades the patient from continuing this habit. After only two months the patient was reviewed and there was a significant improvement in the position of the anterior teeth, in that there was now vertical overlap. The hay-rake is a very efficient and effective device that disrupts the thumb-sucking habit and maximises the chances of achieving a good occlusal result, as by breaking the habit it hopefully enhances the stability of the teeth in the corrected position. An alternative is the Bluegrass appliance, which consists of a palatal arch with a ball or roller of acrylic that can rotate (Figure 11.8). The theory is that as well as preventing digit sucking the patient's tongue will be encouraged to sit forward in the palate as the patient spins the acrylic ball or roller, keeping it out of the anterior open bite.

Lingual Arches and Space Maintainers

There are many methods of providing space maintenance in orthodontics. The problem with removable appliance space maintainers is the fact that they are removable. When the patients remove them, the space available can close down in a matter of weeks, or sometimes even days,

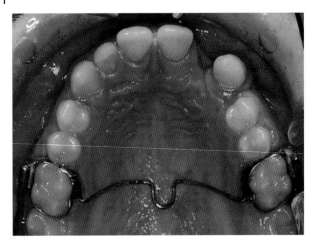 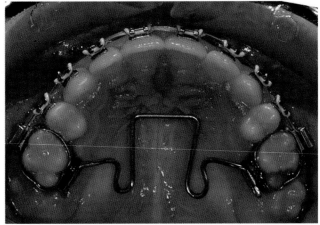

Figure 11.5 Transpalatal arch (*left*) and variation to allow greater activation for expansion (*right*).

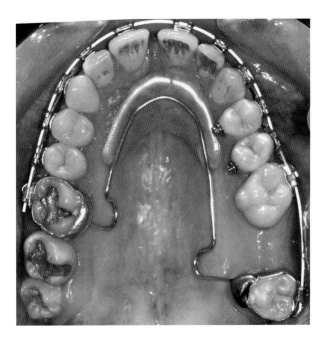

Figure 11.6 Transpalatal arch with Nance acrylic button.

and the patient is then unable to insert the appliance, resulting in even more space being lost.

The alternative is to use the much more reliable fixed space maintainer. This can be simply done by use of a band on the tooth usually posterior to the space being maintained and then a wire loop soldered to the band to engage the distal part of the tooth anterior to the space (Figure 11.9). The advantage of banding posterior teeth is that if the correct size band is selected and fitted well, there is usually no problem leaving these in place for a number of months, and sometimes years, until the impacted tooth erupts. The case shown is a patient who was in the late permanent dentition with retained upper second deciduous molars. Radiographically, the upper second

premolars appeared to be ectopic, lying above the upper second molars and facing mesially. Interceptive extraction of the second primary molars was planned hopefully to normalise the path of eruption of the premolars. To prevent the spontaneous mesial drift of the upper first molars, space maintainers were cemented on both of the upper left and upper right first permanent molars. Within 12 months the upper right second premolar had erupted into the space (Figure 11.10). However, the upper left second premolar failed to erupt and therefore exposure and bonding of this tooth was arranged to allow mechanical traction to be applied to bring it down into the arch.

An alternative for space maintenance in the lower arch is the lingual arch. This is an arch made of 1.0-mm stainless steel that is attached to the lower first molars and which bypasses the premolars and canines and rests on the cingulum of the lower incisors (Figure 11.11). Another use of the lingual arch is to maintain the leeway space, which is the difference in mesiodistal width of the lower primary canines and molars and lower permanent canines and premolars, or more commonly just 'E-space', which is the difference between the second primary molar and the second premolar. In the mandible this can very usefully be up to 2.5 mm on each side of the arch. In cases with mild crowding of the lower labial segment, space can therefore be preserved without extraction by maintenance of the leeway or the E-space in the mixed dentition by placement of a simple lingual arch.[3] This can convert a potential extraction case into a non-extraction case, or change a difficult extraction case into one that can easily be handled with conventional orthodontics.

The case to illustrate this was an 11-year-old boy who presented with a moderately crowded lower labial segment but the lower right D and both lower Es were still in place. A lingual arch was placed to make use of this E-space on

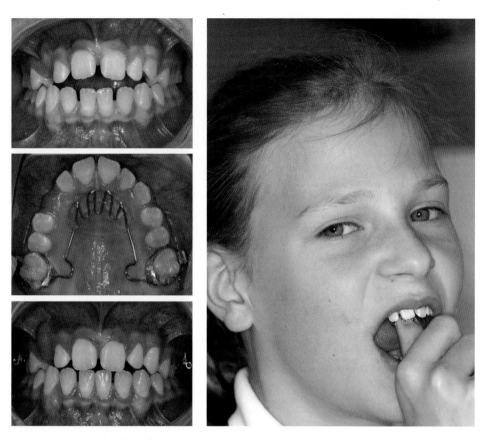

Figure 11.7 Use of a hay-rake palatal arch to discourage a digit-sucking habit.

both sides of the arch (Figure 11.11). Nine months later the premolars had erupted on the right-hand side of the arch and the second premolar was just erupting on the left-hand side of the arch. Once the permanent dentition had erupted, brackets were placed on all teeth anterior to the first molars and the teeth aligned with flexible archwires. The lingual arch had provided the opportunity of gaining 4 mm of space in the lower arch, which provided sufficient space to relieve the anterior crowding without the need for extraction of permanent units.

Headgear and Extraoral Traction

Headgear can be used to reinforce anchorage, create space by distalisation of the buccal segments or exert an orthopaedic effect on the maxilla depending on direction, duration and level of force applied. The force is applied from the back of the neck or head usually to the maxillary first molars via a Kloehn facebow insert into buccal head-gear tubes. The direction of force is determined by its point of application.

- High or occipital pull is applied from the back of the head and has an intrusive effect on the maxillary molars. It is usually used in patients with increased vertical proportions and hyperdivergent growth patterns in order to prevent further bite opening during orthodontic treatment.
- Low or cervical pull is applied from the neck and has an extrusive effect on the maxillary molars, being used in patients with reduced lower face height and hypodivergent growth patterns to assist in bite opening.
- Straight or combination pull headgear provides a direction of force parallel to the occlusal plane and is therefore used in patients with normal vertical proportions, especially if pure molar distalisation is desired.

The main challenge with headgear is patient compliance. Ideally to reinforce anchorage headgear needs to be worn for 10–12 hours per day with a force of 250–350 g per side. When used for molar distalisation or maxillary orthopaedic effects, this increases to 14 hours a day with a force of 450–500 g per side. From studies using timers attached to the appliances, it is known that patients rarely wear headgear for the time prescribed, and in the UK head-gear use has fallen out of favour.[4] In other countries such as Germany and the USA, however, headgear has been proved to be a reliable and successful method of treating maloc-clusion as the patients are 'incentivised' to cooperate with treatment. There are occasionally patients who present

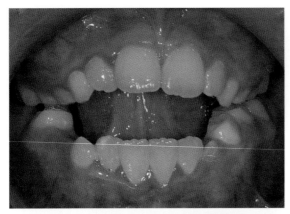

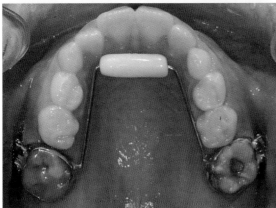

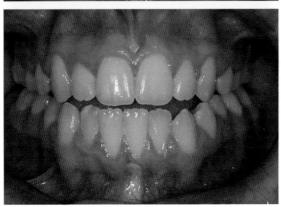

Figure 11.8 Bluegrass appliance.

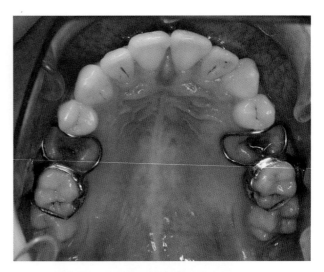

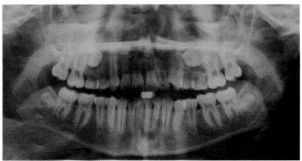

Figure 11.9 Fixed space maintainers to hold space for eruption of ectopic second premolars following extraction of second primary molars.

who insist on being treated on a non-extraction basis, and with a high level of compliance the use of headgear in these situations can prove very effective.

A 13-year-old patient presented with a Class I incisor relationship on a Class I skeletal base. The upper right canine was unerupted and in a reasonable position; however, there was only 4 mm of space within the arch to accommodate this 8-mm tooth (Figure 11.12). All the treatment alternatives were discussed with the patient and parents, including the extraction of an upper second premolar to allow mesialisation of the upper first molar

and distalisation of the upper first premolar, which would then provide sufficient space to accommodate the canine. The patient was keen to be treated without extractions and therefore combination-pull headgear was fitted and a 450-g force applied bilaterally, which she was instructed to wear for a minimum of 14 hours a day. Snap-away springs were used both cervically and occipitally to prevent the risk of catapult injury and a locking inner bow was used to prevent accidental displacement from the molar tubes.[5] The canine erupted spontaneously but was still short of space so the headgear force was continued for a few more months until full molar correction had been achieved and sufficient space created for the canine. Alignment was then carried out with fixed appliances.

Class II Correction

A Class II malocclusion is one of the commonest problems encountered in orthodontics and many ways have been described to treat it. In the USA, treatment modalities were primarily based on fixed appliance systems and use of Class

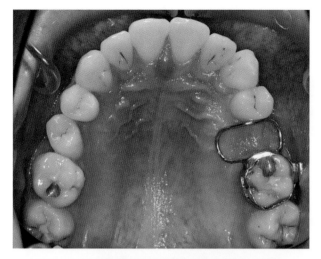

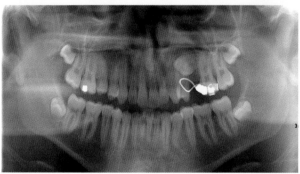

Figure 11.10 Same case as Figure 11.9 showing successful eruption of the upper right second premolar following space maintenance but failure of eruption of the upper left second premolar.

II intermaxillary traction. In Europe, there was the development of functional appliance systems and philosophies that postured the mandible forwards in growing patients, essentially converting a Class II malocclusion into a Class I. While there has been considerable and often acrimonious debate over the decades as to whether these appliances actually have any permanent significant effect on growth (the overwhelming evidence is now that improvements

achieved are largely dentoalveolar movements), they are certainly effective appliances. Most systems and appliances developed were removable, with all the inherent problems of compliance. To overcome this problem, several fixed Class II correctors have been described.

Herbst Appliance

The Herbst appliance is a fixed functional appliance developed early in the twentieth century by Emil Herbst in Germany. It was essentially forgotten until resurrected and further developed by Hans Pancherz in the 1970s, going on to become the most popular functional appliance worldwide especially when its use was promoted in North America by Jim McNamara.[6] Numerous long-term studies have shown it to be an effective appliance, with the advantage of not being dependent on good patient cooperation as the appliance cannot be removed, as opposed to removable functional appliances such as the Twin Block that is the default functional appliance in the UK.

The original Herbst appliance consisted of bands on the first molars and premolars, a lower lingual arch and the piston and rod that posture the mandible forward. However, Hans Pancherz modified the appliance to cobalt chromium cast splints covering the maxillary and mandibular buccal segments, again connected by the piston and rod. While effective, this appliance is expensive and time-consuming to make and can be difficult to remove. Therefore, a more recent development is the cantilever Herbst originally designed to be used in the mixed dentition. The advantage of this is it can be constructed from preformed components.

The case illustrating the cantilever Herbst appliance was a young female patient with a Class II Division I incisor relationship and an overjet of 9 mm for which Twin Block treatment had previously been attempted but her cooperation was not forthcoming (Figure 11.13). The patient claimed that she was still very keen to get a good result and asked if there were any other alternatives. The Herbst appliance used comprised an upper appliance with an

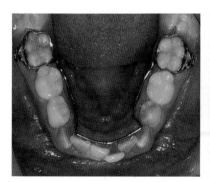 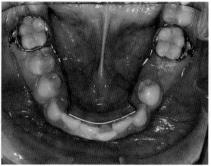 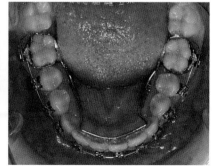

Figure 11.11 Lingual arch used in case with mild to moderate crowding in lower arch to maintain E-space for alignment.

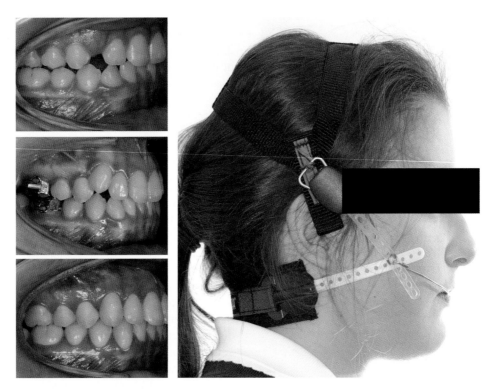

Figure 11.12 Use of headgear to create space for unerupted canine.

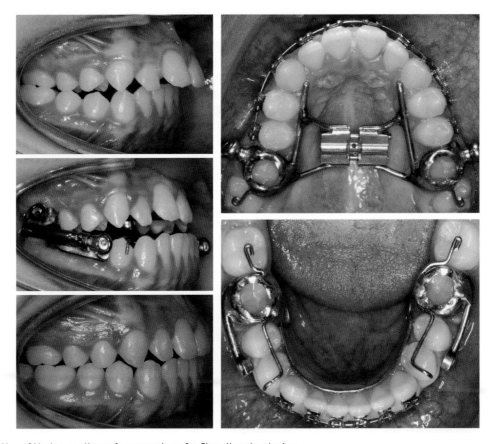

Figure 11.13 Use of Herbst appliance for correction of a Class II malocclusion.

expansion screw soldered onto heavy bands on the upper first molars. The upper first molars also had stops soldered distally to prevent overeruption of the upper second molars and integral threads in the buccal casing into which a piston could be screwed. There was a midline screw that allowed expansion of the upper arch (Figure 11.3) and a metal bar that rested on the palatal surface of the upper premolars and canines which would provide some upper arch expansion.

The lower part of the Herbst appliance comprises heavy bands on the lower first molars to which are soldered occlusal stops for the second molar and the first and second premolars. On the buccal surface of the lower band is an extension arm with an integral thread into which the anterior screw of the piston connecting the upper Herbst to the lower Herbst is screwed. The piston is attached to the upper and lower Herbst by means of screws and 2-mm separators can be placed on the piston arm to advance the lower jaw to the chosen position. With this particular patient the 9-mm overjet was advanced to an edge-to-edge position by using two stops either side on each piston.

The patients will usually then proceed to a comprehensive course of upper and lower straight-wire appliance therapy. Once the overjet is down to zero and the overbite is also down to zero, with overtreated buccal segments, the Herbst appliance is removed. An assessment will be made as to whether the patient needs to continue the Class II effect of treatment with Class II elastics. At the end of treatment this patient had a Class I relationship of the premolars and a 2-mm overjet and 1-mm overbite (Figure 11.13).

The morphological effects of the Herbst appliance have been shown to be similar to those of the Twin Block appliance, namely mainly dentoalveolar.[7] Patients seem to prefer the Herbst appliance and report fewer side effects, but because the breakage rates of the Herbst are significantly higher, it is much more costly and time-consuming and therefore will not be adopted for widespread use in the UK.

Fixed Class II Correctors

Many untested fixed Class II correctors have been described in the literature. Many have come and gone, primarily falling out of favour because of ineffectiveness or high rates of breakage. More recently, with advancing technology and materials, several systems have proved to have greater longevity and are indeed proving both effective and robust for routine clinical use.

The most popular of these is the Forsus™ spring (Figure 11.14). This consists of a rod and a nickel titanium spring that is attached to the maxillary first molar via headgear tube on bands. The appliance is activated by

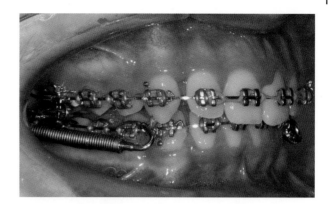

Figure 11.14 Forsus™ appliance.

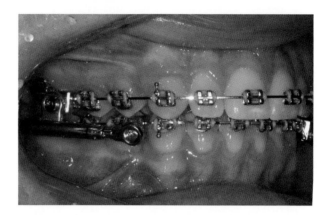

Figure 11.15 Powerscope 2™ appliance.

selection of the correct size rod that is attached directly to the lower archwire either distal to the canine or first premolar. The appliance can be reactivated by the use of split tubing that is attached to the arm on the piston spring. A variation of this principle is the Powerscope™ appliance, which consists of a telescopic piston similar to that used in the cantilever Herbst and which is again attached directly to the archwires mesial to the upper first molar and distal to the lower canine (Figure 11.15).

While useful for Class II correction, the effects of these appliances have shown to be primarily dentoalveolar, proclining the lower incisors and distalising the maxillary first molar.[8]

Tooth Movement

Nickel Titanium Coil Springs

Nickel titanium is very popular for initially aligning archwires due to its superelasticity and shape memory. These properties can also be utilised for space opening and closing using a nickel titanium coil spring. For space opening the

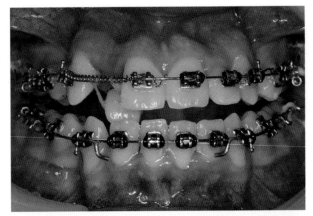

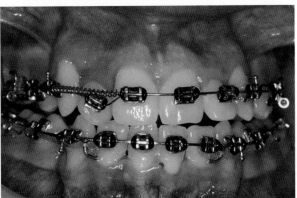

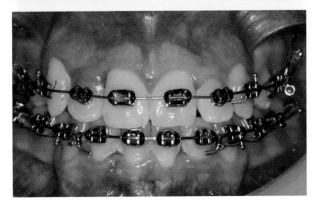

Figure 11.16 Use of nickel titanium push coil to create space for a palatally displaced lateral incisor.

open coil spring is placed on the archwire and compressed between the teeth where space is required (Figure 11.16). To prevent rotation of the teeth and expansion of the arch form, ideally a rigid stainless steel wire should be used and the teeth must be securely tied in with metal ligatures. The coil spring is activated a bracket width, and to prevent any proclination of the incisors the wire should be bent back hard, behind the terminal molar to preserve the arch length.

For space closure, elastomeric force can be used in the form of activated ligatures or power chain (Figure 11.17);

however, elastic chain is subject to rapid force degradation as they absorb moisture and generally become dirty as they collect food and plaque. An effective and much cleaner way to close space is to use a closed nickel titanium coil spring.[9] These come in a variety of sizes and strengths and are usually placed between the first molar and ideally a presoldered hook on the archwire between the canine and lateral incisor. The coils are activated approximately twice their length to deliver a force of 100–150 g, which has been shown to be slightly more effective than elastomeric force for space closure.[10]

Closing Loops

Before the introduction of straight-wire appliances and sliding mechanics, space closure was routinely undertaken with the use of closing loops bent into the archwire between the canine and lateral incisor. While not routinely used today, closing loops can still be very useful to close residual space that is resistant to closure with sliding mechanics.

By introducing vertical loops horizontal flexibility is introduced into the archwire, which can increased by the use of helices: the greater the length of wire, the greater the flexibility. A useful loop therefore for space closure is the Sandusky, which consists of a vertical loop bent into a rectangular steel wire with two helices. It is activated by opening the loop and bending the wire back behind the terminal molar (Figure 11.18).

Vertical flexibility can be also increased in an archwire by introducing more wire horizontally. The double delta can be used to simultaneously close space, reduce a deep overbite, reduce an overjet and provide palatal root torque to the upper incisors. Another loop that is used for some of the previous movements is the 'L' or boot loop (Figures 11.18 and 11.19).

Utility and Intrusion Archwires

The bioprogressive technique developed by R.W. Ricketts used segmental mechanics for anchorage management, overbite control and space closure. While not routinely used with straight-wire appliances, where deep overbites are usually reduced using continuous archwires, the use of utility or intrusion arches can still be very useful, particularly in adult patients with deep bites when specific incisor intrusion is desired.[11]

The utility arch is constructed in either square or rectangular Elgiloy wires (cobalt chromium) or stainless steel. It is vertically stepped down to bypass the premolars and canines and engaged in the bracket slot of the incisors. The wire is activated by placing a vertical bend just mesially to where the wire is placed in the molar tube, resulting in

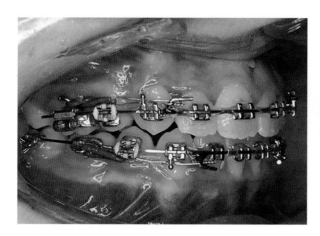
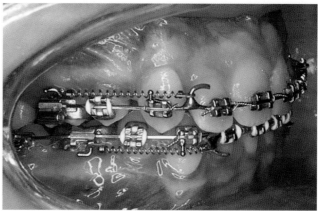

Figure 11.17 An activated elastomeric ligature (*left*) and nickel titanium closing coil (*right*) being used for space closure.

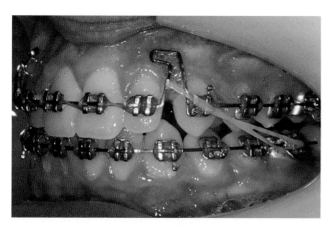
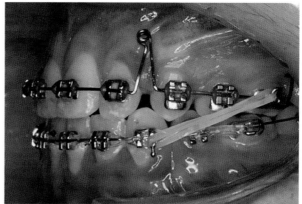

Figure 11.18 L loop (*left*) and Sandusky loop (*right*) for space closure.

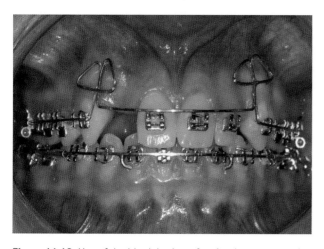
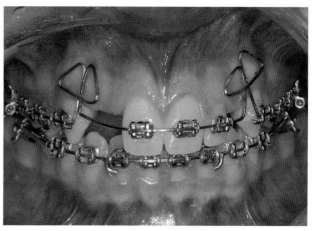

Figure 11.19 Use of double delta loop for simultaneous overjet and overbite reduction.

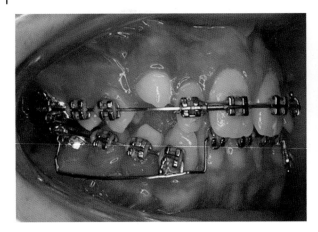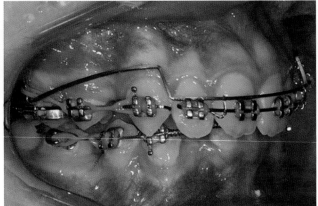

Figure 11.20 Ricketts utility arch (*left*) and Burstone intrusion arch (*right*).

a light intrusive force being applied to the incisors due to the length of wire between the molar and incisor segments (Figure 11.20).

Because the force for intrusion using a utility arch is applied labially to the centre of resistance of the incisors, its use results in both intrusion and proclination which, while it may help with overbite reduction, may be undesirable. The alternative therefore is to use the intrusion arch described by Charles Burstone.[12] This again extends from the molars to incisors, bypassing the premolars and canines, but instead of being placed in the incisor bracket slots directly it is ligated to the archwire. The point of ligation dictates to a degree where the force is directed: the more distal the wire is ligated, the closer the force is to the centre of resistance of the incisors and the less proclination is produced (Figure 11.20). While these were originally made in stainless steel incorporating helices to deliver a low intrusive force to the incisors, beta-titanium or even preformed nickel titanium can be used instead (see Chapter 20).

Sectional Archwires

Sometimes it is desirable or mechanically advantageous to use sectional mechanics. This can be to avoid the direct application of force to teeth where movement is not planned, for example where there is previous evidence of root shortening and resorption (Figure 11.21). This can also be useful in anchorage management in high-anchorage-demanding cases by consolidating simple anchorage in the posterior segments prior to planned movement of the labial segments. Sectional wires can also be used to simplify mechanics and prevent unwanted reciprocal effects of treatment, such as intrusion of adjacent teeth when mechanically extruding a vertically impacted canine (Figure 11.22). To extrude the canines the sectional

archwires, which are constructed of titanium molybdenum alloy (TMA) to increase their range of action, are bent inferiorly and therefore by ligating them to the canines they are activated, applying a light extrusive force to the canines. To prevent tipping of the first molars, these are rigidly fixed together with a transpalatal arch.

Torquing Spurs

Torque control of the upper labial segment can present a challenge, particularly in the treatment of Class II malocclusions and the retraction of the upper labial segment. There will always be a tendency for the upper incisors to upright too much, which is one of the reasons that Lawrence Andrews developed the original straight-wire appliance with positive torque built into the brackets of the upper incisors. Many different prescriptions have been developed since, all with increased torque in the upper incisor brackets. The reason for this is the amount of play between a 0.022 × 0.028-inch slot commonly used and a 0.019 × 0.025-inch archwire, so that the torque in the bracket is never fully expressed. Full dimension archwires can be used, such as 0.021 × 0.025-inch TMA or even stainless steel, but these can be extremely uncomfortable for the patient on placement, and they may prevent any further space closure or tooth movement due to the amount of friction the full engagement creates.

An effective way to apply torque to anterior teeth, particularly upper central incisors, is the use of a torquing spur. This was a technique originally used in the third stage of Begg and Tip-Edge treatment in order to apply torque to the roots of the upper incisors once their crowns had been tipped into the correct position (Figure 11.23). Using a preadjusted edgewise system, a torquing auxiliary can be similarly constructed from Wilcox Australian 0.016-inch regular stainless steel. Carding wax is used to obtain an

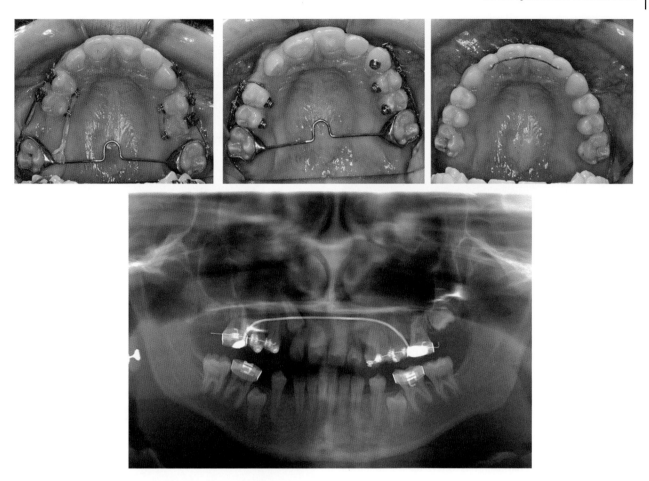

Figure 11.21 Use of sectional mechanics in a case with root resorption of the upper incisors in order to create space for an impacted canine.

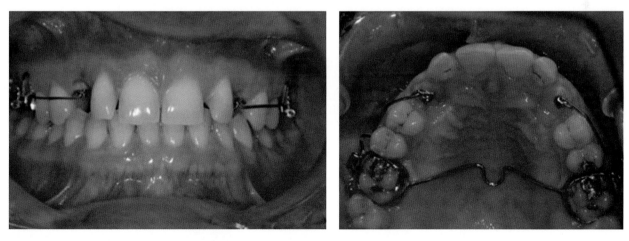

Figure 11.22 Use of TMA sectional archwires to erupt impacted maxillary canines.

impression of the occlusal surfaces of the upper teeth and the exact position of the brackets. The 0.016-inch Australian wire is taken off the reel and bent to an arch form that replicates the arch on the carding wax. The exact position of both mesial and distal bracket wings on the central incisors can be seen in the carding wax, and therefore the torquing spurs, which fit between the wings of the twin brackets, can be placed with precision.

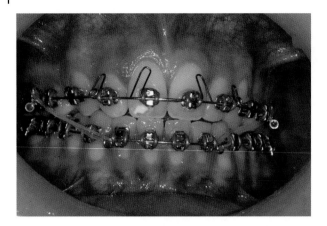

Figure 11.23 Begg-type torquing auxiliary being used in third stage of treatment with Tip-Edge appliance.

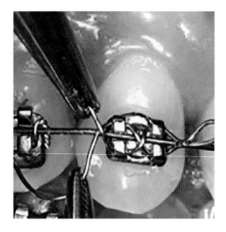

Figure 11.25 Kobayashi hook being ligated with figure-of-eight tie.

Because the torquing spurs are bent in the same horizontal plane as the main archwire, as the wire is engaged they are activated and apply palatal root torque to the incisors (Figure 11.24). To prevent proclination of the incisors the archwire should be bent back hard behind the terminal molar.

Hooks

To allow the use of intramaxillary or intermaxillary traction and sliding mechanics, it is often useful to attach hooks either directly to the brackets or to the archwires. Some brackets, most notably the canines, will come with distogingival hooks. If hooks are needed on other teeth, Kobayashi ligatures which incorporate a hook can be used and the most effective way of applying these is by tying them in a figure-of-eight fashion over both bracket wings (Figure 11.25).

Alternatively, hooks soldered to the archwire or crimpable hooks can be used, although these tend to be much less secure, and if not crimped 100% effectively they will slide up and down the archwires (Figure 11.26).

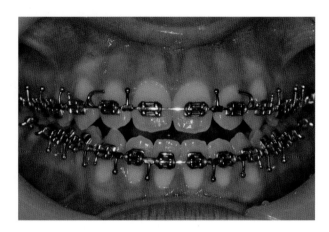

Figure 11.26 Soldered and crimpable hooks used in a case being prepared for orthognathic surgery.

Piggyback Archwires

An effective way to align a severely displaced tooth or an ectopic or impacted tooth is by use of a piggyback archwire (Figure 11.28). This is usually a light 0.016-inch nickel titanium wire tied underneath a rigid stainless

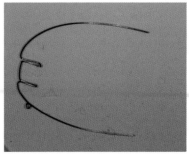
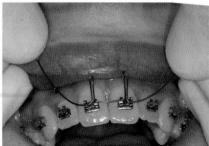
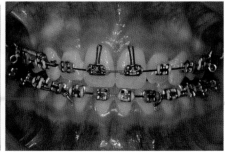

Figure 11.24 Use of torquing spurs to apply palatal root torque to upper central incisors.

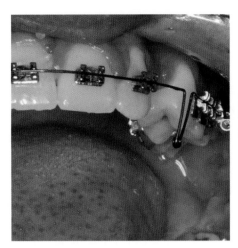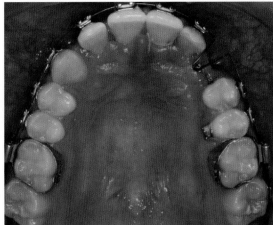

Figure 11.27 Use of ballista spring to mechanically erupt a palatally impacted canine.

steel archwire. The advantages of this approach are that the base archwire maintains the arch form and provides anchorage both vertically and horizontally and allows a stable point of application from which traction to the tooth via the piggyback can be applied. The advantage of a nickel titanium piggyback, as opposed to elastomeric traction, is that it provides continuous force not subject to degradation and can also be fully engaged in the bracket slot to provide better three-dimensional control of the displaced tooth. The base archwire can be either 0.016-inch or 0.018-inch stainless steel while the piggyback should be 0.016-inch nickel titanium so both wires can be relatively well accommodated in the slot of a 0.022 × 0.028-inch bracket. The piggyback sits under the base archwire to reduce the risk of the ends of the wire from displacing and traumatising the gingivae and needs to extend two brackets either side of the displaced tooth to reduce friction. An important point is to create more than enough space before tooth alignment is attempted, otherwise while the crown may align the root will be left displaced.

Ballista Spring

Canines that prove resistant to eruption with traction via a piggyback archwire may benefit from the use of a ballista spring. This is formed from 0.016-inch regular Australian stainless steel wire taken from the reel. The ballista spring when it is passive extends in an occlusal direction at 90° to the occlusal plane. A complete loop is bent in the ballista to allow easy ligation to the gold chain (Figure 11.27). To activate the spring a 0.09-mm metal ligature is passed through the loop on the ballista and also passed through the link of gold chain that is closest to the mucosa. As the ligature is tightened the ballista loop rotates through 90° from its initial vertical position until it is almost in the same horizontal plane as the main archwire. The advantage of

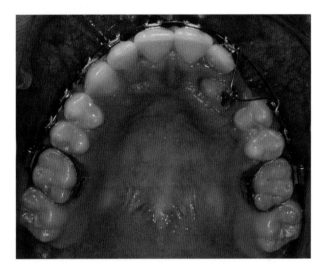

Figure 11.28 Piggyback archwire to align canine once erupted in palate in case shown in Figure 11.27.

the spring is it creates both a vertical and horizontal force, pulling the canine down and towards the arch. Once this has been done and the labial face of the tooth exposed, a piggyback archwire can be used to achieve buccal movement to bring it into the line of the arch before final alignment (see Figure 11.27).

Conclusion

The straight-wire appliance has provided many of the answers to our clinical problems. Together with the judicious use of all the auxiliary devices described in this chapter, even an average clinician should be able to meet all their patients' expectations in an efficient and effective manner. A high standard of treatment finish should be achievable for the majority of patients within a reasonable two-year time frame.

References

1 Gündüz E, Crismani AG, Bantleon HP, et al. An improved transpalatal bar design. Part II. Clinical upper molar derotation: case report. *Angle Orthod.* 2003;73:244–248.

2 Zablocki HL, McNamara JA, Franchi L, Baccetti T. Effect of the transpalatal arch during extraction treatment. *Am. J. Orthod. Dentofacial Orthop.* 2008;133:852–860.

3 Gianelly A. Leeway space and the resolution of crowding in the mixed dentition. *Semin. Orthod.* 1995;1:188–194.

4 Cureton SL, Regennitter FJ, Yancey JM. Clinical versus quantitative assessment of headgear compliance. *Am. J. Orthod. Dentofacial Orthop.* 1993;104:277–284.

5 Samuels RHA, Brezniak N. Orthodontic facebows: safety issues and current management. *J. Orthod.* 2002;29:101–107.

6 Pancherz H. Treatment of class II malocclusion by jumping bite with Herbst appliance: a cephalometric investigation. *Am. J. Orthod.* 1979;76:423–442.

7 O'Brien K, Wright J, Conboy F, et al. Effectiveness of treatment for Class II malocclusion with the Herbst or twin block appliances: a randomized controlled trial. *Am. J. Orthod. Dentofacial Orthop.* 2003;124:128–137.

8 Giuntinin V, Vangelisti A, Masucci C, et al. Treatment effects produced by the Twin Block appliance vs the Forsus Fatique Resistant Device in growing Class II patients. *Angle Orthod.* 2015;85:784–789.

9 Mohammed H, Rizk MZ, Wafaie K, Almuzian M. Effectiveness of nickel–titanium springs vs elastomeric chains in orthodontic space closure: a systematic review and meta analysis. *Orthod. Craniofac. Res.* 2018;21:12–19.

10 Samuels RH, Rudge SJ, Mair LH. A clinical study of space closure with nickel titanium coil springs and elastic module. *Am. J. Orthod. Dentofacial Orthop.* 1998;114:73–79.

11 Ricketts RM. Bioprogressive therapy as an answer to orthodontic needs. *Am. J. Orthod.* 1976;70:359–397.

12 Burstone CR. Deep overbite correction by intrusion. *Am. J. Orthod.* 1977;72:1–22.

12

Optimising Fixed Appliance Treatment with Orthodontic Mini-implants
Richard R. J. Cousley

CHAPTER OUTLINE
Introduction, 219
OMI Advantages, 220
Flexible Timing of Anchorage, 220
No Additional Requirements for Patient Compliance, 220
Predictable Treatment Outcomes and Reduced Treatment Times, 220
Enhanced Control of Target Teeth Movements, 220
Effective Anchorage in all Three Dimensions, 220
OMI Disadvantages, 220
OMI Failure, 220
Root/Periodontal Damage, 220
Pain, 221
Perforation of Nasal and Maxillary Sinus Floors, 221
Damage to Neurovascular Tissues, 221
Mini-implant Fracture, 221
Soft Tissue Problems, 221
Mini-implant Migration, 221
Where Does OMI anchorage Come From?, 221
Anchorage Options: Direct Versus Indirect, 223
Key Clinical Steps Involved in OMI Usage with Fixed Appliances, 226
Clinical and Radiographic Planning, 226
Root Divergence, 226
Pre-insertion Preparation, 226
OMI Insertion, 226
Force Application, 227
Explantation, 227
Three-dimensional Anchorage Applications, 228
Anteroposterior Anchorage, 228
Vertical Anchorage, 228
Transverse Anchorage, 231
References, 231

Introduction

Anchorage loss has been a perpetual problem during fixed appliance treatments, especially when movements involve space closure, incisor root torque and molar distalisation. This may occur in all three dimensions, although the mesial drift of posterior anchor teeth is the archetypal example of anchorage loss. Fortunately, **orthodontic mini-implants (OMIs)**, also known as **miniscrew implants** or **temporary anchorage devices (TADs)**, offer an effective panacea for this problem. Indeed, aside from providing reliable and absolute (bone) anchorage, the integration of OMIs within fixed appliance treatments offers other advantages over conventional anchorage, as outlined in the following section.

OMI Advantages

Flexible Timing of Anchorage

Anchorage control may commence either at the bond-up stage, or more typically once initial alignment has occurred, or even at a later stage (if conventional anchorage loss has occurred).

No Additional Requirements for Patient Compliance

OMI usage is feasible if a patient can tolerate fixed appliance treatment and maintain satisfactory oral hygiene.

Predictable Treatment Outcomes and Reduced Treatment Times

Optimised anchorage control provided by OMIs means that en masse movement of groups of teeth can be performed (rather than two-stage movements) and the orthodontist can be confident that target movements (e.g. overjet reduction in a Class II camouflage case) will be achieved.

Enhanced Control of Target Teeth Movements

Bodily and intrusive movements are achieved, rather than the tipping/extrusive side effects typically associated with straight-wire mechanics.[1–5]

Effective Anchorage in all Three Dimensions

OMI usage has resulted in a significant broadening of the orthodontic (non-surgical) envelope of treatment possibilities. In particular, novel treatments such as molar intrusion (for open bite correction) and skeletal maxillary expansion are now routinely possible, and result in fewer patients requiring maxillofacial surgery.

Consequently, I simply could not envisage trying to offer a modern range of treatments without the option of OMI anchorage in specific indications. However, successful OMI usage requires knowledge of the relevant bone biology and biomechanical nuances. This chapter highlights those factors which influence how OMI usage can optimise fixed appliance treatment processes and outcomes while minimising side effects. It also gives a flavour of the range of fixed appliance applications. For more detailed analysis and technical details, please refer to a contemporary textbook[6] and the wealth of published journal literature.

However, in the first instance it is worth considering potential disadvantages and risks, and debunking any misconceptions.

OMI Disadvantages

OMI Failure

Failure of an OMI is the principal risk since it means that the OMI cannot be used for its intended anchorage purposes. Is this a common occurrence? This depends on multiple factors such as the selected insertion site, but a recent meta-analysis of 3250 mini-implants showed an overall success rate of 86%.[7] When this is broken down according to maxillary and mandibular sites, the success rates are generally reported to be 80% and 90% for alveolar sites in the mandible and maxilla, respectively, and up to 99% in the mid-palate.[8–16] Fortunately, most OMI failures become clinically evident within the first few months of insertion,[9, 12, 13] enabling early replacement or a modification of the treatment plan. Conversely, when an OMI feels clinically firm after two months *in situ*, then normal orthodontic forces may be applied with confidence.

OMI failures are staged according to the time taken for this to manifest. Primary failure occurs occasionally when an OMI is clinically mobile at the time of insertion. This is due to insufficient cortical bone support, close proximity to an adjacent tooth root or incorrect insertion technique. Secondary failure occurs when the OMI was initially stable, but then develops mobility in the subsequent two to three months. This is due to excess bone strain or microscopic necrosis around the endosseous body, which may result from thermal bone damage (during pilot drilling), excessive insertion torque, close proximity to a tooth root, traction overload, or a combination of these.

Root/Periodontal Damage

Multiple clinical and animal studies have consistently shown that traumatised root surfaces are repaired within 12 weeks by cellular cementum and periodontal regeneration, meaning that this is not a clinically significant risk. However, it is unlikely such root trauma will even occur if only superficial local anaesthesia (LA) is used, since the patient will complain of periodontal pain before root contact occurs. If root contact does occur, then the orthodontist is also likely to feel an immediate increase in insertion torque.[17] Therefore, any irreversible effect from close proximity of a mini-implant to a tooth root will impact the mini-implant: it will have an increased risk of failure rather than the tooth being irreversibly damaged.[17–22]

Pain

There is often an expectation that OMI insertion is painful, but the opposite is true, such that some patients feel virtually no discomfort during and after insertion.[23, 24] The majority of patients appear to experience mild pressure-related pain at the time of insertion and up to 24 hours of low-level pain thereafter. This is self-limiting, controlled by simple analgesics and comparable (but of shorter duration) to other orthodontic experiences, such as the effects of separators and aligning archwires,[25] and certainly much less than dental extractions.[26]

When it comes to mini-implant removal, LA is usually not required and indeed patients find that the injection sensation is worse than the actual discomfort of explantation.[27] However, LA may be required for removal of an OMI where it has been inserted in loose mucosa and/or there has been some soft tissue overgrowth of the OMI head.

Perforation of Nasal and Maxillary Sinus Floors

OMI perforation of the nasomaxillary cavities may occur where the maxillary sinus floor has migrated inferiorly.[28] However, the consensus based on dental implant research is that a soft tissue lining rapidly forms over the end of a perforating fixture, and that OMI sites readily heal by bone infill because of the narrow width of the explantation hole. In context, I have never seen signs of either infection or a fistula in several hundred posterior maxillary OMI sites.

Damage to Neurovascular Tissues

Disruption of the inferior dental, mental or greater palatine nerves and blood vessels is highly unlikely given their relative distance from standard insertion sites. The nasopalatine nerve is potentially close to anterior palatal insertion sites, but readily avoidable if the insertion sites are distal to the third palatal rugae.[29]

Mini-implant Fracture

OMI fracture rarely occurs since most materials and designs do not easily fracture within the normal torque limits in clinical practice.[30, 31] Therefore, fracture at the time of insertion is most likely to result from incorrect technique and clinical inexperience. If an OMI fractures on removal, then this is likely to occur flush with the bone surface and the fractured remnant may be left *in situ*, if it will not impede any remaining tooth movements, due to the biocompatibility of titanium alloy.

Soft Tissue Problems

The most common issue is chronic, low-grade, superficial, peri-implant inflammation, analogous to gingivitis around the OMI neck and head. It is more likely if the OMI is inserted into an area of mobile mucosa, over-inserted (partially submerged) in attached gingiva, and/or oral hygiene is inadequate.

Mini-implant Migration

This depends on the head (and neck) to body ratio, on the degree of bone support (stability) and on the relative force level. In effect, OMIs may tip and/or translate bodily in the direction of the applied force.[32–35] This is only problematic if it causes the OMI head to approximate an adjacent bracket or crown, or causes soft tissue impingement or difficulty utilising the OMI head.

Where Does OMI anchorage Come From?

OMI designs originated from maxillofacial bone fixation technology rather than restorative dental implant fixtures. Therefore, OMIs rely on mechanical retention within the bone and not osseointegration. Even when bone-implant contact has been observed in histological studies,[36, 37] it does not equate to a clinically detectable level of OMI–bone ankylosis. This means that OMIs may be loaded immediately (without a latency period) and are removed by simple counterclockwise rotation, even after several years *in situ*. The other key difference from dental implants is that OMIs are much smaller fixtures, enabling their insertion in multiple interproximal alveolar and palate sites.

Most commercially available OMIs are made from grade 5 titanium alloy (Ti-6Al-4V), because of its favourable biocompatibility and reasonable strength. Nowadays, most systems offer self-drilling screws, which means that they are inserted without pilot drilling, in a similar manner that clockwise rotations 'drive' a corkscrew into a cork. The exception occurs in adults in areas of dense and thick cortical bone, but even here a cortical perforation may be performed rather than a full-depth pilot hole. This limited depth (e.g. 2 mm) drilling acts to give the OMI insertion a 'head start' and offset excessive insertion resistance. This resistance, known as insertion torque and measured in Newton centimetres (Ncm), provides an indication of likely success or failure, such that successful OMI insertions typically have a maximum/final insertion torque of 5–20 Ncm. Lower torque values are associated with inadequate primary stability, meaning that the OMI does not have sufficient physical bone engagement to withstand orthodontic loading. Conversely, torque measurements above this range indicate an increased risk of secondary (delayed) failure, where the peri-implant bone strain exceeds its physiological threshold. This initiates excessive bone remodelling (relative to new bone formation) around the OMI threads, leading to loss of (secondary) stability within the first two to three months of insertion.

OMIs are typically inserted in interproximal, mid-palate and mandibular buccal shelf sites. The cortex is usually 1–2 mm thick in adults at most clinically accessible alveolar and mid-palatal sites, and thicker in the posterior mandible.[38–43] Most clinical skeletal anchorage is achieved by engagement of the OMI within this cortical bone. The underlying cancellous bone tends to only provide significant support when the cortical layer is diminutive (e.g. less than 1 mm thick), which may occur in maxillary buccal sites.[44] Consequently, an OMI with a long (e.g. 9 mm) body length may be indicated in the maxilla in order to gain some additional stability from the cancellous bone when the cortex is thin. In contrast, a relatively short OMI (e.g. 6 mm body length) may be stable in adult posterior mandibular sites. The degree of bone support, especially the cortical thickness and density, is indicated clinically by an OMI's maximum insertion torque. However, it is now feasible to gauge cortical thickness before insertion using cone beam computed tomography (CBCT). In addition, I have found a small field of view CBCT increasingly beneficial, immediately prior to insertion, in order to assess the available bone volume (and its anatomical boundaries),

especially where alveolar depth may be limited. This is classically the case in mandibular and anterior alveolar sites (Figure 12.1). Perhaps this is why a recent research study on the use of CBCT for OMI planning purposes concluded that this imaging modality reduces root approximation and hence failure rates.[45]

Table 12.1 summarises the key factors which influence OMI stability, and an awareness of these will maximise your clinical success rates. Many of these factors are interrelated. For example, in terms of patient variables, cortical bone density and thickness tend to increase with patient age (in the transition from adolescence to adulthood),[41, 46, 47] reductions in facial height,[8, 13, 48–50] and relatively higher body mass index (BMI) scores.[51] In design terms, increases in body (endosseous) diameter have more influence on insertion torque than length, because diameter changes affect the OMI–cortex interface (surface area of cortical bone contact) whereas length changes affect the amount of cancellous bone engagement. OMI neck length is relevant because when forces are applied at a 'large' distance from the bone surface it creates a lever effect, causing excessive strain on the cortical rim around the OMI and hence excessive bone remodelling.[52, 53] Finally, the factors within our direct control are the technique ones. In particular, I have found the simple technique of root divergence extremely helpful in preparing alveolar insertion sites prior to OMI insertion. This involves tipping one or both of the teeth adjacent to the planned insertion site,

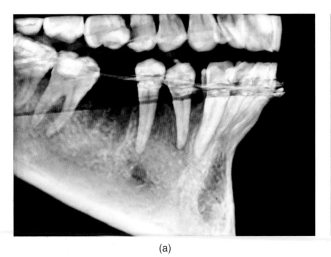

(a)

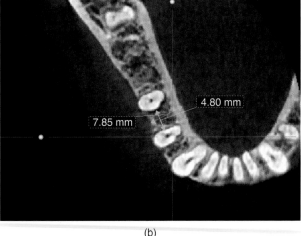

(b)

Figure 12.1 (a) Reformatted CBCT view used to assess the lower premolar root positions and adjacent alveolar height in an adult patient requiring first molar space closure. The first premolar has been distally tipped for root divergence. (b) Axial section of this CBCT with measurements of the interproximal space width (4.8 mm) and depth (7.85 mm). This indicates sufficient bone volume for a 2 mm diameter and 6 mm length OMI (but not a 1.5 × 9 mm version).

Table 12.1 Factors affecting OMI success rates.

Patient factors

Bone volume at insertion site

Cortical thickness and density

Patient age

Facial height

Body mass index

Attached vs. loose mucosa

Oral hygiene

OMI design factors

Body diameter and length

Self-drilling vs. self-tapping threads and insertion

Neck length/head prominence

Neck–soft tissue interface

Material biocompatibility

Ease of clinical use

Technique factors

Root proximity (divergence)

Insertion torque range (within physiological limits)

Cortical perforation

Site (instrument) access

Force application and timing

Operator experience

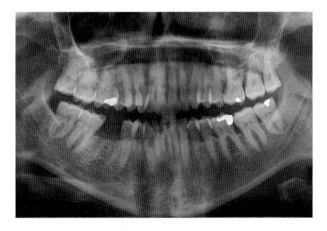

Figure 12.2 Pretreatment panoramic radiograph of the same patient as Figure 12.1. This shows the limited interproximal space between the lower right premolar teeth, and also the insufficient quality of this type of image in terms of root and bone visualisation.

as identified on the pretreatment panoramic radiograph (Figure 12.2) and consequently reduces the risks of unfavourable root proximity by the time of OMI insertion (Figure 12.1). Similarly, correct use of the screwdriver and other instruments may make a fundamental difference

between success and failure, such that attendance on an appropriate hands-on training course is essential for novice OMI orthodontists.

Anchorage Options: Direct Versus Indirect

OMIs may be used to supplement fixed appliance anchorage either directly or indirectly. Direct anchorage involves force application straight from the OMI to the appliance/target teeth. Indirect anchorage involves stabilisation of an anchor tooth/unit by the OMI and then force application between the anchor unit and target teeth. A common example of direct anchorage is when an OMI is inserted in a posterior buccal alveolar site (e.g. mesial to the first molar) and traction applied to the anterior teeth via a powerarm (Figure 12.3). A powerarm is a vertical extension from the archwire or an individual tooth that changes the line of traction from an oblique angle to one which is more parallel to the archwire/occlusal plane, and hence renders the traction application closer to the centre of resistance of the target teeth. This greatly facilitates bodily movement of the target tooth/teeth and overbite reduction. In my experience, such direct anchorage is both simple and effective. It is only a matter of OMI insertion and then immediate loading with elastomeric chain, and this may be undertaken at virtually any stage of fixed appliance treatment.

The simplest forms of indirect anchorage involve connection of a buccal OMI to an anchor tooth using either a metal ligature or a wire strut (Figure 12.4). Alternatively, indirect anchorage may involve stabilisation of the anchor teeth via a transpalatal connecting wire from one or two mid-palatal OMIs. The active force, using either traction or pushing mechanics, is then applied from the anchor teeth to the target teeth. This indirect anchorage approach is particularly suitable in adolescent patients because of the high success rates of parasagittal mini-implants in growing individuals, compared to labile alveolar bone sites.[6] However, although such indirect anchorage provides an anatomical advantage, it carries the risk of hidden anchorage loss through flexing of the intermediary wire connection and tipping or bodily translation of the OMI (especially when heavy distalising forces are applied to a single mid-palatal OMI).[7, 8] It also requires laboratory work (appliance fabrication).

As one might expect, there are advantages and disadvantages with each approach, and these are summarised in Table 12.2. A recent meta-analysis of en masse incisor retraction treatments involving direct (buccal mini-implants) and indirect (palatal) anchorage indicated better anchorage control with direct (than indirect) traction

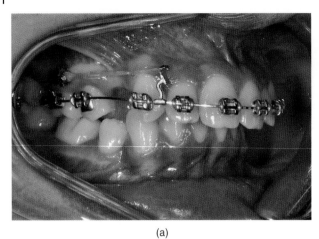

(a)

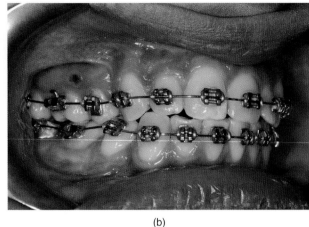

(b)

Figure 12.3 (a) Photograph of elastomeric traction between a buccal OMI (inserted mesial to the first molar) and a crimpable powerarm at the start of traction. (b) View taken after premolar space closure and controlled incisor retraction (with overbite reduction). The OMIs have been removed and the second premolar brackets replaced for correction of their root angulation.

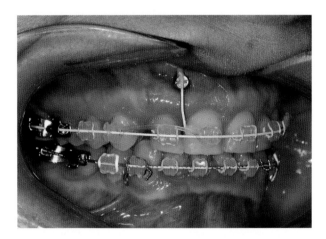

Figure 12.4 Photograph of indirect anchorage of the upper central incisor tooth by an adjacent buccal OMI. A section of 0.019 × 0.025-inch archwire has been used to link this anchor tooth and the OMI, and secured with composite resin at both ends. Elastomeric traction has been applied from the incisor to the ipsilateral first molar for canine space closure by molar protraction.

techniques in both anteroposterior and vertical planes.[54] The authors concluded that direct anchorage provides better outcomes in terms of anchorage control despite the possibility of higher mini-implant stability (success rates) in mid-palate sites. Notably, a comparison of the effectiveness of target tooth movements was not within the remit of this meta-analysis. Therefore, as a generalisation, I prefer to use direct anchorage for standard fixed appliance applications in adults (with normal alveolar bone anatomy), but consider indirect anchorage in young patients where their bone immaturity means that the higher success rates of mid-palate sites offsets the biomechanical limitations of

indirect anchorage. In effect, this is a balancing act where I prioritise biomechanical considerations with direct anchorage but anatomical factors/patient age with indirect anchorage. In addition, there is no palate site option for mandibular anchorage requirements.

Having said that I favour direct anchorage, the potential disadvantage of this approach is that it requires a more careful consideration of force vectors than indirect anchorage (which tends to involve standard fixed appliance biomechanics). Otherwise, undesirable side effects may occur. For example, a steep/oblique vector of traction, from a posteriorly sited OMI, causes either a bowing ('rollercoaster') effect (Figure 12.5) or vertical rotation of the dental arch (when all of the teeth are attached and connected by a rigid archwire). This is because the target teeth rotate or tip and extrude, causing the teeth in the 'passive' part of the arch to intrude. Archwire binding may also occur if the target teeth tip excessively, as a result of the unfavourable traction. This is 'best' exemplified in cases of premolar hypodontia where attempted protraction of the first molar, using oblique traction, causes the molar to tip mesially, the archwire to lock in the molar tube and consequently the whole archwire to be advanced and rotated, and the anterior teeth proclined and intruded (Figure 12.6). Clearly this may be favourable in a Class II deep overbite case, but only to an extent before controlled biomechanics should be utilised to protract the molars with as neutral an effect on the anterior teeth as possible (Figure 12.7). Therefore, in effect, the adjunctive use of OMIs provides more profound anchorage in all three dimensions, but the side effects may also be more strongly expressed than with conventional straight-wire appliance mechanics.

Table 12.2 A comparison of direct and indirect OMI anchorage configurations.

Clinical considerations	Direct anchorage	Indirect anchorage
Method of force application	Simple attachment of force between OMI and target teeth	Auxiliary wire/appliance (laboratory work) required to connect OMI and anchor unit
Typical insertion site	Alveolus: either buccal or palatal aspect	Mid-palate
Optimum patient age	Ideal in adults where failure rates for alveolar sites are low	Potentially higher success rates in adolescent patients due to early mid-palate bone stability
Timing of anchorage	Flexible timing during fixed appliance therapy	Typically added at the start of treatment, if laboratory work needed
Biomechanics	Powerarm connection helps to achieve bodily movements of the target teeth	Conventional biomechanics, i.e. force is applied from the anchor unit to the archwire or target teeth, mimicking standard fixed appliance effects
Anchorage loss	Due to OMI failure or movement	Results from OMI failure, but also wire distortion or loosening of an attachment

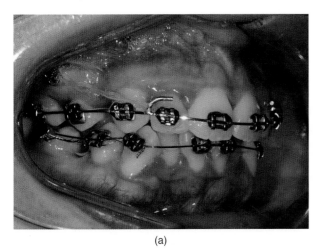 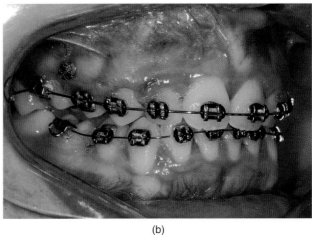

(a) (b)

Figure 12.5 (a) Photograph at the start of 'oblique' elastomeric traction between a buccal OMI (inserted mesial to the first molar) and a short archwire hook. (b) By the end of the traction phase, there has been en masse retraction of the upper anterior teeth, but with incomplete torque and overbite control. In addition, the first molar and second premolar teeth have intruded. The resultant lateral open bite and the vertical step between the first (and just bonded) second molar teeth are evident.

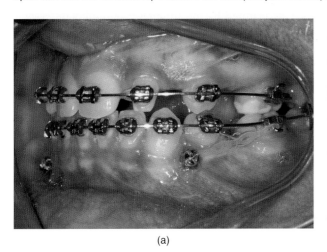 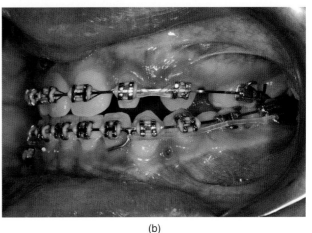

(a) (b)

Figure 12.6 (a) Photographs of a patient with hypodontia requiring protraction of the lower molar teeth for space closure. 'Oblique' traction has been applied to the lower first molar, following distal tipping of the canine crown and insertion of the OMI distal to this canine. (b) Mesial molar tipping (during closure of the deciduous molar space) has resulted in archwire-tube binding and subsequent incisor proclination and intrusion. Consequently, there is a minimal overjet and overbite.

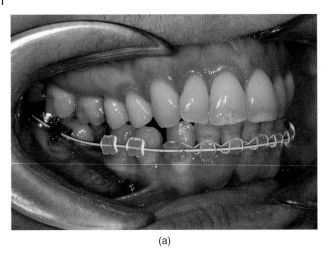
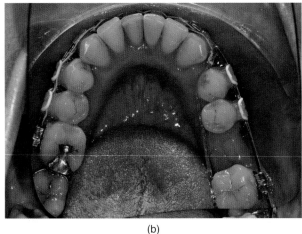

(a)   (b)

Figure 12.7 (a) Photograph of a patient requiring protraction of the second and third molar teeth for space closure. The OMI has been inserted between the premolar roots, and bordering in loose mucosa (resulting in slight bleeding). (b) The side effects of oblique traction are being counteracted by simultaneous traction from the labial segment to a lingual button on the lower second molar.

Key Clinical Steps Involved in OMI Usage with Fixed Appliances

Clinical and Radiographic Planning

Determine the anatomical and biomechanical considerations and hence the optimum OMI insertion site, and both type and timing of anchorage application.

Root Divergence

Many interproximal spaces are limited by close proximity of adjacent tooth roots, especially if the roots are curved and/or the tooth roots are tipped towards one another (see Figure 12.2). Therefore, it makes complete sense to correct this problem at the outset of fixed appliance treatment. Additional interproximal space is readily created, prior to OMI insertion, by altering the tip of one or both of the adjacent brackets in order to move the roots apart. For example, the addition of approximately 30° of mesial bracket tip, on bonding an adjacent premolar, very effectively moves its root mesially during alignment. The insertion site has thus been 'developed' by the time a working archwire has been inserted (see Figure 12.1a).

Pre-insertion Preparation

Once the fixed appliance treatment is reaching the point at which maximum anchorage is required, and a suitable working archwire is *in situ*, then it is time to organise the insertion(s). An up-to-date radiograph is very helpful, especially if tooth movements and root divergence have been performed since the original diagnostic views were

obtained. Classically, this involves taking a periapical view of the insertion site, but with the advent of low-dose, small field of view CBCT imaging I now routinely take a three-dimensional image. This is justified by the increased qualitative data provided and especially by the scope for volumetric assessment. In particular, it is now possible to measure the buccolingual dimension with CBCT (compared to conventional radiographs) and this may alter the OMI selection decision (see Figure 12.1b).

The other key consideration at this stage is whether a guidance stent is indicated. This is particularly helpful for sites which are difficult to access, such as the palate (Figure 12.8). It is also useful for orthodontists who are learning OMI techniques and other clinicians asked to insert them on behalf of an orthodontist. Ideally, the stent should provide truly three-dimensional insertion guidance, as featured by the Infinitas™ mini-implant system with its unique in-house stent fabrication kit (http://www.infinitas-miniimplant.co.uk/guidance-kit.html), rather than very limited guidance based on surface positions only (an 'X marks the spot' approach). At present, we are also on the threshold of CBCT-digital model integrated planning, which will enable optimal virtual positioning of the OMI according to the anchorage needs and individual anatomical features, and then transfer of this to a three-dimensional printed stent (Figure 12.9).

OMI Insertion

OMI insertion, under superficial anaesthesia, typically involves injecting a fraction of 1 ml of LA directly at the insertion site. More profound and widespread anaesthesia is undesirable since this would result in the loss of valuable

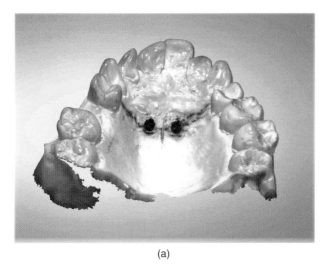

(a)

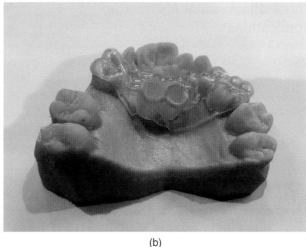

(b)

Figure 12.8 (a) Intraoral scan of a dental model of the maxillary arch including two mid-palate OMI analogues. (b) Photograph of an Infinitas™ system guidance stent fabricated, using the working model and analogues, to locate the insertion instruments and hence the OMIs in all three planes of space.

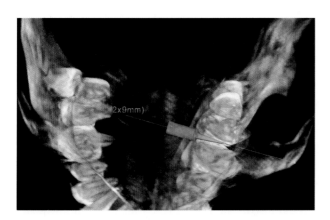

Figure 12.9 Reformatted view of a maxillary CBCT where a virtual OMI (cyan) has been placed in a palatal alveolar site between the molar roots. A virtual abutment (extension) cylinder has been added, which extrapolates the insertion angles, and could be used to form a guidance cylinder.

patient feedback when a pressure sensation is reported from the periodontal receptors surrounding an adjacent tooth root. I have also found it very useful to gauge proximity to adjacent dental roots by the simple test of percussing these teeth. A dull sound indicates close proximity of the OMI to this tooth, and this is relevant if one adjacent tooth has a very different percussion sound to the other one, indicating closer proximity of the mini-implant to the dull-sounding tooth.

Manual (screwdriver) insertion is recommended where access enables this, since full operator control and sensory feedback is provided. However, an appropriate (low speed, variable torque) contra-angle handpiece is required for palatal sites, and ideally this is used with an insertion stent

(guide) in order to reduce positional errors. This 'sacrifices' the sensory feedback from manual screwdriver usage, but the compromise is worthwhile for three-dimensional accuracy in difficult-to-access sites. Finally, care should be taken to avoid over-insertion of the OMI since this will result in soft tissue overgrowth, and it cannot be remedied by partial unscrewing of the OMI (since this loosens it).

Force Application

Light forces (e.g. 50 g for direct anchorage) should be applied for the first four weeks in adults and six weeks in adolescent patients, in order to avoid excessive bone stress and remodelling during this crucial period of the bone healing cycle. This is because the weakest time for the peri-implant bone to withstand OMI loading occurs three weeks after insertion, at the transition between primary and secondary stability phases.[55] In addition, this guideline accounts for the relatively weaker/more labile bone of growing patients by allowing a longer period before standard orthodontic forces are applied.

Explantation

OMIs have the distinct advantage, over conventional anchorage, of allowing the anchorage to be turned 'on' and 'off' during treatment. Hence, an OMI may be left unloaded, but remaining *in situ*, if the orthodontist wishes to test whether anchorage demands have abated prior to explantation. The removal is then easily performed by counterclockwise rotation of the OMI, usually without the need for LA. Healing is uneventful with rapid closure of the circular wound by the surrounding soft tissues.

Three-dimensional Anchorage Applications

Given that OMIs provide anchorage control in all three dimensions, then it is appropriate to consider their uses accordingly. The most common clinical scenarios for each dimension are listed in Table 12.3. The key biomechanical details, as distinct from straight-wire mechanics, are highlighted in the following sections.

Anteroposterior Anchorage

Retraction of anterior teeth requires posterior anchorage reinforcement, using either buccal OMIs sited mesial to the first molar teeth (see Figure 12.3) or mid-palatal OMIs (see Figure 12.8a) for direct and indirect anchorage, respectively. The mid-palate has higher success rates in adolescent patients but the buccal alveolar sites provide more effective biomechanics for bodily retraction or torquing of anterior teeth, as explained earlier in this chapter.

Molar distalisation is most typically warranted, in Caucasian populations, for space creation prior to alignment etc. In this scenario, the mid-palate site offers freedom for the target teeth to move without any approximation of the moving teeth and the OMI(s). Therefore, mid-palatal anchorage of a molar distaliser provides the greatest active range for the appliance. In addition, if the forces are directed at the vertical level of the molar furcations, then better bodily movement is achieved rather than distal crown tipping.[56]

Conversely, molar mesialisation (protraction) requires anterior anchorage reinforcement, using either the mid-palate or buccal alveolar sites. The latter involves fabrication of a customised mesialiser appliance (Figure 12.10). Alveolar sites should be distal to the canine (eminence) to avoid traction from embedding into the soft tissues overlying the 'corner' of the arch. Alternatively, an anterior/labial OMI may be used for indirect anchorage if it anchors a target tooth (e.g. canine) using either a ligature wire or

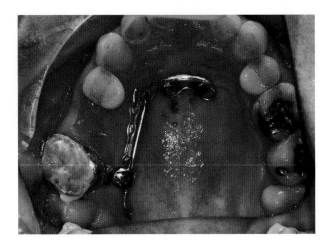

Figure 12.10 Photograph of a mid-palate anchored appliance used to protract the upper right second molar into the first molar space. This is the immediate post-insertion stage, following use of the guidance stent shown in Figure 12.8b. Two parasagittal OMIs have been used to counter any rotational effects (on a single OMI) due to the unilateral traction.

bonded wire strut (see Figure 12.4). Conventional traction is then applied from the anchor teeth to the target tooth.

Vertical Anchorage

Fixed appliance treatment, even when augmented by headgear, has historically provided very poor vertical anchorage control.[57] Therefore, OMIs have revolutionised vertical control, most notably enabling non-surgical anterior open bite correction by molar intrusion from palatal alveolar OMIs, in both adolescent and adult patients (Figure 12.11).[6, 58] Transverse control of the maxillary arch is maintained using a modified transpalatal arch (TPA) or quadhelix (Figure 12.11d), since otherwise the side-effect of palatal traction is molar constriction (and consequently molar crossbites). Conversely, if traction is applied from buccal OMIs then buccal rolling of the molars may occur, resulting in premature contact on the palatal cusps. In my experience, palatal alveolar insertion sites provide better bone volume and cortical support, are reliably accessible (with an appropriate handpiece and ideally a guidance stent), and provide sufficient attached mucosa for the OMI to be inserted at an effective distance from the fixed appliance. While I have seen examples of mid-palate anchorage for molar intrusion, this is not feasible in skeletal anterior open bite cases with high arched palates.

Valuable vertical anchorage control is also achieved using OMIs to avoid anchor tooth intrusion and arch form distortions during extrusion of ectopic teeth. This is especially the case with canine teeth, where their large root surface area and the potential surrounding bone's inertia result in high anchorage demands (Figure 12.12).

Table 12.3 OMI usage according to three planes of anchorage.

Anchorage dimension	Clinical application
Anteroposterior	Incisor retraction and torque
	Molar distalisation
	Molar advancement
Vertical	Single/multiple teeth intrusion
	Tooth extrusion
Transverse	Centreline corrections
	Altering occlusal plane
	Rapid maxillary expansion

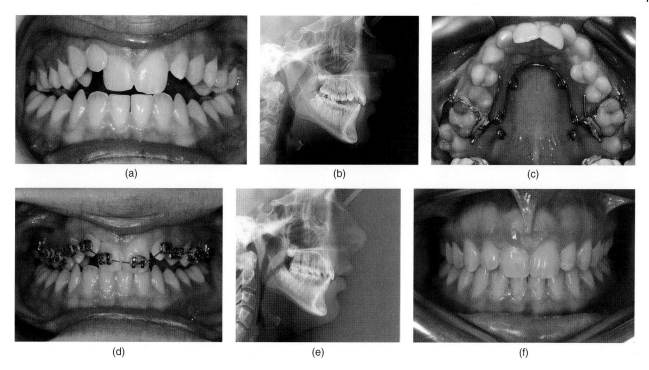

(a)   (b)   (c)

(d)   (e)   (f)

Figure 12.11 (a, b) Pretreatment photograph and lateral cephalogram of an adolescent girl with a compensated skeletal anterior open bite. (c) The start of maxillary molar intrusion, following several months of quadhelix expansion. OMIs have been inserted distal to the first molars and elastomeric traction applied to the molars. (d) A photograph taken once the upper dentition was bonded to correct developing premature occlusal contacts (due to molar intrusion). (e) A lateral cephalogram taken at debond showing a reduction in lower face height Class II corrections. (f) Photograph illustrating stability of the occlusal correction 15 months after debond and despite loss of retainers.

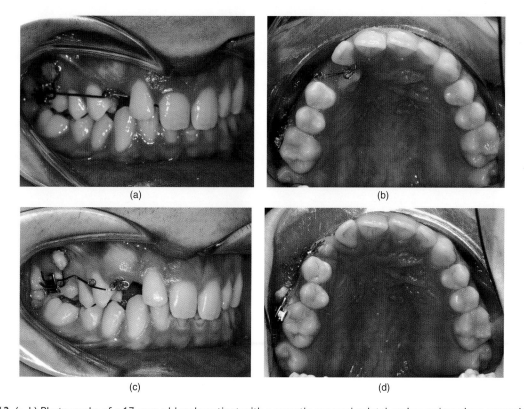

(a)   (b)

(c)   (d)

Figure 12.12 (a, b) Photographs of a 17-year-old male patient with a recently exposed palatal canine and previous resorption of the adjacent lateral incisor root. Distobuccal movement of canine was initiated using indirect anchorage of the right first molar, from a buccal OMI, and a buccal arm form of traction from this anchor unit. (c, d) The right canine had been moved into the line of the arch prior to commencement of 'light' forces fixed appliance treatment for final alignment. Source: reproduced by kind permission from *The Orthodontic Mini-implant Clinical Handbook*, 2nd edn. Wiley Blackwell, 2020.

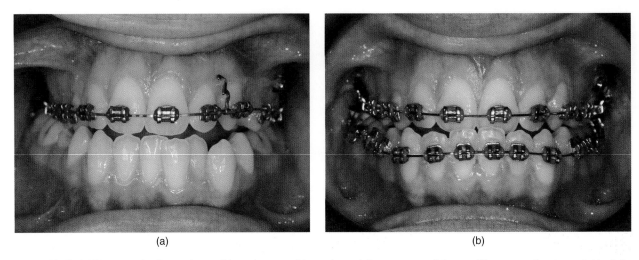

Figure 12.13 (a) Photograph of an orthognathic patient requiring substantial movement of the maxillary centerline towards the left side. A buccal OMI has been inserted mesial to the left first molar and unilateral traction applied to a crimpable powerarm. (b) The traction has been removed following correction of the maxillary centreline and associated incisor decompensation.

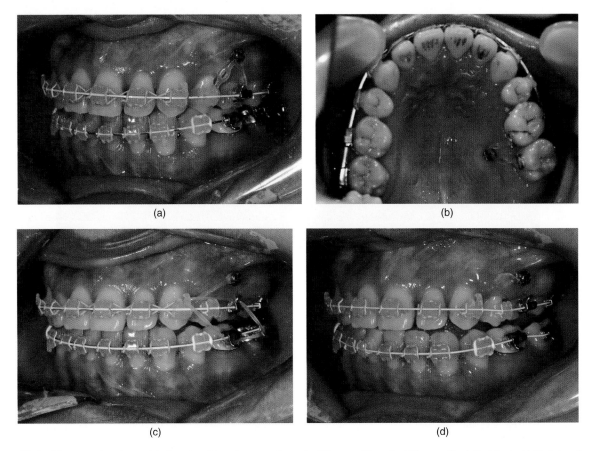

Figure 12.14 Photographs of an adult female with a downwards cant of the maxillary dentition on the left side. (a, b) Unilateral intrusion was commenced to level the maxillary occlusal plane, using a combination of buccal and palatal OMI anchorage and separate elastomeric traction. (c) After six months, a rhomboid intermaxillary elastic has been added to close the resultant lateral open bite by levelling the lower dentition. (d) Traction has ceased, after a further eight weeks, to allow vertical settling (at the same time as bracket repositioning takes effect).

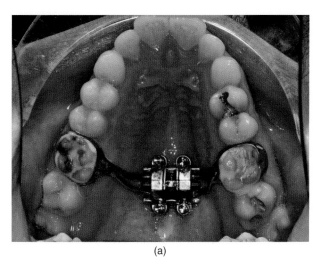
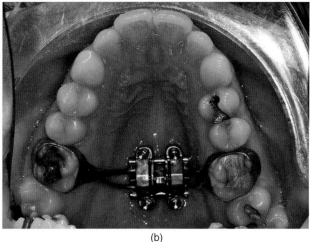

(a) (b)

Figure 12.15 Photographs taken (a) on insertion of a MSE rapid maxillary expander in a 25-year-old male patient and (b) two weeks later. A small midline diastema had developed by one week, so the expansion rate was slowed to 0.27 mm per day. This resulted in spontaneous mesial drift and initial retroclination of the upper central incisors. A conventional upper fixed appliance was bonded one month later.

Transverse Anchorage

Conventional anchorage reinforcement, for large centre-line movements, typically involves bilateral anchorage engagement (e.g. a TPA), but this may be unnecessary or even counterproductive (if relative anchorage loss is required on one side). OMIs readily offer reliable anchorage in only one quadrant, enabling predictable centreline corrections (Figure 12.13), and also vertical control in terms of occlusal cant (Figure 12.14) and scissors bite corrections. The former typically requires both buccal and palatal OMIs in order to achieve true bodily intrusion rather than buccal or palatal tipping.

Finally, bone-anchored maxillary expansion is the latest 'frontier' in OMI anchorage, such that actual basal skeletal expansion may be achieved, even in adult patients and without the assistance of surgical corticotomies (i.e. surgically assisted rapid palatal expansion, or SARPE).[59–62] This may then be followed rapidly by fixed appliance closure of the diastema, and continued orthodontic treatment while the expander remains *in situ* for up to nine months' retention period. Such has been the progress in this field in just the last few years that standardised approaches are still evolving,[6] although it has recently become apparent that posterior mid-palatal insertion sites are optimum, provided that this area is feasible in terms of sufficient palate width and access (Figure 12.15). Such posterior anchorage enhances the chances of non-surgical pterygopalatine disjunction, rather than just separation of the anterior mid-palatal suture (which typically manifests as a midline diastema). At present, the indications are that if physical access is limited to the palatal alveolar shelves (interproximal sites), because of the restricted width and high vault of the posterior palate, then surgical corticotomies may still be required in mature adults.[6] Therefore, referral to the most up-to-date lecture and published journal material is highly recommended for further insight into the latest possibilities in this exciting field.

References

1 Upadhyay M, Yadav S, Nagaraj K, Nanda R. Dentoskeletal and soft tissue effects of mini-implants in Class II division 1 patients. *Angle Orthod.* 2008;79:240–247.

2 Davoody AR, Posada L, Utreja A, et al. A prospective comparative study between differential moments and miniscrews in anchorage control. *Eur. J. Orthod.* 2012;35:568–576.

3 Upadhyay M, Yadav S, Nanda R. Biomechanics of incisor retraction with mini-implant anchorage. *J. Orthod.* 2014;41:S15–S23.

4 Sibaie S, Hajeer MY. Assessment of changes following en-masse retraction with mini-implants anchorage compared to two-step retraction with conventional anchorage in patients with class II division 1 malocclusion: a randomized controlled trial. *Eur. J. Orthod.* 2014;36:275–283.

5 Chen M, Li Z, Liu X, et al. Differences of treatment outcomes between self-ligating brackets with microimplant and headgear anchorages in adults with

bimaxillary protrusion. *Am. J. Orthod. Dentofacial Orthop.* 2015;147:465–471.

6 Cousley RRJ. *The Orthodontic Mini-implant Clinical Handbook*, 2nd edn. Oxford: Wiley Blackwell, 2020.

7 Alharbi F, Almuzian M, Bearn D. Miniscrews failure rate in orthodontics: systematic review and meta-analysis. *Eur. J. Orthod.* 2018;40:519–530.

8 Antoszewska J, Papadopoulos MA, Park HS, Ludwig B. Five-year experience with orthodontic miniscrew implants: a retrospective investigation of factors influencing success rates. *Am. J. Orthod. Dentofacial Orthop.* 2009;136:158.e1–10.

9 Kim YH, Yang S, Kim S, et al. Midpalatal miniscrews for orthodontic anchorage: factors affecting clinical success. *Am. J. Orthod. Dentofacial Orthop.* 2010;137:66–72.

10 Lim HJ, Eun CS, Cho JH, et al. Factors associated with initial stability of miniscrews for orthodontic treatment. *Am. J. Orthod. Dentofacial Orthop.* 2009;136:236–242.

11 Manni A, Cozzani M, Tamborrino F, et al. Factors influencing the stability of miniscrews. A retrospective study on 300 miniscrews. *Eur. J. Orthod.* 2011;33:388–395.

12 Moon C, Lee D, Lee H, et al. Factors associated with the success rate of orthodontic miniscrews placed in the upper and lower posterior buccal region. *Angle Orthod.* 2008;78:101–106.

13 Moon C, Park H, Nam J, et al. Relationship between vertical skeletal pattern and success rate of orthodontic mini-implants. *Am. J. Orthod. Dentofacial Orthop.* 2010;138:51–57.

14 Wu T, Kuang S, Wu C. Factors associated with the stability of mini-implants for orthodontic anchorage: a study of 414 samples in Taiwan. *J. Oral Maxillofac. Surg.* 2009;67:1595–1599.

15 Melo ACM, Andrighetto AR, Hirt SD, et al. Risk factors associated with the failure of miniscrews: a ten-year cross sectional study. *Braz. Oral Res.* 2016;30:e124.

16 Di Leonardo B, Ludwig B, Lisson JA, et al. Insertion torque values and success rates for paramedian insertion of orthodontic miniimplants. *J. Orofac. Orthop.* 2018;79:109–115.

17 Motoyoshi M, Uchida Y, Inaba M, et al. Are assessments of damping capacity and placement torque useful in estimating root proximity of orthodontic anchor screws? *Am. J. Orthod. Dentofacial Orthop.* 2016;150:124–129.

18 Asscherickx K, Vande Vannet B, Wehrbein H, Sabzevar MM. Success rate of miniscrews relative to their position to adjacent roots. *Eur. J. Orthod.* 2008;30:330–335.

19 Dao V, Renjen R, Prasad HS, et al. Cementum, pulp, periodontal ligament, and bone response after direct injury with orthodontic anchorage screws: a histomorphologic study in an animal model. *J. Oral Maxillofac. Surg.* 2009;67:2440–2445.

20 Iwai H, Motoyoshi M, Uchida Y, et al. Effects of tooth root contact on the stability of orthodontic anchor screws in the maxilla: comparison between self-drilling and self-tapping methods. *Am. J. Orthod. Dentofacial Orthop.* 2015;147:483–491.

21 Kang Y, Kang Y, Kim J, et al. Stability of miniscrews invading the dental roots and their impact on the paradental tissues in beagles. *Angle Orthod.* 2008;79:248–255.

22 Motoyoshi M, Uemura M, Ono A, et al. Factors affecting the long-term stability of orthodontic mini-implants. *Am. J. Orthod. Dentofacial Orthop.* 2010;137:588.e1–5.

23 Lee TCK, McGrath CPJ, Wong RWK, Rabie ABM. Patients' perceptions regarding microimplant as anchorage in orthodontics. *Angle Orthod.* 2008;78:228–233.

24 Lehnen S, McDonald F, Bourauel C, Baxmann M. Patient expectations, acceptance and preferences in treatment with orthodontic mini-implants. A randomly controlled study. *Part I: Insertion techniques. J. Orofac. Orthop.* 2011;72:93–102.

25 Kuroda S, Sugawara Y, Deguchi T, et al. Clinical use of miniscrew implants as orthodontic anchorage: success rates and postoperative discomfort. *Am. J. Orthod. Dentofacial Orthop.* 2007;131:9–15.

26 Ganzer N, Feldmann I, Bondemark L. Pain and discomfort following insertion of miniscrews and premolar extractions: a randomized controlled trial. *Angle Orthod.* 2016;86:891–899.

27 Lehnen S, McDonald F, Bourauel C, et al. Expectations, acceptance and preferences of patients in treatment with orthodontic mini-implants. Part II: Implant removal. *J. Orofac. Orthop.* 2011;72:214–222.

28 Motoyoshi M, Sanuki-Suzuki R, Uchida Y, et al. Maxillary sinus perforation by orthodontic anchor screws. *J. Oral Sci.* 2015;57:95–100.

29 Houfar J, Kanavakis G, Bister D, et al. Three dimensional anatomical exploration of the anterior hard palate at the level of the third ruga for the placement of mini-implants: a cone-beam CT study. *Eur. J. Orthod.* 2015;37:589–595.

30 Smith A, Hosein YK, Dunning CE, Tassid A. Fracture resistance of commonly used self-drilling orthodontic mini-implants. *Angle Orthod.* 2015;85:26–32.

31 Assad-Loss TF, Kitahara-Céia FMF, Silveira GS, et al. Fracture strength of orthodontic mini-implants. *Dental Press J. Orthod.* 2017;22:47–54.

32 Alves M, Baratieri C, Nojima LI. Assessment of mini-implant displacement using cone beam computed tomography. *Clin. Oral Implant Res.* 2011;22:1151–1156.

33 El-Beialy AR, Abu-El-Ezz AA, Attia KH, et al. Loss of anchorage of miniscrews: a 3-dimensional assessment. *Am. J. Orthod. Dentofacial Orthop.* 2009;136:700–707.

34 Liou EJW, Pai BCJ, Lin JCY. Do miniscrews remain stationary under orthodontic forces? *Am. J. Orthod. Dentofacial Orthop.* 2004;126:42–47.

35 Liu H, Ly T, Wang N, et al. Drift characteristics of miniscrews and molars for anchorage under orthodontic force: 3-dimensional computed tomography registration evaluation. *Am. J. Orthod. Dentofacial Orthop.* 2011;139:e83–e89.

36 Serra G, Morais LS, Elias CN, et al. Sequential bone healing of immediately loaded mini-implants. *Am. J. Orthod. Dentofacial Orthop.* 2008;134:44–52.

37 Vannet BV, Sabzevar MM, Wehrbein H, Asscherickx K. Osseointegration of miniscrews: a histomorphometric evaluation. *Eur. J. Orthod.* 2007;29:437–442.

38 Laursen MG, Melsen B, Cattaneo PM. An evaluation of insertion sites for mini-implants: a micro-CT study of human autopsy material. *Angle Orthod.* 2013;83:222–229.

39 Baumgaertel S, Hans MG. Buccal cortical bone thickness for mini-implant placement. *Am. J. Orthod. Dentofacial Orthop.* 2009;136:230–235.

40 Deguchi T, Nasu M, Murakami K, et al. Quantitative evaluation of cortical bone thickness with computed tomographic scanning for orthodontic implants. *Am. J. Orthod. Dentofacial Orthop.* 2006;129:721.e7–12.

41 Farnsworth D, Rossouw PE, Ceen F, Buschang PH. Cortical bone thickness at common miniscrew implant placement sites. *Am. J. Orthod. Dentofacial Orthop.* 2011;139:495–503.

42 Martinelli FL, Luiz RR, Faria M, Nojima LI. Anatomic variability in alveolar sites for skeletal anchorage. *Am. J. Orthod. Dentofacial Orthop.* 2010;138:252.e1–9.

43 Park J, Cho HJ. Three-dimensional evaluation of interradicular spaces and cortical bone thickness for the placement and initial stability of microimplants in adults. *Am. J. Orthod. Dentofacial Orthop.* 2009;136:314.e1–12.

44 Marquezan M, Lima I, Lopes RT, et al. Is trabecular bone related to primary stability of miniscrews? *Angle Orthod.* 2014;84:500–507.

45 Landin M, Jadhav A, Yadav S, Tadinada A. A comparative study between currently used methods and small volume-cone beam tomography for surgical placement of mini implants. *Angle Orthod.* 2015;85:446–453.

46 Cassetta M, Sofan A, Altieri F, Barbato E. Evaluation of alveolar cortical bone thickness and density for orthodontic mini-implant placement. *J. Clin. Exp. Dent.* 2013;5:e245–e252.

47 Ohiomoba H, Sonis A, Yansane A, Friedland B. Quantitative evaluation of maxillary alveolar cortical bone thickness and density using computed tomography imaging. *Am. J. Orthod. Dentofacial Orthop.* 2017;151:82–91.

48 Horner KA, Behrents RG, Kim K, Buschang PH. Cortical bone and ridge thickness of hyperdivergent and hypodivergent adults. *Am. J. Orthod. Dentofacial Orthop.* 2012;142:170–178.

49 Ozdemir F, Tozlu M, Germec-Cakan D. Cortical bone thickness of the alveolar process measured with cone beam computed tomography in patients with different facial types. *Am. J. Orthod. Dentofacial Orthop.* 2013;143:190–196.

50 Veli I, Uysal T, Baysal A, Karadede I. Buccal cortical bone thickness at miniscrew placement sites in patients with different vertical skeletal patterns. *J. Orofac. Orthop.* 2014;74:417–429.

51 Ohiomoba H, Sonis A, Yansane A, Friedland B. Quantitative evaluation of maxillary alveolar cortical bone thickness and density using computed tomography imaging. *Am. J. Orthod. Dentofacial Orthop.* 2017;151:82–91.

52 Kuroda S, Nishii Y, Okano S, Sueishi K. Stress distribution in the mini-screw and alveolar bone during orthodontic treatment: a finite element study analysis. *J. Orthod.* 2014;41:275–284.

53 Lin T, Tsai F, Chen C, Lin D. Factorial analysis of variables affecting bone stress adjacent to the orthodontic anchorage mini-implant with finite element analysis. *Am. J. Orthod. Dentofacial Orthop.* 2013;143:182–189.

54 Becker K, Pliska A, Busch C, et al. Efficacy of orthodontic mini implants for en masse retraction in the maxilla: a systematic review and meta-analysis. *Int. J. Implant Dent.* 2018;4:35.

55 Ure DS, Oliver DR, Kim KB, et al. Stability changes of miniscrew implants over time. A pilot resonance frequency analysis. *Angle Orthod.* 2011;81:994–1000.

56 Gelgor IE, Karaman AI, Buyukyilmaz T. Comparison of 2 distalization systems supported by intraosseous screws. *Am. J. Orthod. Dentofacial Orthop.* 2007;131:161.e1–8.

57 Li F, Hu HK, Chen JW, et al. Comparison of anchorage capacity between implant and headgear during anterior segment retraction. A systematic review. *Angle Orthod.* 2011;81:915–922.

58 Hart TR, Cousley RRJ, Fishman LS, Tallents RH. Dentoskeletal changes following mini-implant molar intrusion in anterior open bite patients. *Angle Orthod.* 2015;85:941–948.

59 Cantarella D, Dominguez-Mompell R, Mallya SM, et al. Changes in the midpalatal and pterygopalatine sutures

induced by microimplant-supported skeletal expander analyzed with a novel 3D method based on CBCT imaging. *Prog. Orthod.* 2017;18:34.

60 Celenk-Koca T, Erdinc AE, Hazara S, et al. Evaluation of miniscrew-supported rapid maxillary expansion in adolescents: a prospective randomized clinical trial. *Angle Orthod.* 2018;88:702–709.

61 Choi S, Shi K, Cha J, et al. Nonsurgical miniscrew-assisted rapid maxillary expansion results in acceptable stability in young adults. *Angle Orthod.* 2016;86:713–720.

62 Song K, Park J, Moon W, et al. Three-dimensional changes of the zygomaticomaxillary complex after mini-implant assisted rapid maxillary expansion. *Am. J. Orthod. Dentofacial Orthop.* 2019;56:653–662.

13

Care of Fixed Appliances

Nazan Adali, Daljit S. Gill, and Farhad B. Naini

CHAPTER OUTLINE

Introduction, 235
Before Fixed Appliance Treatment, 236
During Fixed Appliance Treatment, 237
   Dental Plaque Biofilm Control Methods, 238
   Strengthening of the Enamel Surfaces, 241
   Dietary Control, 244
   Management of Orthodontic Discomfort, 244
After Fixed Appliance Treatment, 245
Conclusions, 245
References, 245

Introduction

Primum non nocere (First, do no harm)

The care of fixed appliances requires a regime that encompasses both the best available evidence base and addresses each patient's specific needs in order to optimise the time invested for the regime and the benefits derived from treatment whilst minimising risks. A good oral care regime consists mainly of a tetrad of plaque biofilm control, strengthening of the enamel surfaces, and dietary and discomfort control. For fixed appliance patients, the aim of an effective oral care regime is to lower the risk of permanent damage to the oral structures during treatment. Prior to treatment, patients should demonstrate a good oral health status. On commencing treatment, patients are tasked with a new care regime to sustain throughout treatment. Maintaining lifelong good oral care habits may be a bonus after treatment.

The tendency for plaque entrapment and accumulation around the fixed appliance, and the shift towards anaerobic pathological microbial species are a known challenge.[1] This type of flora disrupts the natural cycle of enamel demineralisation and remineralisation, leading to *subsurface demineralisation*. The localised reduced mineral density has a different refractive index to adjacent areas, so the eye detects a colour difference called a **white spot lesion** (Figures 13.1 and 13.2). The incidence of visible white spot lesions during fixed appliance treatment is between 15 and 85%,[2] and they are most often seen at sites difficult to clean where stagnation of food and dental plaque can occur, i.e. bracket bases of lower canines/first premolars, upper canines/lateral incisors, and gingival margins. They can appear within only four weeks so prevention and early diagnosis is critical.[3] Left untreated, the progression to a cavitated carious lesion is rapid,[4] predisposing to enamel fracture at debond. The risk factors for white spot lesion development, essentially a *high frequency of sugar in the diet* combined with poor oral hygiene and dental plaque deposits, should be identified before treatment and addressed in the tailored care regime. *It should be noted that excessive dental plaque deposits lead to gingivitis, but for the development of white spot lesions a high-frequency sugar diet is required.*

The plaque flora predisposes to gingivitis, presenting with bleeding gingivae during home or professional oral hygiene procedures. Gingival inflammation often develops at sites of stagnation, creating further plaque traps and perpetuating the cycle (Figure 13.3) and this may progress to periodontal disease in susceptible individuals. With more adults seeking orthodontic treatment, their tailored

Preadjusted Edgewise Fixed Orthodontic Appliances: Principles and Practice, First Edition. Edited by Farhad B. Naini and Daljit S. Gill.
© 2022 John Wiley & Sons Ltd. Published 2022 by John Wiley & Sons Ltd.

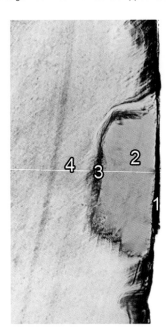

Figure 13.1 The anatomy of a smooth surface enamel white spot lesion (early carious lesion). The four zones making up a white spot lesion are as follows. (1) Surface zone: the surface layer is intact. There is 1% mineral loss. This is a zone of potential remineralisation. Cavitation is the loss of this layer. (2) Body: the body of the lesion has 5–25% loss of mineral content. (3) Dark zone: the porous dark zone surrounding the body has 2–4% mineral loss overall but a zone of remineralisation just behind the advancing front. (4) Translucent zone: this is the earliest and deepest demineralisation, with 1% mineral loss.

care regime should take the periodontal history into account.

This chapter details how the prudent clinician can address the key considerations of the care regime before, during and after fixed appliance treatment.

Before Fixed Appliance Treatment

At the initial consultation, the clinician assesses the oral health risk factors for the patient, detects any active disease and obtains baseline clinical records. These risk factors should be assessed as follows.

Motivation

- External sources of motivation are associated with poorer outcomes.

Medical and Social History

- Changes to systemic health or mental health status or to medication.
- Endocrine disease, e.g. poorly controlled diabetes mellitus as a risk for periodontal disease.
- Smoking history and alcohol intake, as an indicator of risk of oral dysplasia and periodontal disease.

Dental History

- Inconsistent attendance record for dental health check-ups.
- High dietary sugar and acidic food/drink intake.
- Previous orthodontic treatment.
- Previous periodontal disease and dental or restorative treatment.

Intraoral

- Diagnosis of active primary or secondary carious lesions.
- Diagnosis of active gingival or periodontal disease.
- Leaking margins, cracks and overhangs in existing restorations.
- Inadequate contact points, resulting in food packing and inflammation.
- Pre-existing white spot lesions.
- Intraoral piercings, which may cause local trauma and which are discouraged.

The clinician should seek evidence of any changes in medical history, mental health, pattern of attendance and dietary histories. Active disease should be stabilised by the general dentist or periodontist before embarking on orthodontic treatment. Monitoring for reactivation of primary disease, such as inactive carious lesions, should form part of the care regime during active treatment and the general dental practitioner should be requested to replace the restorations deemed significantly defective.

Baseline clinical records allow for future comparisons. High-quality photographs are used to record and monitor minor restoration defects and existing enamel opacities in order to differentiate existing from new ones. Correct photographic technique requires drying of the tooth surface, appropriate magnification and reduction of flash reflection.

Clinical indices are used to monitor risks factors. Many plaque indices are not suitable for orthodontic patients as they do not score the most at-risk sites. The **Orthodontic Plaque Index**[5] scores the plaque present around the bracket bases from 0 to 4 in each sextant, and a score over 3 indicates the need for prophylaxis (Figure 13.4).

The **Basic Periodontal Examination (BPE)** should be carried out for all patients. The standardised technique uses the World Health Organization probe with a 0.5-mm ball and banding at 3.5–5.5 mm (see Appendix I). Children aged 7–11 years should have the six permanent first molar teeth and incisors assessed using BPE codes 0–2 (Tables 13.1 and 13.2). Those aged 12 years and over can have the full BPE code applied with the mouth divided into sextants,[6] and adult patients should have a full periodontal pocket charting.

The **Gingival Bleeding Index**[7] scores six points on each tooth with a binary score and is expressed as a percentage. **Miller's classification of gingival recession**

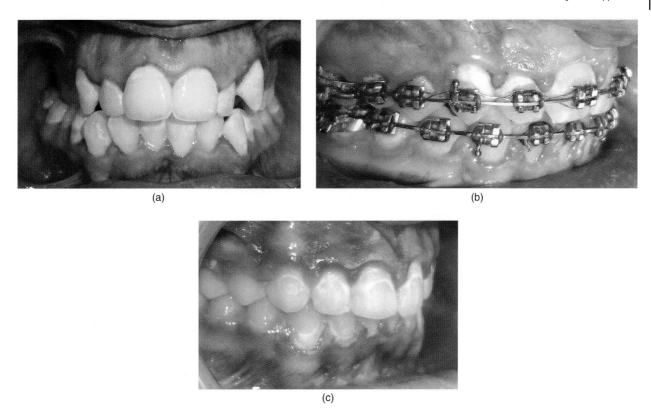

(a)

(b)

(c)

Figure 13.2 (a–c) Extensive white spot lesions with poor oral hygiene, following removal of a fixed appliance.

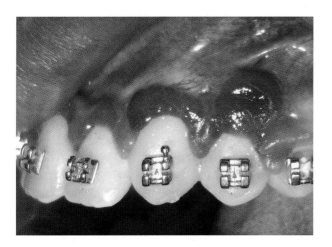

Figure 13.3 Gingival inflammation with fixed appliances *in situ*.

(Figure 13.5) identifies the extent of periodontal attachment loss and can help to guide treatment planning.[8] **DMFT scores** refer to the number of Decayed, Missing (due to caries), and Filled permanent Teeth, and are widely used. Zimmer and Rottwinkel[9] showed a positive correlation between DMFT scores and decalcification incidence within their teenage orthodontic group. This group demonstrated the most benefit from the targeted prevention programme, highlighting the importance of assessing risk factors when planning the care regime.

During Fixed Appliance Treatment

Routine general dental check-ups, including review of the restorations being monitored, should continue during treatment. At the orthodontic appointments, oral health scores will be monitored, together with dietary and smoking status, and appearance of new white spot lesions. If new disease or reactivation of previous disease should appear, treatment should be paused to allow the necessary intervention to occur, which is likely to delay orthodontic progress.

The ideal regime should be evidence-based and effective, tailored to the patient's risk factors, simple and easy to comply with and thereby sustainable throughout treatment. Key components to deliver this message are effective communication and the use of reminders. Verbal instruction is best supported with written and visual information, including chairside demonstrations.

In school-age children, a practical demonstration of plaque control techniques by an experienced professional, with regular reinforcement, appears effective in maintaining adequate oral hygiene standards. For adolescent orthodontic patients, automated daily text message reminders may be an effective approach to improve oral hygiene status,[10] as may smartphone apps with real-time feedback (Figures 13.6 and 13.7).[11]

OPI score	Example	Description
0		Brackets are plaque-free
1		Isolated plaque islands on one surface at bracket base
2		Plaque on two surfaces at bracket base
3		Plaque on three surfaces at bracket base
4		Plaque on all surfaces at bracket base
		and/or gingival inflammation

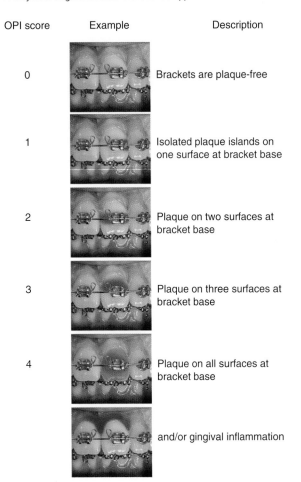

Figure 13.4 Orthodontic Plaque Index (OPI) scores (after Berberhold et al.[5]).

Table 13.1 Basic Periodontal Index (BPE) scoring codes.

0	No pockets >3.5 mm, no calculus/overhangs, no bleeding after probing (black band completely visible)
1	No pockets >3.5 mm, no calculus/overhangs, but bleeding after probing (black band completely visible)
2	No pockets >3.5 mm, but supra- or sub-gingival calculus/overhangs (black band completely visible)
3	Probing depth 3.5–5.5 mm (black band partially visible, indicating pocket of 4–5 mm)
4	Probing depth >5.5 mm (black band entirely within the pocket, indicating pocket of 6 mm or more)

Both the number and the furcation involvement (*) should be recorded if a furcation is detected, e.g. the score for a sextant could be 3* (i.e. indicating probing depth 3.5–5.5 mm *and* furcation involvement in the sextant).

Dental Plaque Biofilm Control Methods

Mechanical Cleaning

Home Cleaning The Department of Health Dental Toolkit, *Delivering Better Oral Health: Evidence Based Toolkit for*

Table 13.2 Guidance on interpretation of BPE scores.

0	No need for periodontal treatment
1	Oral hygiene instruction (OHI)
2	OHI
	Removal of plaque retentive factors, including all supra- and sub-gingival calculus
3	OHI
	Root surface debridement (RSD)
4	OHI and RSD
	Assess the need for more complex treatment; referral to a specialist may be indicated
*	OHI and RSD
	Assess the need for more complex treatment; referral to a specialist may be indicated

As a general rule, radiographs to assess alveolar bone levels should be obtained for teeth or sextants where BPE codes 3 or 4 are found.

Prevention,[12] gives clear guidance for maintaining good oral health. For plaque control, the advice for adults and patients aged seven years and over is as follows.

- Brush at least twice a day with fluoridated toothpaste (1350–1500 ppm). Brush last thing at night and at least on one other occasion and spit out rather than rinse after brushing to maintain fluoride concentration levels.
- Daily cleaning between the teeth and below the gumline, using the methods demonstrated by dental professionals.
- Behaviour change techniques should be used with oral hygiene instructions.

Mechanical plaque removal from the tooth surfaces can be carried out with either a manual or electric toothbrush. Introduced in the 1960s, electric toothbrushes, with their improved design and lower costs, have become very popular. Design changes include different speed settings, pressure sensors to prevent excess force application, and timers with smartphone connectivity. The brush head motions may be side to side, circular, ultrasonic vibration, rotation–oscillation or counter-oscillation and the selection is influenced by user preference, marketing, cost or by professional recommendation (Figures 13.6 and 13.7).

In a randomised clinical trial, Erbe et al.[13] reinforced earlier findings that the rotation–oscillation brushes were more effective in plaque removal for young orthodontic patients than manual brushes. A smaller orthodontic attachment brush was used, giving good access around the stagnation areas of the bracket bases and tie-wings.

For patients who prefer a manual toothbrush, a plethora of designs are available. Some guidance for effectiveness in plaque removal is helpful, for example the triple-headed

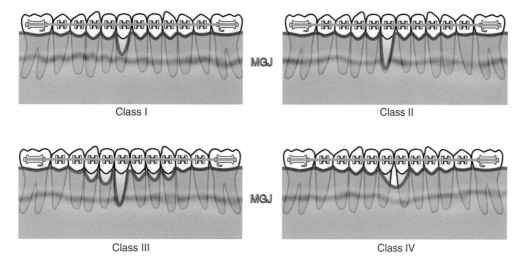

Figure 13.5 Miller's classification of recession defects. Class I: recession that does not extend to the mucogingival junction (MGJ), with no periodontal bone loss in the interdental areas. Class II: recession that extends to or beyond the MGJ, with no interdental bone loss. Class III: recession that extends to or beyond the MGJ, with some periodontal attachment loss in the interdental area or malpositioning of teeth. Class IV: recession that extends to or beyond the MGJ, with severe bone and/or soft tissue loss in the interdental area and/or severe malpositioning of the teeth. Source: Adapted and redrawn from Miller PD Jr. A classification of marginal tissue recession. *Int. J. Periodontics Restorative Dent.* 1985;5(2):8–13. © 1985, Quintessence Publishing Co, Inc.

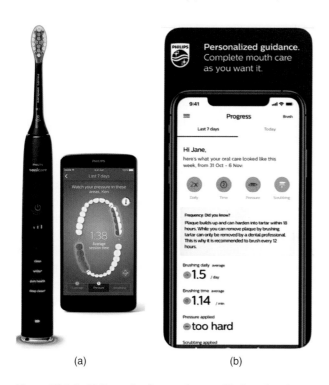

(a) (b)

Figure 13.6 (a, b) Example of a rotation–oscillation electric toothbrush for adults, with smartphone app. Source: Koninklijke Philips.

brushes or brushes with a 'bracket groove' (Figure 13.8) have been shown to be more effective than conventional brushes in reducing the plaque score.[14]

Whichever system is chosen, it is important to emphasise the importance of applying an effective brushing technique. The **modified Bass technique** has long been held to be effective. The bristles of the toothbrush are held at approximately 45° to the tooth surface, angled towards the gingival margins. The bristles should thereby project towards and slightly into the gingival sulcus or any pockets. The technique focuses on plaque removal at the gingival margin with added small circular toothbrush movements.[15] The patient should be instructed to brush all surfaces of the teeth and above and below each bracket (Figure 13.9). A travel toothbrush should also be recommended to patients, which may be taken to school or work as required (Figure 13.10). Visible feedback of brushing effectiveness can be provided with the use of chewable disclosing tablets (Figure 13.11), where the organic microbiological stains show the location of any residual plaque.

Effective toothbrushing alone is insufficient for orthodontic patients, as the most challenging are the interdental sites that can only be accessed from beneath the wire. Many devices are available to help orthodontic patients to access these sites, including interdental brushes, single-tufted brushes, rubber interdental sticks, water irrigators and dental floss (Figure 13.12). The choice is often a matter of professional recommendation, patient dexterity and personal preference. Cleaning frequency following each food intake is advisable but often hard to sustain.

The challenge facing clinical researchers studying the efficacy of these devices has been the elimination of research bias. Bias can be introduced by the non-standardised duration of device use, loss to follow-up

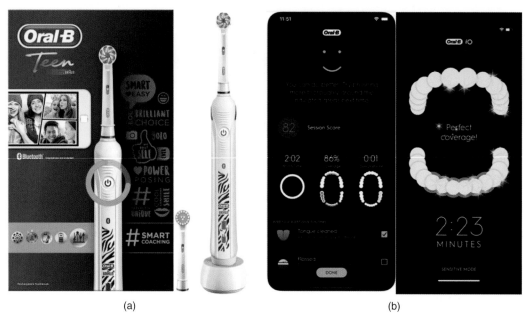

(a)   (b)

Figure 13.7 (a, b) Example of rotation–oscillation electric toothbrush aimed at teenagers, with smartphone app. Source: The Procter & Gamble Company.

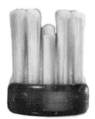

Figure 13.8 Toothbrush incorporating a 'bracket groove', a special groove designed in the brush head for the cleaning of teeth fitted with fixed orthodontic appliances.

and insufficient power to support stated benefits. By attempting to standardise the cleaning duration, a randomised clinical trial reported no difference between the sonic toothbrush and manual toothbrush with or without interdental brushing in their ability to remove plaque or to prevent gingivitis.[16]

Professional Cleaning Regular appointments with a dental hygienist during fixed appliance treatment may be effective in sustaining a low plaque level. When this forms part of a periodontal maintenance plan, it is important for the patient to adhere to the schedule carefully. Treatment includes professional prophylaxis, hygiene instruction and targeted motivation for the required home care. The two main types of prophylaxis methods are conventional rubber cup prophylaxis and air powder polishing systems, both of which are effective at removing plaque for orthodontic patients. The frequency of appointments may vary according to need, though a monthly hygiene evaluation and three- to six-monthly prophylaxis protocol has been suggested.[17]

Some patients develop dental calculus deposits very rapidly, particularly on the lingual aspect of their mandibular incisors. Professional removal of calculus deposits regularly will be required in such cases.

Chemotherapeutic Cleaning
The adjunctive use of topical antimicrobial agents during fixed appliance treatment can help to control plaque levels. Of these, chlorhexidine gluconate mouthwash is the most effective and widely used. It inhibits plaque growth by disrupting the cell membranes of a broad range of microbes and has good *substantivity* (binding to the oral tissues to retain a longer duration of action) (Figure 13.13). Short-term use is recommended due to the side effects of perturbance of taste, surface discoloration of teeth and margins of adhesive resin restoration, and less commonly parotid swelling and mucosal erosion. For local problem areas, 1% gel can be applied to reduce the side effects (Figure 13.13). The 0.2% mouthwash is particularly helpful after orthognathic surgery when mechanical cleaning is limited,[18] and can also be used in oral irrigation devices for direct interdental site access.

Other mouthwashes include Listerine®, cetylpyridinium compounds, povidone-iodine and octenidine, all of which inhibit plaque formation but are less effective than chlorhexidine, with similar drawbacks, and have not been shown to reduce white spot lesions.[19]

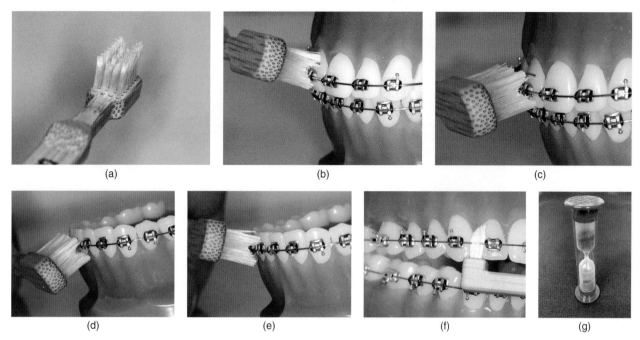

(a)   (b)   (c)

(d)   (e)   (f)   (g)

Figure 13.9 (a) A toothbrush with the bristles arranged into a V-shape can facilitate cleaning both above and beneath the archwire. (b) Patients should be instructed to clean above the maxillary brackets, paying particular attention to the gingival margins. They can be instructed to roll the brush in circular movements, 'massaging the gum margins'. (c) Then they should clean below the maxillary archwire to clean the opposite half of the teeth, occlusal to the archwire. (d, e) The same is technique is used in the lower arch. Particular attention needs to be given to the gingival margins in the incisor region, which are frequently missed. (f) Finally, a single tufted or spiral interspace brush is used the clean beneath the archwire adjacent to each bracket side. Because of the reduced interbracket span in the lower arch, a smaller-sized brush may be required to clean beneath the archwire. (g) A sand hourglass timer (in this case, adapted for approximately two to three minutes) may be used to ensure enough time is spent brushing the teeth. It is otherwise easy to overestimate the amount of time spent on oral hygiene maintenance. *Note*: Patients should be informed of the environmental benefits of using toothbrushes with a wooden (usually bamboo) handle, rather than a plastic handle.

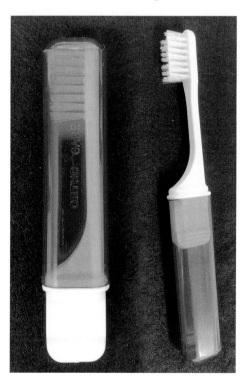

Figure 13.10 Travel toothbrush.

If these methods to control plaque levels prove unsuccessful, removal of the archwires for one visit to allow direct access can be considered. A last resort is early removal of the appliances in order to stop further detriment to oral health.[20]

Strengthening of the Enamel Surfaces

Topical Fluoride Agents

Both the protective and strengthening effects of fluoride ions on surface enamel is well established. The Department of Health Dental Toolkit[12] recommends the following regime during orthodontic treatment.

- Daily fluoride mouthwash (0.05% NaF).
- Professional application of fluoride varnish (2.2%) twice a year.
- If history of active caries: 10–16 year olds to use 2800 ppm fluoride toothpaste; over 16 year olds to use 5000 ppm formulation.

Many formulations of topical fluoride compounds are available (sodium fluoride, stannous fluoride, sodium monofluorophosphate) at varying concentrations and modes of delivery (toothpaste, varnish, gel, mouthwash,

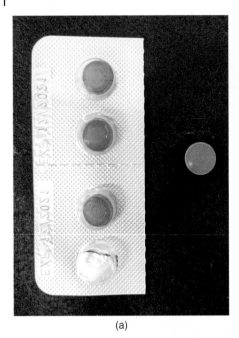
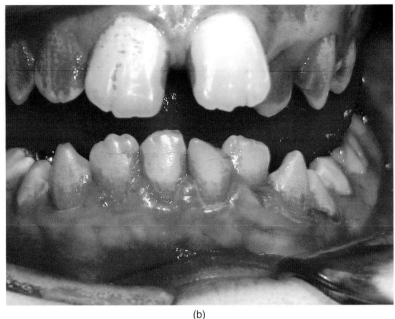

(a)   (b)

Figure 13.11 (a) Disclosing tablets. (b) Visible feedback of brushing effectiveness can be provided with the use of chewable disclosing tablets, where the organic microbiological stains show the location of any residual plaque.

foam) (Figure 13.14). Despite the plethora of investigations into the efficacy of different formulations, delivery and regimes in the prevention of white spot lesions for orthodontic patients, the limitations of study design, such as detection bias, inadequate control methods and underpowered designs, restrict any conclusion that any one regime may be most effective. Importantly, studies have highlighted the patient perceptions of the negative aesthetic impact of white spot lesions.[21]

In summary, a standard regime recommended by orthodontists is a daily 0.05% fluoride mouthwash with twice-daily use of 1450 ppm fluoride toothpaste. Fluoride mouthwash should be used at a time different to brushing for a more even replenishment, and release, of salivary fluoride ion reserves. Application of fluoride varnish can help reverse existing white spot lesions, though the ideal frequency is unclear.[22]

An area of potential benefit are fluoride-releasing components of fixed appliances. Use of fluoride-releasing glass ionomer cements for adhesion of molar bands may result in fewer white spot lesions than with use of resin-bonded molar tubes. The greater protective effect of resin-modified glass ionomer cement over composite material for the

bonding of brackets is generally accepted, although there is a lack of high-quality evidence to support any true benefit of this protection from white spot lesions at the expense of bond strength.[21] The role of fluoride-releasing sealants, or those applied to the full enamel surface as an adjunct for protection, needs to be further investigated. Fluoride-containing elastomeric ligatures have not been shown to provide sustained fluoride release. However, modern smaller bracket designs and attention to composite flash removal and using sealants to cover the labial surface may have a more significant indirect impact on removing plaque traps and improving enamel protection.

Topical Non-fluoride Agents

As the surface layer of the white spot lesions remineralise in the presence of fluoride ions, if the local calcium and phosphate ion concentration is too low, the deeper enamel within the lesion remains unaffected and the aesthetic problem remains. Absorbable calcium and phosphate ions are available in formulations such as casein phosphopeptide amorphous calcium phosphate (CPP-ACP) (Figure 13.15) and tricalcium phosphate. When these are present in the environment of a white spot lesion, the

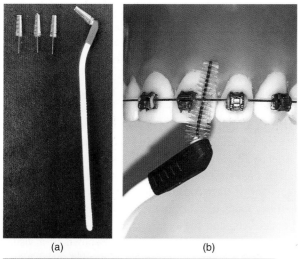

(a)   (b)

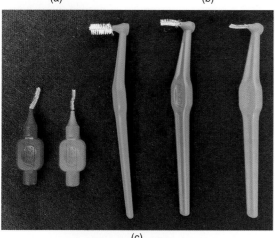

(c)

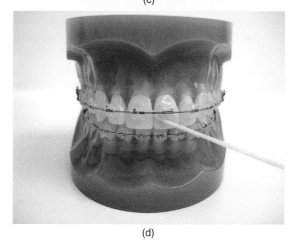

(d)

Figure 13.12 Interdental cleaning aids, such as interdental brushes (a, b), Tepe brushes (c) and Superfloss (d).

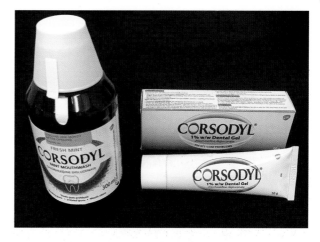

Figure 13.13 Various chlorhexidine formulations. Source: GSK Group of Companies.

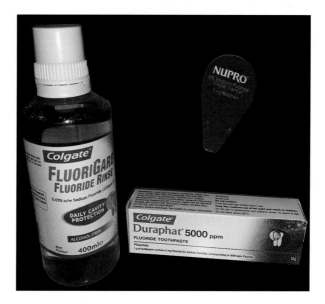

Figure 13.14 Duraphat high-fluoride toothpaste (2800 or 5000 ppm), Fluorigard mouthwash and 5% sodium fluoride varnish. Source: Colgate-Palmolive.

calcium phosphate crystals precipitate deep within the lesion and a deeper more complete reversal of the white spot lesion is thought to occur. This may also improve the aesthetic outcome.

These agents may be used as an alternative to fluoride in young children in order to reduce the fluoride exposure risks. It has been postulated that these agents can be combined with fluoride for a more effective and

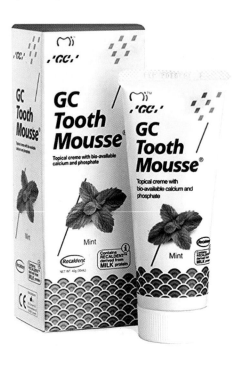

Figure 13.15 GC Tooth Mousse (CPP-ACP for application twice a day after brushing). These are available in a variety of flavours. Source: GC America Inc.

homogeneous remineralisation of white spot lesions. In a randomised clinical trial, Smyth and Noar[23] reported that topical tricalcium phosphate paste with high levels of fluoride appeared to be more effective in a 12-year-old patient group than both a tricalcium phosphate paste with low fluoride and the CPP-ACP paste only group. Further high-quality clinical trials will give clarity as to the most effective formulation for prevention of white spot lesions during treatment.

Dietary Control

Dietary recommendations from the Department of Health Dental Toolkit[12] includes the following.

- Frequency and amount of consumption of sugars should be reduced, particularly at bedtime.
- Added sugars should provide less than 10% of total energy in the diet or 60 g per person (30 g for young children). One teaspoon of sugar equates to approximately 5–6 g.
- Assistance to adopt good dietary practice in line with the 'Eat Well Guide'.

When describing these dietary recommendations to patients, special emphasis on the heightened risks with fixed appliances should be explained. The consumption of carbonated drinks (not simple carbonated water, but carbonated 'fizzy' soft drinks that contain a plethora of unhealthy ingredients, including acids such as phosphoric acid) and foods with added or natural simple sugars create an acidic environment in the mouth, resulting in enamel demineralisation. These extrinsic sugars are the main microbial substrate and the fastest to be metabolised. In the microenvironments created by fixed appliances, the buffering action of saliva is less effective, creating greater opportunity for progression of enamel demineralisation.[24]

Dietary advice should include the avoidance of consumption of high-sugar foods, particularly a reduction in the frequency of their consumption. Also, avoidance of hard or sticky foods in order to avoid the debonding of tubes and brackets, and the breakage and distortion of wires. Alternatives to popular foods can be shown in a visual format and regular reinforcement is needed, particularly after repair of breakages, to be most effective.

Management of Orthodontic Discomfort

Ulceration

Most patients will experience some discomfort from the disturbance of the oral mucosa adjacent to the fixed appliance at some stage of treatment. In the space closure phase of treatment, the excess archwire may begin to protrude from the terminal molar tube end. Cinching or bending back the archwire ends is important to prevent irritation to the patient's intraoral soft tissues (see Chapter 14). The use of orthodontic relief products can be very helpful if brackets are rubbing against the inside of the lips and cheeks. The area causing the irritation may be dried and wax moulded over the bracket or attachment, reducing the problem until the patient is seen at their subsequent appointment. These products may be natural wax (Figure 13.16) or silicone based and their use should be demonstrated to patients at the start of treatment. Traumatic ulcers should heal within a few days. Non-healing ulcers should be investigated further, with the suspicion of possible haematinic deficiencies.

Orthodontic Pain

Dental discomfort following the placement or adjustment of the appliances is frequently reported, and often increases in intensity until the third day. This can be effectively remedied with simple analgesia and both ibuprofen and paracetamol appear equal in effectiveness in pain control.[25] Anecdotal reports of non-pharmacological methods to reduce pain, such as low-level laser, have not been shown to be clinically effective. However, informing patients prior to the placement of appliances about the type of pain that may be experienced will manage the perception of the pain experience later.

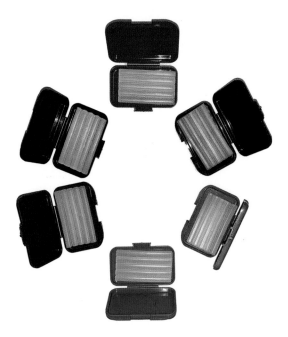

Figure 13.16 Orthodontic relief wax. These are available in different flavours. If part of a fixed appliance is rubbing against the oral mucosa, e.g. a canine bracket hook, the area may be dried with a tissue and a small amount of relief wax moulded onto the offending area of the appliance.

It is important to exclude dental or periodontal origins of any reported pain, in particular if there is a restorative or periodontal history related to the teeth in question, or if there are stagnation sites where food packing and local inflammation can occur. The recent pain history can reveal the diagnosis, and periapical radiographic investigations, vitality testing and comparison with the original record of any restoration defects can also be helpful in the diagnosis of these cases. A non-vital tooth will need to be referred to an endodontist and removed from the archwire during any intervention.

Mouthguards

Mouthguard use during contact sports are recommended for all patients. The types available include stock mouthguards, mouth-moulding and custom-made mouthguards.

The latter provide the highest level of protection by dissipating the energy on impact away from the appliance and teeth.[26] Custom-made mouthguards are close-fitting, made with ethylene vinyl acetate with additional fit-surface layers for additional protection but can be more costly as remakes are needed as the tooth positions change to ensure fit. A CE mark is required from the laboratory constructing these mouthguards to confirm that the required standards set by the Personal Protective Equipment Regulation (EU) 2016/425[27] have been met.

After Fixed Appliance Treatment

Long-term good oral hygiene and dietary habits may continue after the end of treatment. Any new white spot lesions should be noted prior to debond to help reduce the risk of enamel fractures. Beerens et al.[28] studied existing lesions after debond, observing that many improved without treatment. Older, deeper lesions may be more resistant to natural remineralisation. Monthly targeted fluoride varnish can improve the white spot lesion area.[29] Remaining lesions should be assessed after six months. Possible treatment options are erosion-resin infiltration, bleaching or microabrasion. Further clinical studies are required to clarify the optimum protocols for these new developments.[30]

Conclusions

When we ask patients to learn, adopt and sustain a new oral care regime throughout the duration of fixed appliance treatment, these efforts can only be worthwhile if they are backed by evidence. The identification of risk factors for each patient and tailoring of a regime to simultaneously reduce the microbial load, strengthen enamel surfaces and reduce available microbial substrate with dietary control are the most effective approaches when combined.[31] The benefits then outweigh the risks of the orthodontic intervention.

References

1 Ireland AJ, Soro V, Sprague SV, et al. The effects of different orthodontic appliances upon microbial communities. *Orthod. Craniofac. Res.* 2014;17(2):115–123.

2 Tufekci E, Dixon JS, Gunsolley JC, Lindauer SJ. Prevalence of white spot lesions during orthodontic treatment with fixed appliances. *Angle Orthod.* 2011;81(2): 206–210.

3 Lucchese A, Gherlone E. Prevalence of white-spot lesions before and during orthodontic treatment with fixed appliances. *Eur. J. Orthod.* 2013;35(5): 664–668.

4 Gorlick L, Geiger AM, Gwinnett AJ. Incidence of white spot formation after bonding and banding. *Am. J. Orthod.* 1982;81(2):93–98.

5 Beberhold K, Sachse-Kulp A, Schwestka-Polly R, et al. The Orthodontic Plaque Index: an oral hygiene index for patients with multibracket appliances. *Orthodontics (Chic.)* 2012;13(1):94–99.

6 Clerehugh V, Kindelan S. Guidelines for periodontal screening and management of children and adolescents under 18 years of age. Available at www.bsperio.org.uk

7 Ainamo J, Bay I. Problems and proposals for recording gingivitis and plaque. *Int. Dent. J.* 1975;25(4):229–235.

8 Miller PD Jr. A classification of marginal tissue recession. *Int. J. Periodontics Restorative Dent.* 1985;5(2):8–13.

9 Zimmer BW, Rottwinkel Y. Assessing patient-specific decalcification risk in fixed orthodontic treatment and its impact on prophylactic procedures. *Am. J. Orthod. Dentofacial Orthop.* 2004;126(3):318–324

10 Ross MC, Campbell PM, Tadlock LP, et al. Effect of automated messaging on oral hygiene in adolescent orthodontic patients: a randomized controlled trial. *Angle Orthod.* 2019;89(2):262–267.

11 Alkadhi OH, Zahid MN, Almanea RS, et al. The effect of using mobile applications for improving oral hygiene in patients with orthodontic fixed appliances: a randomised controlled trial. *J. Orthod.* 2017;44(3):157–163.

12 Public Health England. Delivering Better Oral Health: An Evidence-based Toolkit for Prevention, 3rd edn. London: PHE, 2017. Available at www.gov.uk/government/publications/delivering-better-oral-health-an-evidence-based-toolkit-for-prevention

13 Erbe C, Klees V, Braunbeck F, et al. Comparative assessment of plaque removal and motivation between a manual toothbrush and an interactive power toothbrush in adolescents with fixed orthodontic appliances: a single-center, examiner-blind randomized controlled trial. *Am. J. Orthod. Dentofacial Orthop.* 2019;155(4):462–472.

14 Terrana A, Rinchuse D, Zullo T, Marrone M. Comparing the plaque-removal ability of a triple-headed toothbrush versus a conventional manual toothbrush in adolescents with fixed orthodontic appliances: a single-center, randomized controlled clinical trial. *Int. Orthod.* 2019;17(4):719–725.

15 Ganss C, Schlueter N, Preiss S, Klimek J. Tooth brushing habits in uninstructed adults: frequency, technique, duration and force. *Clin. Oral Investig.* 2009;13(2):203–208.

16 Zingler S, Pritsch M, Wrede DJ, et al. A randomized clinical trial comparing the impact of different oral hygiene protocols and sealant applications on plaque, gingival, and caries index scores. *Eur. J. Orthod.* 2014;36(2):150–163.

17 Migliorati M, Isaia L, Cassaro A, et al. Efficacy of professional hygiene and prophylaxis on preventing plaque increase in orthodontic patients with multi-bracket appliances: a systematic review. *Eur. J. Orthod.* 2015;37(3):297–307.

18 James P, Worthington HV, Parnell C, et al. Chlorhexidine mouthrinse as an adjunctive treatment for gingival health. *Cochrane Database Syst. Rev.* 2017;(3):CD008676.

19 Pithon MM, Sant'Anna LI, Baião FC, et al. Assessment of the effectiveness of mouthwashes in reducing cariogenic biofilm in orthodontic patients: a systematic review. *J. Dent.* 2015;43(3):297–308.

20 Machen DE. Legal aspects of orthodontic practice: risk management concepts. Periodontal evaluation and updates: don't abdicate your duty to diagnose and supervise. *Am. J. Orthod. Dentofacial Orthop.* 1990;98(1):84–85.

21 Benson PE, Parkin N, Dyer F, et al. Fluorides for preventing early tooth decay (demineralised lesions) during fixed brace treatment. *Cochrane Database Syst. Rev.* 2019;(11):CD003809.

22 Stafford GL. Fluoride varnish may improve white spot lesions. *Evid. Based Dent.* 2011;12(4):104–105.

23 Smyth RSD, Noar JH. Preventing white spot lesions with fluoride pastes. *Evid. Based Dent.* 2019;20(3):88–89.

24 Richards D. Impact of diet on tooth erosion. *Evid. Based Dent.* 2016;17(2):40.

25 Monk AB, Harrison JE, Worthington HV, Teague A. Pharmacological interventions for pain relief during orthodontic treatment. *Cochrane Database Syst. Rev.* 2017;(11):CD003976.

26 Salam S, Caldwell S. Mouthguards and orthodontic patients. *J. Orthod.* 2008;35(4):270–275.

27 Personal Protective Equipment Regulation (EU Directive) 2016/425 of 9 March 2016. https://eur-lex.europa.eu/legal-content/EN/TXT/?uri=CELEX%3A32016R0425

28 Beerens MW, Ten Cate JM, Buijs MJ, van der Veen MH. Long-term remineralizing effect of MI Paste Plus on regression of early caries after orthodontic fixed appliance treatment: a 12-month follow-up randomized controlled trial. *Eur. J. Orthod.* 2018;40(5):457–464.

29 Höchli D, Hersberger-Zurfluh M, Papageorgiou SN, Eliades T. Interventions for orthodontically induced white spot lesions: a systematic review and meta-analysis. *Eur. J. Orthod.* 2017;39(2):122–133.

30 Khoroushi M, Kachuie M. Prevention and treatment of white spot lesions in orthodontic patients. *Contemp. Clin. Dent.* 2017;8(1):11–19.

31 Laing E, Ashley P, Gill D, Naini FB. An update on oral hygiene products. *Dent. Update* 2008;35:270–279.

Section III

Stages of Treatment with Preadjusted Edgewise Appliances

14

Alignment and Levelling

Farhad B. Naini and Daljit S. Gill

CHAPTER OUTLINE

Introduction, 249
Anchorage Requirements and Preparation, 250
  Anchorage Reinforcement with Headgear, 252
Arch Form, 255
Tooth Movement with Preadjusted Fixed Appliances, 256
Alignment, 257
  Bracket Positioning Variations, 258
  Initial Alignment, 258
  Choice of Archwire Size and Material, 263
  Placement of Lacebacks, 264
  Methods of Archwire Ligation, 267
  Cinching versus Bend Backs, 269
  Step-by-Step Archwire Placement, 271
  Archwire Removal, 273
  Space Creation and Redistribution, 277
  Crossbite Correction, 282
  Ectopic and Impacted Canines and Incisors, 283
  Impacted Mandibular Second Molars, 286
  Intrusion of Overerupted Maxillary Second Molars, 286
  Diastema Closure and Frenectomy, 287
  Wire Bending, 288
  Pain from Initial Archwires, 291
  Accelerated Tooth Movement, 292
Levelling, 293
Conclusion, 294
References, 294

Introduction

For didactic purposes and ease of technical description, preadjusted edgewise appliance orthodontic treatment is usually described as being divided into successive stages (Table 14.1). Alignment is usually, but not always, the first stage of treatment (e.g. arch expansion is sometimes undertaken prior to alignment, as is distal movement of the maxillary molars).

Following comprehensive clinical diagnosis and the formulation of a thorough treatment plan with clear treatment aims (where you are planning to move the teeth), the step-by-step road map of treatment required for the successive stages of treatment (i.e. how you are planning to move the teeth), referred to as **treatment mechanics**, are decided (see Chapter 1, Figure 1.1). The clinician should have a clear plan for where each tooth within each dental arch is to be positioned, in relation to the three planes of space and the three axes of rotation,[1] and how these movements are to be accomplished.

The aims of the alignment stage of treatment are as follows.

- To bring the malaligned teeth within each dental arch into alignment within the planned arch form.

Preadjusted Edgewise Fixed Orthodontic Appliances: Principles and Practice, First Edition. Edited by Farhad B. Naini and Daljit S. Gill.
© 2022 John Wiley & Sons Ltd. Published 2022 by John Wiley & Sons Ltd.

Table 14.1 Stages of preadjusted edgewise appliance treatment.

Stage I
Alignment
Levelling
Initiate incisor (overjet and overbite) and buccal segment correction
Initiate arch width coordination
Stage II
Space redistribution and closure
Completion of incisor and buccal segment correction
Completion of arch width coordination
Stage III
Finishing[a]
Detailing[b]
Stage IV
Retention

(a) Finishing refers to the positions and relations of teeth within each dental arch, i.e. achieving ideal alignment.
(b) Detailing refers to the interdigitation of the teeth and dental occlusion. However, the terms 'finishing' and 'detailing' are often used interchangeably.

- To begin the expansion or contraction of the dental arches as required to obtain the desired arch widths.
- To initiate the correction of the sagittal position of the incisors as far as possible. Some of this may be planned to be undertaken in the space closure stage of treatment, particularly in extraction cases or patients with spaced dental arches. It is worthwhile noting that prior to the placement of the fixed appliances, removable appliances may be very useful in initiating the correction of incisor inclinations whilst preserving anchorage (Figures 14.1 and 14.2). The value of removable appliances should not be underestimated in such situations, and can make subsequent fixed appliance treatment easier and reduce its duration.

Alignment may be considered as two often relatively seamless stages in fixed appliance orthodontic treatment. Initial alignment is either the first, or one of the first, stages of overall treatment, and involves predominantly the alignment of the teeth into the planned arch form. However, subsequent alignment may be required during any of the following stages of treatment, including space closure and finishing, and includes the ideal three-dimensional positioning of individual teeth.

Though usually the first stage of treatment, alignment continues throughout treatment; the clinician should constantly monitor tooth positions and bracket positions throughout the treatment process. Alignment may be said to be the first stage of treatment that carries through to the end of treatment.

Anchorage Requirements and Preparation

The principles of orthodontic anchorage have been described in Chapter 3. Treatment planning, including space analysis and space planning, has been described in Chapter 1. These form the basis of, and help to determine, the anchorage considerations for a proposed patient's treatment with fixed orthodontic appliances. It is worth reviewing the information in Chapters 1–3 before continuing with the rest of this chapter. However, this short section summarises the salient points regarding anchorage requirements and preparation.

It is worth remembering that single isolated tooth movements with orthodontic appliances are almost impossible

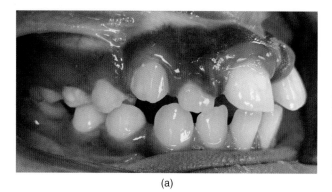

(a)

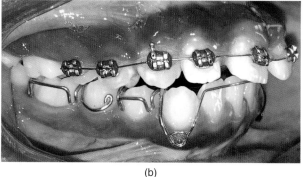

(b)

Figure 14.1 (a) Bimaxillary dental proclination with spacing in the dental arches. The proclined position of the mandibular incisors prevents retroclination of the maxillary incisors. (b) Retroclination of the mandibular incisors with a lower removable appliance and a modified Roberts' retractor (the term 'retractor' is a misnomer here, as the spring retroclines the incisor teeth rather than bodily retracting them) has retroclined the mandibular incisors and created an incisor overjet, which will permit retroclination of the maxillary incisors.

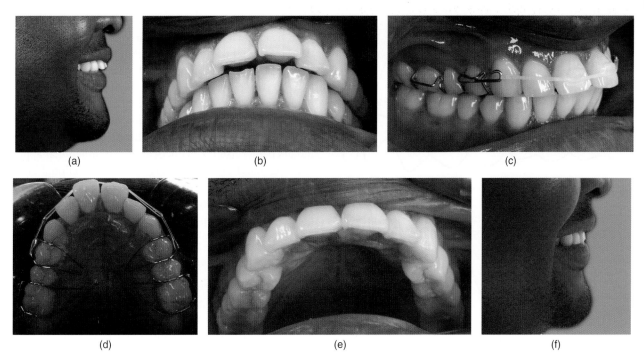

Figure 14.2 (a, b) Pretreatment views demonstrating proclined maxillary central incisors. (c, d) Upper removable appliance with light elastic force to retrocline the maxillary central incisors. Small beads of composite are bonded to the labial surface of the incisor crowns to prevent the elastic from riding up on the teeth. Acrylic palatal to the maxillary incisors must be removed in order to provide space for the retroclining maxillary incisors. (e, f) Following retroclination just with the upper removable appliance.

to achieve. Every single intentional orthodontic tooth movement will be accompanied by one or more undesirable tooth movements, affecting the tooth being moved (e.g. the desired retraction of an incisor may also lead to its unwanted intrusion or extrusion), adjacent teeth, or the anchor teeth from which the force is being applied. Much of the thought required in planning the application of orthodontic biomechanics to any given situation is in permitting efficient desirable tooth movements whilst preventing, or at least limiting, the undesirable consequences. This can only be achieved if the undesirable tooth movements have been anticipated, which requires a thorough understanding of orthodontic biomechanics and anchorage.

Anchorage describes the resistance to undesirable tooth movement, provided either by the teeth that the clinician wants to keep stationary or by non-dental structures such as the palate, screws placed in intraoral bone, or by using an extraoral source (e.g. the head or neck). The active forces causing desirable tooth movements will have potentially undesirable reactive consequences on other teeth, according to Newton's Third Law. For example, a force between tooth A and tooth B will move both teeth an equal amount in opposite directions, if everything about the teeth is otherwise identical. However, if tooth A has three times the root surface area of tooth B, the latter is likely

to move the greater distance. The tooth or teeth that the clinician would like to move are known as the **active unit**. The teeth that the clinician does not want to move are referred to as the **reactive unit**, or **anchor/anchorage unit**. Immobilisation of the teeth in the anchor unit is, to all intents and purposes, impossible (unless they are ankylosed). The purpose of anchorage preparation in the planning phase of treatment is to prepare the appliance and mechanics in such a way as to maximise the desirable tooth movements whilst minimising the undesirable tooth movements.

The **anchorage value** of a tooth may be defined as its *capacity to resist movement* when a force is applied to it. The higher the anchorage value of a tooth, the better it will resist being moved. For example, an ankylosed tooth will have a very high anchorage value, because even exceptionally high forces will be unlikely to move it. Conversely, a lower incisor with significant loss of periodontal support will have a very low anchorage value. One of the most important parameters pertaining to the anchorage value of each tooth is its effective root surface area. The comparative root surface area of each tooth attached to the periodontal ligament is provided in Figure 14.3.[2]

The **optimum force** for orthodontic tooth movement is defined as the lightest force capable of most efficiently producing the desired movement. The magnitude of the

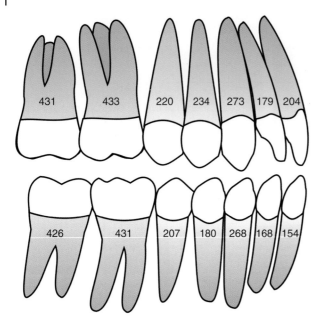

Figure 14.3 Comparative root surface area (mm²) of the permanent dentition, which provides an indication of the relative anchorage value of teeth of average size with normal periodontal support.

optimum force will vary depending on the type of tooth movement (e.g. simple crown tipping requires lower forces compared with bodily movement) and the root surface area of the tooth or teeth to be moved (see Chapter 3, Table 3.1).

The concept of anchorage preparation may be described using the example of a first premolar extraction case. Treatment planning may demonstrate that, following alignment and levelling, approximately half the amount of premolar extraction space still remaining will be required for incisor retraction and the other half can be closed with protraction of the posterior teeth. In such a situation, some forward movement of the posterior teeth is desirable, otherwise excess premolar extraction space will remain at the end of treatment. Therefore, anchorage reinforcement is not required, although the requirements must be re-checked following initial alignment and levelling, prior to space closure. However, if another case requires a considerable amount of the premolar extraction spaces for alignment, leaving just enough space for the desired amount of incisor retraction, the clinician cannot afford any forward movement of the posterior anchor unit. Where such differential incisor retraction is planned, **anchorage reinforcement** will be required to prevent **anchorage loss**, i.e. the undesirable forward movement of the posterior anchor teeth.

If anchorage reinforcement is required, it may be achieved by increasing the root surface area of the posterior anchor unit, for example by including the second molar

teeth, by using intermaxillary elastics, using extraoral force from headgear to the anchor unit, or by using orthodontic mini-implants/temporary anchorage devices (TADs), which are temporary attachments placed in the alveolar bone to provide anchorage (see Chapter 12). Other forms of anchorage preparation and reinforcement that may be employed with fixed appliance orthodontic treatment include removable appliances with headgear to distalise molars before fixed appliances are fitted, functional appliance treatment (see Chapter 18), and fixed-functional Class II correctors (see Chapter 18).

Anchorage planning for space closure is discussed in greater depth in Chapter 15.

Anchorage Reinforcement with Headgear

Anchorage reinforcement may be provided using some intraoral appliances, such as the Nance palatal arch (see later), and the use of TADs has been described in Chapter 12. Another method that may be used for anchorage reinforcement with fixed appliances is headgear. Headgear is the term given to a range of extraoral appliances using a cranial or cervical strap to apply forces to the teeth. The term **extraoral anchorage reinforcement** describes the use of headgear to prevent the undesirable movement of the anchor teeth, whereas the term **extraoral traction** refers to the use of headgear to actively distalise the anchor teeth. Headgear may also be used to apply forces to the jaws for potential jaw growth modification treatment.

The components of headgear are the head-cap or neckstrap, elastics or springs that provide the force, and a facebow, which attaches both to the teeth, via its inner bow, and to the elastics/springs via its outer bow to the head-cap or neckstrap (Figure 14.4a). The inner, intraoral part of the facebow usually fits into the headgear tubes attached to bands cemented onto the maxillary first permanent molar teeth.

The direction of pull of the headgear is usually dependent on the patient's vertical facial pattern, i.e. the greater the vertical growth pattern or facial type, the higher the direction of pull of the headgear, in order to prevent overeruption of the maxillary molars and thereby prevent undesirable vertical changes (Figure 14.4b). Therefore, some patients with reduced lower anterior face height and deep incisor overbite may have cervical-pull (Kloehn-type) headgear to actively extrude the maxillary molars, help to reduce the incisor overbite and potentially increase the lower anterior face height.

When using high-pull (occipital-pull) or straight-pull headgear, it is common practice to place a transpalatal arch (TPA) between the maxillary first molars. This is to prevent the upward and outward force from the headgear to the buccal aspect of the molars from buccally flaring the maxillary molars.

Preformed headgear facebows may be obtained in a variety of sizes. The inner bow also has bilateral adjustment loops, which may be adjusted to move the insertion part forward or back (Figure 14.4c). Keeping the inner bow adjustment loops facing downward relative to the maxillary arch will prevent the loops from potentially damaging the brackets on the premolar teeth during facebow placement and removal (Figure 14.4d). The width of the inner bow should be checked against the maxillary dental study model for the patient. When the appropriate size of facebow has been chosen, minor adjustments to the

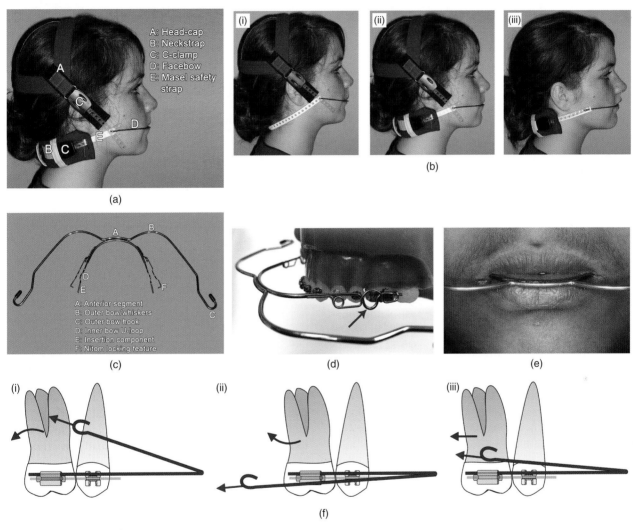

Figure 14.4 Headgear, including safety features. (a) Headgear components: head-cap and/or neckstrap, facebow and safety features, including steel C-clamp with snap-away safety release system, and Masel safety strap under the cervical component. (b) Types of headgear: (i) Occipital- or high-pull headgear applies a distal and an intrusive force on the first permanent maxillary molars. The figure also demonstrates the Masel safety strap. (ii) Combination- or straight-pull headgear applies a distal force to the maxillary first permanent molars. (iii) Cervical-pull headgear applies a distal and extrusive force to the maxillary first permanent molars. (c) Facebow component parts. (d) Keeping the inner bow adjustment loops facing downward relative to the maxillary arch will prevent the loops from potentially damaging the brackets on the premolar teeth during facebow placement and removal. (e) The anterior part of the facebow is resting slightly too low. The inner bow arms may be adjusted with Adams pliers to slightly elevate the anterior part so that it rests between the lips, without encroaching on either lip. (f) Length and position of outer bow can theoretically affect tipping of the first permanent maxillary molars. (i) A short outer bow, and/or one that is tipped upwards, can lead to distal tipping of the molar roots. (ii) A long outer bow, and/or one that is tipped downwards, may tend to distal tipping of the molar crowns. (iii) If the outer arm hook is kept adjacent to the first molar teeth and approximately level with the centre of resistance, a straight direction of pull should not lead to rotation of the molars. (g) Nitom locking safety facebow: (i) open; (ii) locked. (h) Hamill safety facebow. (i) The force delivery attachment part of the appliance should include a safety-release spring with snap-away mechanism, such as this steel C-clamp and safety self-releasing springs.

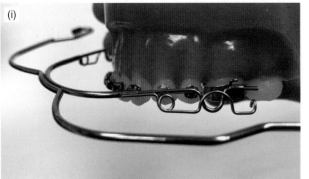
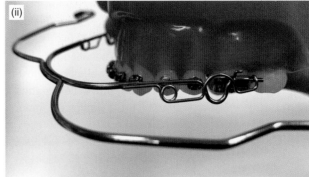

(i) (ii)

(g)

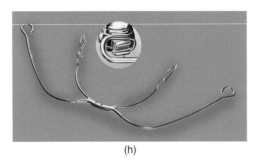
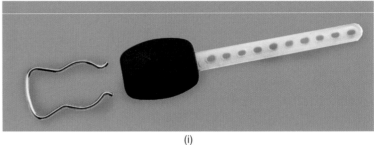

(h) (i)

Figure 14.4 (*Continued*)

inner bow loops may be made using Adams pliers. The inner bow should insert into the first molar headgear tubes relatively easily and passively, but the rest of the inner bow should lie at least 3–4 mm from the buccal/labial surface of the teeth and brackets. The inner bow loops also limit penetration into the headgear tubes. The anterior part of the facebow should rest between the lips, without encroaching on either lip (Figure 14.4e). The outer bow, or whiskers, should rest a few millimetres from the cheeks. Its end hooks should usually lie adjacent to the skin overlying the first molar teeth. The activating force from the head or neckstrap, via active springs, is applied to the hooks formed at the end of the outer bow. Variations in the length and vertical position of the outer bow may be required in patients undergoing growth modification treatment, but are usually not required for orthodontic anchorage reinforcement (Figure 14.4f). The facebow must have some form of safety feature, preventing its accidental removal (see below).

The appropriate size of head-cap or neckstrap is selected. The force delivery attachment part of the appliance should include a safety-release spring with snap-away mechanism, which releases the force from the facebow if it is pulled (see below). The degree of force per side may be checked using a force gauge. For anchorage reinforcement, between 250 and 300 g per side for 10–12 hours per day is usually required, though somewhat lighter forces may be used with cervical-pull headgear. For extraoral traction, between 400 and 500 g per side for 14 hours per day is recommended. Once the forces have been applied from the strap to the facebow, the position of the facebow should be re-checked to ensure patient comfort. Patients should be instructed to always support the anterior part of the facebow with one hand whilst applying the spring force to the hook of the outer bow. A final safety feature is an additional safety neckstrap, which may be worn under the rest of the headgear passively (see below). The patient should be able to place and remove the headgear under the clinician's supervision to ensure safe use. Headgear should usually be worn only at home and during sleep.

Safety with headgear wear is paramount. Younger patients and their parents should be warned that no form of rough activity or play is permitted when wearing headgear in order to prevent injury. If the facebow is pulled by someone during boisterous play, there is a risk of the facebow disengaging from the molar tubes whilst still attached to the head-cap or neckstrap, and potentially springing back into the mouth, facial soft tissues or eyes. This is referred to as a *catapult injury*. Ocular injury is potentially extremely serious, due to the risk of the transfer of oral microorganisms into the eye from the facebow ends, infection and potential sympathetic ophthalmitis of the unaffected eye. However small the risk, the potentially devastating consequences make safety features mandatory and patient compliance imperative. Therefore, avoidance of play whilst wearing the appliance is of paramount importance. The facebow safety features are either a locking-type safety facebow (Figure 14.4g) or other safety facebow design (Figure 14.4h), and snap-away self-releasing springs (Figure 14.4i), which detach from the head or neckstrap if the force exceeds a certain amount. These two safety features also help to prevent accidental *nocturnal disengagement*. We recommend the use of a third safety mechanism in the form of an additional safety strap, such as the Masel safety strap. The risk of harm from not following instructions should be discussed unequivocally as part of informed consent. Headgear wear requires excellent patient compliance. Any lack of motivation or signs of immaturity on the part of a patient or their parents should prohibit the use of headgear.

There is no doubt that the rise in popularity of orthodontic mini-implants/TADs has resulted in a reduction in the use of headgear in orthodontics. However, it is possible that some younger patients may prefer to avoid TADs, or their use may be deemed inappropriate, e.g. palatal TADs in young patients. There are situations where the use of headgear may be beneficial and clinicians should be familiar with their use.

Arch Form

Arch form refers to the shape of an individual dental arch as viewed from the occlusal surfaces of the dentition (i.e. dental arch form), or to the shape of an archwire formed to fit or alter the form of that arch. It is presumed that the morphology of each dental arch forms in relation to the shape of the underlying bone, and following dental eruption, the dental arch form alters due to the forces from the surrounding oral musculature. This may partly explain the variation in dental arch form.

The initial aligning archwire in modern orthodontics is almost exclusively a thin, round nickel titanium alloy (NiTi) and these wires cannot be shaped to a specific arch form at the chairside. *There is individual variability in dental arch form and dimensions.* Therefore, manufacturers make **preformed archwires** with several different shapes, from which the clinician must select the archwire form they wish to use.

Other than in specific situations (e.g. significant expansion with rapid maxillary expansion), the patient's original dental arch form should be maintained, or at least not altered significantly. As a general rule, preservation of the original arch form appears to improve stability of treatment results.[3] In addition, when the maxillary and mandibular dental arches are not coordinated, it is the mandibular dental arch form that is usually used as a template around

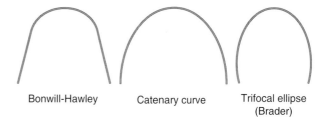

Figure 14.5 The three standard arch forms: Bonwill–Hawley, catenary, and trifocal ellipse (Brader).

which to form the maxillary arch. Needless to say, this guideline does not apply if the mandibular dental arch is distorted.

There are two classifications of arch form. The three basic arch forms in the standard classification are as follows (Figure 14.5).

- **Bonwill–Hawley**: this was described by Charles Hawley in 1905,[4] before the origin of the edgewise appliance. Hawley named it after William G.A. Bonwill and himself and it is still used by some manufacturers today. The wire from canine to canine is curved but distal to the canines the archwire is straight.
- **Catenary curve**: this is the shape formed by a segment of chain suspended from two hooks a certain distance apart at equal height. Clearly the precise shape depends on the chain length and the distance between the hooks from which it is suspended. The position of the hooks is akin to the intermolar width of the first permanent molar teeth, and the curve of the hanging chain approximates the dental arch form from the premolars through to the incisors. However, distal to the first molars the fit of this curve is usually too broad, as the second and third molar teeth commonly curve somewhat lingually relative to the first molars.
- **Trifocal ellipse (Brader)**: this is an alternative geometrical model, described by Brader in 1972.[5] The anterior part of this arch form is similar to the catenary curve, but the posterior part, distal to the first molar teeth, gradually narrows. The inward taper distal to the first molars gives the overall arch an egg-shaped morphology. The rationale for the use of archwires based on the Brader arch form is that they provide greater expansion in the premolar regions, potentially increasing the interpremolar width and thereby broadening the smile, yet take into account the relative lingual position of the second and third molars relative to the first molars.

Another early classification of dental arch form was described by Chuck in 1932.[6] This classification is used by some manufacturers. Based on this, the usual types

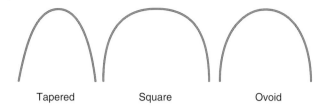

Figure 14.6 Arch forms described by Chuck: tapered, square, and ovoid.

of arch form used in preformed archwires are as follows (Figure 14.6).

- **Ovoid**: this is usually the standard type of arch form used and it is based on the catenary curve.
- **Tapered**: this is useful for patients with narrow dental arch forms, narrow intercanine width and thin gingival biotype, in order to avoid excessive buccal expansion and potential gingival recession.
- **Square**: this arch form may be indicated in patients with broad arch forms, and when greater degrees of expansion are desired.

These arch forms are usually available in archwires of different sizes and shapes (i.e. round, square or rectangular in cross-section). It is important to bear in mind that for any patient the preformed flexible archwires are only the starting point. As a general guideline, the longer the period of time that the patient will be in initial aligning archwires or the larger and stiffer the archwire, the more important that it is customised to the patient's planned arch form.

Whichever arch form is employed in the early alignment stage of treatment, when moving to stainless steel archwires later in treatment the clinician should customise the arch form for each patient to conform to their original planned arch form rather than a preformed shape. Pre-treatment dental study models may be used as a reference against which these archwire forms may be shaped. These archwires may also require adjustment bends in order to move the teeth into their appropriate positions within the dental arch and into a functional occlusion.

It is important to realise that in clinical treatment the arch form is established by the shape of the archwires, and is not related to the preadjusted bracket prescription system. With the variety of archwires in different arch forms available, the clinician may choose the appropriate arch form for each patient that respects their original dental arch form and alveolar process morphology, and where possible customise the arch form for each individual patient.

Tooth Movement with Preadjusted Fixed Appliances

Tooth movement occurs when a prolonged or continuous force is applied to a tooth via a bracket, which initiates the biological process of tooth movement, i.e. bone resorption on the compression/pressure side and bone deposition on the tension side within the periodontal ligament. **Tipping movement** occurs from single point forces applied to the crown that produce compressive loads that are greatest at the alveolar crest and root apex on diagonally opposite sides of the root. **Bodily movement** from force couples results in even compressive loads along one side of the periodontal ligament (Figure 14.7).

The magnitude of the force delivered is important in determining the tissue response. Ideally, orthodontic forces should not exceed **capillary pressure** within the periodontal ligament, in order to avoid ischaemia and tissue necrosis. The optimum force for tooth movement also depends on the type of tooth movement planned and the root surface area of the teeth to be moved (see Chapter 2). Teeth with smaller roots will require less force to produce movement than teeth with larger roots. Force levels required for different tooth movements have been described in Chapter 3, Table 3.1. Forces required for bodily movement or root uprighting and torquing are approximately double those required for tipping as double the root surface area is compressed on one side during such movements. Forces for intrusion are the lightest as

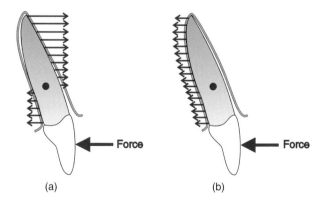

(a)   (b)

Figure 14.7 (a) Tipping movements result from compressive forces on diagonally opposite ends of the periodontal ligament. These are greatest at the alveolar crest and root apex and reduce to zero adjacent to the centre of resistance. Tension is created in other areas of the periodontal ligament. (b) Bodily movement results from approximately even compressive forces along one side of the periodontal ligament and tension on the opposite side.

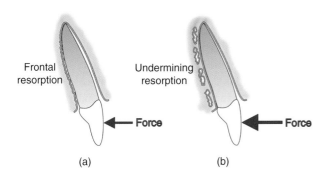

Figure 14.8 (a) Frontal resorption occurs when using light orthodontic forces that do not exceed capillary pressure within the periodontal ligament. (b) Undermining resorption occurs when capillary pressure is exceeded and hyalinisation occurs within the periodontal ligament.

all the force is concentrated at the root apex, which has a small surface area.

Light orthodontic forces that do not exceed capillary pressure result in **frontal resorption** of the alveolar bone in areas of compression, and bone deposition in areas of tension. Forces that exceed capillary pressure result in sterile necrosis of the affected area of the periodontal ligament; this process is termed **hyalinisation**, as the area appears translucent when viewed under a light microscope. Orthodontic tooth movement is delayed and bone resorption commences from within the alveolar bone, beneath the area of necrosis, within a few days. This is termed **undermining resorption** because the cellular response occurs from within the alveolar bone on the undersurface of the area of necrosis (Figure 14.8). It can take approximately 7–14 days for the process of undermining resorption to remove the lamina dura next to the necrotic periodontal ligament, which is the point when tooth movement begins.

Based on the above, a *light force* may be defined as a force that can move a tooth or group of teeth without producing undermining resorption and hyalinisation areas in the periodontal ligament for that type of tooth movement. Therefore, light forces are preferable to heavy forces in order to avoid undermining resorption. However, this is not always possible, as certain orthodontic mechanics may result in the concentration of forces in certain areas of the periodontal ligament. A time period of six to eight weeks is recommended between appliance reactivation appointments, depending on the mechanics being used, to allow adequate time for repair of damaged tissues following decline in the active forces. The rate of tooth movement is approximately 1 mm/month, under ideal conditions, but there is individual variability as the rate

depends on the efficiency of the appliance, the magnitude of the cellular response and the density of the alveolar bone. The initiation of tooth movement may be slower in adults due to the reduced cellularity and vascularity of the periodontal ligament and the greater density of the alveolar bone compared with children.

It is impossible to place a force directly perpendicular to the centre of resistance of a tooth, which is located approximately one-third of the distance between the alveolar crest and root apex of single-rooted teeth (see Chapter 2). A theoretical situation where direct finger pressure could be placed perpendicular to the centre of resistance would lead to bodily translation of the tooth (see Chapter 2, Figure 2.8). However, in reality, forces are placed via brackets bonded to the crowns of the teeth, at some distance from the centre of resistance. As such, these forces create moments (effectively the tendency of a force to produce rotation) resulting from the distance of the applied force to the centre of resistance of the tooth (see Chapter 2, Figure 2.12). The type of tooth movement depends on the significance of the created moments (see Chapter 2). With initial round aligning archwires, the movements occur by contact of the archwire with the bracket slot, predominantly resulting in tipping and rotational movements of the crowns.

Alignment

The term *alignment*, though frequently used in orthodontic parlance, is rarely adequately defined. To the layperson it may be thought to mean simple *straightening* of the teeth; however, in orthodontics the term has a more comprehensive meaning. **Alignment** may be defined as the movement of the teeth into their correct relative positions in relation to a planned dental arch form in order to achieve the desired/planned facial and smile aesthetics and optimal dental-occlusal function.

Alignment thereby involves movement of the teeth *horizontally/radially* and *vertically*, predominantly by forces generated by the archwire engaged in the brackets, and in terms of correcting three-dimensional crown and root angulation, inclination and rotational position by *rotational* movements. That is, alignment involves all the following types of tooth movement.

- Horizontal/radial: in–out movements.
- Vertical: up–down movement.
- Rotational: tip, torque, and rotation round the tooth's long axis.

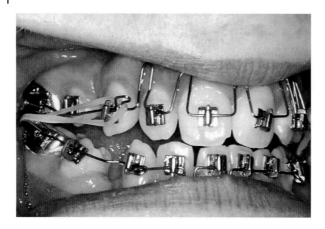

Figure 14.9 Multiloop archwire: this image shows classic Begg treatment. Source: courtesy of Dr David Spary.

In the early days of fixed appliance orthodontics, even thin, round, stainless steel archwires were too rigid and could not be engaged in misaligned teeth. Therefore, the flexibility of the system was increased by the incorporation of loops into the archwire at appropriate locations (Figure 14.9). The looped sections were more flexible radially to the dental arch than vertically, and bending loops into the archwires was rather time-consuming and required skill. The generated forces were rather complex with unforeseen adverse tooth movements sometimes occurring. These problems were circumvented by advances in archwire materials technology, particularly the advent of flexible nickel titanium alloy (NiTi) and titanium molybdenum alloy (TMA), which led to a move away from looped archwires to plain flexible archwires of **low flexural rigidity** for the initial alignment phase of treatment. Thin and thereby more flexible round archwires are used initially and as the dental alignment progressively improves the orthodontist works up through progressively thicker wires until a full-size archwire can be engaged; alternatively, somewhat thicker archwires of low flexural rigidity (such as braided steel, NiTi or TMA) may be used, though this is generally not recommended as it may place unnecessarily large forces on the roots, which at this crown aligning stage is not required.

Bracket Positioning Variations

The importance of accurate bracket positioning has been discussed in Chapter 7, but cannot be emphasised enough. It is worth checking dental study models at the chairside before bracket placement in order to improve the accuracy of bracket positioning. It may also be worth checking panoramic radiographs which, though not particularly accurate, provide an indication of root angulations, and this may aid bracket positioning.

Following a thorough diagnosis and establishment of a treatment plan, and depending on the prescription of the bracket system to be used, there are a number of local bracket variations which may be useful (Table 14.2). Such bracket variations can make treatment more straightforward and reduce the requirement for additional mechanics and wire bending later in treatment. It is important to state that *the appliance system and bracket prescriptions are not as important as the clinician's understanding of their utilisation.* Experienced orthodontists may sometimes mix brackets from different systems, taking advantage of local variations, depending on the desired tooth movements.

Initial Alignment

Initial alignment may begin once the brackets and molar tubes or bands have been positioned as accurately as possible. The initial archwire should be flexible enough to be fully or at least partially engaged and tied into most of the bracket slots. Whether using elastomeric modules or steel ligatures to ligate the archwire into position, it is important that the wire is not excessively deflected in order to avoid its permanent deformation. The size, material and degree of deflection of the archwire should be such as to place a *light continuous force* to each of the teeth in order to initiate and sustain tooth movement into the planned positions.

Dental development is such that tooth buds tend to develop in relatively normal positions and it is often during the eruptive process that the crowns of teeth begin to become displaced. As such, unless a tooth bud begins developing in an ectopic position, even in severely displaced teeth, the root apices tend to be closer to the correct position than the crowns. Therefore, the purpose of the initial aligning archwires is usually predominantly to move the crowns of displaced teeth into better positions, which is the reason that thin flexible round archwires are ideal. It is not necessary or even advisable to use flexible rectangular archwires for initial alignment, as they may place untoward forces on root apices, potentially causing greater patient discomfort, damage to the root apices and, as labial crown torque will begin to express in the maxillary incisors, potentially facilitating a loss of posterior anchorage. As the desired initial tooth movement is essentially crown tipping in a horizontal or mesiodistal direction, or slight vertical repositioning of displaced teeth, no more than approximately 50 g of force is required.

As far as is practical, the interaction of the archwire and bracket slot should be free from **binding** (i.e. the archwire binding against a bracket, then being released, usually under the forces of occlusion and mastication, moving a little, then binding again) and **friction** (see Chapter 2).

Table 14.2 Local variations in bracket positioning.

Clinical situation	Bracket positioning variation	Justification
Maxillary lateral incisors palatally in-standing (crowns and root apices)	Inverting (bonding upside down) maxillary lateral incisors	Assists in providing labial root torque in the rectangular archwire stage
Maxillary canine lateralisation, i.e. canines in missing lateral incisor position	Inverting maxillary canine	Reverses the torque from original labial root torque to palatal root torque (e.g. from $-7°$ to $+7°$ in Andrews' prescription brackets). First- and second-order values are unaffected. This does not work effectively in brackets with low torque prescriptions
		The integrated hook on canine brackets, when the bracket is inverted, may catch the patient's upper lip
	Bond maxillary lateral incisor brackets on lateralised canines	This is an alternative option, but potential difficulties are the greater labiopalatal thickness of the lateral incisor brackets and incorrect contour of the bracket base (as it is designed for a lateral incisor)
Maxillary canines buccally positioned or prominent, especially if combined with thin gingival biotype +/− recession	Inverting maxillary canine	Reverses the torque from original labial root torque to palatal root torque (e.g. from $-7°$ to $+7°$ in Andrews' prescription brackets)
		Alternatively, use $0°$ or $+7°$ (i.e. inverted) torque MBT prescription canine brackets
Maxillary canine mesiopalatally bulbous, in Class III orthognathic surgical preparation[7]	0.5–0.75 mm mesial bonding of maxillary canine	Leads to slight mesiolabial rotation of the canine, thereby rotating the mesiopalatal prominence of the canine away from the tip of the mandibular canine in occlusion, permitting better interdigitation
Maxillary canines upright or distally angulated in Class II orthodontic patient	Maxillary first premolar brackets on canines	Reduces the mesial tip (e.g. Andrews' prescription reduces from $11°$ to $2°$)
		Alternatively, use $0°$ tip MBT prescription canine bracket
Class III camouflage, i.e. the requirement to maintain or increase the compensated retroclination of the mandibular incisors in order to maintain or improve the incisor relationship	Contralateral mandibular canines (sometimes referred to as 'reversing' the brackets)	To maintain or increase Class III compensation in the lower labial segment, bonding contralateral mandibular canine brackets reverses their tip from a mesial to a distal direction. First- and third-order values are unaffected. This also helps to keep or increase lower incisor retroclination
During space closure in the lower arch, if there is a need to protract the posterior teeth (i.e. 'burn' posterior anchorage) and limit retroclination of the lower incisors	Inversion of mandibular incisor brackets (with rectangular archwires)	Reverses labial root torque to lingual. This is more effective in MBT prescription (changing root torque from labial $-6°$ to lingual $+6°$, with zero angulation) compared with Andrews' or Roth prescriptions, changing from only $-1°$ to $+1°$)

The term **clearance** refers to the size difference between an archwire diameter and shape relative to the size of the bracket slot. This clearance or *play* of the archwire within the bracket slot, together with the method of ligation, determine how freely the archwire can move within the brackets. *The greater the freedom of the archwire within the bracket slot, the greater its manoeuvrability and the lighter the force that will be able to initiate and sustain tooth movement.* It follows that the lighter the forces used for tooth movement, the more biologically healthy the system. The forces should be light enough to stimulate cellular activity without crushing the blood supply around the roots, periodontal ligament and surrounding alveolar bone. As such, some ligatureless and passive self-ligating bracket systems may be better at this initial stage of treatment as the archwire has excellent clearance within the bracket

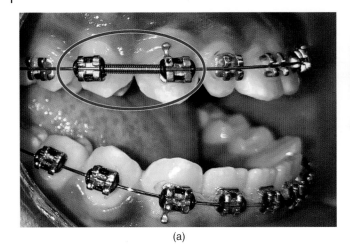
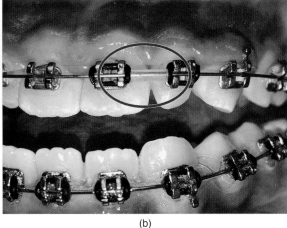

(a)   (b)

Figure 14.10 Archwire reinforcing sleeves. (a) Closed coil spring is very thin orthodontic wire (0.010–0.012 inch) wound into a coil whose helices are in contact, thereby rendering it incompressible. It is usually delivered as a length of coil spring wound round a spool, and is cut to the appropriate length depending on the intended application, which is usually to reinforce flexible archwires over long spans and/or maintain a space. (b) Plastic tubing is also delivered as a long length wound round a spool, which may be cut to the required length and may be used instead of closed coil spring, though inevitably it has less rigidity.

slot, and there is no pressure from an elastomeric or steel ligature pushing the archwire into the bracket slots. Alternatively, the brackets may be tied *loosely* with steel ligatures, which may work in a similar way to self-ligation, but may be more time-consuming as each tooth has to be ligated individually.

When using thin, flexible, initial aligning archwires, particularly where the wire is traversing an extraction space, a large interbracket span or bypassing a severely displaced tooth, an additional stainless steel wire (see section Placement of lacebacks), or **reinforcing sleeves**, such as closed coil spring or plastic tubing cut to size, may be used to reinforce the wire in the interbracket span. Reinforcing sleeves reduce the likelihood of accidental archwire disengagement or deformation, particularly under the forces of mastication (Figure 14.10).

Individual teeth that are severely displaced from the line of the arch, or ectopic teeth such as unerupted canines or incisors, should usually not be ligated with the initial archwire, as their ligation would lead to uncontrolled arch form alteration with such flexible archwires. Ideally, such teeth should be bypassed until the rest of the dental arch is relatively well aligned and a stiffer base archwire has been placed, following which forces may be applied to the severely displaced tooth via elastomeric thread (Figure 14.11) or chain, or via a flexible **piggyback (overlay) archwire**, which is a flexible auxiliary archwire ligated in addition to the base archwire (Figure 14.12). The base archwire maintains arch form while the piggyback wire aligns the displaced tooth. When the displaced tooth is nearly aligned, the base wire may be removed and

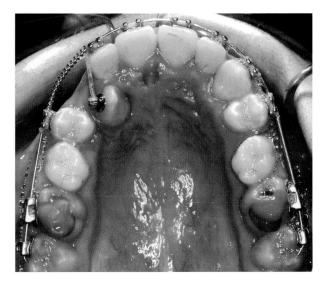

Figure 14.11 The maxillary dental arch is relatively well aligned and a stiff base archwire is in situ. Force is applied to the displaced maxillary right canine using elastomeric thread.

the entire dental arch ligated with the flexible aligning archwire.

Bracket size is an important consideration in initial alignment and should be sufficient to permit effective control of tooth movement. Mesiodistally narrow brackets will increase the **interbracket span**, making rotational correction around the long axis of a tooth difficult. Brackets that are excessively wide will tend to reduce the interbracket span, which thereby increases the stiffness of even the most flexible archwire in that interbracket region, potentially reducing the effectiveness of tooth movement. Brackets

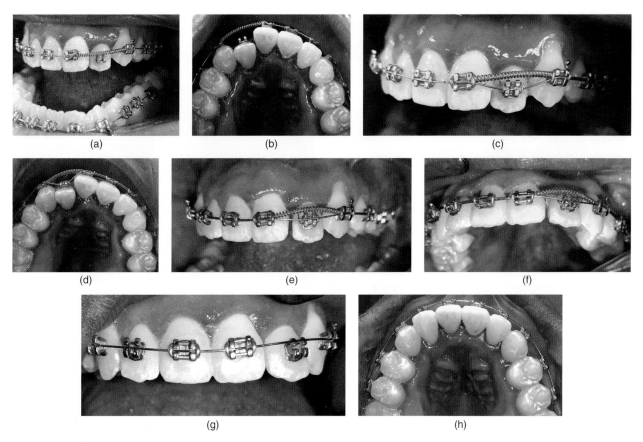

(a)   (b)   (c)

(d)   (e)   (f)

(g)   (h)

Figure 14.12 (a, b) A stiff 0.018-inch stainless steel base archwire has been placed and space opened for the in-standing maxillary lateral incisor using active compressed coil spring. With the space created, the lateral incisor bracket is bonded. (c, d) Force applied to the severely displaced tooth via a flexible piggyback (overlay) NiTi archwire, which is a flexible auxiliary archwire ligated in addition to the base archwire. The base archwire maintains arch form while the piggyback wire aligns the displaced tooth. (e, f) The displaced tooth is nearly aligned. (g, h) The base wire may now be removed and the entire dental arch ligated with the flexible aligning archwire.

ideally should be wide enough to provide rotational control, but not excessively wide; from a practical point of view, brackets should not be wider than approximately half the tooth width (see Chapter 2).

Initial flexible archwires tend to migrate laterally along the dental arch, which means that even if they are cut exactly to the correct length distal to the terminal molar teeth, their lateral movement, possibly due to the forces of mastication over time, means the wire will protrude from one side while simultaneously coming out of the opposite side molar tube. On the side that the wire is protruding, it may cause ulceration of the soft tissues, sometimes leading to considerable patient discomfort. Such unwanted **archwire migration** may be prevented by placing a stop on the wire between two brackets that are relatively close together. Some wires have crimpable stops on them, referred to as **crimpable split tubes**, which just need to be crimped into the required position (Figure 14.13). Alternatively, a small bead of flowable composite resin, known as a **composite stop**, may be run onto the archwire in an interbracket span

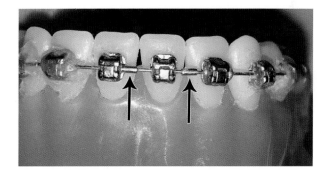

Figure 14.13 Crimpable split tubes, which may be crimped onto the archwire with Weingart pliers.

and light cured (Figure 14.14). Neither of these manoeuvres is necessary if the archwire is either cinched or bend backs are placed distal to the terminal molars (see below).

In some patients, particularly those with deep bites, well-interdigitated occlusion and potentially strong jaw musculature, the interdigitation of the dental occlusion

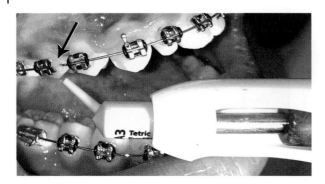

Figure 14.14 A small bead of flowable composite resin, known as a composite stop, may be run onto the archwire in an interbracket span and light cured.

itself may be a hindrance to initial alignment. In such situations, *the posterior teeth may be separated just beyond the resting vertical dimension and freeway space.* Such **temporary bite opening** may be achieved by placing a removable clip-over anterior bite plane, bonding a composite resin anterior bite plane or bite opening turbo props bonded palatal to the maxillary central incisors (Figure 14.15). Anterior bite opening with a removable or fixed bite plane permits vertical clearance to bond the mandibular arch and permits easier levelling of the mandibular dental arch. However, if there is an increased incisor overjet, posterior bite opening may be required. This may be achieved by placing glass ionomer cement over the occlusal surfaces of the posterior molars, usually the upper molars, which makes their subsequent removal easier (Figure 14.16). With this latter posterior bite opening approach, it is important that the mandibular dental arch

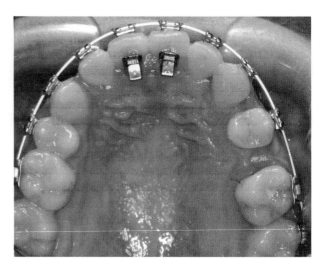

Figure 14.15 Anterior bite opening turbos (turbo props).

is bonded in order to avoid uncontrolled overeruption of the mandibular incisors (Figure 14.17).

Sometimes brackets cannot be ideally positioned during initial placement, e.g. partially erupted teeth, severe imbrication or severely rotated teeth. In subsequent appointments, *as the brackets become better aligned on the archwire, any initial bracket positioning discrepancies become more apparent.* Therefore, reassessment of dental alignment and bracket positions should be undertaken at each subsequent visit, as bracket positioning errors can be better elicited once the dental arches are better aligned. Missed bracket positioning errors result in incorrect tooth positions even though the archwire may be passive within the bracket

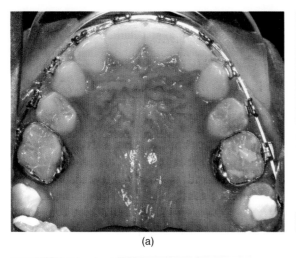

(a)

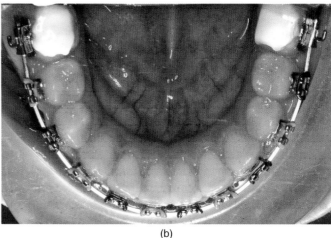

(b)

Figure 14.16 Glass ionomer cement bonded to (a) occlusal surfaces of maxillary molars or (b) mandibular molars, to open the anterior bite.

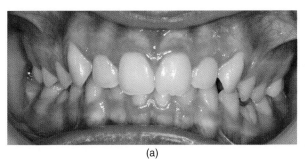
(a)

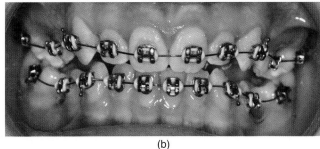
(b)

Figure 14.17 (a) Deep incisor overbite malocclusion. (b) Mandibular arch has been bonded, with glass ionomer cement on the occlusal surfaces of maxillary first molars providing the required anterior bite opening.

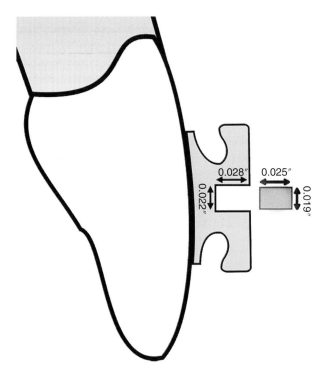

Figure 14.18 Bracket slot dimensions and rectangular archwire dimensions in cross-section. A 0.022 × 0.028-inch bracket slot is shown, with a 0.019 × 0.025-inch rectangular archwire. Source: Naini FB, Gill DS (eds). *Orthognathic Surgery: Principles, Planning and Practice*. Oxford: Wiley Blackwell, 2017; reprinted with permission.

Table 14.3 Archwire cross-sectional dimensions.

Archwire cross-sectional shape	Imperial unit measurements (inches)	Metric measurements (mm)
Round	0.008	0.2
	0.010	0.25
	0.012	0.3
	0.014	0.35
	0.016	0.4
	0.018	0.45
	0.020	0.5
Square	0.016 × 0.016	0.4 × 0.4
	0.018 × 0.018	0.45 × 0.45
	0.020 × 0.020	0.5 × 0.5
Rectangular	0.016 × 0.022	0.4 × 0.55
	0.017 × 0.025	0.43 × 0.64
	0.018 × 0.025	0.45 × 0.64
	0.019 × 0.025	0.48 × 0.64
	0.021 × 0.025	0.53 × 0.64
	0.0215 × 0.028	0.55 × 0.7

Note: A useful technique for *approximate conversion* from imperial to metric units is to divide the last two digits of the imperial measurement by 4 and move the decimal point in front of the resulting number. For example, 0.018-inch wire, divide 18 by 4, which gives 4.5, and move the decimal point, giving 0.45 mm.

slots. At this stage the clinician must decide whether to reposition the brackets more accurately, or alternatively to place bends in subsequent steel wires to compensate for any inaccurate bracket positions. As a general guideline, the earlier it is in the treatment process, the more efficient it will be to reposition the brackets rather than placing bends in every subsequent archwire. A convenient time to reposition brackets is when undertaking repairs or picking up second molars during treatment, as the clinician may need to drop down to lighter archwires anyway.

Choice of Archwire Size and Material

Although metric measurements are commonly used in orthodontic practice, archwire and bracket slot dimensions (Figure 14.18) are still described in imperial units (Table 14.3).

As described above, initial alignment requires low friction and good bracket clearance that allow relatively free movement of the archwire within the bracket slots. When using an 0.022 × 0.028-inch bracket slot, the initial archwire is usually one of the following.

- **Superelastic nickel titanium**: this is the most commonly used initial round archwire. The extended flat load–deflection curve for this material makes it theoretically very useful for initial alignment, as it places a relatively low, continuous force over a considerable range of deflection (see Chapter 10, Figures 10.4 and 10.5). Sizes vary from 0.012 inch (in severely crowded/rotated teeth, in adults and in more anxious children where the discomfort of the first archwire is to be kept as mild as possible), 0.014 inch (the most commonly used initial archwire), or 0.016 inch (when the teeth are not excessively crowded or rotated). Attempting to place too large an archwire too early will result in excessive patient discomfort and increase the likelihood of brackets debonding or deformation of the archwire.

- **Thermally active nickel titanium**: these heat-activated NiTi archwires may be larger round (e.g. 0.018 inch), square (0.016 × 0.016 inch) or rectangular (0.016 × 0.022 inch) in cross-section. Although some manufacturers recommend use of these square or rectangular archwires for initial alignment, we would recommend round archwires for this stage, due to the reasons already discussed. These wires may be relatively passive when cold, allowing easier ligation of chilled wires, and begin delivering the required forces only when they reach mouth temperature. Therefore, they may be kept in a refrigerator prior to use, or local ice may be applied to the region of the archwire to be ligated most fully (e.g. ethyl chloride or a form of cold spray onto cotton wool pellets, with the frosted pellets applied to the archwire).

- **Titanium molybdenum alloy (also known as beta-titanium)**: this wire material, developed by Charles Burstone specifically for orthodontics, has a stiffness and springiness between stainless steel and NiTi, but is formable, i.e. the clinician can bend loops in TMA if required. However, it has relatively high friction.

- **Multistrand stainless steel**: prior to the advent of flexible NiTi archwires, multiple thin stainless steel wires were wrapped together to form multistrand or braided archwires. These wires are either three or more wires of similar dimensions twisted together, or coaxial, i.e. three or more wires of similar dimensions twisted around a central core of wire (Figure 14.19). The purpose is to have the elastic deformability of the individual small wires combined with the flexural rigidity of the sum of the wires. These wires work relatively well so long as the dental irregularity is not significant. When used, these are usually 0.015 or 0.0175 inch in cross-section. These wires may have lower cost compared with NiTi wires, but they would need to be removed at each visit and adjusted to ensure removal of any distortions.

Placement of Lacebacks

A standard **laceback** is a stainless steel ligature (usually 0.010 inch) tied passively in a 'figure-of-eight' fashion from the terminal molar hook to the canine bracket in the same quadrant. Lacebacks are usually placed under the archwire (Figure 14.20). In the alignment stage of treatment, the potential purpose of the laceback is as follows.

- **Prevention or reduction of canine mesial crown tip**: if the canine tooth is either upright or distally angulated, the engagement of the initial archwire into the canine bracket will lead to mesial crown angulation as the mesial tip in the canine bracket is expressed. Inevitably, this will also procline incisors engaged with the same wire. To counteract this effect, the laceback

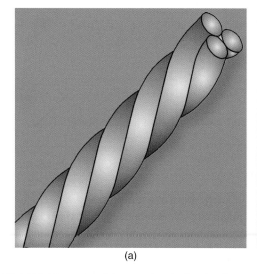
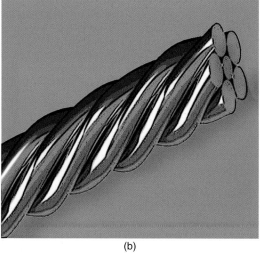

(a)   (b)

Figure 14.19 (a) Multistrand stainless steel archwire showing cross-section. (b) Coaxial stainless steel archwire showing cross-section.

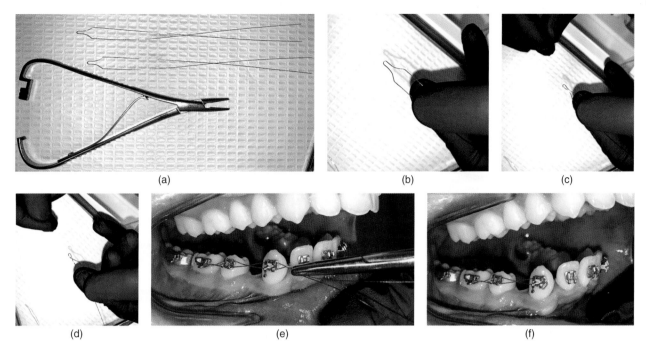

Figure 14.20 Laceback placement. (a) Long ligatures are used, and tied with Mathieu pliers. (b–d) The end of the long ligature is squeezed together and twisted to form a small loop. (e) The loop is placed over the first molar hook, and the wire is tied in a figure-of-eight mode over the premolar bracket and again over the canine bracket. It is then twisted with Mathieu pliers and the end is cut with a ligature cutter, leaving approximately 3 mm of twisted wire (f) which is tucked under the canine bracket with a ligature tucker.

serves to tie the canine crown back to the terminal molar, maintaining its sagittal position such that the change in angulation of the canine is encouraged to occur by distal root movement rather than mesial crown tip (Figure 14.21). Whether this occurs in practice to the desired theoretical extent is subject to debate (see below).

- **Dental midline correction**: unilateral lacebacks may be used to restrict mesial canine crown movement on one side, thereby allowing the expression of the mesial tip of the contralateral canine to aid in dental midline correction. The dental midline will thereby move towards the side with the laceback.
- **Archwire protection from masticatory forces**: masticatory forces, particularly over a bolus of food, may lead to vertical forces on thin initial archwires causing them to disengage from the brackets or molar tubes. The laceback provides some protection against this occurring, particularly in premolar extraction sites where the initial archwire is unsupported for a greater interbracket span.
- **Canine retraction**: theoretically, tight lacebacks may be used to begin canine retraction in cases with severe lower incisor crowding. However, they are unlikely to be very effective as they will not be active over anything more than a very short range. Elastomeric chain may be more beneficial in such situations (see below).

Fully Twisted Tie-back/Laceback

The standard laceback described has the disadvantage of loosening over time. Although it can be tightened at subsequent visits, when the requirement to avoid mesial tipping of the canine crown is greater, the laceback may be placed as a fully twisted tie-back. The molar, premolar(s) and canine are tied together tightly by twisting the stainless steel ligature continuously between the interbracket spans. The tie-back wire is usually placed and twisted with Mathieu pliers, which twists the wire from the engaged beaks of the pliers towards the bracket (Figure 14.22). An alternative but more technically challenging method is to tie the stainless steel wire using Coon's ligature-locking pliers, which have a reverse action to conventional 'outside-in' ligature tying methods, i.e. the initial twist of the wire occurs at the bracket, with the continued rotation of the pliers twisting away from the bracket (Figure 14.23). This gives the ligature a very tight fit around the brackets.

Elastomeric Chain 'Laceback'

Another alternative to the standard stainless steel wire laceback is to 'laceback' the canine bracket to the molar tube using elastomeric chain. This should not be active in the sense of moving the canine crown distally, but just active enough to counteract the mesial crown movement of the canine. It is preferable to use 'open', i.e. spaced elastomeric

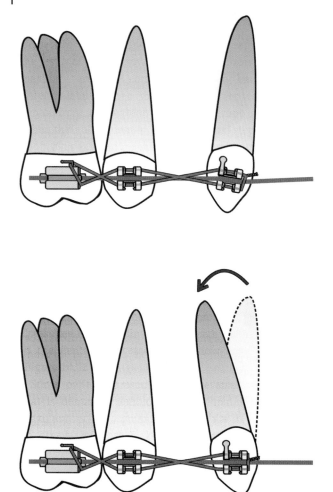

Figure 14.21 A laceback will serve to maintain the sagittal position of the canine crown, so that the mesial tip expression of the canine bracket tip will correct the angulation of the tooth by distal root movement rather than mesial crown tipping.

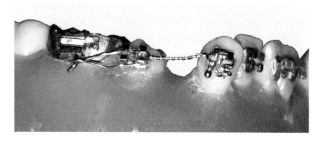

Figure 14.22 A twisted tie-back.

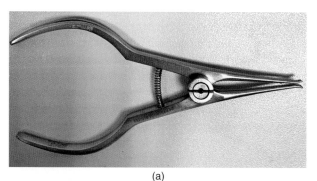

(a)

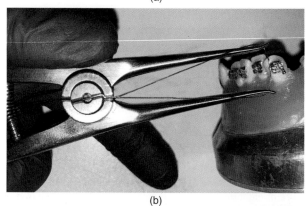

(b)

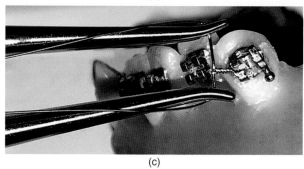

(c)

Figure 14.23 (a) Coon's ligature-locking pliers. (b) These have a reverse action to conventional 'outside-in' ligature tying methods, i.e. the initial twist of the wire occurs at the bracket, with continued rotation of the pliers twisting away from the bracket. (c) This gives the ligature a very tight fit around the brackets.

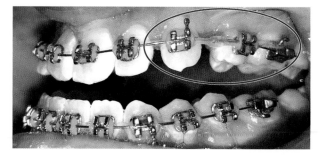

Figure 14.24 Elastomeric chain that is slightly active may be used to tie back the canine crown to the first molar.

chain, which is placed from the hook on the first molar tube, engages the premolars as required, but should only engage the distal wings of the canine brackets. This will prevent unwanted mesiobuccal rotation of the canine tooth (Figure 14.24). Elastomeric chain lacebacks may be placed under or over the initial archwire.

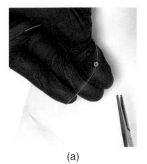
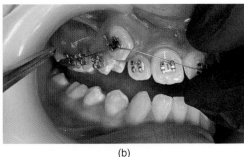
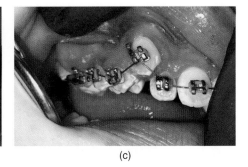

(a) (b) (c)

Figure 14.25 (a) To align teeth that are vertically out of position, an elastomeric module is first placed onto the aligning archwire. (b) The archwire is subsequently placed into the molar tube, and with the wire maintained occlusal to the bracket on the vertically displaced tooth, the elastomeric module is stretched and ligated over the entire bracket. This limits archwire deflection. (c) The other teeth are subsequently ligated as required; the maxillary lateral incisor is shown partially engaged.

Methods of Archwire Ligation

A **ligature** is a tie that secures an archwire, or sometimes other auxiliaries, into bracket slots. Placement of ligatures is referred to as **ligation**, or **tying-in** of an archwire. Ligatures are usually tied under and around a bracket's tie-wings.

With initial aligning archwires, lightly pre-stretched **elastomeric ligatures (modules or rings)** may be used to ligate the archwire at the first visit. Elastomeric modules are available under a variety of proprietary names, but essentially they are small round bands of elastomeric material that is stretched around a bracket's tie-wings to hold an archwire in position. They are usually held in mosquito pliers (also termed haemostats), which have a mechanical locking mechanism located between the handles. *It is not essential for the initial aligning archwire to be fully engaged into every bracket slot at this visit*, which could potentially cause considerable patient discomfort in the first few days following archwire placement. Teeth that are severely malaligned or rotated may be **partially engaged** over the required number of bracket wings, and teeth that are vertically out of position may be engaged occlusal to the bracket slot in order to limit archwire deflection (Figure 14.25). At the first adjustment visit, usually approximately six to eight weeks following initial archwire placement, and at subsequent adjustment visits for continued alignment, it will usually be possible gradually to more fully ligate any teeth where the archwire was not completely seated in the bracket slot.

The major advantage of elastomeric modules is their ease of use and speed of placement. However, their use carries significant drawbacks. They may fail to fully engage an archwire when such engagement is intended. One way around this is to use a 'figure-of-eight' ligation method (see below), though this will significantly increase friction. Another disadvantage is the substantial degradation of their mechanical properties in the oral environment, with significant **force relaxation** occurring within days of ligation,[8] potentially leading to reduced wire engagement over time.

The use of elastomeric modules can work relatively well in situations where the desired movement of the teeth is by the brackets being pulled along with the archwire as it is returning to its original shape. However, where greater sliding of teeth is desired, it may be better to ligate the archwire *lightly* with **stainless steel ligatures** (see below). The pivotal word here is 'lightly', as excessive tightening of steel ligatures will have the opposite effect, potentially hindering initial alignment. Inevitably, steel ligatures take longer to place and remove than elastomeric ligatures, which is their main drawback. Steel ligatures are made from annealed stainless steel wire, usually 0.010 inch, although sometimes 0.012 inch may be used, such as in Kobayashi ligatures (Figure 14.26). These ligatures are usually held with Mathieu pliers (which have a positive-locking ratchet and spring for easy opening and closing) and are engaged under the bracket tie-wings and twisted around the bracket until they are as tight as required. The excess wire is cut with ligature cutters and the twisted end is tucked under the archwire and bracket wings with a ligature director (wire tucker) (see below). It is important that care is taken at this stage in order to prevent sharp ligature ends untwisting and causing trauma to the patient's mucosa between appointments.

When a tooth is severely rotated, the bracket should be bonded as far as possible into the rotation. At subsequent adjustment visits, if full engagement of an aligning archwire into a severely rotated tooth is difficult, a useful technique is to place a length of dental floss around the archwire and thereby pull the wire lingually into position while simultaneously ligating it with a steel ligature (Figure 14.27).

Alternatively, **self-ligating brackets** may be employed, which may be very useful at this initial alignment stage of

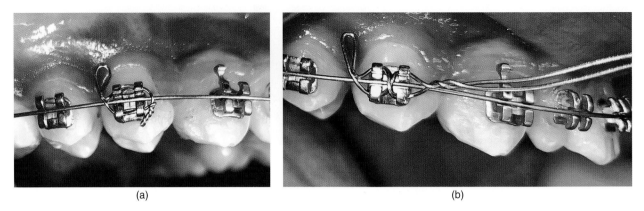

(a) (b)

Figure 14.26 The Kobayashi ligature's legs are welded together to form a helical hook at its end, permitting attachment of orthodontic elastics. (a) Standard ligation of a Kobayashi ligature. (b) Figure-of-eight ligation of a Kobayashi ligature.

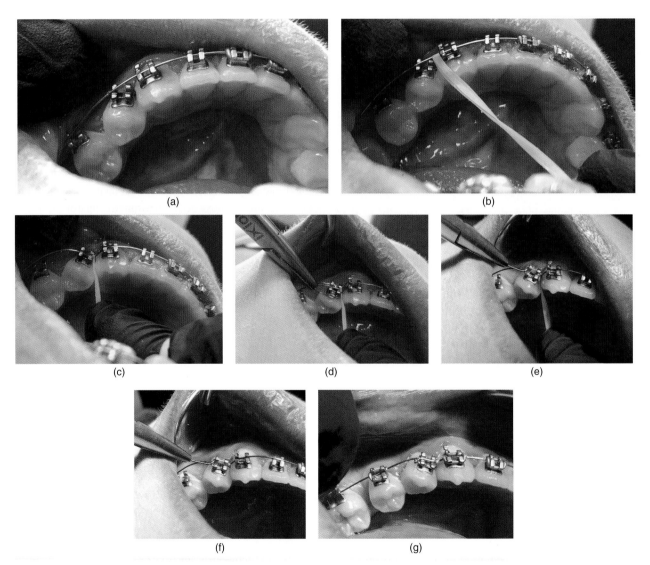

(a) (b)

(c) (d) (e)

(f) (g)

Figure 14.27 (a) A severely rotated lower left first premolar, with the bracket positioned as far into the rotation as possible. (b, c) A length of dental floss is tied around the archwire and pulls it lingually into position, while (d–f) simultaneously ligating it with a steel ligature. (g) Finally, the surrounding teeth are ligated.

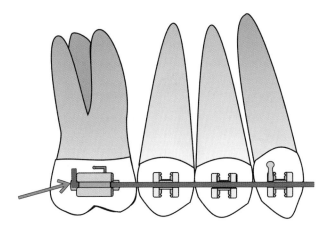

Figure 14.28 A cinch refers to the placement of an acute bend (usually at approximately 90° to the archwire in a gingival direction) on the archwire exactly as it exits distal to the terminal attachment in an orthodontic arch, usually the most distal molar tube. It serves to limit incisor proclination during alignment and levelling, and prevents archwire migration in the interval between patient appointments.

treatment due to the reduced friction and relatively unhindered play of the archwire within the brackets. Any obstruction of the relatively free movement between the archwire and bracket slots in preadjusted edgewise systems will delay the progress of initial alignment and may lead to anchorage loss.

Cinching versus Bend Backs

Cinching of an archwire refers to the placement of an acute bend (usually at approximately 90° to the archwire in a gingival direction) on the archwire *exactly as it exits distal to the terminal attachment* in an orthodontic arch, usually the most distal molar tube (Figure 14.28). If the acute bend on the archwire is not exactly as it exits the molar tube or other distal attachment, then it is not a cinch. The purpose of a cinch is to reduce, as far as possible, the tendency to increase in the arch length, and to limit incisor proclination in the alignment and levelling stages of treatment; the evidence for their effectiveness in this regard requires further investigation.

Technically, it is possible to place a cinch in a NiTi archwire by bending it beyond the point of elastic deformation. This may be undertaken using a Weingart plier (Figure 14.29).

Alternatively, exposing the 3–4 mm ends of a NiTi archwire to an open flame with a miniature orthodontic gas

blowtorch for a few seconds (the wire will appear orange to red-hot in the approximately 650°C heat) will significantly reduce the shape memory and permit a cinch or bend back to be placed (Figure 14.30). Thinner archwires, i.e. 0.012- and 0.014-inch NiTi wires, tend to fracture with bending after such flame exposure, but NiTi archwires of 0.016 inch or larger usually maintain their bends relatively well after such flame exposure. This exposure of an archwire end to an open flame is sometimes termed 'annealing', but this is an incorrect use of the term and should be avoided. The term **annealing** (from Old English *onælan*, to set on fire or subject to fire) refers to a form of carefully controlled heat treatment followed by a specified rate and type of cooling employed in the manufacturing process of archwires, used to reduce hardness and increase the ductility of a metal by eliminating the residual stresses induced in the wire-making process.

Titanium appears to be well tolerated by the tissues in the biological environment, which explains its biomedical and dental applications. Nickel ions have been classified as carcinogenic chemicals,[9] though it may be that not all forms of nickel are carcinogenic, and there is no supportive evidence in the implication of nickel released from biomedical materials as being unsafe (much larger prostheses with higher nickel content are used routinely by orthopaedic surgeons). However, exposing an archwire end to an open flame is uncontrolled, the extent of the process along the length of the wire is unknown, and the wire becomes brittle and susceptible to fracture. Therefore, cinching without exposure to an open flame may be considered more appropriate.

A **distal-end bend back** is a bend made on the archwire, usually in a gingival or medial direction, *one or more millimetres distal to the terminal attachment* (usually the molar tube) (Figure 14.31). Bend backs serve to secure the archwire in position and prevent or limit lateral sliding and mesial migration of the archwire and potential disengagement from the most distal molar tubes or brackets, in the intervals between patient appointments, thereby preventing soft tissue trauma from a disengaged archwire end. Bend backs will permit a degree of arch lengthening and incisor proclination, depending on the planned number of millimetres the archwire extends distal to the molar tubes before the bend back.

An alternative to distal-end bend backs that is available is known as the 'split stop', which is essentially a wire stop that is crimped onto the archwire distal to the terminal molar tube (Figure 14.32).

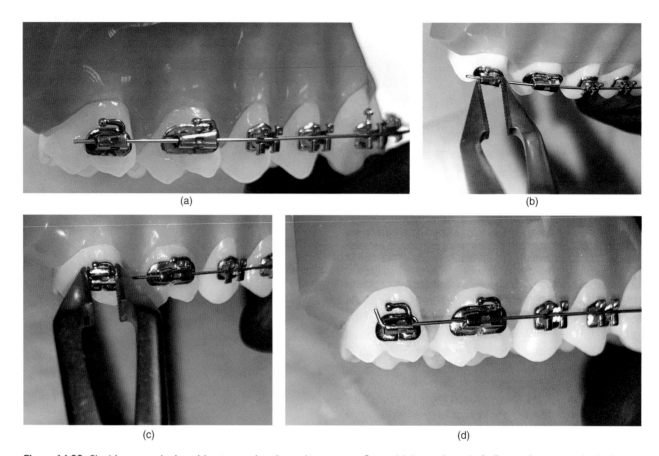

(a)

(b)

(c)

(d)

Figure 14.29 Cinching an archwire without exposing the end to an open flame. (a) Approximately 2–3 mm of excess archwire is maintained distal to the terminal molar tube. (b) The beaks of Weingart pliers are placed such that the mesial beak holds the attachment away from the base. This is important to avoid inadvertent debonding of the tube. (c) Squeezing the pliers places the cinch on the archwire as it exits the tube. (d) Cinch in position.

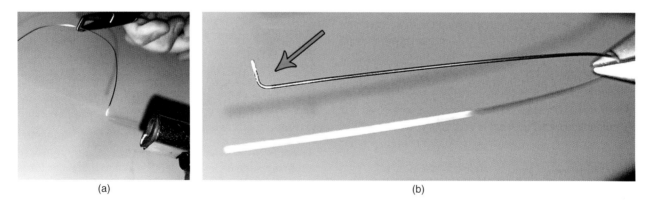

(a)

(b)

Figure 14.30 Cinching an archwire with exposure of the end to an open flame. (a) Flame exposure of the 3–4 mm ends of a NiTi archwire with a miniature orthodontic gas blowtorch for a few seconds. Gloves should not be worn near the blowtorch. (b) Flame exposure significantly reduces the shape memory and permits a cinch or bend back to be placed. However, the wire becomes brittle, and thinner wires may fracture when the bend is being placed. Overall, the technique described in Figure 14.29 is preferred.

Figure 14.31 (a) A distal-end bend back in a vertical and gingival direction. (b) A distal-end bend back in a medial direction.

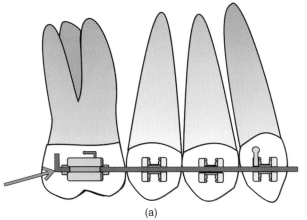

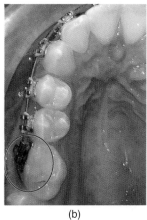

(a)   (b)

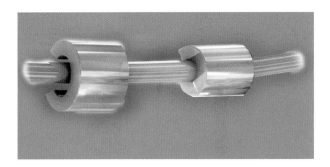

Figure 14.32 A split stop, which may be crimped onto the archwire as it exits the most distal attachment.

Step-by-Step Archwire Placement

- Check the accuracy of bracket placement in the mouth and using the dental study models as a reference and guide.
- Select the appropriate archwire size, shape and material.
- Using the pretreatment study models at the chairside, cut the distal ends of the archwire to the appropriate length with distal-end cutting pliers (Figure 14.33) in relation to the study models. The archwire length is then checked in the patient's mouth.
- An appropriate excess of distal length is often left on the archwire to permit either cinching or placement of bend backs. The wire ends may be heated to facilitate cinching, although it may be preferable to use an alternative approach not requiring heating of the wire, as described above.
- Tie lacebacks if required.
- Introduce the archwire into the molar tubes on either side, taking care that neither end cuts the patient's soft tissues. The clinician may direct the wire with their fingers or using Weingart pliers. The midline identifying marks on the archwire should be positioned in the midline of the dental arch (Figure 14.34).

- Before the first ligature is placed, inform the patient that they may get a 'tight' feeling as the 'wire is about to the tied'.
- The most displaced tooth is usually ligated first, although it may be useful to ligate one of the incisors first just to stabilise the archwire. Proceed to ligate all the teeth, either fully or partially.
- If using elastomeric modules, the patient may choose their favourite colour (Figure 14.35). The modules are usually pre-stretched (Figure 14.36), which increases their laxity, both for ease of engagement and potentially placing lighter forces whilst engaging the archwire. Each module is held securely in the mosquito pliers, enclosing one border edge of the module while leaving enough of the lumen exposed in order to permit easy ligation (Figure 14.37). Each elastomeric module is placed around one gingival bracket tie-wing, then both occlusal tie-wings and finally the other gingival tie-wing (Figure 14.38). Care should be taken not to slip, particularly as elastomeric modules sometimes snap during placement. If greater engagement is required, the elastomeric modules may be ligated in a **figure-of-eight** configuration. The module is placed over one gingival tie-wing, stretched down over and under the opposing occlusal tie-wing, stretched laterally under the adjacent occlusal tie-wing, and finally rotated round itself and stretched up and over the other gingival tie-wing (Figure 14.39).
- If using stainless steel ligatures, the archwire may be directed in position using a wire tucker. The steel ligatures are held in Mathieu pliers, and the narrow projecting loop of wire is squeezed between one's fingers to narrow it, and the loop is then turned up at 90°. This will make it easier to slide the steel ligature over and around each bracket (Figure 14.40). Steel ligatures, so long as not excessively tightened, provide less

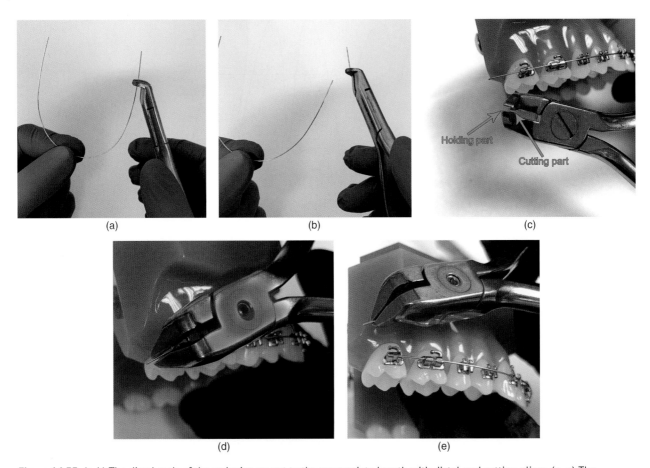

Figure 14.33 (a, b) The distal ends of the archwire are cut to the appropriate length with distal-end cutting pliers. (c–e) The distal-end wire cutter has juxtaposed cutting edges set at right angles to the long axis of the instrument. As the inner *cutting* part cuts the distal end of an archwire, the outer *holding* part grips the wire allowing its easy removal from the mouth.

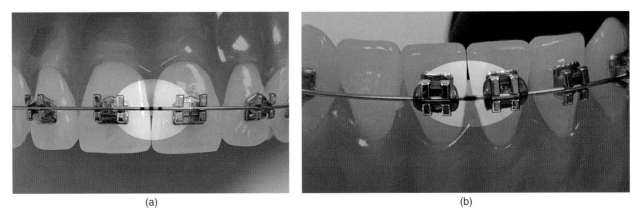

Figure 14.34 (a) Upper archwires tend to have three identifying marks, with the middle mark indicating the middle of the wire. (b) Lower archwires tend to have one midline identifying mark.

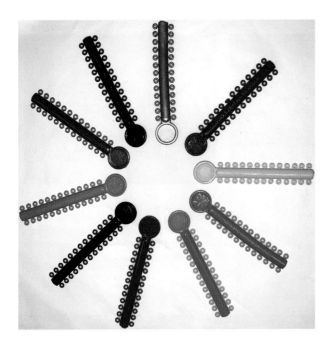

Figure 14.35 Elastomeric modules are available in different colours. Silver is the least noticeable with stainless steel brackets. Clear modules are available, but tend to pick up stain between patient visits.

friction and less resistance to sliding than elastomeric modules. Excessive tightening of steel ligatures may also notch and damage the archwire, potentially inhibiting the sliding of teeth. The excess wire is cut with ligature cutters and the twisted end is tucked under the archwire and bracket wings with a wire tucker (Figure 14.41).

- If using self-ligating brackets, the requirement for elastomeric modules or steel ligatures is obviated. It is important that the self-ligating mechanism is secure.
- The ends of the archwire are either cinched or bent back if required, or some other form of mechanism to limit archwire migration is employed.

Archwire Removal

When archwires need to be changed, removal of the ligatures is required. Elastomeric modules may be removed carefully using a dental probe (Figure 14.42) and stainless steel ligatures may be cut with a ligature cutter and removed (Figure 14.43), or alternatively the twisted end may be held in Mathieu pliers and unwound.

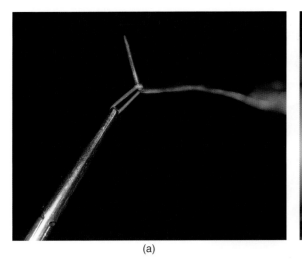

(a)

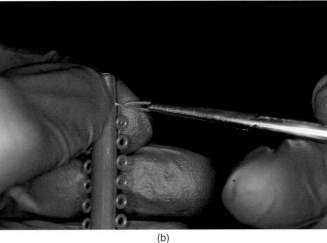

(b)

Figure 14.36 Pre-stretching elastomeric modules. (a) Whilst holding the module firmly with mosquito pliers, a dental probe may be used to stretch it. (b) Alternatively, the modules may be lightly stretched as they are removed from their holder.

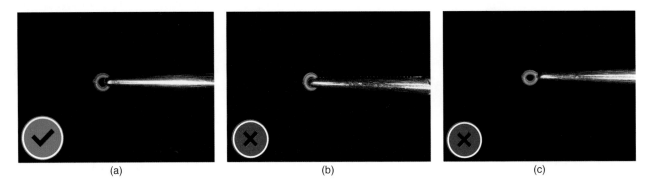

(a) (b) (c)

Figure 14.37 (a) Correct holding of an elastomeric module requires the mosquito pliers to enclose one border edge of the module while leaving enough of the lumen exposed in order to permit easy ligation. (b) Incorrect holding of an elastomeric module without exposing the lumen, which will prevent the module being placed around the bracket tie-wings. (c) Incorrect holding of an elastomeric module by insecure pinching of the edge, which will lead to the mosquito pliers coming off during attempted placement of the module.

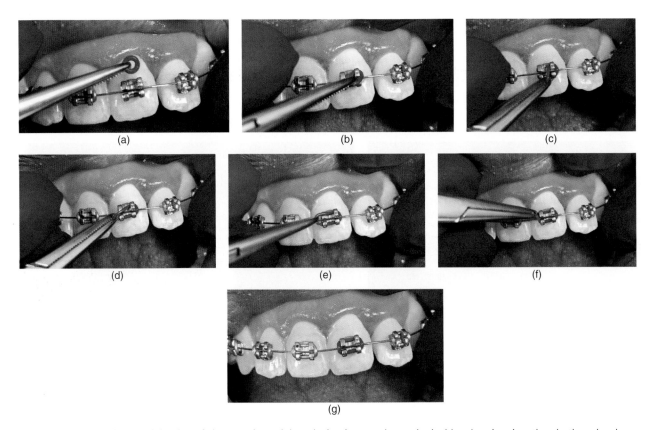

(a) (b) (c)
(d) (e) (f)
(g)

Figure 14.38 (a–g) Standard ligation of elastomeric modules, placing it around one gingival bracket tie-wing, then both occlusal tie-wings and finally the other gingival tie-wing.

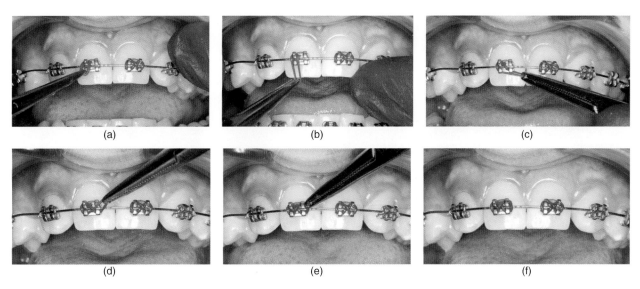

(a)   (b)   (c)

(d)   (e)   (f)

Figure 14.39 (a–f) Figure-of-eight ligation of elastomeric module.

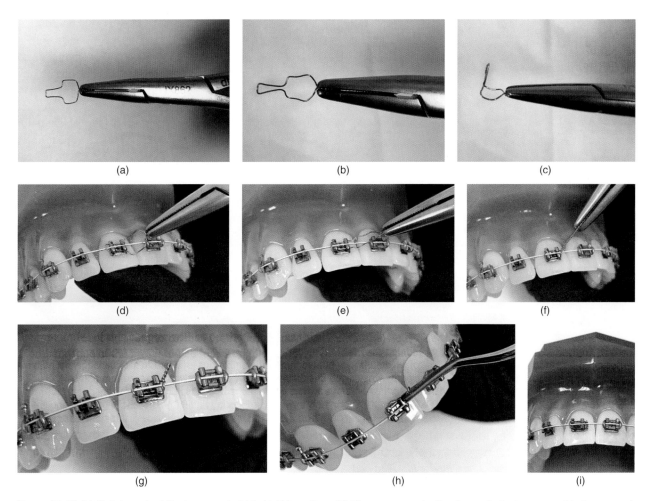

(a)   (b)   (c)

(d)   (e)   (f)

(g)   (h)   (i)

Figure 14.40 (a) Stainless steel ligatures are held in Mathieu pliers. (b) The narrow projecting loop of wire is squeezed between one's fingers to narrow it, and (c) the loop is then turned up at 90°, which will facilitate sliding the steel ligature over and around each bracket. (d–f) The ligature is tightened by twisting the Mathieu pliers. (g) The excess wire is cut with ligature cutters leaving approximately 3 mm of the twisted end. (h) The twisted end is tucked under the archwire and bracket wings with a wire tucker. (i) Steel ligature in situ. The clinician should gently run her finger over the bracket to ensure that there are no sharp ends of ligature wire.

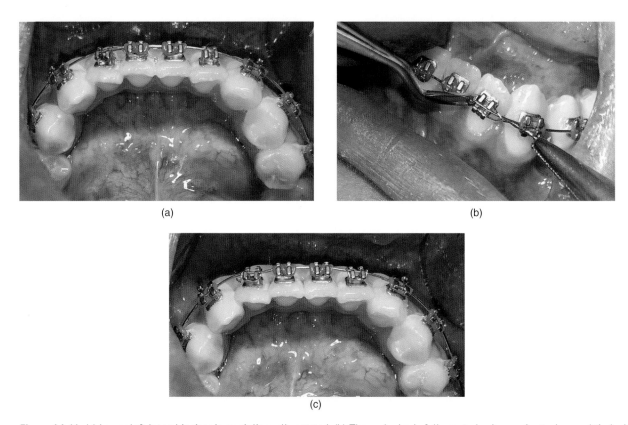

(a)

(b)

(c)

Figure 14.41 (a) Lower left lateral incisor is mesiolingually rotated. (b) The archwire is fully seated using a wire tucker, and tied with the steel ligature while held in position by the tucker. (c) Archwire fully engaged in lower left lateral incisor.

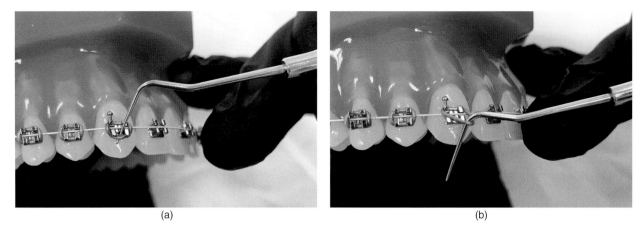

(a)

(b)

Figure 14.42 (a, b) Elastomeric modules may be removed carefully using a dental probe.

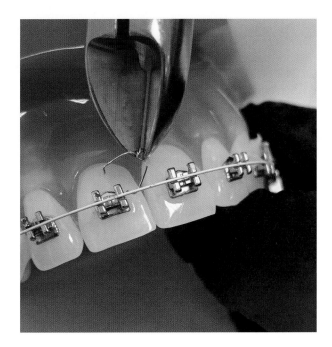

Figure 14.43 Stainless steel ligatures may be removed by cutting the plain side with wire cutters, then holding the twisted side with the same cutters and removing the ligature.

Removal of round or thin rectangular archwires is relatively straightforward and usually accomplished using a tool such as Weingart pliers. However, in the later stages of treatment when using a 0.022 × 0.028-inch bracket slot, a working archwire of 0.019 × 0.025-inch or even 0.0215 × 0.025-inch dimensions may be required. The removal of such archwires, particularly stainless steel archwires, from

molar tubes may be rather difficult if a traditional *pulling* force is applied to the archwire. The archwire often seems reluctant to move, leading to quite considerable discomfort for the patient. This is particularly relevant when changing the surgical archwires in the early postoperative period in the orthognathic surgery patient.[7]

A simple method to remove a heavy archwire without causing discomfort to the patient requires utilisation of the concept of leverage.[10] Having made sure that the archwire is not cinched or kinked in any way, Weingart pliers are placed on the archwire between the terminal molars, or between the terminal molar and premolar (Figure 14.44a). Contrary to the traditional method of archwire removal, the wire is *not pulled* out from the molar tubes. The pliers act as a lever arm with the pivot point being the embrasure between the teeth. While gripping the archwire firmly, the clinician moves the pliers mesially in an arc-type motion, gently *pushing* the archwire out of the buccal tubes (Figure 14.44b). The action is repeated until the archwire is free from the tubes.

Space Creation and Redistribution

There are a number of **methods of space creation** in orthodontics, and the clinician should be aware of the advantages and drawbacks of each approach (Table 14.4).

Dental extractions are deliberately at the bottom of this list. When a decision to extract teeth is taken, the clinician should be confident that it is in the best interest of the patient and is a justifiable requirement to achieve the best aesthetic, functional and

Figure 14.44 (a, b) With the pivot point between the posterior teeth, the pliers act as a lever arm, which is moved in a mesial arc-type motion and gently *pushes* the archwire out of the buccal tube.

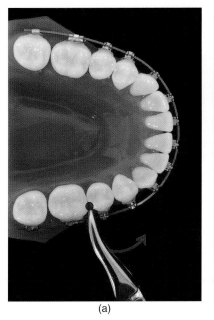

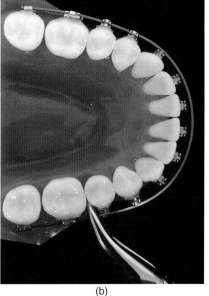

(a) (b)

Table 14.4 Methods of space creation in orthodontics.

Method of space creation	Advantages	Disadvantages
Increasing arch length by incisor proclination	Relatively easy technically	Must be controlled; excessive, uncontrolled incisor proclination has potentially severe deleterious aesthetic and functional consequences
Increasing arch length by distal movement, e.g. using headgear, removable appliances, or temporary anchorage devices (TADs)	Distal movement of molars may provide considerable space without the deleterious aesthetic consequences	Technically more difficult
		Requires considerable patient cooperation if using headgear or removable appliances
Increasing arch width dentally, e.g. expanded archwires, quadhelix, removable appliances with expansion screws	Relatively easy technically	Can lead to buccal flaring of molars and premolars
		May lead to root dehiscence through the buccal cortical plate, or may increase risk of gingival recession
Increasing arch width dentoskeletally, e.g. RME or SARPE	RME may be relatively straightforward to undertake	SARPE is a surgical procedure with postoperative morbidity
	Space provision is useful if there is pre-expansion dental crowding	Space provision is detrimental if there is no pre-expansion dental crowding
Interdental (interproximal) enamel reduction	Avoids dental extractions	Involves removal of tooth tissue, although small amounts appear to be acceptable, with no apparent long-term damage to the teeth
	Useful if incisors are triangular in shape, potentially reducing or eliminating interdental black triangles that often result when triangular incisors are aligned	This is usually undertaken following alignment
Dental extractions, e.g. premolars, molars, incisors or canines	Provides space, often close to where it is required, e.g. first premolar extractions if incisor retraction desired	Patients (and their parents) generally do not like the idea of dental extractions
	Can reduce treatment time, e.g. extraction of in-standing lateral incisor, or ectopic canine, as opposed to attempts at space creation and their alignment	Irreversible: if an incorrect extraction decision has been made, treatment time may be prolonged in attempts to close extraction spaces, and mechanics and anchorage control would need to be employed to avoid undesirable incisor retraction
	Very useful for:	
	Extreme crowding	
	Severe crowding in a dental arch not appropriate for arch expansion (e.g. normal arch width and no posterior crossbites, or thin gingival biotype and tendency to gingival recession)	
	Bimaxillary dental proclination	

RME, rapid maxillary expansion; SARPE, surgically assisted rapid palatal/maxillary expansion.

stable outcome (see Chapter 1). If in doubt, treatment may be undertaken with a **therapeutic diagnosis** approach, i.e. begin treatment on a non-extraction basis but inform the patient from the outset that a decision to extract dental units may be required during treatment.

Alignment in non-extraction cases often requires increasing the arch length, i.e. increasing the sagittal distance between the incisors and the molars (Figure 14.45). In situations where incisor proclination is acceptable or desirable, and depending on the extent of forward movement of the incisors that is required, a planned length of archwire may be left protruding from the distal part of the terminal molar tubes before being bent back. Therefore, theoretically the incisors will procline until the bend backs reach the distal part of the terminal molar tubes. Such bend backs in the archwire are important to prevent uncontrolled forward movement of the incisor teeth, e.g. if the patient misses subsequent appointments. The impetus for the forward movement of the incisors is predominantly from the mesial tip in the canine brackets, i.e. as the mesial tip in the canine bracket is expressed and

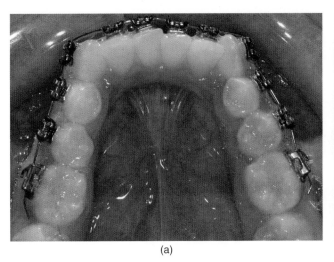
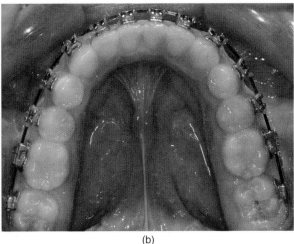

(a)   (b)

Figure 14.45 (a) Non-extraction alignment of the lower arch on initial bonding appointment with a NiTi archwire. Note that 2-mm length of archwire has been left protruding from the distal part of the terminal molar tubes before being bent back, in order to accommodate the planned increase in arch length. (b) Alignment has occurred predominantly by incisor proclination and concomitant increase in the arch length.

the canine crown tips mesially, the archwire will carry the ligated incisor teeth forward with it.

Non-extraction treatment where incisor proclination is undesirable will require an increase in arch length from **distal movement** of the posterior dentition (using headgear or miniscrew anchorage) and/or **interdental enamel reduction** (Figure 14.46).[11] Space for alignment may also be gained from increasing the arch width through dental and/or dentoskeletal arch expansion. From an aesthetic-centred perspective, non-extraction treatment

should be carefully planned and managed by the clinician in order not to produce excessive incisor protrusion or proclination.[12]

In patients with extremely severe crowding (greater than 9 mm per arch) where an increase in arch length is not desirable or sufficient to create space for alignment, and/or where there is significant incisor proclination that is an aesthetic concern for the patient, **dental extractions** (usually premolars) may be required. In such situations, the canines need to be retracted into the available

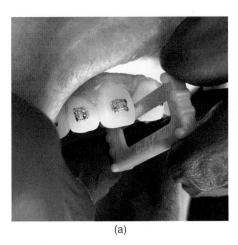
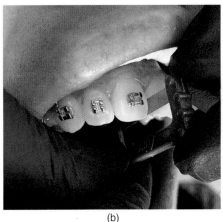

(a)   (b)

Figure 14.46 Interproximal or interdental enamel reduction (IPR or IDR), also termed enamel *stripping*, involves removal of enamel from the interproximal regions. The technique may be used to generate variable degrees of space per contact point depending on the thickness of enamel and tooth morphology. Up to approximately 0.5 mm of enamel per tooth (i.e. 1 mm per contact point) may be removed in the buccal segments, and up to 0.75 mm per contact point in the labial segments. Different methods of enamel reduction are available, including (a, b) handheld or (c, d) automated polishing strips, (e) discs with a slow handpiece (shown here with a guard), or very fine tungsten carbide or diamond burs with an air rotor (combined with water cooling to prevent rise in pulp temperature). (f) An incremental thickness gauge may be used to measure the amount of enamel removal required; these are usually available in thicknesses of 0.1, 0.2, 0.25, 0.3, 0.4 and 0.5 mm. The newly exposed enamel does not appear to be more susceptible to caries, but the application of topical fluoride varnish is advisable following enamel reduction.

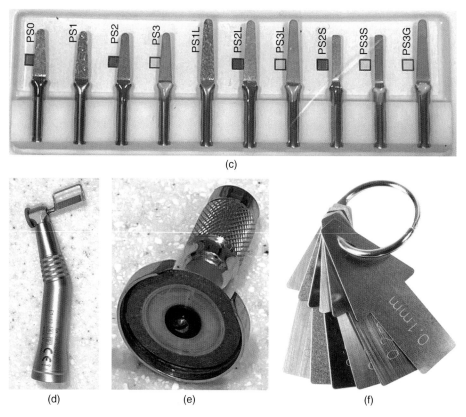

(c)

(d)   (e)   (f)

Figure 14.46 (*Continued*)

spaces to allow for alignment of the incisors. In extreme cases of crowding, the canines may need to be retracted independently (possibly with a sectional appliance before the incisors are bonded) in order to avoid excessive proclination of the incisors. This may require posterior **anchorage reinforcement** to prevent forward movement of the anchor teeth distal to the extracted premolars, for example using a Nance palatal arch, a combined TPA and Nance palatal arch (Figure 14.47), a lingual arch for the mandibular dental arch (Figure 14.48), TADs (see Chapter 12) or headgear (see Chapter 3). The canines may be retracted and/or distally tipped using elastic forces, which in some circumstances, such as forward positioned buccal canines, may be undertaken prior to engaging the archwire (Figure 14.49). Another useful technique is the use of **stopped arches**, although this would require

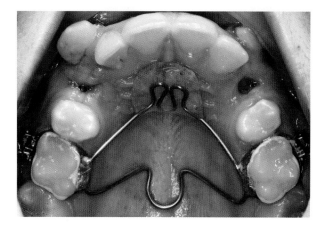

Figure 14.47 A transpalatal arch (TPA) with an omega loop is shown combined with a Nance arch, which has a palatal acrylic button that rests against the most superior–anterior aspect of the palatal vault. A TPA or Nance button may be used independently or combined for potentially greater posterior anchorage reinforcement.

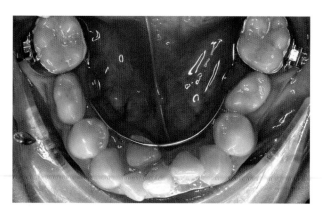

Figure 14.48 A lingual arch.

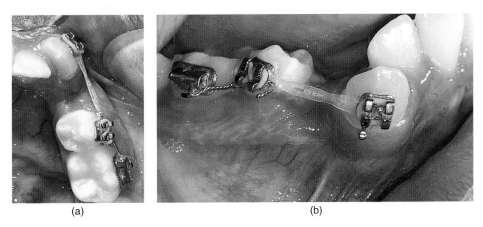

(a)   (b)

Figure 14.49 (a, b) Sectional lower fixed appliance to retract the forward and buccally positioned lower right canine tooth, prior to bonding the rest of the mandibular dental arch. This will avoid excessive proclination of the lower incisor teeth. The elastomeric chain is attached only to the distal wings of the canine bracket in order to reduce the tendency for mesiobuccal rotation. Once the canine is retracted at least partly into the first premolar space, the rest of the mandibular arch may be bonded.

an 0.018-inch stainless steel archwire, and thereby can only be undertaken when this archwire can be placed (Figure 14.50). From an aesthetic-centred perspective, extraction treatment should be carefully planned and managed by the clinician in order not to produce excessive incisor retraction; this is more pertinent to the space closure phase of treatment, but must also be considered during alignment.[12]

In cases of moderate to severe crowding (5–8 mm per arch) where extractions are required, it is possible to retract the canines whilst simultaneously aligning the incisor teeth, i.e. to avoid separate canine retraction.

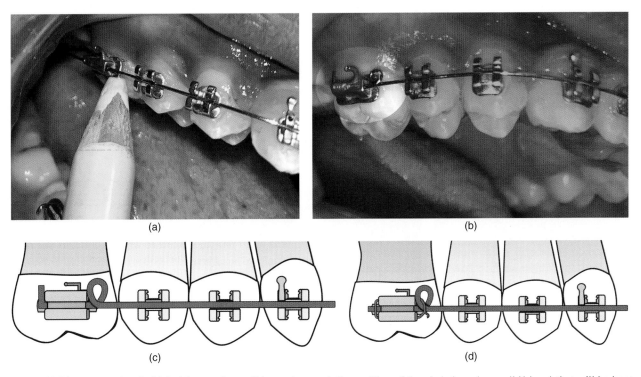

(a)   (b)

(c)   (d)

Figure 14.50 A stopped arch. (a) A chinagraph pencil is used to mark the position of the circle loop (or small U-loop) that will be bent into an 0.018-inch round stainless steel archwire. (b) A circle loop has been bent into position using light-wire pliers. (c) When the archwire is inserted into the molar tube, it is placed such that the circle loop is tight against the mesial aspect of the tube, and the wire is tightly cinched on exiting the molar tube. (d) The alternative to cinching the archwire is to tie the circle loop tightly with a stainless steel ligature to the molar tube or its hook. The techniques shown in (c) and (d) will effectively lock the molar against retracting forces to the anterior dentition, preventing mesial molar movement.

Crossbite Correction

Crossbites affecting individual incisor teeth are usually the result of severe crowding. Lateral incisors, particularly maxillary, are most commonly affected, being forced to erupt palatally when there is insufficient space in the dental arch, although any tooth may erupt into crossbite. When their alignment is desired, the first step is space creation. This is usually achieved by a combination of lightly active compressed coil spring (push-coil) between the teeth on either side of the in-standing tooth, sometimes combined with elastic pulling forces to distalise the same teeth (referred to as 'push–pull' mechanics). Usually slightly more space than is required is created (1–2 mm). This is followed by opening the bite if required, bearing in mind that patients have a freeway space, which in some patients may be enough to permit an in-standing tooth to be moved 'over the bite'. Either elastic forces or a piggyback NiTi may be used to align the incisor in crossbite (Figure 14.51). Crossbites involving in-standing teeth further posteriorly in the dental arch essentially follow a similar process (Figure 14.52).

Some patients present with a reverse incisor overjet that is dental in aetiology, rather than skeletal. If the maxillary incisor segment is in crossbite in a patient with an otherwise Class I skeletal pattern, with retroclined upper incisors, the ability to achieve an edge-to-edge incisor relationship, and an obvious forward mandibular displacement into a reverse incisor overjet, crossbite correction involves correcting the incisor inclinations, i.e. proclining the upper incisors and sometimes retroclining

the lower incisors (Figure 14.53). However, if the patient has signs of a moderate to severe Class III skeletal pattern or compensated retroclined mandibular incisors, crossbite correction of the incisor segment should not be attempted, as it is most likely to require subsequent orthognathic correction.

Posterior crossbites of skeletal aetiology, i.e. resulting from a narrow maxilla, usually benefit from skeletal widening of the maxilla. This may be achieved by rapid maxillary expansion (RME) if undertaken prior to maturation of the palatal midline suture (Figure 14.54), or possibly with surgical expansion in later years. In some patients, the severity of crowding may be such that premolar extractions may still be required, even after such expansion (Figure 14.55). Once such expansion has been achieved, the RME appliance should be kept in situ for approximately three months, allowing time for bony infill of the opened palatal suture. Following removal of the RME appliance, maintaining the widened arch may be achieved with placement of a heavy auxiliary archwire constructed at the chairside. This may be made from an expanded 0.019 × 0.025-inch stainless steel or a larger round steel wire with a diameter of 1–1.13 mm, which runs over the main archwire and is inserted into the headgear or auxiliary tubes of the first molar bands and secured anteriorly with a ligature.

Posterior dental crossbites may be corrected with expanded archwires, a quadhelix or cross elastics. Cross elastics usually extend from the palatal cleats on upper molar bands, or bonded buttons on the palatal aspect of upper premolars, to the buccal attachment of the opposing

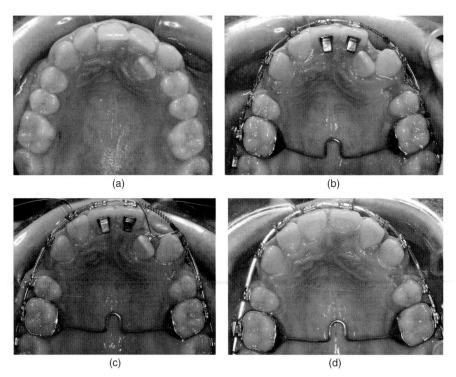

(a) (b)

(c) (d)

Figure 14.51 (a) Space creation for upper left lateral incisor, which was in crossbite. (b) Space has been created by extraction of first premolar teeth, and a transpalatal arch placed for anchorage reinforcement. Sliding mechanics are being undertaken on a 0.018-inch round stainless steel archwire, which is useful for sliding the teeth along the archwire. Active compressed coil spring, also known as a 'push-coil' (a coil whose helices are spaced, allowing it to be compressed along its long axis; it is cut to a length greater than the interbracket span between the teeth that are to be moved apart, and is compressed prior to insertion), is being used between the central incisor and canine to push these teeth apart, and the canines are also being retracted simultaneously. (c) The bite has been opened with bite turbos, and a piggyback NiTi is being used to align the lateral incisor and move it 'over the bite'. (d) The lateral incisor has been aligned.

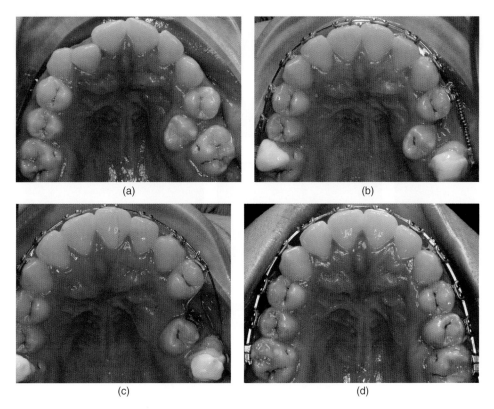

Figure 14.52 (a) Upper second premolar crowded palatally and in crossbite. (b) Space creation with active compressed coil spring. (c) Alignment with piggyback NiTi archwire and bite opening with glass ionomer cement on occlusal surfaces of molars. (d) Second premolar aligned.

lower teeth (see Chapter 11, Figure 11.3). The extrusive component of these elastics must be borne in mind, which has a tendency to open the bite anteriorly. Their use is often short term and must be monitored closely.

Ectopic and Impacted Canines and Incisors

The terms 'ectopic' and 'impacted' are not interchangeable. An **ectopic tooth** is one that has developed in an abnormal position. This may be due to an abnormal initial position of the developing tooth bud or from a developing tooth going off course during its development and possibly eruption. An **impacted tooth** is one whose path of eruption has been impeded by another structure, e.g. other teeth in a crowded dental arch, a supernumerary tooth, or excessively thick gingival soft tissues.

In either situation, the treatment plan may dictate alignment rather than surgical removal of an ectopic or impacted tooth. With impacted teeth, they may well erupt if the impediment to their eruption is removed and if space is created for them in the dental arch. However, particularly with maxillary canines and incisors, they often need orthodontic force to guide their eruption into the correct position.

The first step in orthodontic alignment of ectopic or severely impacted teeth is **precise localisation**. The traditional **tube-shift** or **parallax technique**,[13] using two radiographs taken at different angles, may be employed, particularly for maxillary canines. The **vertical parallax** technique uses a panoramic radiograph and an upper occlusal radiograph, whereas the **horizontal parallax** technique is usually undertaken with two periapical radiographs taken at two different horizontal X-ray tube positions. Either way, if the unerupted canine is palatal in position, it will appear to move between the two radiographs in the direction of the X-ray tube shift. However, with more difficult cases, the most accurate three-dimensional localisation of unerupted teeth is with **cone beam computed tomography (CBCT)**.

The next step in preparatory orthodontics is **space creation**. A TPA is placed to provide some vertical anchorage support for when vertical traction is applied to a high canine, and transverse anchorage for when moving palatally erupted canines buccally. Space is created in the appropriate position within the dental arch for the unerupted tooth. If not already established, once space has been created, the clinician should work up to a relatively heavy base archwire, at least a 0.018-inch stainless steel, if not a rectangular steel archwire. Once surgical exposure has been undertaken, this will permit active forces to be placed on the unerupted tooth as soon as a point of application has been established.

Surgical exposure of an unerupted tooth may be undertaken with an open or closed exposure. An **open exposure**

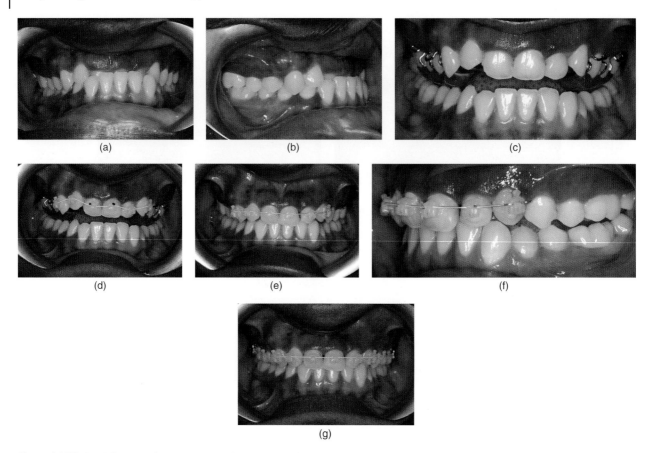

Figure 14.53 (a–g) Some patients present with a reverse incisor overjet that is dental in aetiology, rather than skeletal. If the maxillary incisor segment is in crossbite in a patient with an otherwise Class I skeletal pattern, with retroclined upper incisors, the ability to achieve an edge-to-edge incisor relationship, and an obvious forward mandibular displacement into a reverse incisor overjet, crossbite correction involves correcting the incisor inclinations. In this patient, the bite was opened with an upper removable appliance with posterior bite planes. The maxillary incisors were proclined initially with a sectional fixed appliance.

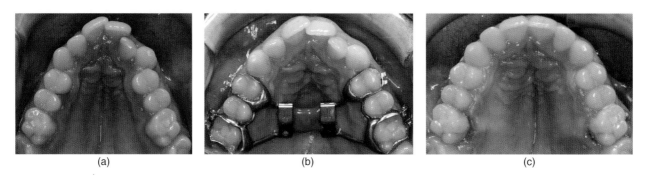

Figure 14.54 (a) Narrow V-shaped maxillary arch. (b) Following active rapid maxillary expansion (RME) for two weeks, the screw is stabilised with glass ionomer cement to prevent it turning backwards, and the appliance is maintained in situ for three months to allow for bony infill of the opened midpalatal suture. (c) At debond, a broader U-shaped maxillary arch.

may be undertaken, particularly for palatal canines, which involves the surgical removal of a window of palatal mucosa and overlying bone to create a channel through which the canine erupts unaided. A surgical pack is usually sutured into the exposed area for a week following the surgery to prevent the mucosa growing over the exposed site. Although given time these teeth often erupt spontaneously, or if an attachment is bonded at a later date, excessive mucosal removal in creation of the channel may result in the less than ideal attachment of gingiva and an elongated canine crown appearance.[14, 15] Alternatively, and more routinely, a **closed exposure** is undertaken,

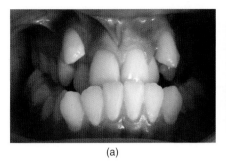
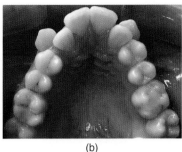
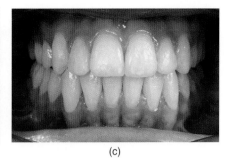

(a)   (b)   (c)

Figure 14.55 (a, b) Hypoplastic maxilla in a severe skeletal Class III with severe crowding. Following RME, upper first premolars were extracted to create further space for alignment and correct incisor positioning. (c) Following bimaxillary surgery, at debond.

which involves surgical reflection of a flap, removal of a small section of overlying alveolar bone, and bonding of a **gold chain attachment** to the crown.[16] The flap is sutured back in position, but with the gold chain drawn through into the mouth *along the proposed path of eruption*, allowing traction to be placed to the unerupted tooth.

Palatal canines which have developed close to the roots of the incisor teeth should first be moved further palatally, away from the roots of the incisors, before being moved laterally into the line of the arch. The palatal movement may be achieved using **elastomeric thread/string**, a stretchable thread, that is available in a variety of cross-sectional thicknesses and which may be used as a force-producing mechanism for the application of forces to these teeth. The elastomeric thread is tied from the gold chain to a hook soldered to the arm of a TPA (Figure 14.56). Once some palatal movement has occurred, lateral and eruptive movements may be achieved with elastic thread from the gold chain to the base archwire.

With buccally impacted canines, it is vital that their created path of eruption is through attached gingiva, not alveolar mucosa. If a gold chain has been bonded subgingivally, it should be brought through the attached gingiva.

Alternatively, if the canine is not vertically too far from the arch, an **apically repositioned flap** may be reflected, suturing the attached gingiva where the crown has been exposed, and allowing the tooth to erupt through attached gingiva. If a buccal canine is not too far out of position and there is a relatively wide band of attached gingiva, a window may be excised such as to leave a band of attached gingiva covering the cervical area of the canine crown. This will ensure that the eventually well-aligned canine will be invested with attached gingiva.

Orthodontic traction should begin as soon as possible after surgical exposure, ideally immediately following the procedure. Traction may be applied to the canine tooth via the attached gold chain using elastomeric thread (Figure 14.57). Alternatively, a piggyback NiTi may be threaded through the gold chains (see Figure 14.56).

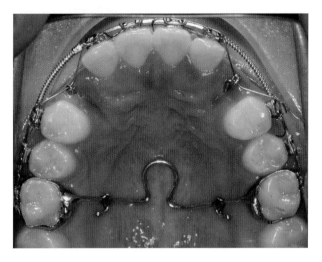

Figure 14.56 Transpalatal arch (TPA) with hooks soldered to its arms, which were used to pull the unerupted canines palatally away from the incisor roots. The canines are now being aligned with piggyback NiTi archwires threaded through the gold chains attached to the unerupted canines.

Another technique is the ballista-type spring, which is a vertical spring constructed from an auxiliary 0.014-inch stainless steel archwire.[17] The ballista spring is a loop bent into the wire, which passively lies at 90° occlusally to the dental arch. Activation involves rotating the loop through approximately 90° palatally to be ligated to the gold chain (see Chapter 11, Figure 11.27). Once the canine is sufficiently erupted, it may be aligned using elastomeric thread or a piggyback NiTi.

A potential problem with attempts to align impacted teeth is their **ankylosis**. Ankylosed teeth will not move, and orthodontic traction will lead to undesirable tilting and potentially intrusion of the anchor teeth adjacent to the space. Sometimes canines begin to move and their ankylosis occurs during traction. In such situations the area of ankylosis may be small, and it may be possible to lightly luxate the tooth to free the ankylosis, under local anaesthesia, although traction would have to be reapplied

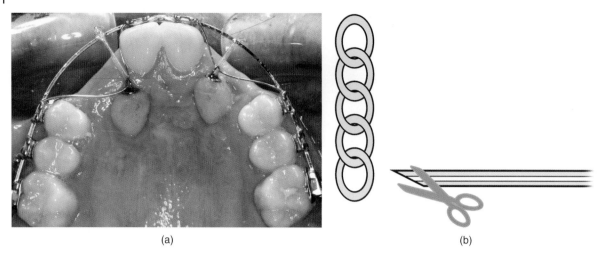

(a)   (b)

Figure 14.57 (a) Maxillary canines being aligned with elastomeric thread/string as well as piggyback NiTi archwires. (b) In order to more easily thread the elastomeric string through a small diameter link of a gold chain or any other attachment, the tip of the elastomeric thread should be cut at an oblique angle. The sharper end is easier to thread.

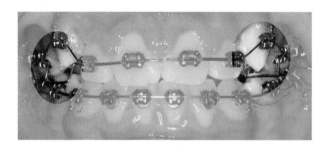

Figure 14.58 Vertical steps bent into the base archwire adjacent to the brackets on either side of the space in order to reduce the potential unwanted movement of anchor teeth (in this case intrusion of the lateral incisor and first premolar teeth).

immediately, before re-ankylosis occurs. In order to prevent or at least limit unwanted movement of anchor teeth, vertical steps may be bent into the base archwire, adjacent to the brackets on either side of the space (Figure 14.58). The vertical legs of the stepped archwire will provide some impediment to unwanted tilting and vertical movement of the anchor teeth (in this case the lateral incisor and first premolar), and the step will permit a greater range of movement for the tooth and the applied traction.

Most of this information is pertinent to impacted maxillary incisors. However, it is imperative to assess preoperative radiographs for root dilaceration. A lateral cephalometric radiograph or CBCT may be required. The placement of the gold chain attachment may be better near or potentially customised for the incisal edge.[18]

Impacted Mandibular Second Molars

Impaction of mesioangular mandibular second molars occurs when their mesial marginal ridge becomes trapped against the distal aspect of the first molar. In early adolescence, mild mesial impaction of mandibular second molars often spontaneously corrects following loss of the second deciduous molars and subsequent mesial drift of the first molars. In such patients, monitoring the dental development is often the best course of action.

In older patients, or more significant impaction, the second molar needs to be distally tipped in order to disimpact from the first molar. In milder impactions, a separator may be placed between the first and second molar teeth, and may be enough to permit the second molar to disimpact and erupt into position. In more severe impactions, active appliance treatment may be required. If a developing third molar is present close to the distal aspect of the second molar, it may need to be surgically removed. At this stage of development, third molar removal is relatively straightforward as significant root formation has not yet taken place. If the second molar can be bonded with a buccal tube in as close to the correct position as possible, an auxiliary spring may be designed, either to be placed in the auxiliary tube of the first molar or alternatively simply clipped over a rigid base archwire as a cantilever spring (Figure 14.59). Either way, the effect is to distally angulate and extrude the second molar. Once disimpacted, a flexible rectangular archwire may be placed to achieve full alignment.

Intrusion of Overerupted Maxillary Second Molars

A conventional method for intruding overerupted maxillary second molars is to place a convertible molar band on the first molar tooth, and a step-up bend in a rectangular archwire to intrude the second molar (Figure 14.60).

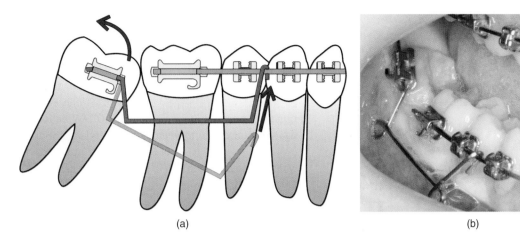

(a) (b)

Figure 14.59 (a) An auxiliary cantilever spring may be used to generate the force required to disimpact a mesioangular impaction of a mandibular second molar tooth. (b) A clinical case using a 0.019 × 0.025-inch stainless steel base archwire and a 0.017 × 0.025 TMA cantilever spring.

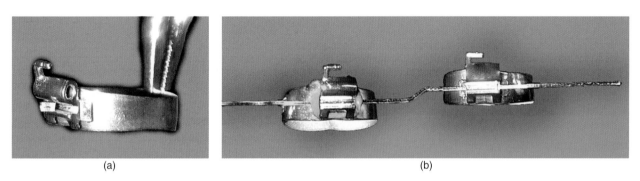

(a) (b)

Figure 14.60 (a) Ligature cutters may be used to peel back and remove the buccal cap from a convertible molar tube, which converts the tube into a bracket. (b) Converting the first molar tube into a bracket permits insertion of a continuous archwire with a step between the first and second molars, which would otherwise not be possible. Source: Naini FB, Gill DS (eds). *Orthognathic Surgery: Principles, Planning and Practice.* Oxford: Wiley Blackwell, 2017. Reprinted with permission.

Alternatively, TADs such as miniscrews/mini-implants may be used to help intrude maxillary second molars.

Diastema Closure and Frenectomy

The simple presence of a labial frenum, or a maxillary dental midline diastema, should not be an unconsidered indication for frenectomy. The principal indications, all relatively uncommon, for an upper labial frenectomy are as follows.[19]

- The presence of a low (inferiorly attached, towards the gingival margin), thick and fleshy frenal attachment, which may be unattractive and a concern for the patient (Figure 14.61).
- The frenum is a potential obstruction to the maintenance of good oral hygiene, or causing recurrent trauma with toothbrushing.
- Tethering of the upper lip by the frenum, leading to hypomobility of the philtrum of the upper lip.

The presence of a diastema less than approximately 2 mm may be considered normal in the mixed dentition stage of dental development (referred to as physiological spacing), with the diastema often closing spontaneously upon eruption of the maxillary canines.

As already mentioned, neither the presence of an upper labial frenum nor a maxillary dental midline diastema is in itself an indication for a frenectomy. This is the case even when pulling the upper lip away from the dentoalveolus leads to visualisation of blanching in the palatal mucosa. This blanching is an indication that fibrous tissue from the labial frenum is passing between the central incisors, usually through an alveolar notch in the region of the diastema, and inserting into the palatal mucosa. Maintenance of orthodontic closure of a significant diastema would require a palatal bonded retainer regardless of whether a frenectomy has been undertaken, owing to the fact that such space closure is predominantly unstable. As

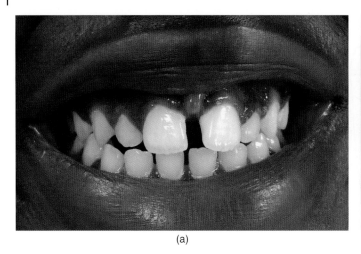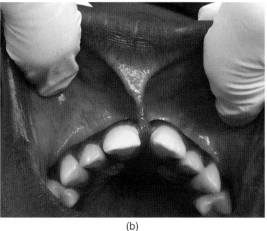

(a) (b)

Figure 14.61 (a, b) A low (inferiorly attached), thick and fleshy frenal attachment, which is evident on smiling and a concern for the patient.

such, there is no automatic requirement for an additional frenectomy. Furthermore, undertaking a frenectomy too early and removing the interdental fibres leads to scar tissue formation, generating an obstacle which may lead to difficulties in subsequent diastema closure. Therefore, frenectomy is almost always contraindicated prior to orthodontic treatment. When a frenectomy is indicated, the timing should be agreed between the orthodontist and surgeon.

The frenectomy may be undertaken when the incisor teeth are orthodontically aligned and space closure is imminent or partial space closure has been undertaken, i.e. during orthodontic treatment. As such, the surgeon has interdental space to carry out the procedure safely, and space closure may be instigated or resumed immediately following surgery. Theoretically, the subsequent scar tissue formation may help to keep the diastema closed (Figure 14.62). However, it is imperative to point out that as stability remains an issue, a palatal bonded retainer will still be indicated.

Wire Bending

Preadjusted edgewise appliances have significantly reduced the requirement for wire bending, and in simpler cases may obviate their need. However, dental morphology and size is variable, as are jaw relationships. As such, inevitably, for some patients the bracket prescriptions will not take the clinician from the A to Z of planned treatment, leaving the final part of the journey to artistic wire bending in order to achieve the optimal outcome. Although artistic bends are often required during the finishing stages of treatment, they may nevertheless also be considered as part of final alignment.

Clinicians should be familiar with certain wire bends, which include first-, second- and third-order bends (Figures 14.63 and 14.64), loops (such as the ballista-type spring or circle loops) (Figure 14.65), the incorporation of progressive or continuous torque for the buccal segments (Figures 14.66 and 14.67), and the incorporation of accentuated or reverse curves of Spee (Figure 14.68).

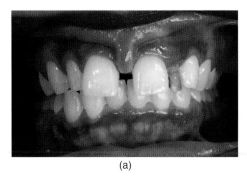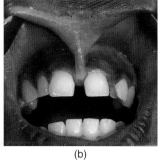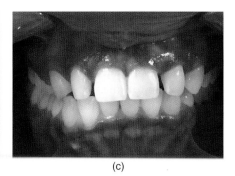

(a) (b) (c)

Figure 14.62 (a, b) A low, thick frenal attachment with maxillary dental midline diastema. (c) Frenectomy was undertaken after partial closure of the diastema, following which the diastema was closed. A palatal bonded retainer was placed to maintain the space closure.

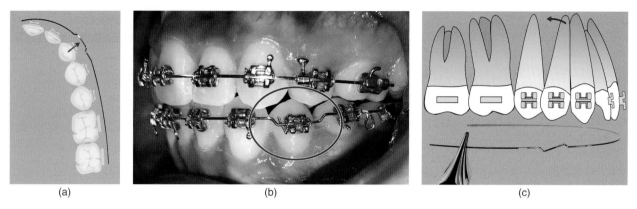

(a) (b) (c)

Figure 14.63 (a) First-order horizontal bend to buccally offset a maxillary canine tooth. (b) First-order vertical bend to intrude a mandibular premolar tooth. (c) Second-order 'angulation' or 'tip' bend to correct the first premolar angulation. First- and second-order bends are usually placed with light-wire pliers. After such archwire bends have been placed, it is important to test the archwire on a flat piece of glass or table top in order to detect and thereby correct any unwanted deflections from the horizontal plane.

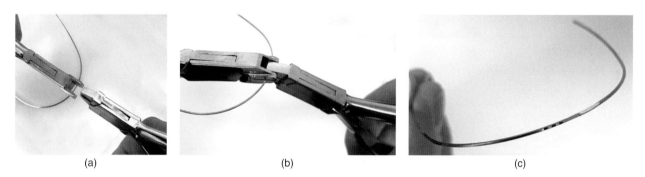

(a) (b) (c)

Figure 14.64 (a–c) Third-order 'torquing' bends for individual teeth may be placed with individual torquing pliers. The archwire should be marked with a chinagraph pencil in the mouth, ensuring the accuracy of the bends. After such archwire bends have been placed, it is important to test the archwire on a flat piece of glass or table top in order to detect and thereby correct any unwanted deflections from the horizontal plane.

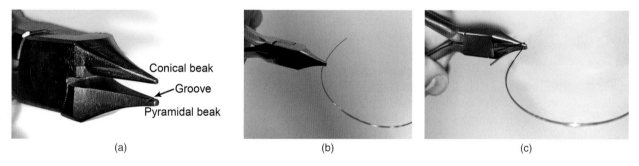

(a) (b) (c)

Figure 14.65 (a) Light-wire pliers. These pliers have two slender beaks, one conical and an opposing pyramidal beak, and are very useful for bending small circle and U-loops and springs. Ideally, they should have one or more grooves near the tip of the pyramidal beak, which aid in making reproducible loops and helices. (b) To bend a circle loop: first mark the archwire with a chinagraph pencil based on study models or in the mouth, in order for the loop to be in the correct position. Hold the wire (here, an 0.018-inch round stainless steel archwire) positioned in the groove on the pyramidal beak, with the conical beak on top. (c) Use the thumb of your free hand to turn the free end of the archwire through almost half a circle. (d) Change your thumb position to the other side and continue turning the free end until it is approximately turned through three-quarters of a circle. (e) Keeping the wire position stationary, rotate the pliers through 45°. (f) Place the thumb of your free hand underneath the wire and continue turning the wire as far as possible, changing the position of the pliers as required until a rotation has been achieved through a complete 360°. (g) Finally, check that the wire arms are both symmetrical and flat.

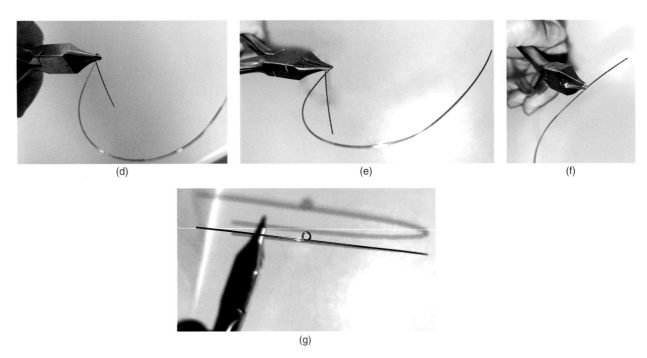

(d) (e) (f)

(g)

Figure 14.65 (*Continued*)

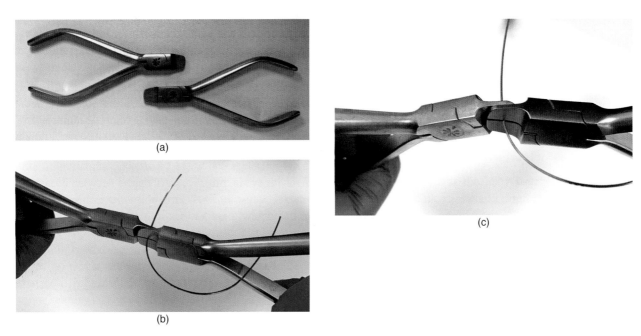

(a)

(b)

(c)

Figure 14.66 Continuous buccal segment torque. (a) Tweed torquing pliers are used to place torque in square or rectangular archwires. The pair of pliers have symmetrically flattened blades that fit parallel to one another at a separation of 0.020 inch (0.5 mm). (b) This torquing activation may be placed by holding the archwire with one of the pair of pliers distal to the canine, and holding the other pliers very closely from the opposite side and (c) twisting in the appropriate direction, depending on whether continuous buccal or lingual/palatal torque is desired. In terms of biomechanics, the tooth immediately distal to the position of the pliers inevitably will get more torque activation, so it is not accurately a continuous effect for the entire buccal segment.

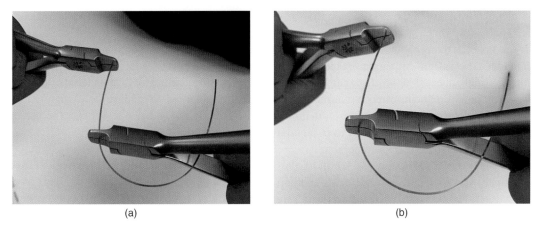

(a) (b)

Figure 14.67 Progressive buccal segment torque. (a) This torquing activation is undertaken by holding the archwire with one of the pair of Tweed torquing pliers distal to the canine and the other pair of pliers close to the end of the wire. (b) The latter is twisted in the appropriate direction, depending on whether progressive buccal or lingual/palatal torque is desired.

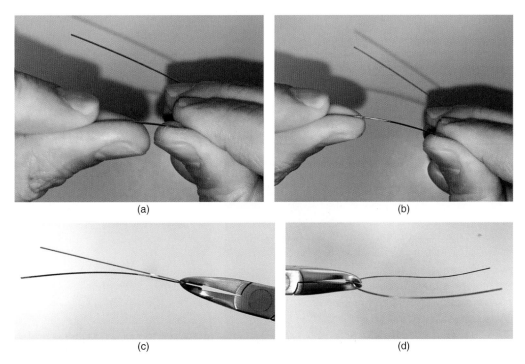

(a) (b)

(c) (d)

Figure 14.68 Bending a reverse curve of Spee in mandibular steel archwire. (a) Hold the archwire in the region of the canine on one side between your right thumb and index finger, with the free ends of the wire pointing to your left. Place the index finger of your left hand on the upper surface of the wire, approximately 15 mm behind your thumb, which is on the lower surface of the wire. (b) In a gradual sweeping motion, press upwards with your left thumb and downwards with your left index finger whilst pulling the archwire with your right hand. (c) Check the curve in that leg of the archwire relative to the contralateral straight leg. This process is repeated for the opposite leg of the wire. (d) Finally, check the archwire from the lateral aspect to ensure that both legs of the wire have the same degree of curvature.

Pain from Initial Archwires

Evidence for pain from initial archwires is minimal and difficult to obtain, as it is primarily reliant on patient-reported pain experiences.[20] However, there does appear to be relatively wide individual variation in the degree of pain experienced, with many patients comparing the sensation to the tight feeling when getting used to new shoes, whilst others can experience quite considerable discomfort. Either way, discomfort usually begins a few hours after initial archwire engagement, progressively escalates reaching a peak 24–72 hours later, then gradually diminishes over the next few days. Patients should be informed of this general trend and the wide individual variation in the level of pain they may experience. Analgesics may be started prior to the onset of discomfort and taken as required thereafter. It may be prudent to avoid non-steroidal anti-inflammatory medications (e.g. aspirin, ibuprofen) due to their prostaglandin secretion inhibitory effects, thereby reducing osteoclast numbers and potentially decreasing the speed of orthodontic tooth movement; however, reducing patient discomfort over the first few days may be considered more important.

Some patients may develop pulpal-type discomfort, possibly from pulpal hyperaemia, as opposed or in addition to the expected periodontal pain.[21] There have been rare reports of severe pain from single teeth, which continued following archwire removal and all but immediately disappeared upon removal of the bracket, which may therefore be postulated to have been due to deformation of the crown from a bonded bracket.[21]

Accelerated Tooth Movement

A number of surgical and non-surgical methods have been described with the intended benefit of accelerating orthodontic tooth movement. **Non-surgical methods** include low-level laser therapy, pulsed electromagnetic fields, vibrational forces and even the potential bone regeneration enhancement of relaxin injections. A prospective randomised clinical trial found no evidence to support the use of supplemental vibrational forces with preadjusted edgewise fixed appliances in order to accelerate the rate of initial tooth movement or reduce the amount of time required to achieve final alignment,[22] and there is currently no evidence to support the use of any of the described non-surgical methods.[23]

A number of methods have also been described involving different types of **adjunctive surgical interventions**. The theoretical background is that these procedures may accelerate regional orthodontic tooth movement by stimulation of bone metabolism resulting from controlled surgical trauma. The orthopaedic surgeon Herald Frost first described how controlled osseous surgical trauma results in restructuring activity adjacent to the surgical site, thereby coining the term **regional acceleratory phenomenon (RAP)** to describe the subsequent cascade of physiological healing.[24–26] This forms the basis of the concept of accelerating orthodontic tooth movement by undertaking small surgical perforations in the buccal cortical plate in the region requiring the most tooth movement (Figure 14.69).

A systematic review of adjunctive surgical interventions to accelerate tooth movement found limited research

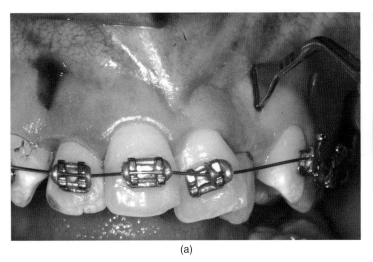

(a)

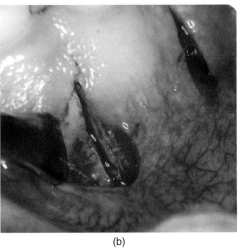

(b)

Figure 14.69 (a) Piezo-cut in the buccal cortical plate. (b) Piezo-cuts in the mandibular buccal cortical plate. Source: courtesy of Dr Elif Keser. The piezoelectric effect was discovered by Paul-Jacques Curie together with his younger brother Pierre Curie (husband of Marie Sklodowska-Curie) in 1880 and it has had multiple applications, one of which has been in surgery. Piezosurgery (piezoelectric bone surgery) involves piezoelectric ultrasonic microvibrations for precise and selective cutting of bone without injuring surrounding soft tissues. The ultrasonic frequency is modulated in the range 25–50 kHz, causing microvibrations of 60–210 µm. The low frequency enables the cutting of mineralised tissues but not soft tissues. Piezocision is performed after the placement of orthodontic appliances. The patient is anaesthetised with local anaesthetic infiltration; once a complete anaesthesia is achieved a small vertical incision is performed buccally and interproximally in the attached gingiva or mucosa. A mid-root level incision is made between the roots of the teeth involved. The soft tissues and the periosteum need to be cut to create access for the insertion of the piezoelectric knife. The tip of the piezotome is inserted in the opening and a 3-mm depth piezoelectrical corticotomy is performed. The depth of the corticotomy is extremely important. The decortication has to pass through the cortical layer and reach the medullary bone in order to achieve the full effect of the regional acceleratory phenomenon (RAP). Hard and soft tissue grafts can be added via a tunnelling procedure in areas with thin gingivae, recession, thin cortical bone or dehiscences.

concerning their effectiveness, with the available evidence being of low quality.[27] Nevertheless, the conclusion reached was that these procedures appear to show some promise as a means of accelerating tooth movement and may prove useful; however, further prospective research with longer follow-up is required to confirm potential benefits.

Orthodontists with considerable experience in treating orthognathic surgical patients will often attest to the clinical observation that the patient's teeth often move faster in the six to eight weeks following surgery. Therefore, the concept of accelerating tooth movement deserves further investigation. Other potential situations where this concept may be useful include planning the surgical exposure of impacted teeth to permit the immediate postoperative application of traction, and undertaking dental extractions near the time of space closure, if the space is not needed sooner, which may accelerate subsequent tooth movement. However, logic and common sense would dictate that there are certain specific situations, e.g. extreme difficulty in moving teeth or attempts to close large spaces, where acceleration of tooth movement would be particularly advantageous. In most instances, 'patience is a virtue' and orthodontic treatment may be safely undertaken without the need for additional speed.

Levelling

Dental arch levelling may be defined as the stage of treatment which aims to flatten, or almost flatten, the curve of Spee (i.e. the sagittal curve of the occlusion) by permitting the relative vertical movement of the teeth in each arch in order to bring their marginal ridges to lie approximately in the same horizontal plane. A relatively flat (i.e. 'level') curve of Spee is one of the prerequisites to a normal dental occlusion.

Comprehensive planning permits the clinician to determine whether levelling of the dental arches will be undertaken by maxillary and/or mandibular incisor intrusion, by molar and premolar extrusion, or a combination of the two.

The treatment planning decision is primarily based on aesthetic considerations.[1] If the maxillary incisor exposure at rest is acceptable, maxillary incisor intrusion should be avoided. In such situations, absolute or relative mandibular incisor intrusion is recommended. In a *growing patient* with a reduced lower anterior face height (LAFH), vertical extrusion of the mandibular molars will *relatively* intrude the incisors, i.e. the mandibular incisors do not actually intrude into the alveolus, but the incisor overbite reduces due to extrusion of the posterior teeth. In an adult patient with no vertical growth potential, absolute intrusion of

the mandibular incisors is required. Conversely, if the maxillary incisor exposure in relation to the upper lip is increased (e.g. overerupted maxillary incisors), intrusion of the maxillary incisors would be beneficial. Combinations of these approaches may be required depending on the clinical presentation.

In the vast majority of patients, arch levelling occurs by working through progressively stiffer continuous flat archwires. A typical archwire sequence of progression is as follows.

- **Initial wire (round NiTi):** this is predominantly for alignment, though it will begin gentle levelling of the bracket slots relative to one another. The usual initial archwire is 0.014-inch NiTi (0.012 inch in adults or patients with severe imbrication), followed by 0.016-inch NiTi or 0.018-inch heat-activated NiTi.
- **Interim wire**
  - **Round stainless steel:** usually an 0.018-inch stainless steel, although an 0.016-inch steel may be used if there is difficulty engaging the larger wire. This wire will begin levelling in cases where sliding mechanics are required, or retroclination/proclination of incisors, or possibly maintenance of arch expansion.
  - **Rectangular NiTi:** alternatively, in patients where a round stainless steel wire is not required, the clinician may progress to a rectangular NiTi, using 0.017 × 0.025-inch, 0.018 × 0.025-inch or 0.019 × 0.025-inch wire. This is essentially a transition wire to the subsequent rectangular stainless steel wires. The largest wire that can be engaged without causing patient discomfort should be used.
- **Rectangular stainless steel:** this is the working archwire, which in most patients will be a 0.019 × 0.025-inch steel. Because of its stiffness this is a useful continuous archwire for levelling, but patience is required in providing time for such levelling to occur.

When using flat continuous archwires, a larger bracket slot (i.e. a 0.022 × 0.028-inch as opposed to a 0.018 × 0.025-inch bracket slot) may be beneficial, as it permits the use of heavier steel archwires and thereby potentially better arch levelling.

In the mandibular arch, it is advisable to band the second molars as early as possible in alignment, and to cinch the archwires to reduce the tendency to incisor proclination while the arch is levelling (i.e. the flat continuous archwire is trying to flatten itself, thereby vertically levelling the teeth in the dental arch). Despite even tight cinching of archwires, an element of incisor proclination is an inevitable consequence of arch levelling. Clinical situations which call for restriction on incisor proclination may require segmental mechanics to level the arch (see

Chapter 20). Alternatives include aiding arch levelling with an anterior bite plane, perhaps prior to fixed appliance treatment, or the use of lingual brackets, which due to their position closer to the centre of resistance of the mandibular incisors may have a tendency to level with less proclination (see Chapter 20).

Some authorities advocate placing a reverse curve of Spee in the initial round steel mandibular archwire, presumably in order to place extrusive forces on the premolars. However, placing a reverse curve into a mandibular archwire ideally should not be undertaken until the arch is relatively flat, otherwise the downward vector of forces on the brackets labial to the incisor crowns will tend to produce proclination rather than intrusion. Such curves in round archwires also tend to buccally flare the molars. In most patients, it is not necessary to place curves in the archwires. However, once a rectangular steel archwire is flat, but the mandibular arch requires further levelling, a gentle reverse curve may be wiped into the rectangular steel archwire. This will tend to procline the lower incisors. If this is to be avoided, before placement of the curve, labial root torque should be added to the incisor region of the lower archwire, which removes or reduces the proclining effect of the curve.

If there is difficulty placing a large rectangular stainless steel archwire, the clinician can place a 0.020-inch round archwire for one visit, and the following visit the 0.019 × 0.025-inch archwire or even larger archwire will usually fit relatively easily.

This section should be read in conjunction with Chapter 20, which discusses in more depth the different techniques for arch levelling and overbite reduction.

Conclusion

The duration of the alignment and levelling stage of treatment is variable, and depends on the severity of the initial malocclusion as well as other factors discussed in this chapter. The clinician should be patient and not rush into the second stage of treatment until the objectives of the first stage have been met.

References

1 Naini FB. *Facial Aesthetics: Concepts and Clinical Diagnosis*. Oxford: Wiley Blackwell, 2011.
2 Jepsen A. Root surface measurement and a method for X-ray determination of root surface area. *Acta Odontol. Scand.* 1963;21:35–46.
3 de La Cruz A, Sampson P, Little RM, et al. Long-term changes in arch form after orthodontic treatment and retention. *Am. J. Orthod. Dentofacial Orthop.* 1995;107:518–530.
4 Hawley CA. Determination of the normal arch and its application in orthodontia. *Dent. Cosmos* 1905;47:541–552.
5 Brader AC. Dental arch form related to intra-oral forces. *Am. J. Orthod.* 1972;61:541–561.
6 Chuck GC. Ideal arch form. *Angle Orthod.* 1934;4:312–327.
7 Naini FB, Gill DS. Preparatory and postoperative orthodontics: principles, techniques and mechanics. In: Naini FB, Gill DS (eds). *Orthognathic Surgery: Principles, Planning and Practice*. Oxford: Wiley Blackwell, 2017.
8 Taloumis LJ, Smith TM, Hondrum SO, Lorton L. Force decay and deformation of orthodontic elastomeric ligatures. *Am. J. Orthod. Dentofacial Orthop.* 1997;111:1–11.
9 World Health Organization, International Agency for Research on Cancer. *Chromium, Nickel and Welding. IARC Monographs on the Evaluation of Carcinogenic Risks to Humans* Vol. 49. Lyon: IARC, 1990.
10 Naini FB, Gill DS. Painless removal of full thickness rectangular stainless steel archwires. *Orthod. Update* 2020;13:41.
11 Sheridan JJ. Air-rotor stripping. *J. Clin. Orthod.* 1985;19:43–59.
12 Naini FB, Manouchehri S, Al-Bitar ZB, et al. The maxillary incisor labial face tangent: clinical evaluation of maxillary incisor inclination in profile smiling view and idealized aesthetics. *Maxillofac. Plast. Reconstr. Surg.* 2019;41:31.
13 Clark CA. A method of ascertaining the relative position of unerupted teeth by means of film radiographs. *Proc. R. Soc. Med. (Odontol. Section)* 1910;3:87–90.
14 Kohavi D, Becker A, Zilberman Y. Surgical exposure, orthodontic movement and final tooth position as factors in periodontal breakdown of treated palatally impacted canines. *Am. J. Orthod.* 1984;85:72–77.
15 Chaushu S, Brin I, Ben-Bassat Y, et al. Periodontal status following surgical-orthodontic alignment of impacted central incisors by an open-eruption technique. *Eur. J. Orthod.* 2003;25:579–584.
16 Hunt NP. Direct traction applied to unerupted teeth using the acid-etch technique. *Br. J. Orthod.* 1977;4:211–212.

17 Becker A, Chaushu S. Impacted teeth and their orthodontic management. In: Gill DS, Naini FB (eds). *Orthodontics: Principles and Practice.* Oxford: Wiley Blackwell, 2011.

18 Noar JH, Gaukroger MJ. Customized metal coping for elastic traction of an ectopic maxillary central incisor. *J. Clin. Orthod.* 2000;34:585–589.

19 Naini FB, Gill DS. Oral surgery: labial frenectomy. Indications and practical implications. *Br. Dent. J.* 2018;225:199–200.

20 Otasevic M, Naini FB, Gill DS, Lee RT. Prospective randomized clinical trial comparing the effects of a masticatory bite wafer and avoidance of hard food on pain associated with initial orthodontic tooth movement. *Am. J. Orthod. Dentofacial Orthop.* 2006;130:6.e9–15.

21 Gulabivala K, Naini FB. Orthodontic–endodontic interface. In: *Gulabivala K, Yuan-Ling Ng (eds) Endodontics, 4th edn. Mosby Elsevier*, 2014.

22 Woodhouse NR, DiBiase AT, Johnson N, et al. Supplemental vibrational force during orthodontic alignment: a randomized trial. *J. Dent. Res.* 2015;94:682–689.

23 El-Angbawi A, McIntyre GT, Fleming PS, Bearn DR. Non-surgical adjunctive interventions for accelerating tooth movement in patients undergoing fixed orthodontic treatment. *Cochrane Database Syst. Rev.* 2015;(11):CD010887.

24 Frost HM. The biology of fracture healing. An overview for clinicians. Part I. *Clin. Orthop. Relat. Res.* 1989;248:283–293.

25 Frost HM. The biology of fracture healing. An overview for clinicians. Part II. *Clin. Orthop. Relat. Res.* 1989;248:294–309.

26 Frost HM. The regional acceleratory phenomenon: a review. *Henry Ford Hosp. Med. J.* 1983;31:3–9.

27 Fleming PS, Federowicz Z, Johal A, et al. Surgical adjunctive procedures for accelerating orthodontic treatment. *Cochrane Database Syst. Rev.* 2015;(6): CD010572.

15

Controlled Space Closure

Daljit S. Gill and Farhad B. Naini

CHAPTER OUTLINE

Introduction, 297
At Completion of Alignment and Levelling, 298
Objectives during Space Closure, 298
Classification of Anchorage, 299
Types of Space Closure, 299
Sliding Mechanics with the Preadjusted Edgewise Appliance, 300
  The 0.018-inch versus 0.022-inch Slot, 300
  Working Archwires, 300
  Method of Force Application, 303
  Force Levels, 304
  Incorporation of Second Molars, 304
  Two-stage Space Closure versus En Masse Retraction, 305
Frictionless Mechanics with the Preadjusted Edgewise Appliance, 306
  Generation of Forces, 306
  Generation of Moments, 307
  Loop Designs, 307
  T-Loop, 307
  Segmented Arch Mechanics, 308
Monitoring Space Closure, 308
Conclusion, 309
References, 309

'A goal without a plan is just a wish.'
Antoine de Saint-Exupéry

Introduction

It has already been mentioned that the stages of orthodontic treatment with fixed appliances can be conveniently divided into a number of successive phases to help plan the treatment sequence. Following diagnosis and treatment planning (including informed consent), these are:

1. alignment and levelling
2. space closure
3. finishing
4. retention and follow-up
5. normal visits to the general dentist during orthodontic treatment.

Controlled space closure is an important objective in fixed appliance treatment, particularly when teeth have been extracted or where there is spacing present (e.g. microdontia, hypodontia). Teeth are often extracted for the management of dentoalveolar disproportion (i.e. crowding) and for dentoalveolar compensation to manage mild to moderate skeletal discrepancies. A comprehensive **space analysis** should be undertaken when planning treatment, as has already been outlined in Chapter 1. Maxillary incisor retraction, and space closure, will often commence while a deep overbite is reducing, or has been reduced in the case

Preadjusted Edgewise Fixed Orthodontic Appliances: Principles and Practice, First Edition. Edited by Farhad B. Naini and Daljit S. Gill.
© 2022 John Wiley & Sons Ltd. Published 2022 by John Wiley & Sons Ltd.

of complete overbites, and typically when spacing within the labial segments (2-2 or 3-3) has been consolidated.

The aim of this chapter is to discuss the space closure phase of treatment with the preadjusted edgewise appliance. It has already been mentioned that there is overlap between the above-mentioned treatment stages (see Chapter 14). Extraction space closure can occur during the alignment and levelling phase as some space may be needed for the relief of crowding and levelling of the arches.

It is important that space closure is controlled, as uncontrolled space closure can lead to a failure to achieve a number of important treatment objectives.

- Poor incisor positioning leading to an unfavourable facial profile and smile aesthetic changes.
- Failure to correct the incisor occlusion: overjet, overbite and centrelines.
- Failure to correct the molar occlusion: anteroposterior, transverse and vertical.

At Completion of Alignment and Levelling

Once the arches have been aligned and levelled, it is important to undertake a comprehensive case re-evaluation, including reassessment of:

- patient concerns
- facial profile and smile aesthetics
- space available within each quadrant
- estimation of remaining facial growth based on pubertal stage
- overjet, overbite and centreline position
- molar and canine relationship
- compliance with treatment to date.

All these factors combine to determine the treatment mechanics that may be most appropriate from this stage forwards. It may be worthwhile at this stage to document treatment progress by taking a full set of extraoral and intraoral photographs. These are relatively inexpensive records to take, with no patient risk, and can help to confirm the plan for the next stage of treatment and to justify why certain mechanics were used from that point of record taking.

Objectives during Space Closure

There are a number of important objectives that we should aim to achieve during space closure. It is useful to review patient concerns before commencing space closure as these may have changed during alignment and levelling. It is particularly important to identify new concerns that may be

unrealistic to manage and a frank discussion at this stage can help to reset patient expectations, which will help to improve satisfaction at the end of treatment.

A reassessment of the facial profile will also help determine how much upper incisor retraction is advisable when correcting an increased overjet in Class II malocclusions. In cases where the lips are retrusive relative to the facial profile, the nasolabial angle is increased, particularly with a backward inclination of the upper lip, and it may be advisable to only partially correct an increased overjet. In cases were the patient feels that the upper lip has been pushed forward excessively during alignment and levelling, it would be sensible to plan for more incisor retraction.

Concerning the smile, an assessment of the incisor inclination in profile view can help to determine if this needs to be maintained during upper incisor retraction or whether some retroclination or proclination is required to achieve the best aesthetic outcome. A tangent to the labial face of the central incisor crown should be approximately parallel to the true vertical with the patient in natural head position (Figure 15.1).[1] A clinical assessment is important as cephalometric analysis alone does not provide all the required information about the most aesthetic appearance and can be misleading. Where the upper incisor display

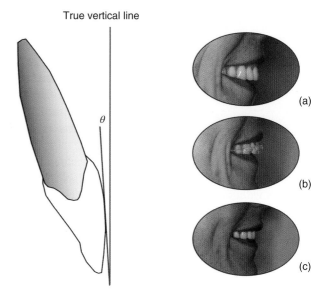

Figure 15.1 Ideal aesthetic upper incisor inclination. Judged clinically, with the patient's head in their natural head position, a tangent to the labial face of the upper central incisor crown (red line) should be 0–5° to the true vertical (green line). The inset photos show aesthetically pleasing (a), proclined (b) and slightly upright (c) incisors. This assessment cannot be made cephalometrically and should be made clinically. Source: based on Naini FB, Manouchehri S, Al-Bitar ZB, et al. The maxillary incisor labial face tangent: clinical evaluation of maxillary incisor inclination in profile smiling view and idealized aesthetics. *Maxillofac. Plast. Reconstr. Surg.* 2019;41(1)31.

is reduced at rest and during smiling, particularly when the overbite is reduced, consideration may be given to some (1–2 mm) extrusion of the upper incisors to help improve the incisor show and increase the overbite. Where the incisor show is increased at rest and during smiling, care has to be taken to minimise any mechanics that may extrude the upper incisors further (e.g. Class II intermaxillary elastics) and consideration can be given to reducing a deep overbite by upper as well as lower incisor intrusion.

An assessment of the amount of space remaining within each quadrant, measurement of the overjet, overbite, centreline positions, molar relationship and likely remaining anteroposterior mandibular growth will give an indication of the likely anchorage requirements in order to achieve the desired occlusal outcome. This will then allow an assessment of how much space within each arch should be closed by incisor retraction or molar protraction (i.e. differential space closure). In Class II malocclusion, the aim is often to maximise maxillary incisor retraction and mandibular molar protraction in order to facilitate molar and incisor anteroposterior correction to achieve dentoalveolar compensation for the skeletal discrepancy. In Class III malocclusion, the opposite is usually the case (i.e. maximum lower incisor retraction and maximum upper molar protraction). It should be remembered that there is a limit to how much the inclination of incisors can be changed for dentoalveolar compensation. Excessive change may lead to **non-axial loading**, with concomitant risk to periodontal health, roots protruding outside of the labial plate of alveolar bone, poor smile aesthetics and reduced access to oral hygiene on the lingual surfaces of excessively retroclined lower incisors.

Another important aim of space closure is to achieve the desired aesthetic and occlusal objectives by maximising bodily tooth movement, achieving root parallelism and controlling the arch form. An important principle of treatment is often to maintain the lower incisor position as the pretreatment position is considered the most stable position.[2] However, there is no guarantee that this position will automatically confer stability and retention is still necessary (see Chapter 17). One can then argue that if there is no guarantee of stability, and retention is still required, small changes in lower incisor position may be acceptable. In cases where the lower incisors have been held back by abnormal soft tissue activity (e.g. lip trap, significant digit sucking) that is removed as part of treatment, where it is thought that the lower incisors have been trapped by a deep and complete overbite (e.g. Class II division 2 malocclusion) and in Class III camouflage cases where the lower incisors are retroclined and positioned behind the upper incisors, it may be more acceptable to produce larger changes in lower incisor inclination. If the aims of

treatment are to maintain the lower incisor position, it can be useful to take a lateral cephalometric radiograph when a few millimetres of space are still left to close in the lower arch. In this way the final mechanics of space closure can be planned to achieve the desired goal.

Classification of Anchorage

Anchorage may be classified according to Burstone's Classification.[3]

- Group A: space closure by predominantly incisor retraction (75%) with some allowance for molar protraction (25%).
- Group B: approximately equal amounts of incisor retraction and molar protraction.
- Group C: space closure by predominantly molar protraction (75%) with some allowance for incisor retraction (25%).

A number of factors affect anchorage loss, so it is difficult to make hard and fast rules; however, Table 15.1 outlines some of the principles of anchorage management during space closure. On some occasions, anchorage requirements may be asymmetrical, so treatment mechanics may vary between the left and right sides. For a more detailed discussion of anchorage management, please refer to Chapter 3.

Types of Space Closure

Space can be closed using **loop (frictionless)** or **sliding (friction)** mechanics. Closing loops were used for space closure with the standard edgewise technique because the presence of archwire bends (i.e. first-, second- and third-order bends) did not allow sliding mechanics. Loop mechanics involves incorporation of loops, within a continuous or segmented archwire, and the springback properties of the activated loop generate the required forces to move groups of teeth without resistance from frictional forces. Design features within the loop are required to produce the necessary counterbalancing moments to control the type of tooth movement (i.e. bodily movement versus tipping) (see Chapter 2). Generating differential moment-to-force ratios between the active and anchorage units facilitate the delivery of differential tooth movement (i.e. tipping versus bodily movement), which will facilitate differential space closure. With a properly designed loop, a good range of activation can also be generated.

The introduction of the preadjusted edgewise appliance by Lawrence Andrews[4] largely eliminated the need for

Table 15.1 Some principles of anchorage management where the molar position is to be largely maintained, movement of molars and incisors is desired and where the incisor position is largely to be maintained.

	Upper arch	Lower arch
Group A (75% incisor retraction)	Extract 4's rather than 5's if possible	Extract 4's rather than 5's if possible
	Increase number of posterior anchor teeth	Intermaxillary elastics (Class III)
	Nance palatal arch	TADs
	Intermaxillary elastics (Class II)	J-hook headgear
	Stopped arch	
	Altering moment–force ratios between active and anchorage units (loop mechanics)	
	Skeletal anchorage, e.g. TADs	
	Supplemental forces: headgear to support the molars or J-hook headgear to retract incisors	
Group B (equal molar/incisor movement)	Extract 4's rather than 5's if possible	Extract 4's rather than 5's if possible
	Incorporate second molars if necessary	Incorporate second molars if necessary
	Intermaxillary elastics if necessary	Intermaxillary elastics if necessary
	Skeletal anchorage if anchorage loss unexpectedly rapid	Skeletal anchorage if anchorage loss unexpectedly rapid
Group C (75% molar protraction)	Class III elastics	Class II elastics
	Single tooth protraction	Single tooth protraction
	Labial crown torque	Labial crown torque
	TADs	TADs

TADs, temporary anchorage devices; 4's, first premolar teeth; 5's, second premolar teeth.

archwire bends, giving rise to the *straight-wire technique*, which allows for the use of sliding mechanics, where the archwire and bracket slots slide past each other with resistance from friction, binding and possibly notching.[5] Forces are delivered using elastics or coil springs (closed or open) and the guiding archwire generates the necessary counterbalancing moment necessary for bodily tooth movement (see Chapter 2). The forces applied must overcome frictional resistance and provide the necessary force for tooth movement. Frictional forces are variable within the cycle of tooth movement, as teeth tip and then upright, so the forces applied to the periodontal ligament also vary and are unknown. Because the applied force within the periodontal ligament is unknown and the interbracket distance between the canine and second premolar bracket is short, the ability for differential space closure by applying differential moment-to-force ratios between the anchorage and active units is small and mainly Group B anchorage is achieved unless additional anchorage reinforcement techniques are employed, for example headgear, intermaxillary elastics or temporary anchorage devices (TADs).[6]

The advantages and disadvantages of sliding and loop mechanics for space closure are outlined in Table 15.2.

Sliding Mechanics with the Preadjusted Edgewise Appliance

The 0.018-inch versus 0.022-inch Slot

Globally, the majority of orthodontists use the 0.022-inch dimension bracket (working archwire 0.019 × 0.025-inch stainless steel) compared to the 0.018-inch dimension bracket (working archwire 0.016 × 0.022-inch stainless steel). This dimension refers to the height of the bracket slot. A perceived advantage of the 0.022-inch slot is that it allows a larger-dimension working archwire to be used which may be mechanically more efficient. There is good evidence that no one slot size is superior to another in terms of treatment duration, quality of occlusal outcomes, patient satisfaction, root resorption and pain experience.[7–9] Therefore, the choice is due to operator preference as both systems can produce good results.

Working Archwires

0.019 × 0.025-inch Stainless Steel
In the majority of cases a customised 0.019 × 0.025-inch stainless steel archwire is used for space closure within

Table 15.2 Advantages and disadvantages of loop and sliding mechanics.

	Advantages	Disadvantages
Sliding (friction) mechanics	• Minimal archwire manipulation helping to reduce chairside time • Patient comfort as no extending archwires • Good control of arch form	• Larger forces required to overcome friction • Requirement for anchorage reinforcement may be higher
Loop (frictionless) mechanics	• Reduced friction • Better anchorage control? • Differential tooth movement by varying moment-to-force ratios between anchorage and active units (but technique sensitive)	• Increased chairside time in constructing loops • Loops may hinder oral hygiene and cause soft tissue trauma • Control of arch form may be reduced as loops increase flexibility and greater reliance on beta-titanium wires rather than stainless steel • Complex forces and greater understanding of force systems required or risk of uncontrolled tooth movement

a 0.022-inch dimension bracket system. This dimension of archwire theoretically provides 0.003 inch (approximately 0.08 mm) of vertical clearance to help reduce frictional forces and allow sliding mechanics to occur whilst providing sufficient rigidity to allow bodily tooth movement and good control of arch form during space closure. Stainless steel also has favourable surface characteristics due to the low level of asperities (microscopic peaks), which also helps to reduce frictional forces to facilitate sliding mechanics (see Chapter 2). The vertical clearance is theoretical because there is good evidence that archwire and bracket slot dimensions are not accurate due to manufacturing errors.[10] The 0.003 inch of theoretical vertical clearance also introduces approximately 10° of *slop* into the system. The degree of slop may be less in reality, and archwires may perform better than expected, because of residual tip that may remain uncorrected when the archwire is first placed (Figure 15.2) and which may occur during treatment as teeth move.[11] If any degree of slop is undesirable during maxillary incisor retraction, this can be compensated for by using a high torque bracket

prescription (e.g. MBT > Roth > Andrews) or by placing palatal root torque into the archwire anteriorly. Use of light retraction forces will also help to lessen the moment that causes incisor retroclination as the size of the moment is proportional to the force applied.

Extension arms/hooks (also termed **power arms**) (Figure 15.3) of varying heights can also be used to control movement of the anterior segment during en masse incisor retraction. When an extension arm is placed mesial to the canine at the level of 0 mm (bracket slot level), palatal tipping of the incisors is observed as well as downward deflection of the wire (extrusion), but when a extension arm of 5.5 mm is used bodily tooth movement with minimal deflection of the archwire may be achieved.[12] In the treatment of Class II division 1 malocclusion with excessively proclined upper incisors but with their root apices in a relatively good position, controlled palatal crown tipping, in which the incisor retroclines around its apex as the centre of rotation, is required. In this case, the use of an extension arm height of 4–5 mm is recommended. For Class II division 2, lingual root tipping of the incisors is

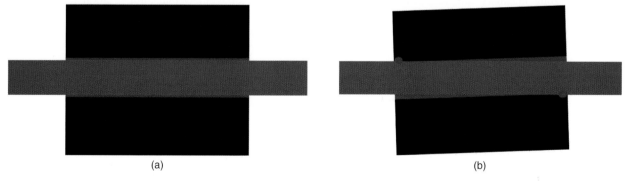

(a)   (b)

Figure 15.2 A 0.19 × 0.025-inch archwire in a 0.022-inch slot. (a) Theoretically, the 0.003 inch (0.08 mm) of vertical clearance (red area) would introduce approximately 10° of slop (play in the third dimension). (b) In reality there may be less slop as teeth may be slightly tipped so the archwire does make contact in some areas (red spots).

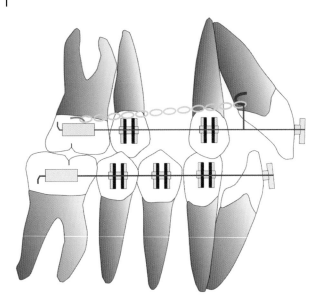

Figure 15.3 Extension hooks, shown anteriorly on the maxillary archwire, are available in variable lengths. Space closing forces applied to an extension hook help to facilitate bodily incisor retraction.

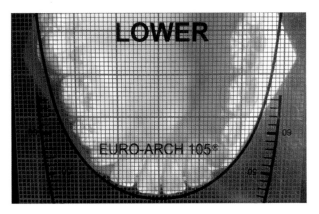

Figure 15.5 Customisation of the arch form is facilitated by the use of clear arch form templates. The correct size template is selected first for the lower arch, in this case the 105% Euro arch template. The arch form should be held over the dental model in the position of the archwire. The lower arch wire is then customised to this and the upper arch wire to the corresponding upper 105% template. In this way the arch form is 'customised' to minimise changes in arch dimension and maximise stability.

desirable, which could be carried out by raising the height of the extension arm to above 5.5 mm. To achieve bodily anterior tooth movement, an extension arm of 5.5 mm can be used.[12]

The 0.025-inch depth of the archwire is important for providing sufficient torque control by helping to create a counterbalancing moment that reduces tipping and facilitates bodily incisor retraction. The counterbalancing moment is created by engagement of the rectangular archwire with the opposing walls (gingival and occlusal) of the bracket slot (Figure 15.4).

It is important that the lower archwire is customised in width in order to produce minimal changes in lower intercanine and intermolar width, as this is known to be prone to relapse.[13] The maxillary archwire is then customised using the corresponding maxillary template. Customisation is facilitated by using clear templates that can be placed over the pretreatment lower study model (Figure 15.5).

If at the time of archwire placement the 0.019 × 0.025-inch wire slides freely through the slots, then space closure can commence immediately. If there is resistance to insertion due to friction, usually as a consequence of inadequate torque or molar rotation control, then the archwire should be ligated and allowed to become passive for six to eight weeks before space closure is commenced.

0.018-inch or 0.017 × 0.025-inch Stainless Steel Archwires

In certain situations, an undersized archwire may be used for space closure.

- In Class III cases, an undersized archwire may be used in the lower arch where retroclination of the lower incisors is desired for dentoalveolar compensation. In such cases,

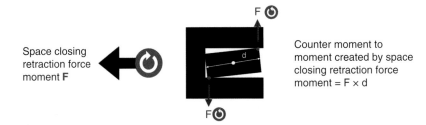

Figure 15.4 A central incisor bracket viewed in profile view with an engaged 0.019 × 0.025-inch stainless steel archwire. As the incisor is retracted it tips backwards, because of the clockwise space closing retraction force moment (F) and slop present, until the archwire makes contact with the bracket (red circles). An anticlockwise counter-moment is generated (F), which prevents further tipping and allows for bodily retraction. The 0.025-inch dimension of the archwire is important in creating a sufficient counter-moment as the size of the moment is proportional to the depth of the wire.

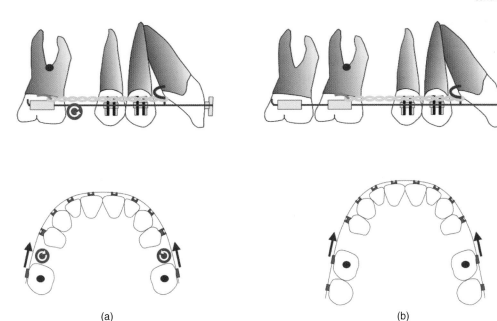

(a)   (b)

Figure 15.6 (a) Rigid archwires help to control mesial molar tipping and mesiolingual rotation because of the moments generated when a force is not passed through the centre of resistance. (b) If smaller dimension archwires are used for space closure, or where second premolars have been extracted, incorporation of the second molars will help to control the movement of the first molar by preventing tipping and rotation.

a circle-loop or U-bend can be placed mesial to the space to be closed for the application of intra-arch space closing forces or use of Class III intermaxillary elastics. It is important that the archwire is customised after placement of a circle-loop or U-bend as these do distort the arch form.

- To close final spaces (1–2 mm) where space closure has been very slow, an undersized archwire may be used to reduce friction, aid sliding and facilitate final space closure.

Care must be taken when using smaller archwires with reduced rigidity for space closure as there is greater likelihood of tooth tipping and loss of arch form (e.g. distobuccal rotation of the molars), particularly if space closing forces are high, as high forces generate bigger moments (moment = force × distance). Greater first molar control, for tipping and rotation, can be achieved by incorporating the second molars into the appliance in such cases (Figure 15.6).

Method of Force Application

Space closing forces are usually applied between a hook on the archwire, between the lateral incisor and canine bracket, and the first or second molar tube hook (Figure 15.7). Either a soldered or crimpable hook is placed mesial to the canine in case separate canine retraction is required. Soldered hooks tend to be more secure than crimpable hooks but they have the downside that a greater

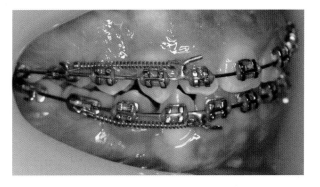

Figure 15.7 Space closing forces are usually applied between a hook on the archwire (crimpable or soldered), between the lateral incisor and canine, and a hook on the first or second molar tube. In this case a space closing NiTi coil is being used for space closure.

inventory of archwires is needed with differing hook positions.

Space closing forces can be applied using a number of different methods (Figure 15.8):

- elastomeric chain (e.g. power chain, E-Links) (see Appendix II)
- closed coil springs (NiTi or stainless steel)
- active ligature tie-backs (o-ligs)
- elastics (e.g. $^{3}/_{16}$-inch diameter) (see Appendix II).

Evidence would suggest that NiTi closing springs may result in more rapid space closure compared to elastomeric

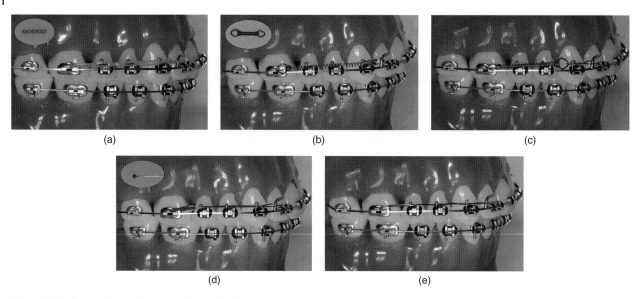

(a) (b) (c)

(d) (e)

Figure 15.8 Space closing forces can be applied using a number of methods. (a) Power chain, which is usually stretched between 50 and 100% of its length. (b) Closed coil springs (NiTi), which are available in a variety of lengths and force levels. (c) Closed coil springs can also be attached using ligature wire anteriorly to prevent them from being overstretched in some cases. (d) Active ligature tie-backs (o-ligs), which are made by threading a elastomeric module onto 0.010-inch ligature wire. The forces are applied to either the first or second molar depending on how much posterior anchorage is required. (e) Once space closure is complete a passive ligature wire can be used to maintain the space closure and this is also facilitated by gently bending the end of the archwire distal to the last molar, which helps maintain the arch length.

chain, with a mean difference of 0.2 mm per month.[14] Active ligature tie-backs appear to be least effective.[15] Elastomeric techniques may be less efficient because of the rapid decay of elastic forces within the oral environment (see Chapter 11). There does not appear to be any difference in anchorage loss between elastomeric chain and closed coil springs.[14] There are no studies comparing root resorption, pain difference and cost-effectiveness between the two techniques. Elastics ($^3/_{16}$ inch) may be less effective than springs but this may be related to patient compliance in wearing them.[16]

Force Levels

Although there is no definitive evidence for the optimal force required during space closure, a force delivery system that generates 150–200 g of orthodontic force is usually prescribed.[17, 18] It would appear that 150 or 200 g forces are equally effective.[19] Lower forces are probably preferable in those with periodontal disease as the centre of resistance for tooth movement is moved apically, because of bone loss, which creates bigger moments that will also translate into greater tipping per unit of applied force. Force levels can be measured using a force measuring gauge (Figure 15.9).

Incorporation of Second Molars

Second molars are incorporated into fixed appliances for a number of reasons, as outlined in Box 15.0. For space

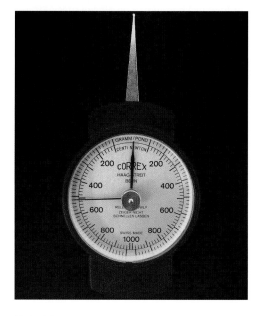

Figure 15.9 A force measuring gauge. This device can be used to measure the magnitude of applied forces to ensure correct amounts are applied. A number of gauge sizes are available for different force ranges (see also Appendix II).

closure, the main reasons for incorporating second molars into a fixed appliance are:

- to provide more anchorage
- to help control movement of the first permanent molars
- to close space mesial to the second molar.

Box 15.1 Reasons for incorporating second molars into a fixed appliance

- Poorly aligned second molars (e.g. rotation)
- Poor occlusion (e.g. crossbite)
- Non-working side interferences (e.g. low palatal cusp)
- Anchorage
- Control of mesial tipping of first molars (second premolar extraction)
- To assist in overbite reduction
- Extraction of first molars

Anchorage

The second molars may be bonded or banded in order to provide anchorage support for greater incisor retraction. Incorporation of second molars will increase anchorage by increasing the root surface area of the anchorage unit and also by reducing mesial tipping of the first permanent molar. For the second molar to be incorporated into the anchorage unit, space closing forces can be applied directly to it, or the molars can be tied together as a block with a stainless steel undertie, and the forces can be applied to the first molar hook. Incorporation of second molars does increase frictional resistance to space closure so it is often wise to leave a 0.019 × 0.025-inch archwire ligated in position for one visit without placing space closing forces to allow greatest passivity. Debonding of the second molar tube can be a particular concern and it may be wise to consider banding rather than bonding to reduce breakages.[20]

Control of the First Molar

Incorporation of the second molar helps to provide the necessary anchorage to prevent mesial tipping and mesiolingual rotation of the first molar, particularly when the second premolars have been extracted or are missing or when an undersized archwire is used for space closure (see Figure 15.6). This will also help to fully express the torque in the first molar tube by providing the necessary anchorage. In second premolar extraction cases,

incorporating the second molar will maximise space closure by bodily tooth movement of the first permanent molar, which will help to achieve good root parallelism at the completion of treatment.

Because of these principles, when the first permanent molar has been extracted, incorporation of the third molar, if it has erupted, will help to better control the second molar. A problem can arise when the third molar is absent, which is the case in most children. In such cases, unwanted rotation of the second molar during space closure can be minimised by using the double traction technique where space closing forces are applied both buccally and lingually to the second molar to minimise moments tending to cause rotation (Figure 15.10). Mesial tipping in such cases can also be reduced by sweeping a gentle curve into the posterior part of the archwire.

Close Space Mesial to the Second Molar

In many cases, when applying space closing forces to the first molar, when the second molar is not bonded, the pull from the trans-septal fibres will pull the second molar forward and maintain contact between the two teeth. Occasionally the second molar will not follow, for example if there is an occlusal interference, and the tooth must be incorporated into the appliance to encourage its mesial movement.

Two-stage Space Closure versus En Masse Retraction

Space closure, using sliding or loop mechanics, can be achieved either by separately retracting the maxillary canines followed by the four incisors (two-step) or by en masse retraction of the whole anterior canine-to-canine segment simultaneously. It has been claimed that the two-step technique may be superior in anchorage preservation as smaller forces may be used for separate canine and incisor retraction, which may reduce the strain on the anchorage unit. In reality, clinicians are unlikely to control the forces used with such accuracy. The evidence would suggest that two-stage space closure does not result in less anchorage loss.[21] The two-stage technique may also be less

Figure 15.10 (a) The single traction technique. (b) The double traction technique.

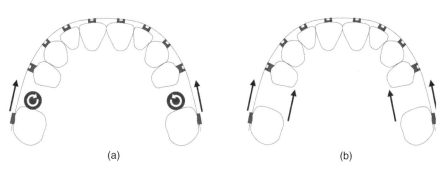

(a)   (b)

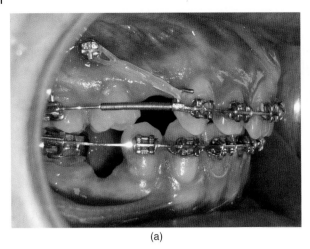
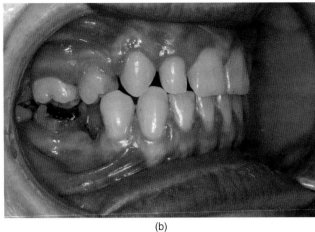

(a)   (b)

Figure 15.11 (a) A TAD has been placed high to generate a larger component of vertical force to cause incisor intrusion as well as retraction in this patient who was unhappy with her 'gummy' smile. (b) End of treatment.

patient friendly as it produces unaesthetic spaces mesial to the canines before incisor retraction can commence.

Evidence also suggests that the en masse/TAD combination is superior to the two-stage technique with regard to anchorage preservation and amount of incisor retraction.[22] Limited evidence suggests that en masse retraction requires less treatment time and that no significant differences exist in the amount of root resorption between the two techniques.[22]

If using TADS for anchorage for en masse retraction, it should be remembered that altering the vertical positioning of a TAD placed between the first and second premolar roots can alter the vertical component of force to the incisors during en masse retraction to produce differing outcomes (Figure 15.11). If space closing forces are placed between a high TAD (>10 mm above the archwire) and a 6-mm extension arm, retraction, anticlockwise rotation as well as intrusion are achieved, which can be useful for improving excessive upper incisor display during rest/smiling. Placing the TAD lower (<8 mm from the archwire) would cause retraction, clockwise rotation and extrusion. Intermediate positioning (8–10 mm from the archwire) may produce bodily retraction.[23]

Frictionless Mechanics with the Preadjusted Edgewise Appliance

Loops can be placed into continuous archwires to generate opening and closing forces and moments to control tooth movement (i.e. bodily movement versus tipping).

Generation of Forces

When placed into a stainless steel archwire and activated, a loop will obey Hooke's law (see Chapter 10) and display characteristics such as elastic deformation and a proportional limit beyond which permanent deformation will occur. The ideal properties of a loop are:

- a large range of activation
- a high proportional limit to reduce the risk of permanent deformation
- a low load (force)–deflection rate, so that light constant forces are delivered over as large a range as possible.

The load (force)–deflection characteristics are dependent on a number of factors, including the following.

1. Young's modulus of the alloy used (stainless steel > cobalt chromium > beta-titanium > NiTi), which is calculated from the gradient of the stress–strain graph. The greater the modulus of elasticity, the higher the load (force)–deflection rate.
2. Wire cross-section: rectangular wires have a higher load (force)–deflection rate than round wires.
3. Wire dimension: thicker wires have a higher load (force)–deflection rate than thinner wires. However, reducing wire dimensions reduces wire strength, so an increase in wire length can be used to reduce the force–deflection rate of thicker wires.
4. Length of wire: force varies inversely to the third power of the length. Helical coils can be used to increase the effective length of a wire and reduce the load (force)–deflection rate.

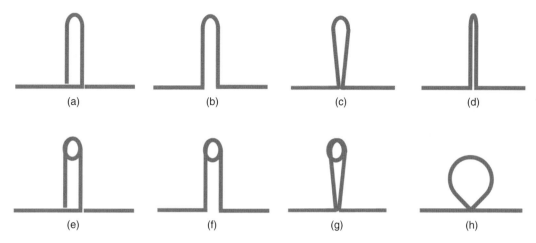

Figure 15.12 Various loop designs, other than the T-loop, exist: (a) reverse vertical loop, (b) open vertical loop, (c) closed vertical loop, (d) bull loop, (e) reverse vertical loop with helix, (f) open vertical loop with helix, (g) closed vertical loop with helix and (h) tear drop loop.

Generation of Moments

Because force cannot be delivered directly through the centre of resistance of teeth, application of forces will create moments, or a force tending to cause rotation, which will lead to tipping movements. The generation of a counterbalancing moment to these forces, by careful loop design, helps to control tooth movement. Creating different degrees of counterbalancing moments between **anchorage** and **active units** can help to control anchorage balance and the degree of tipping within each unit (see Chapter 2).

Loop Designs

Many designs of loop exist (Figure 15.12) because no single loop has all the ideal properties. The simplest form of loop, the open vertical loop (U-loop), does not have good force–deflection characteristics and cannot generate sufficient counterbalancing moments to control tooth movement, so variations on its design exist. The focus of the remainder of this chapter will be on the T-loop, as this is probably one of the most studied loop designs.

T-Loop

The T-loop was first described in 1976 by Burstone and Koenig.[3] Incorporating a horizontal section of wire at the apex of an open vertical loop (U-loop) was found to be more biomechanically favourable in terms of load–deflection characteristics and comfort than incorporating multiple helices at the apex. Increasing the horizontal width of the T-loop, within anatomical limits, also improved the

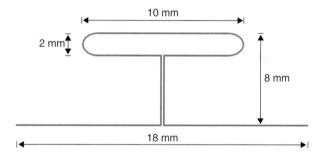

Figure 15.13 The shape and size of a simple T-loop made from 0.017 × 0.025-inch beta-titanium wire.

load–deflection characteristics as well as increasing the moment-to-force ratio. Figure 15.13 shows the shape and dimensions of a clinically useful passive T-loop made from 0.017 × 0.025-inch beta-titanium wire.[6] Stainless steel is less preferable as it exerts approximately 40% greater force.

The T-loop is activated by pulling the archwire through the molar tube and cinching it back. This has the effect of expanding the loop and as long as it is not deformed beyond the proportional limit it will spring back and deliver a space closing force. As well as a horizontal force, an 'activation moment' will also be created (as outlined in Figure 15.14) as the base of the spring becomes angled upwards upon activation. This form of spring will only produce a moment-to-force ratio of 4–5 mm which is only adequate to tip the teeth, so gable bends also need to be placed into the loop (Figure 15.15) in order to achieve ratios of 10 : 1 which are necessary for translation. These moments, termed *residual moments*, are generated when the archwire is engaged and are not dependent on spring activation. Differential tooth movement can be created

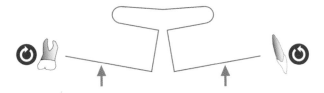

Figure 15.14 Activation of a T-loop is achieved by pulling the wire through the buccal tube and cinching. This will deform the spring and create a space closing force. The base of the spring (arrows) are also angled upwards to generate activation moments, in the direction shown by the curved arrows, which will reduce the degree of tipping during incisor retraction and also tip back the molars producing greater anchorage.

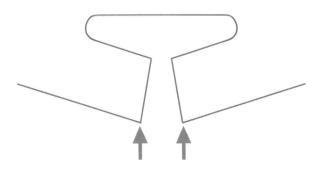

Figure 15.15 If gable bends (arrows) are placed into a passive T-loop as shown in Figure 15.13, residual moments are created which can be sufficient to produce incisor retraction by bodily movement.

by placing asymmetrical gable bends, which produce asymmetrical residual moments between the active and anchorage units, and positioning the spring asymmetrically across an extraction space.[6]

Segmented Arch Mechanics

In the segmented arch technique, the arch is segmented into an anterior and posterior unit (Figure 15.16). The

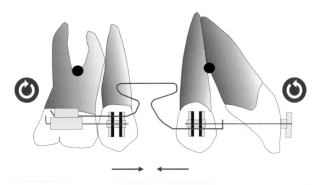

Figure 15.16 If gable bends (arrows) are placed into a passive T-loop as shown in Figure 15.13, residual moments are created which can be sufficient to produce incisor retraction by bodily movement.

posterior teeth can be connected with a transpalatal arch to create a single posterior anchorage unit. A T-loop can be used to apply space closing forces and differential space closure can be achieved by placing asymmetrical gable bends and positioning the T-loop asymmetrically where it will create greater moments closer to the side that it is positioned. There is no evidence that this technique is more conservative of anchorage than sliding mechanics for space closure and it has the drawbacks of segmental mechanics as outlined in Table 15.2.

Monitoring Space Closure

The normal rate of space closure is variable during sliding mechanics, with figures ranging from 0.5 to 2 mm per month for NiTi coil springs and elastomeric chain, with NiTi coil springs appearing to be slightly more efficient.[14] Many **appliance and patient-related** factors probably contribute to this variability, including the force delivery system, friction and bone biology. There is evidence that the bracket type (self-ligating versus conventional) does not affect rate of space closure.[24] There is good evidence that space closure occurs more rapidly during the pubertal growth spurt, which occurs at age 14 (±2) years in males and 12 (±2) in females.[25] Delaying dental extractions as close as possible to the time of space closure may accelerate the rate of closure by the **regional acceleratory phenomenon** and by reducing the bone density (see Chapter 14).

The rate of space closure should be monitored. This may be undertaken by measuring the size of the extraction space at each visit, or by measuring the decrease in arch length by measuring the excess archwire protruding through the distal tube at each visit. Small asymmetries in the rate of space closure are normal; however, if the asymmetry is significant (>25%) this may indicate a local problem.

The most common local problem that may hinder sliding mechanics, and therefore space closure, is frictional resistance. If the archwire cannot be removed or inserted with minimal force, then friction is likely to be a cause. There are numerous causes of elevated friction:

- poor alignment (e.g. torque discrepancies, rotated second molars)
- kinked archwire
- distorted bracket or tube (e.g. molar tubes)
- calculus deposits on archwire and/or bracket.

If friction is thought to be the main factor, then often changing to a new archwire or placing a slightly undersized archwire (0.017 × 0.025 inch), and waiting a visit before reapplying forces, will often help. If it does not then other factors should be considered, such as:

- occlusal or appliance interferences
- deep overbite
- retained roots
- root clash
- dense bone island
- low maxillary sinus
- thick gingival tissue
- ankylosis
- late-forming supernumeraries at the site of space closure.

Once space closure is complete it is necessary to maintain the closed space. This can be achieved with a passive ligature tie and turning the end of the archwire gingivally (see Figure 15.8e).

Conclusion

The clinician should be clear about the objectives of treatment and plan the mechanics of space closure accordingly. The single most important factor is controlling anchorage so that the desired tooth movements can occur. Space closure utilising sliding mechanics can produce predictable results. Space closing forces in the range of 150–200 g appear to be optimal.

References

1 Naini FB, Manouchehri S, Al-Bitar ZB, et al. The maxillary incisor labial face tangent: clinical evaluation of maxillary incisor inclination in profile smiling view and idealized aesthetics. *Maxillofac. Plast. Reconstr. Surg.* 2019;41(1):31.

2 Mills JR. Stability of the lower labial segment. A cephalometric survey. *Dent. Pract. Dent. Rec.* 1968;18(8):293–306.

3 Burstone CJ, Koenig HA. Optimizing anterior and canine retraction. *Am. J. Orthod.* 1976;70(1):1–19.

4 Andrews LF. The straight-wire appliance. *Explained and compared. J. Clin. Orthod.* 1976;10:174–195.

5 Burrow SJ. Friction and resistance to sliding in orthodontics: a critical review. *Am. J. Orthod. Dentofacial Orthop.* 2009;135:442–447.

6 Burstone CJ, Choy K. *The Biomechanical Foundation of Clinical Orthodontics.* Chicago: Quintessence Publishing, 2015.

7 Yassir YA, El-Angbawi AM, McIntyre GT, et al. A randomized clinical trial of the effectiveness of 0.018-inch and 0.022-inch slot orthodontic bracket systems. Part 1: duration of treatment. *Eur. J. Orthod.* 2019;41(2):133–142.

8 Yassir YA, El-Angbawi AM, McIntyre GT, et al. A randomized clinical trial of the effectiveness of 0.018-inch and 0.022-inch slot orthodontic bracket systems. Part 2: quality of treatment. *Eur. J. Orthod.* 2019;41(2):143–153.

9 El-Angbawi AM, Yassir YA, McIntyre GT, et al. A randomized clinical trial of the effectiveness of 0.018-inch and 0.022-inch slot orthodontic bracket systems. Part 3: biological side-effects of treatment. *Eur. J. Orthod.* 2019;41(2):154–164.

10 Joch A, Pichelmayer M, Weiland F. Bracket slot and archwire dimensions: manufacturing precision and third order clearance. *J. Orthod.* 2010;37(4):241–249.

11 McLaughlin RP, Bennett JC, Trevisi HJ. *Systemized Orthodontic Treatment Mechanics*, 2nd edn. Edinburgh: Mosby, 2001.

12 Tominaga JY, Tanaka M, Koga Y, et al. Optimal loading conditions for controlled movement of anterior teeth in sliding mechanics. A 3D finite element study. *Angle Orthod.* 2009;79:1102–1107.

13 Lee RT. Arch width and form: a review. *Am. J. Orthod. Dentofacial Orthop.* 1999;115(3):305–313.

14 Mohammed H, Rizk MZ, Wafaie K, Almuzian M. Effectiveness of nickel-titanium springs vs elastomeric chains in orthodontic space closure: a systematic review and meta-analysis. *Orthod. Craniofac. Res.* 2018;21(1):12–19.

15 Dixon V, Read MJF, O'Brien KD, et al. A randomized clinical trial to compare three methods of orthodontic space closure. *J. Orthod.* 2002;29:31–36.

16 Sonis AL. Comparison of NiTi coil springs vs. elastics in canine retraction. *J. Clin. Orthod.* 1994;28:293–295.

17 Samuels RHA, Orth M, Rudge SJ, Mair LH. A comparison of the rate of space closure using a nickel-titanium spring and an elastic module: a clinical study. *Am. J. Orthod. Dentofacial Orthop.* 1993;103:464–467.

18 Samuels RHA, Rudge SJ, Mair LH. A clinical study of space closure with nickel-titanium closed coil springs and an elastic module. *Am. J. Orthod. Dentofacial Orthop.* 1998;114:73–79.

19 Barlow M, Kula K. Factors influencing efficiency of sliding mechanics to close extraction space: a systematic review. *Orthod. Craniofac. Res.* 2008;11:65–73.

20 Nazir M, Walsh T, Mandall NA, et al. Banding versus bonding of first permanent molars: a multi-centre randomized controlled trial. *J. Orthod.* 2011;38:81–89.

21 Heo W, Nahm DS, Baek SH. En masse retraction and two-step retraction of maxillary anterior teeth in adult

Class I women. A comparison of anchorage loss. *Angle Orthod.* 2007;77(6):973–978.

22 Rizk MZ, Mohammed H, Ismael O, Bearn DR. Effectiveness of en masse versus two step retraction: a systematic review and meta-analysis. *Prog. Orthod.* 2017;18:41.

23 Sung JH, Kyung HM, Bae SM, et al. *Microimplants in Orthodontics. Daegu*, Korea: Dentos, 2006: 15–32.

24 Songra G, Clover M, Atack NE, et al. A comparative assessment of alignment efficiency and space closure of active and passive self-ligating vs. conventional appliances in adolescents: a single center randomised controlled trial. *Am. J. Orthod. Dentofacial Orthop.* 2014;145:569–578.

25 Ireland AJ, Songra G, Clover M, et al. Effect of gender and Frankfort mandibular plane angle on orthodontic space closure: a randomized controlled trial. *Orthod. Craniofac. Res.* 2016;19:74–82.

16

Finishing
Mohammad Owaise Sharif and Stephen M. Chadwick

CHAPTER OUTLINE

Introduction, 311
Aims and Objectives of Orthodontic Treatment, 312
Common Errors Encountered at the Finishing Stages of Treatment, 312
    Alignment, 312
    Marginal Ridge Discrepancies and Occlusal Contacts, 313
    Interproximal Contacts (Spacing), 314
    Centreline (Dental Midline), 314
    Root Angulation, 315
    Buccolingual Inclination, 316
    Occlusal Relationship and Overjet, 317
Efficient Finishing: the Importance of Diagnosis and Treatment Planning, 317
    Tooth Size Discrepancies, 317
    Bracket Alterations to Maximise the Efficiency of Treatment and Finishing, 318
    Personalisation of Appliances, 318
    Indirect Bonding, 318
    Incisal Edge Recontouring and Interproximal Reduction, 318
Conclusion, 318
References, 318

Introduction

The introduction of the preadjusted edgewise appliance in the 1970s revolutionised orthodontics by bringing together earlier attempts at bracket design and producing a concept on which prescription could be based.[1] Over the last four decades this appliance has stood the test of time and a plethora of different bracket prescriptions and treatment philosophies utilising the preadjusted edgewise appliance principle have been introduced. The aims of orthodontic treatment generally include some or all of the following stages: relief of crowding, alignment of the arches, correction of the dental centrelines, correction of overbite, correction of overjet, closure of residual space, and finishing and detailing the occlusion. As the experience of the orthodontic profession in using the preadjusted edgewise appliance has increased, so too has the efficiency in progressing through the various stages of fixed appliance treatment. With the correct diagnosis and treatment plan,

careful monitoring of anchorage and the patient's response to mechanotherapy, it is now possible for the orthodontist using a preadjusted edgewise appliance to obtain a predictably good outcome. However, inherent shortfalls of the preadjusted edgewise appliance and individual patient variations mean that regardless of the complexity of the presenting malocclusion, finishing and detailing of the occlusion is almost always needed. The shortfalls of the preadjusted edgewise appliance include the following.

- Tooth size discrepancies are not automatically taken into account.
- Anatomical variation of crown and root will affect expression of the bracket prescription.
- Dimensional discrepancies: a typical working archwire in the 0.022 × 0.028-inch bracket slot measures 0.019 × 0.025 inch, and therefore the bracket slot is underfilled and there is approximately 10° of slop.

- Force application can produce undesirable tooth movement as forces cannot be delivered directly to the centre of resistance of a tooth.
- Brackets are made for each tooth but are not designed to account for individual variation.

Operator factors can also contribute to the need for finishing and include:

- Inaccurate bracket placement.
- inadequate anchorage control.
- Failure to recognise poor progress in treatment.
- Failure to close space.

The aim of this chapter is to provide an overview of ideal orthodontic treatment and the common features that need addressing in the finishing stage of treatment. In addition, the clinical relevance and influence of a tooth size discrepancy (TSD), the role of personalised appliances, and enamel reduction in finishing orthodontic cases are discussed.

Aims and Objectives of Orthodontic Treatment

The aim of orthodontic treatment is to provide an aesthetic and functional occlusion whilst causing minimal harm to the patient. There have been many methods proposed to describe the ideal tooth arrangement. One of the earliest proposed arrangements was Angle's molar classification, based on the position of the first permanent molars.[2]

Subsequent to this, Andrews' Six Keys of Occlusion were identified from his collection of 120 non-orthodontic examples of naturally ideal dentition.[3] This study became the foundation for the development of the preadjusted edgewise appliance as the prescription in the brackets was based on producing a correction of the malocclusion to become as close as possible to the ideal. The Six Keys of Occlusion as described from Andrews' research are as follows.

- Molar relationship: the distal surface of the distobuccal cusp of the upper first permanent molar occludes with the mesial surface of the mesiobuccal cusp of the lower second molar.
- Crown angulation (tip): the gingival part of the long axis of the crown is distal to the incisal part of the axis. The extent of angulation varies according to tooth type.
- Crown inclination (labiolingual or buccolingual inclination): the labiolingual or buccolingual inclination of the long axis of the crown.
  - The crown inclination of upper and lower anterior teeth is sufficient to resist overeruption of anterior

teeth and sufficient also to allow proper distal positioning of the contact points of the upper teeth in their relationship to the lower teeth; this permits proper occlusion of the posterior crowns.
  - The crowns of upper posterior teeth (canines through molars) have a lingual inclination. This is constant and similar from the canines through the second premolars and slightly more pronounced in the molars.
  - The crowns of the lower posterior (canines through molars) have a lingual inclination, which increases progressively from the canines through to the second molars.
- Rotations are not present.
- There are no interdental spaces and contact points are tight.
- There is a flat plane of occlusion.

The Six Keys of Occlusion came from the description of consistent features identified in the 120 non-orthodontically treated ideal occlusions. However, finishing orthodontic treatment cannot always conform to all six keys. Therefore, the American Board of Orthodontics (ABO) *Grading System for Cast and Radiographic Evaluation*[4] will be used as a reference for the ideal orthodontic outcome (Table 16.1).

In terms of the functional dynamic occlusion it is proposed that orthodontic treatment should ideally produce a mutually protected occlusion (MPO). This is an occlusal arrangement where the posterior and anterior teeth provide protection for each other during function. This is usually described as an occlusal scheme where *canine guidance* or *group function* is seen on the working side and the non-working side is free from occlusal interferences on lateral excursions. In addition, occlusal interferences are not seen in protrusion and there is a smooth glide seen between the retruded contact position and the intercuspal position.

Common Errors Encountered at the Finishing Stages of Treatment

Alignment

Alignment errors in both the anterior and posterior segments are readily identifiable (Figure 16.1). These may occur due to bracket/band positioning errors, uneven thickness of bracket adhesive across an individual bracket base, or a failure to allow for full expression of aligning archwires. Bracket slot deformation or blockage (e.g. by composite or calculus) can also result in errors of alignment. In the molar regions, space closure in undersized archwires can result in excessive rotation.

Table 16.1 Parameters assessed in the ABO Grading System for Cast and Radiographic Evaluation.

Criteria	Features assessed
Alignment	**Anterior (3-3)**: coordination of incisal edges, lingual and labial incisal surfaces
	Posterior (4-7)
	Mandible: mesiobuccal and distobuccal cusps in the same mesiodistal alignment *Maxilla*: central grooves in the same plane/alignment
Marginal ridges	Marginal ridges of adjacent posterior teeth should be at the same level or within 0.5 mm of the same level
	The canine–premolar contact and distal aspect of the mandibular first premolar is not included in the assessment
Buccolingual inclination	**Mandible**: a flat surface across contralateral molars and premolars should contact the buccal cusps
	Maxilla: a flat surface across contralateral molars and premolars should contact the lingual cusps
	The mandibular first premolar and the distal cusps of the second molars are not included in the assessment
Occlusal contacts	Buccal cusps of mandibular and lingual cusps of maxillary molars and premolars should contact the occlusal surfaces of opposing teeth
	If the distolingual maxillary cusp is short, it is not included in the assessment
Occlusal relationship	The maxillary canine cusp tip should align within 1 mm of the embrasure between the mandibular canine and adjacent premolar
	Class I molar finish: the mesiobuccal cusp of the maxillary first permanent molar should align within the embrasure between the mesial and middle cusps of the lower first permanent molar
	Class II molar finish: the buccal cusp of the maxillary first molar should align within the embrasure between the mandibular second premolar and first molar. The buccal cusp of the maxillary second molar should align within the embrasure between the mandibular first and second molar
	Class III molar finish: the buccal cusp of the maxillary second premolar should align with the buccal groove of the mandibular first molar
Overjet	**Anterior**: the mandibular canines and incisors will contact the lingual surfaces of the maxillary canines and incisors
	Posterior: the buccal cusps of the mandibular molars and premolars will contact in the centre (buccolingually) of the maxillary premolars and molars
Interproximal contacts	The mesial and distal surfaces of the teeth should be in contact with one another
Root angulation	**Panoramic radiograph**: roots of the maxillary and mandibular teeth should be parallel to one another and perpendicular to the occlusal plane
	Omit the canine relationship with adjacent tooth root

Source: based on The American Board of Orthodontics (ABO) Grading System for Cast and Radiographic Evaluation, 2012.

In the finishing stages of treatment, the most straightforward method of correcting these errors is by placing an aligning archwire with or without bracket/bond repositioning (the need for repositioning depends on the cause of the malalignment). However, this is not always possible or desirable, and therefore other methods that can be utilised include the placement of archwire finishing bends (see Chapter 14). In order to correct rotational errors in molar teeth it may be necessary to convert the molar tube to allow archwires with bends to be seated. A further option for correcting rotational errors is the placement of rotation wedges (these are particularly useful for teeth with flat labial surfaces, i.e. incisors).

Marginal Ridge Discrepancies and Occlusal Contacts

Marginal ridge height and occlusal contact discrepancies often affect the premolars and second molars. One reason for this in the adolescent population is that these teeth are not fully erupted or the gingival margins have not matured at the time of fixed appliance placement. Gingivally offset premolar brackets are helpful, as is the availability of height gauges that have been proposed for use at appliance placement to help reduce vertical positioning errors (see Chapter 7).

Methods for correcting these discrepancies in the finishing stages of treatment include bracket repositioning, placing archwire bends, the use of intermaxillary elastics

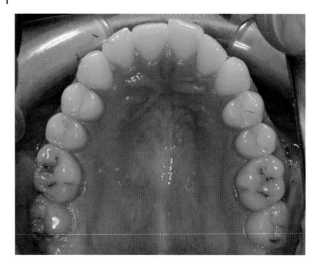

Figure 16.1 Alignment errors evident, especially the incisor and premolar regions.

(with settling archwires), or bypassing an aligning archwire under the brackets to move the teeth into occlusion.

Interproximal Contacts (Spacing)

Managing spacing is generally straightforward; however, identifying the cause is key to its effective management. Table 16.2 summarises the common causes of problematic space closure. It is important to appreciate that there may

Table 16.2 Common causes of impaired space closure.

Cause	Example
Intraosseous	Sclerotic bone
	Necking of bone
Tooth related	Retained root
	Ankylosis
	Abnormally shaped roots
Appliance related	Occlusal interferences
	Inadequate force
	Excessive force
	Archwire deformation
	Slot/tube deformation
	Calculus deposits on archwire/brackets
	Root contact with cortical bone (inappropriate torque expression)
Patient related	Inadequate compliance (e.g. with elastics)
	Medications: bisphosphonates

be situations when the occlusal relationship is correct but space remains within one arch; this is often as a result of a TSD. The elimination of space may result in a compromise of the overjet or occlusal relationship. If these compromises are not desirable, then adjustment to torque, tip and rotations should be considered before the use of adhesive restorations to build up narrow teeth in one arch with or without interproximal enamel reduction in the opposing arch to optimise tooth fit.

Finishing in Class II camouflage cases where the posterior molar is brought into a full unit Class II position often necessitates the closure of residual space; this is because the extractions can introduce a TSD and therefore affect the occlusal fit. Often, the placement of a *toe-out* bend to rotate the upper molar distolabially is sufficient to eliminate this residual space. This is because the dimensions of a rotated upper molar mean that it will take up more space in the arch than a non-rotated molar. The supplemental use of Class III elastics to aid molar protraction may be an alternative approach to consider. The likelihood of introducing a TSD with extractions can be investigated during the treatment planning stage by obtaining a Kesling set-up of the end occlusion, or alternatively with digital planning software.

Occasionally, sliding mechanics on a full-size working archwire may prove ineffective in closing residual space. One option is the placement of an undersized archwire to aid space closure (e.g. 0.018-inch stainless steel). However, the associated loss of tooth control in all three dimensions and axes of rotation (in–out, tip, rotation and torque) needs to be appreciated and there may be a need to advance to a full-size rectangular archwire following space closure. In difficult cases alternatives such as looped mechanics may need to be employed to close residual space (see Chapters 2 and 14).

Centreline (Dental Midline)

The management of the dental centreline should be considered at the diagnosis stage of treatment and may influence the creation of space, the management of microdontia and hypodontia, and the choice of dental extractions (see Chapters 1 and 14). Space may be needed to correct the centreline by moving the two central incisors, although this movement will create space on the other side of the arch, which is often needed due to the presence of crowding. The centreline is also considered during space closure when elastics may help to manage or maintain the upper dental centreline whilst also helping to close the buccal segment space. Figure 16.2 highlights the use of asymmetrical elastics to help manage a centreline discrepancy.

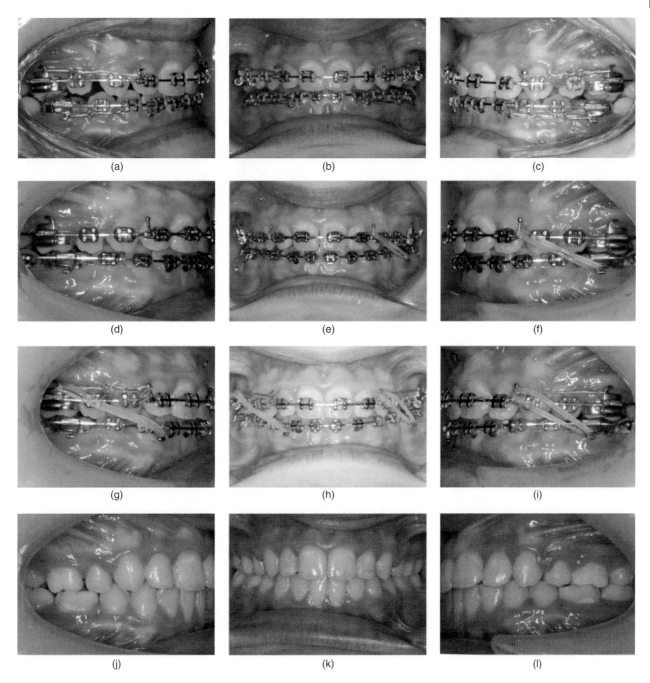

Figure 16.2 Case photographs demonstrating the successful use of asymmetrical elastics to help manage a dental centreline discrepancy. (a–c) Upper and lower 0.019 × 0.025-inch stainless steel archwires. Space closure with elastomeric ligatures in all quadrants. (d–f) Upper and lower 0.019 × 0.025-inch stainless steel archwires. It is evident that the upper centreline is to the right in comparison to the lower. A Class II intermaxillary elastic on left side is being used to aid centreline correction. (g–i) Upper and lower 0.019 × 0.025-inch stainless steel archwires. There has been some improvement in the centreline after two months; asymmetrical intermaxillary elastics (Class III right side and Class II left side) have been utilised to further aid centreline correction. (j–l) End of treatment photographs showing the centreline discrepancy corrected.

Root Angulation

In contemporary dental practice, root parallelism is particularly important in cases where appliances are being used to maintain or open space for future prosthetic replacement.

If implant placement is planned or may be pursued at a later date, then sufficient space needs to be available between the roots of teeth adjacent to the potential placement site.

Figure 16.3 highlights a case where sufficient space was created for implant placement. Sometimes brackets need

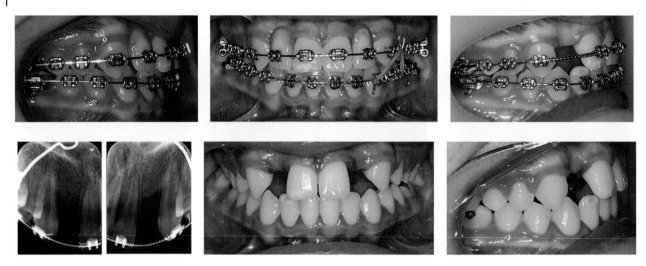

Figure 16.3 Sufficient space has been created in the upper lateral incisor regions both coronally and apically.

to be positioned in a non-ideal position in order to create sufficient space between the roots of the teeth for dental implants to be an option for the long-term replacement of missing units. However, it is important to note that over-correcting root angulation may adversely affect coronal aesthetics.

It is important to appreciate that correct root angulation is also important to help optimise bone thickness around a root.

Buccolingual Inclination

Discrepancies of buccolingual inclination are due to errors in the application of torque. Reasons for this include incorrect bracket positioning, anatomical variation in crown form, and slop between the archwire and bracket, but may also result from excessive use of elastics. Methods for improving the inclination include using full-sized archwires, for example a 0.021 × 0.025-inch archwire in a 0.022 × 0.028-inch bracket slot. In addition, torque can be placed in an archwire or auxiliaries used to increase torque expression. Figure 16.4 shows an example of a simple torquing auxiliary that can be fabricated at the chairside.

Torque control of the upper labial segment in Class II division 2 malocclusions is particularly challenging. One approach to increasing palatal root torque in the upper labial segment efficiently would be to select a bracket prescription with increased palatal root torque in this region (e.g. MBT prescription).

The assessment of inclination is often subjective; however, it can be judged cephalometrically using the upper incisor to maxillary plane inclination and the inter-incisor

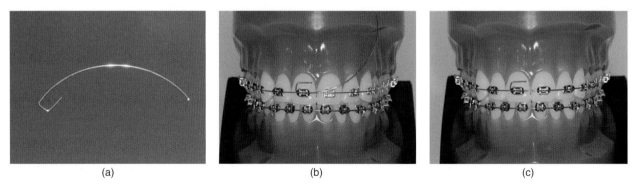

(a) (b) (c)

Figure 16.4 (a) An incisor or canine torquing auxiliary can be formed at the chairside from a 0.018-inch stainless steel archwire. (b) The torquing auxiliary ligated passively to the tooth to which the torquing force is to be applied. (c) The outer arm has to be moved downwards to be ligated. This will in turn place palatal pressure on the smaller inner arm, above the central incisor bracket, resulting in a palatally directed root torquing force. If the auxiliary is inverted, with the inner arm incisal to the central incisor bracket, torque will be placed in the opposite direction. We find this a very effective technique when large amounts of torquing force must be applied. The auxiliary delivers gentle consistent forces over a long range, unlike a third-order bend in a rectangular archwire. The auxiliary should be kept *in situ* until the time of debond, when retainers can be quickly placed, as in our experience the changes are prone to rapid relapse. Source: courtesy of Daljit Gill.

angle. Other methods to assess torque include the use of a tooth inclination protractor,[5] a simple protractor with an additional rotating arm that may be used to check crown inclination on dental study casts. As mentioned in previous chapters, maxillary incisor inclination should be assessed clinically and it is the aesthetic appearance rather than cephalometric angle that is the most important factor. The labial face of the tooth should be approximately vertical, with the head in natural head position (see Chapter 1 and Figure 1.8).

Occlusal Relationship and Overjet

In the absence of a TSD or errors in angulation and inclination, a Class I buccal segment (including the canine) will result in a Class I incisor relationship and a normal overjet. If, however, the buccal segment relationship alters from a Class I relationship, then this will result in variations in the centreline or the incisor relationship, including the overjet. Any variation from a Class I buccal segment towards the end of treatment, in the absence of space, may be the result of anchorage loss. Frequently, anchorage loss in the maxillary arch results in the buccal segment tending towards a Class II relationship, and consequently the overjet is increased. Strategies that can be employed to overcome this problem include the use of intermaxillary elastics or distalisation of the upper buccal segments. Practically speaking, with good compliance, intermaxillary elastics will not generally correct a molar discrepancy greater than one-quarter unit in the absence of spacing. Anchorage loss in the mandibular arch results in the buccal segment tending towards a Class III relationship, and subsequently the overjet is reduced. Methods that can be used to overcome this problem include intermaxillary elastics or a revision of the original aims of treatment.

If there is an overjet outside the range of 2–4 mm in the presence of a Class I buccal segment, the cause of this may be a TSD. This can be accepted or corrected by tooth tissue reduction (enamel stripping) often of the lower labial segment. The microdont upper lateral incisor is a common cause of this problem that is often resolved by the addition of acid etch composite and a long-term restorative plan.

Efficient Finishing: the Importance of Diagnosis and Treatment Planning

Orthodontic finishing is arguably the lengthiest phase of active orthodontic treatment. It commences with the initial assessment, is considered during the placement of the orthodontic appliance and should inform all decisions about retention. It is therefore important to identify potential challenges for finishing during the diagnostic stage, allowing for appropriate selection of bracket prescription and modifications, bracket positioning and use of bracket variations at the start of treatment. The identification of a TSD is particularly important before commencing treatment. This will allow for either patient expectations to be managed concerning the end result at an early stage or the use of other strategies such as interproximal enamel reduction and/or restorative treatment to be discussed.

Tooth Size Discrepancies

Tooth size discrepancies have the potential to cause significant difficulties in obtaining an excellent occlusal result. Bolton proposed two ratios for assessment of a TSD, the overall and anterior ratio.[6] The overall ratio is ascertained by dividing the sum of mesiodistal widths of the mandibular 12 teeth (first molar to first molar) by the sum of mesiodistal widths of the maxillary 12 teeth (first molar to first molar). He ascertained that a mean value 91.3 ± 1.91 was predictive of an excellent occlusion. The anterior ratio is ascertained by dividing the sum of mesiodistal widths of the mandibular six anterior teeth (canine to canine) by the sum of mesiodistal widths of the maxillary six teeth (canine to canine). Bolton ascertained that a mean value 77.2 ± 1.65 was predictive of an excellent occlusion. However, a literature review by Othman and Harradine[7] revealed that 20–30% of the orthodontic population have a significant anterior TSD and 11–14% have an overall TSD according to the Bolton ratio. The authors argue that Bolton's original sample was based on individuals with excellent occlusions and so it is not likely to be appropriate for determining the discrepancy required to preclude an excellent occlusal result at the end of orthodontic treatment. One suggestion therefore is to quantify the size of such a discrepancy. Bernabé et al.[8] suggested that a figure of 1.5 mm or greater is clinically significant, although currently there is no agreed figure.

Clinical experience suggests there is likely to be an influence on occlusal fit if maxillary lateral incisors are smaller than the mandibular lateral incisors and if maxillary and mandibular second premolars are of differing sizes (this would be identified by an increased anterior ratio). Conversely, an excess of tooth tissue in the maxillary arch in relation to the mandibular arch can lead to a residual overjet at the end of treatment (this would be identified by a reduced anterior ratio).

If a TSD is highlighted in the initial assessment, then this can avoid lengthy attempts at managing its consequences in the finishing stage of treatment. Instead, a plan can be developed at the outset to manage the TSD by tooth tissue reduction, increase, or a combination of the two.

Alternatively, the patient may opt to accept spacing or even a compromised occlusal result.

Bracket Alterations to Maximise the Efficiency of Treatment and Finishing

For options relating to local bracket alterations please refer to Chapter 14.

Personalisation of Appliances

The preadjusted edgewise appliance was developed from Andrews' unique concept of every tooth having a pre-scribed angulation, inclination, in–out and rotation within the construction of the bracket. This would theoretically eliminate the need for archwire bends to produce the desired tooth movement. However, the brackets, though specific for each tooth, were not individualised for each patient. Technology now exists for appliances to be con-structed from impressions or scans of the tooth surface and recently there has been an argument for the use of customised appliance systems to reduce treatment time and make finishing more efficient. These appliances utilise the concept of reverse-engineering brackets from a vir-tual design of a finalised treatment result. Retrospective studies have demonstrated a reduction in ABO score for customised labial appliances when compared to conven-tional preadjusted bracket systems; however, there are no randomised controlled trials comparing the effectiveness and efficiency of customised appliances.[9]

Indirect Bonding

Another approach that has been utilised to improve finish-ing and treatment efficiency is the use of indirect bonding (see Chapter 7). However, a recent systematic review and meta-analysis concluded that there appears to be no difference in terms of bracket placement accuracy or oral hygiene status when comparing direct and indirect bonding.[10] Furthermore, the authors reported that total chairside time may be reduced with an indirect approach, but that total working time was increased.

Incisal Edge Recontouring and Interproximal Reduction

Changing the shape of the incisal edge may be necessary as part of orthodontic treatment. The incisal edge can suf-fer trauma or wear, mamelons may persist where incisors have no occlusal contact, or adjacent teeth may be differ-ent sizes. The enamel surface should be reshaped to pro-duce the most aesthetic outcome for the patient. This may involve the addition of acid etch composite material to build up small teeth (liaison with the dentist is required to decide on the timing of such restorations) or reshaping to disguise the effects of trauma or attrition on the enamel surface.

Black triangles are often seen in patients where teeth with triangular-shaped crowns or those teeth affected by recession are aligned. A triangular shape may be a reflec-tion of inadequate interproximal wear, often seen when imbricated incisors are aligned. Interproximal enamel reduction allows the size of the black triangles to be reduced or eliminated by stripping the proximal enamel surface. This reshaping of the tooth can be achieved either mechanically or manually using diamond strips (see Chapter 14). Careful attention must be paid to produce the smoothest enamel surface possible and the use of fluorides to strengthen the enamel following the procedure is recommended.

Conclusion

The key to excellence in finishing is accurate diagnosis, treatment planning, monitoring the patient's response to mechanotherapy, and retention. Challenges particularly in relation to tooth morphology, anchorage demands and TSDs should be appreciated prior to commencing treat-ment. Patients may opt not to proceed with the adjunctive procedures required to achieve high levels of finishing according to the ABO criteria; moreover, the additional time required to achieve 'ideal' goals may be dispropor-tionate to the potential gain. Any potential compromises in the outcome should be clearly outlined in the consent process prior to starting treatment.

References

1 Andrews LF. The straight wire appliance: origin, controversy, commentary. *J. Clin. Orthod.* 1976;10(2): 99–114.
2 Angle EH. *Treatment of Malocclusion of the Teeth. Angle's System.* Philadelphia: S.S. White Dental Manu-facturing Company, 1907.

3 Andrews LF. The six keys to normal occlusion. *Am. J. Orthod.* 1972;62(3):296–309.
4 American Board of Orthodontics (ABO). Grading sys-tem for cast and radiographic evaluation. https://www .americanboardortho.com/orthodontic-professionals/ about-board-certification/clinical-examination/

certification-renewal-examinations/mail-in-cre-submission-procedure/case-report-examination/case-report-preparation/cast-radiograph-evaluation/

5 Richmond S, Klufas ML, Sywanyk M. Assessing incisor inclination: a non-invasive technique. *Eur. J. Orthod.* 1998;20(6):721–726.

6 Bolton WA. Disharmony in tooth size and its relation to the analysis and treatment of malocclusion. *Angle Orthod.* 1958;28(3):113–130.

7 Othman SA, Harradine NW. Tooth-size discrepancy and Bolton's ratios: a literature review. *J. Orthod.* 2006;33(1):45–51; discussion 29.

8 Bernabé E, Major PW, Flores-Mir C. Tooth-width ratio discrepancies in a sample of Peruvian adolescents. *Am. J. Orthod. Dentofacial Orthop.* 2004;125(3):361–365.

9 Weber DJ II, Koroluk LD, Phillips C, et al. Clinical effectiveness and efficiency of customized vs. conventional preadjusted bracket systems. *J. Clin. Orthod.* 2013;47(4):261–266.

10 Li Y, Mei L, Wei J, et al. Effectiveness, efficiency and adverse effects of using direct or indirect bonding technique in orthodontic patients: a systematic review and meta-analysis. *BMC Oral Health* 2019;19(1):137.

17

Retention

Simon J. Littlewood

CHAPTER OUTLINE

Introduction, 321
Historical background, 322
Aetiology of Post-treatment Changes, 323
    Post-treatment Changes due to Relapse, 323
    Post-treatment Changes due to the Ageing Process, 323
    Consent and Retainers, 323
    Third Molars and Relapse, 324
Reducing Relapse During Treatment, 324
Choice of Retainers, 324
Fixed Retainers, 324
    Placement of a Fixed Retainer, 325
    Problems and Complications with Bonded Retainers, 326
    Maintenance of Bonded Retainers, 326
Removable Retainers, 327
    How Often Should they be Worn?, 327
    Adherence with Removable Retainers, 327
    Hawley-type Retainer, 327
    Clear Plastic Retainers, 328
    Positioners, 328
Responsibilities in Retention, 329
    Responsibilities of the Orthodontist, 329
    Responsibility of the Patient, 329
    Responsibility of the General Dentist, 329
Conclusions, 329
Acknowledgements, 329
References, 329

Introduction

Orthodontic retention is a vital part of any treatment plan involving fixed orthodontic appliances. Post-treatment changes in the position of teeth are unpredictable. These changes are due to relapse of the teeth moving back towards their initial position, but they are also due to the effects of growth and ageing, which can lead to irregularity of the teeth.

Orthodontic retainers, either removable or fixed, can be used to reduce these unwanted changes, and should be worn for as long as the patient wants to keep their teeth straight. The choice of retainers should be tailored to the individual patient according to the likely stability of the result, and the original malocclusion. The choice is also influenced by the patient's preference and expectations. The aim of retention is to reduce post-treatment changes to a level that maintains the favourable changes achieved during treatment to the satisfaction of the patient.

Planning for stability at the end of treatment with fixed orthodontic appliances should be an integral part of the initial treatment plan. In many ways it is the most important part. Absolute stability will never be possible, as the occlusion sits within a biological environment that is constantly changing throughout life.

Preadjusted Edgewise Fixed Orthodontic Appliances: Principles and Practice, First Edition. Edited by Farhad B. Naini and Daljit S. Gill.
© 2022 John Wiley & Sons Ltd. Published 2022 by John Wiley & Sons Ltd.

This chapter discusses the historical background to retention, the aetiology of post-treatment changes, approaches used during treatment to reduce instability, as well as the practical and safe use of different types of retainers, including the evidence for their use.

Historical background

This section provides a historical background to the use of orthodontic retainers, helping to explain how many of the retainers and techniques we use in modern-day orthodontics have developed.

As early as 1860 it was noted that orthodontic retention was needed to stabilise the result after orthodontic treatment.[1] Edward Angle is often referred to as the Father of Modern Orthodontics, and in his seminal textbook in 1900 he described using a combination of a removable and a fixed retainer for a period after orthodontics to allow the supporting tissues around the teeth to adapt to their new positions.[2] His removable retainer was a vulcanite palate, retained by spurs engaging the necks of the crowns of the premolars and molars. The fixed retainer consisted of bands on the canines connected by a lingual bar. Bands were used as direct bonding to teeth was not possible in this era.

In 1919 Hawley described his retainer,[3] which became the most popular removable retainer for the next 80 years (Figure 17.1). Initially it consisted of a vulcanite palate and labial bow made with gold wire, but it was later constructed with a combination of acrylic and stainless steel wire, the materials we still use today.

In the 1940s it became clear that it was only possible to treat patients to a certain degree of accuracy, with cases often finished with minor residual irregularities and small interdental spaces left after removing the bands that were used on every tooth. This led to the development of positioners.[4] Near the end of treatment, impressions were taken. The teeth were removed from the model and repositioned in ideal positions, using wax to hold them in this corrected position. Elastomeric positioners were then made to fit over each corrected arch and the upper and lower parts were sealed together. Patients then 'chewed' into the positioner to move the teeth into the final, more ideal position. The positioner could then be worn as an orthodontic retainer.

Vacuum-formed plastics in orthodontics were first described in the 1964,[5] but the original materials that were used were unreliable and unsuited to the role of retainers, often cracking and breaking. It was Jack Sheridan who developed the **'Essix' retainer**,[6] using plastic with physical properties that made them much more reliable and helped to popularise the use of clear plastic materials as retainers (Figure 17.2).

The discovery of the acid-etch technique,[7] allowing direct bonding to the teeth, meant that **fixed retainers** could now be directly bonded to the palatal aspect of teeth and also became known also as **bonded retainers**. This led to the use of bonded retainers fixed to the palatal and lingual surfaces of the upper and lower labial segments.

Before the 1990s, orthodontists typically asked patients to wear retainers for one to two years, with the aim of allowing the teeth and supporting periodontal tissues to adapt to the new tooth positions. This relatively short retention period began to be challenged as a result of the ground-breaking work undertaken at the University of Washington, Seattle, in the 1970s and 1980s.[8] Over 900 cases were followed up for at least 10 years after traditional retention had

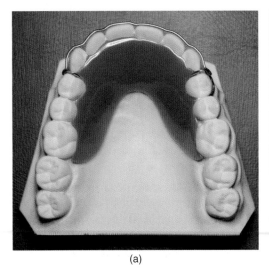
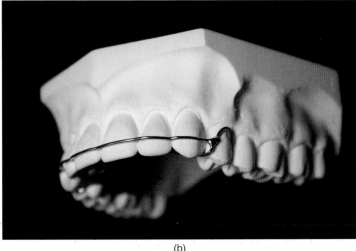

(a) (b)

Figure 17.1 Original Hawley design: (a) occlusal view; (b) anterior view to show fitted labial bow.

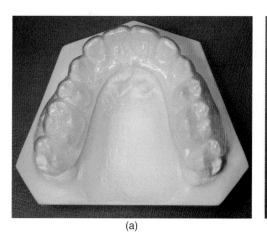
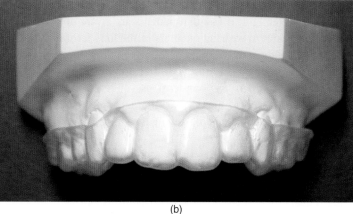

Figure 17.2 Clear plastic retainer: (a) occlusal view; (b) anterior view.

been stopped. It became clear that post-treatment changes continued long after the retainers had been discontinued, and that a significant number of the cases would need retreatment due to the unwanted changes in alignment that were observed. They noted that maxillary teeth were generally less likely to relapse, but overall the arch length and width constricted over time, particularly the lower intercanine width. Perhaps the most disappointing finding was that post-treatment changes were unpredictable, making it difficult to identify which patients were most likely to relapse. Subsequent research has found different levels of relapse, but a common finding in various long-term studies on stability is that relapse is unpredictable. Not all patients relapse, although most do, and because it is difficult to identify who will remain stable and who will relapse, we have to presume everyone has the potential to relapse. This changed the approach to retention, with a recognition that long-term use of retainers is advisable. This has implications for our choice and maintenance of retainers, and is an important consideration for patients when deciding whether to go ahead with orthodontic treatment.

Aetiology of Post-treatment Changes

Understanding the reasons for post-treatment changes should help us understand how to reduce the chances of these unwanted changes occurring.[9] Post-treatment changes are due to two different processes and it is important that the clinician explains this to the patient.

Post-treatment Changes due to Relapse

Relapse is the movement of teeth back towards their initial position. There is a tendency for teeth to move back to their pretreatment position due to tension in the periodontal fibres around the neck of the teeth, i.e. the **dentogingival** and **interdental fibres**. The majority of these fibres will reorganise into the new tooth position within the first 12 months after treatment, although some elastic fibres may take a little longer. Wearing retainers during the first few years after treatment should be considered part of the healing and adaptive stage of retention, allowing the periodontal fibres to reorganise into the final tooth position.

Uneven or deflecting occlusal contacts at the end of treatment may also cause tooth movement, resulting in unwanted post-treatment changes. It is therefore important, where possible, to ensure that a good occlusion is achieved at the end of treatment.

Post-treatment Changes due to the Ageing Process

The teeth are in a biological environment that is constantly changing. As with all parts of the body, ongoing growth and age changes occur throughout life. Subtle changes in the relationship between the maxilla and mandible can affect the occlusion, as well as changing soft tissue pressures on the dentition. These age changes manifest themselves in reduced arch length and width, and increased crowding and irregularity, particularly in the lower labial segment. Even patients who have never had orthodontics show these same types of changes.[10] Wearing retainers long term to reduce age changes should be considered the maintenance stage of retention.

Consent and Retainers

When patients are consented for treatment, it is important that they not only understand the risks, benefits, options and commitments of orthodontic treatment, but also the long-term implications for the retention phase of treatment (see Chapter 1). It is key that patients are aware of the need to commit to wearing retainers in the long term if they want to reduce the chances of the irregularity that is part of the normal ageing process. If they are unwilling or unable to commit to the long-term use of retainers, then they need to accept there is an unpredictable risk of unwanted post-treatment changes in the positions of the teeth.

Third Molars and Relapse

For many years there was a presumption that third molars had the capacity to apply a mesial force on the occlusion, leading to crowding of the anterior teeth, particularly in the lower arch. However, the best available evidence suggests that this irregularity occurs whether the third molars are present or not.[11] As a result, third molars should not be removed purely on the grounds of reducing relapse.

Reducing Relapse During Treatment

The teeth sit in an area known as the 'neutral zone', found between the tongue on the lingual side, and the lips and cheeks on the buccal side. Keeping teeth within this neutral zone reduces the chances of relapse. However, the challenge for the clinician is that the neutral zone cannot be seen, is likely to be different for every patient, and may change throughout life. Anything that moves teeth out of this neutral zone is likely to be unstable. Examples include changes made to the lower arch form, particularly in the intercanine region, or significant labial or lingual movement of lower incisors. If major changes to the lower arch form or lower incisor position are needed to correct a malocclusion, then the final result may be more unstable, and permanent full-time retention should be considered.

Rotated teeth are particularly prone to relapse due to the periodontal fibres around the neck of rotated teeth pulling the teeth back to their original position. During treatment it is advisable to start derotating them as early as possible in order to give the fibres longer to reorganise and adapt to the new position. Overcorrecting the rotation, before aligning the tooth to the final position, is also advisable. Finally, there is a very minor surgical procedure that can be done under local anaesthesia to cut the fibres around the neck of the teeth. This process is called **circumferential supracrestal fiberotomy**, or **pericision**. After a local anaesthetic is given, the blade of a scalpel is inserted down the gingival sulcus, cutting the fibres around the tooth just

above the alveolar bone. This has been shown to reduce the relapse of significantly rotated teeth by up to 30%, and is particularly effective in the maxilla.

Choice of Retainers

Retainers can be either removable, so patients can take them in and out, or fixed, which are bonded to the teeth. The choice of retainer depends on a number of factors, including the preference of the patient, the preference of the operator, the final malocclusion, the presenting malocclusion, the degree of relapse the patient is able to accept, costs, compliance of the patient, and the type of maintenance the patient can commit to.[9] Table 17.1 summarises the advantages and disadvantages of removable and fixed retainers.

Sometimes both removable and fixed retainers can be used in combination, known as dual retention. Asking a patient to wear a removable retainer in addition to the fixed retainer provides a back-up if the fixed retainer becomes loose or fails.

Research comparing removable and fixed retainers tends to show a patient preference for bonded retainers, as patients do not need to remember to wear them[13] and stability is better in the long term as some patients stop wearing their removable retainers.[14] However, there is the potential for periodontal disease unless oral hygiene is maintained around the fixed retainers[13] and fixed retainers are more expensive due to the increased clinical time needed to place them.

Fixed Retainers

Fixed (bonded) retainers are bonded to the palatal aspect of teeth, and are typically attached to the labial segment only using composite resin. There are many different types (Figures 17.3–17.6). There are certain situations where the final result is so unstable that a fixed retainer is recommended. Examples include the following.

- After closure of naturally spaced dentition, including midline diastemas.
- Teeth with a compromised periodontal support.
- Following alignment of severely rotated teeth.
- Following treatment in a cleft palate patient where surgical scar tissue may increase instability.
- Significant changes in the lower arch form, or labiolingual position of lower incisors.
- Correction of anterior open bite.
- Teeth with no opposing teeth in order to prevent over-eruption.

Table 17.1 Advantages and disadvantages of removable and fixed retainers.

	Advantages	Disadvantages
Removable	Patient can remove for cleaning their teeth	Patients need to commit to and remember to wear them as advised
	Does not need to be worn full-time	They can fracture and need replacing
	Cheaper to fit	Can be dangerous if worn while drinking cariogenic drinks
	Covers all teeth, so offers stability across the arch	As not fixed in place, they may not be sufficient to reduce unwanted movement in very unstable cases
		Can affect speech
		Patient may not like aesthetics
		May slow down posterior settling of the occlusion if there is occlusal coverage
Fixed	Patient does not need to remember to wear it	Can fail by debonding from the tooth or by wire fracture, requiring professional repair
	Aesthetic	
	Permanently fixed so good at reducing relapse in very unstable cases	May partially debond without the patient realising, leading to relapse
		Time-consuming and therefore expensive to place
	Good at reducing rotational relapse	Can cause unwanted tooth movement if not placed passively or becomes active during wear
	Allows settling of posterior teeth	In the absence of good oral hygiene can lead to plaque accumulation with the risk of gingivitis, periodontal disease and caries
		Does not maintain posterior expansion
		Requires long-term maintenance and checks by clinician

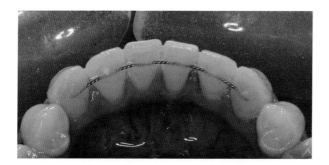

Figure 17.3 Twistflex retainer bonded to every tooth. This is a flexible retainer that maintains stability of all bonded teeth, but can be difficult to clean around and if one composite fails the patient may not notice until the tooth has already relapsed.

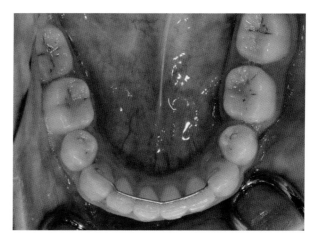

Figure 17.4 Canine and canine-only retainer: a stiffer stainless-steel wire bonded only to the canine teeth. If one attachment fails, the patient will realise and seek advice. It is also a little easier to clean around. However, it does not maintain the stability of the non-bonded incisors as well.

Placement of a Fixed Retainer

A method to place a bonded retainer is described here. For ease of description the placement of a laboratory constructed bonded wire is discussed.

1. A bonded wire can be customised at the chairside or within the laboratory. For laboratory-made retainers, the laboratory can construct the retainer on a study model made from an alginate impression taken at the time of debond, or from a three-dimensional model printed from a scan.
2. Ideally, a bonded wire should be positioned so that it is clear of the gingival margins, does not obstruct the path of an interdental brush beneath the contact point,

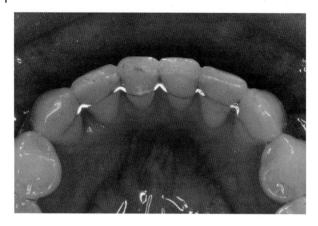

Figure 17.5 Nickel titanium CADCAM retainer. This is very well customised to the tooth surface, but is expensive and not fully tested yet.

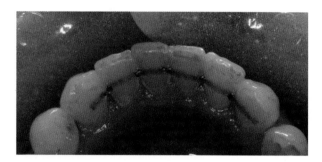

Figure 17.6 Articulated stainless steel chain. This is easy to place at chairside and low profile, but is not recommended for keeping spaces closed.

is non-visible (away from an embrasure space) and is out of traumatic occlusion. The clinician's instructions on the laboratory sheet should be detailed regarding positioning. It is simpler to fulfil these criteria with a lower bonded wire. An upper bonded wire may be in traumatic occlusion and then the operator is forced to place it more gingivally, which can then lead to problems with oral hygiene. The risk of this can be reduced by ensuring that the incisor overbite is fully reduced, and even overcorrected to a small degree, at the end of treatment. Sending a scan of the teeth in occlusion, or an impression and a bite registration will aid the laboratory in positioning the wire away from the occlusion. Positioning a wire on the incisal side of the contact area helps to keep it away from the gingival margin and to allow use of an interdental brush gingival to the contact area.

3. It is important to check the oral hygiene on the lingual surfaces on the visit prior to debond. To minimise the risk of gingival bleeding during bonding of the wire there should be no gingivitis or calculus deposits

present. If there is, the patient should be given strict oral hygiene instructions and advised to visit a hygienist at least two to three weeks before debond to provide time for the gingival inflammation to subside.

4. When fitting the retainer, it is important to have excellent moisture control.

5. Before etching, it may be useful to sandblast the lingual surfaces to be bonded with 50-μm aluminium oxide particles using an intraoral sandblaster, or to run over the enamel surface with a debonding bur. Not only does this clean the enamel surface and remove the hard pellicle, but it may also improve the bond strength.

6. Following this, the surfaces are washed, dried, etched and coated with bonding agent. The clean bonded wire is positioned in a passive position, before bonding with composite resin. One method of positioning is using a transfer jig, and composite resin is placed over the wire and enamel surface over the central third of each tooth and light cured.

7. Following placement, the patient should be asked to check for any roughness; for upper retainers the occlusion should be checked.

8. A vacuum-formed retainer can then be constructed and fitted over the bonded wire. As tooth movement can still occur with a bonded wire, a supplementary removable retainer worn a few nights a week helps to further reduce the risk of tooth movement.

Problems and Complications with Bonded Retainers

There are a number of reasons why bonded retainers can fail.

- Bond failures, with the composite separating from the enamel. This is usually due to moisture contamination during the bonding process.
- Wire fracture.
- Failure of bond between wire and composite.
- Gingivitis and potential for periodontal problems.
- Unwanted tooth movement as a result of movement in the wire. This may be due to the wire not being passive when it was placed or becoming active once *in situ*. This can cause significant problems, potentially moving teeth out of their periodontal support.[15]

Maintenance of Bonded Retainers

Patients who are fitted with bonded retainers need to be willing and able to look after them, and have them checked by a dentist or orthodontist on a regular basis. They need to learn how to clean around the wire, often using small interdental brushes or by threading floss under the wire. All bonded retainers will fail in some way eventually, so patients need to be aware of the costs and maintenance required when consenting to having a bonded retainer fitted.

Removable Retainers

There are broadly three types of removable retainers:

- Hawley-type (based on acrylic and stainless-steel wire)
- clear plastic
- positioners.

How Often Should they be Worn?

There is evidence to suggest that removable retainers only need to be worn at night.[16–18] This reduces the amount of compliance required from a patient, and helps to extend the longevity of the appliance.

Adherence with Removable Retainers

Relapse is slightly higher with removable retainers than fixed retainers, as patients do not always wear them as often as they should.[14] One of the most important roles of the treating clinician is to educate and motivate patients in the importance of wearing retainers. This involves explaining the risks of relapse, and helping patients to establish the regular habit of wearing the removable retainers, and ensuring that if there are any problems the patient knows where to seek professional advice.

Hawley-type Retainer

The Hawley-type retainer (Figure 17.7) typically consists of a stainless-steel labial bow and clasps connected to

an acrylic baseplate. It provides transverse stability after expansion, and in cases of hypodontia prosthetic teeth can easily be added to the retainer (Figure 17.8). Unlike the clear plastic retainer, it can be worn while eating and drinking, so is particularly useful for patients with prosthetic teeth on their retainers.

Research shows that patients may not be as keen on wearing Hawley retainers as clear plastic retainers, partly related to comfort but principally related to aesthetics.[19] A variation with a more aesthetic bow has been developed to improve the visual appeal of the Hawley retainer (Figure 17.9).

A variation called a spring retainer was developed to apply a gentle force from the labial and lingual aspects in order to keep the anterior teeth aligned (Figure 17.10).

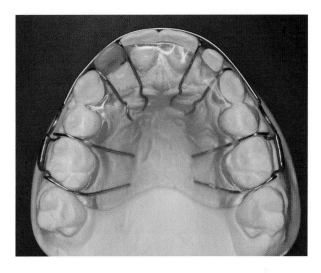

Figure 17.8 Hawley retainer with prosthetic tooth replacing the upper right lateral incisor

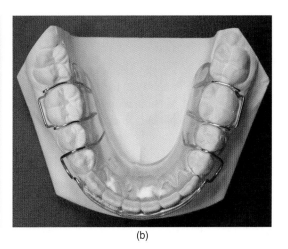

(a) (b)

Figure 17.7 Hawley retainer: (a) upper; (b) lower.

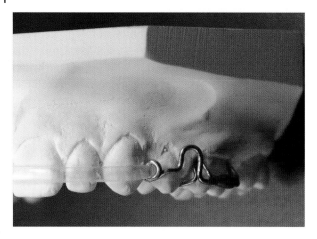

Figure 17.9 Hawley retainer with aesthetic Clearbow®.

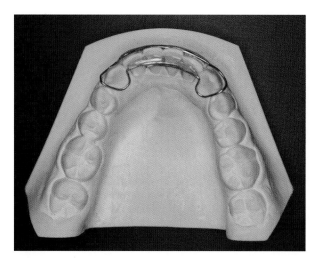

Figure 17.10 Spring-type retainer called a 'barrer appliance' with active force labially and lingually on the labial segment.

It can also be used to align teeth where there has been minor relapse.

Clear Plastic Retainers

Clear plastic retainers (see Figure 17.2) have the advantage over Hawley-type retainers of being more aesthetic, making them more popular with patients, and as a consequence they have been shown to maintain better stability, at least in the short term.[19, 20]

They are usually made from sheets of plastic that are heated using a thermoforming process. These plastic sheets are shaped over a cast of the teeth using either pressure or vacuum forces. It is useful to make two sets for each patient, so that the patient always has a spare set.

Box 17.0 shows the information provided for patients wearing clear plastic retainers.

Box 17.1 Information for patients wearing clear plastic retainers

Your retainers are as important as your braces
If you do not wear your retainers, your teeth will start to go crooked again. If for any reason you can't wear your retainers, contact your orthodontist.

Do not eat or drink with your retainer in
Take your retainer our for eating or drinking as there is a risk of damage to your teeth.

How often do I wear them?
Every night in bed.

How long do I have to wear them?
For as long as you want to keep your teeth straight. We know that as we get older our teeth begin to get more crooked as a natural ageing process so we advise you to keep wearing your retainers.

How do I keep them clean?
Clean your retainers with a toothbrush and water, but do not use toothpaste as this can damage the retainer. You can freshen up the retainer with a special retainer cleaner that your orthodontist can recommend.

Keep the retainer safe
When you are not wearing your retainer, keep it safely in a protective box, away from heat.

What do I do if I miss a night?
You must try and wear the retainer every night. If you forget, then wear the retainer full-time except meals for two days. This is often enough to squeeze the teeth back into place.

What do I do if I lose a retainer?
If you lose a retainer, use the spare you were provided with. Then contact your orthodontist or dentist to get a new one made. There will be a charge for this.

What do I do if my retainer rubs?
You can smooth it with an emery board that you would use to file your nails. If this does not work, contact your orthodontist.

Bring your retainers to all your check-ups
It is important to bring your retainers to all your check-ups with your orthodontist and dentist, so they can check if they need adjusting or replacing.

Positioners

As discussed in the historical background at the start of this chapter, positioners were initially designed to fine detail the occlusion (Figure 17.11). However, they have also been used as retainers.[21] The patients are advised to wear the positioners only at night. They have the advantage of maintaining not only alignment but also inter-arch stability.

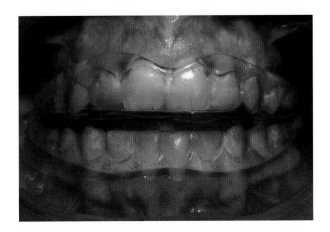

Figure 17.11 Positioner.

They also offer the potential to make minor corrections if there is some degree of relapse, but the disadvantage is that they can be quite bulky and may be a problem for patients to wear in the long term.

Responsibilities in Retention

The long-term commitment to retention should not be underestimated, and brings responsibilities for the orthodontist, the patient and the general dental practitioner.[22]

Responsibilities of the Orthodontist

The orthodontist needs to inform the patient of the need and importance of retainers, choose the appropriate type of retainer, and inform them how to look after retainers to minimise any risks and possible complications. The orthodontist needs to motivate the patient to wear and maintain their retainers, making appropriate arrangements for long-term maintenance and replacement, and ensure the patient understands the costs and commitment involved before starting the course of orthodontic treatment. The orthodontist also needs to liaise with the patient's general dentist to inform them about the retainers that have been fitted.

Responsibility of the Patient

The patient has to take responsibility for wearing the retainer, following the instructions, maintaining it and seeking advice if there are any problems. They will also need to take responsibility for the long-term costs of any maintenance or replacements.

Responsibility of the General Dentist

As patients are now advised to wear their retainer long term, it is helpful if general dentists can review retainers as part of a patient's normal dental check-up. If a dentist is suitably trained and appropriately remunerated for this, they could replace removable retainers if required, detect loose bonded retainers and repair and replace if indicated, and motivate patients to continue wearing and looking after their retainers.

Conclusions

Retention is arguably the most important aspect of any course of orthodontic treatment. Retention is required to resist the unwanted post-treatment changes caused by relapse of the teeth back towards their initial position, but also to reduce the normal unwanted age changes that lead to an increase in irregularity of the teeth. Removable and fixed retainers are available and have different advantages and disadvantages. The choice of retainer should be tailored to the individual patient according to the likely stability of the result, the original malocclusion, and also considering patient preference and expectations.

Acknowledgements

Thanks to Dr Gudrun Edman Tynelius for kindly providing the photos for Figures 17.4 and 17.11, and to Elizabeth Thorpe for the orthodontic laboratory work.

References

1 Angell EC. Treatment of irregularities of the permanent or adult teeth. *Dent. Cosmos* 1860;1:540–544.

2 Angle EH. Retention. In: *Treatment of Malocclusion of the Teeth and Fractures of the Maxillae*, 6th edn. Philadelphia: S.S. White Dental Manufacturing Company, 1900: 150–166.

3 Hawley CA. A removable retainer. *Int. J. Orthod. Oral Surg.* 1919;5:291–305.

4 Kesling HD. The philosophy of the tooth positioning appliance. *Am. J. Orthod.* 1945;31:297–304.

5 Nahoum HI. The vacuum-formed dental contour appliance. *New York State Dent. J.* 1964;9:385–390.

6 Sheridan JJ, Le Doux W, McMinn R. Essix retainers: fabrication and supervision for permanent retention. *J. Clin. Orthod.* 1993;27:37–45.

7 Buonocore MG. A simple method of increasing the adhesion of acrylic filling materials to enamel surfaces. *J. Dent. Res.* 1955;34:849–853.

8 Little RM, Riedel RA, Artun J. An evaluation of changes in mandibular anterior alignment from 10–20 years post-retention. *Am. J. Orthod. Dentofacial Orthop.* 1988;93:423–428.

9 Littlewood SJ. Retention. In: Littlewood SJ, Mitchell L (eds). *An Introduction to Orthodontics*, 5th edn. Oxford: Oxford University Press, 2019: 204–213.

10 Schütz-Fransson U, Lindsten R, Bjerklin K, Bondemark L. Mandibular incisor alignment in untreated subjects compared with long-term changes after orthodontic treatment with or without retainers. *Am. J. Orthod. Dentofacial Orthop.* 2019;155:234–242.

11 Pithon MM, Baiao FCS, Sant'Anna L, et al. Influence of the presence, congenital absence, or prior removal of third molars on recurrence of mandibular incisor crowding after orthodontic treatment: systematic review and meta-analysis. *J. World Fed. Orthod.* 2017;6: 50–56.

12 Edwards JG. A long-term prospective evaluation of the circumferential supracrestal fiberotomy in alleviating orthodontic relapse. *Am. J. Orthod. Dentofacial Orthop.* 1988;93:380–387.

13 Forde K, Storey M, Littlewood SJ, et al. Bonded versus vacuum-formed retainers: a randomized controlled trial. Part 1: stability, retainer survival, and patient satisfaction outcomes after 12 months. *Eur. J. Orthod.* 2018;40:387–398.

14 Al-Moghrabi D, Johal A, O'Rourke N, et al. Effects of fixed vs removable orthodontic retainers on stability and periodontal health: 4-year follow-up of a randomized controlled trial. *Am. J. Orthod. Dentofacial Orthop.* 2018;154:167–174.

15 Kučera J, Marek I. Unexpected complications associated with mandibular fixed retainers: a retrospective study. *Am. J. Orthod. Dentofacial Orthop.* 2016;149:202–211.

16 Littlewood SJ, Millett DT, Doubleday B, et al. Retention procedures for stabilising tooth position after treatment with orthodontic braces. *Cochrane Database Syst. Rev.* 2016;(1):CD002283.

17 Gill DS, Naini FB, Jones A, Tredwin CJ. Part-time versus full-time retainer wear following fixed appliance therapy: a randomized prospective controlled trial. *World J. Orthod.* 2007;8:300–306.

18 Shawesh M, Bhatti B, Usmani T, Mandall N. Hawley retainers full or part time? A randomized clinical trial. *Eur. J. Orthod.* 2010;32:165–170.

19 Hichens L, Rowland H, Williams A, et al. Cost-effectiveness and patient satisfaction: Hawley and vacuum-formed retainers. *Eur. J. Orthod.* 2007;29:372–378.

20 Rowland H, Hichens L, Williams A, et al. The effectiveness of Hawley and vacuum-formed retainers: a single-center randomized controlled trial. *Am. J. Orthod. Dentofacial Orthop.* 2007;132:730–737.

21 Edman Tynelius G, Bondemark L, Lilja-Karlander E. Evaluation of orthodontic treatment after 1 year of retention: a randomized controlled trial. *Eur. J. Orthod.* 2010;32:542–547.

22 Littlewood SJ. Responsibilities and retention. *APOS Trends Orthod.* 2017;7:211–214.

Section IV

Management of Malocclusions with Preadjusted Edgewise Appliances

18

Management of Class II Malocclusions

Martyn T. Cobourne and Mithran S. Goonewardene

CHAPTER OUTLINE

Introduction, 333
Management Options, 334
    Growth Modification, 334
    Orthodontic Camouflage, 335
    Orthodontics and Orthognathic Surgery, 336
Growth Modification, 336
    Removable Functional Appliances, 336
    Fixed Functional Appliances (Class II Correctors), 338
Orthodontic Camouflage, 342
    Molar Distalisation Strategies, 344
Orthodontics and Orthognathic Surgery, 356
References, 356

Introduction

Class II malocclusion represents a relatively common post-normal sagittal discrepancy between the maxillary and mandibular dental arches. There is prominence of the upper incisors, with the lower incisor edges situated behind the upper incisor cingulum plateaux, and this feature defines the Class II incisor relationship. In the majority of cases, the upper incisors are proclined or of normal inclination and the overjet is increased, i.e. a Class II division 1 relationship. Alternatively, the upper (often central) incisors can be retroclined and the overjet minimal whilst the overbite is increased, i.e. a Class II division 2 incisor relationship (Figure 18.1). In the buccal segments, there is generally a Class II relationship although considerable variation can exist, and the size of this discrepancy is often a good indicator of severity, particularly if it is accompanied by underlying dentoalveolar compensation. Occasionally, a Class I incisor relationship can exist in the presence of a Class II buccal segment relationship associated with space loss and crowding.

The skeletal pattern is generally Class II and the presence of mandibular retrognathia is a common finding.[1] Indeed, a retrusive mandible is often the defining aetiological factor, although maxillary prognathism or some combination of the two is also seen. The vertical skeletal pattern reflected in the maxillary–mandibular plane angle can also play a significant role in Class II malocclusion. In general, a Class II division 1 incisor relationship is associated with average or increased vertical proportions, whilst Class II division 2 is more commonly seen in combination with reduced vertical proportions. The size of the sagittal discrepancy can further influence the incisor relationship depending on the underlying vertical proportions and lip morphology. In the presence of reduced vertical proportions, if the mandibular deficiency is substantial, the lower lip will tend to sit behind the upper incisors at rest and procline them, producing a Class II division 1 relationship and often an increased overbite. If the mandibular deficiency is less significant, in the presence of reduced vertical proportions the upper lip will tend to sit in front of the upper incisors and retrocline them. In this scenario, the incisor relationship will be Class II division 2 and the overbite will also be increased. In reality, significant clinical variation is seen amongst Class II individuals and the features are influenced overall by the combined effects of skeletal pattern, dentoalveolar compensation and soft tissue function.

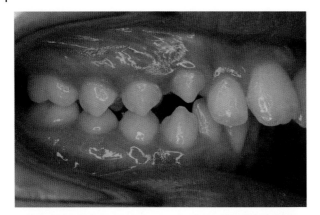

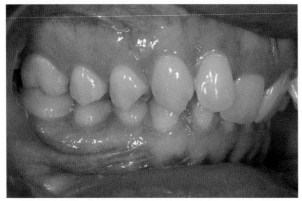

Figure 18.1 Class II division 1 (*top*) and Class II division 2 (*bottom*) malocclusion.

The morphological variation that is seen in Class II cases is in many instances a reflection of the underlying mandibular growth pattern. In Class II division 1 malocclusion there can be a downward and backward rotation associated with increased vertical proportions and potential unfavourable increase in the overjet with facial growth. Conversely, an upward and forward rotation associated with less severe mandibular retrognathia as seen in Class II division 2 cases can undergo more favourable growth and aid correction of the sagittal discrepancy.[2]

Management Options

The management of Class II cases will depend primarily on the age of the patient and severity of the underlying malocclusion. The essential goals of treatment are to correct the incisor relationship, obtain a symmetrical Class I canine relationship and align the teeth. Correction of the malocclusion should be achieved in harmony with the underlying facial features and smile aesthetics, and care needs to be taken in relation to this, particularly when planning extraction-based camouflage in the presence of a more severe Class II skeletal pattern. It is important for the clinician and patient to clearly outline the goals of treatment that will define a successful outcome. Clinicians often feel the necessity to establish efficient systems in their offices and can be tempted to select a universal strategy for all Class II management. If these systems are managing issues through a 'one size fits all' approach and the goals are simply to fit the teeth together without considering patient-centred goals, then it has been said that 'everything works' and 'nothing really matters' when it comes to choice of strategy.[3] In simple terms, Class II discrepancies can be managed with some form of growth modification, or at least an attempt to utilise facial and dentoalveolar maturation during sagittal correction, with orthodontic camouflage utilising tooth movement within the existing skeletal envelope or with orthodontics and orthognathic surgery to correct the malocclusion in conjunction with surgical correction of the jaw position (Figure 18.2).

Growth Modification

For those cases with a moderate to severe skeletal discrepancy and inherent growth potential, an initial phase of functional appliance therapy is often indicated. The aim of growth modification is to improve the skeletal relationship and correct the post-normal occlusion, although in practice the occlusal change achieved by these appliances is far more impressive than the skeletal.[4] This type of treatment often focuses on mandibular advancement and can be provided with an initial stand-alone functional appliance phase prior to treatment with fixed appliances; or in conjunction with the fixed appliance therapy itself, usually with a fixed functional Class II corrector. Removable functional appliances or fixed Class II correctors effectively hold the mandible forward in a corrected occlusal position, distracting the mandibular condyle from the fossa. In theory, the mandible then expresses its innate capacity to grow at an earlier stage than originally patterned.[5] If the individual grows favourably in magnitude and direction, there is the possibility for significant dentoalveolar compensation. Ideally, this phase of treatment will coincide with the pubertal growth spurt to maximise any potential skeletal change, although evidence to suggest significant long-term alteration in the skeletal pattern is weak.[6] It is generally more practical to focus on starting treatment in the late mixed dentition of a growing child, with the expectation that the overjet will be corrected and the occlusion stabilised by the time that the child is in the early permanent dentition and ready to proceed with fixed appliances. Indeed, Class II patients have been reported to exhibit favourable patterns of growth where the mandible can outgrow the maxilla,[7] although the maxillary dentition can compensate forward with the growing mandible which, in effect, means that the skeletal changes are often minimal due to this dentoalveolar compensatory mechanism.[8] It appears therefore

Figure 18.2 Treatment strategies in the management of Class II malocclusion. Growth modification involves the use of removable or fixed functional appliances to correct the sagittal discrepancy through mandibular advancement in a growing child. Orthodontic camouflage involves the distal movement of posterior teeth or extraction-based mechanotherapy. Orthodontic/surgical correction involves orthognathic surgery to definitively correct the skeletal relationship, either with mandibular advancement surgery (shown) or combined maxillary and mandibular surgery.

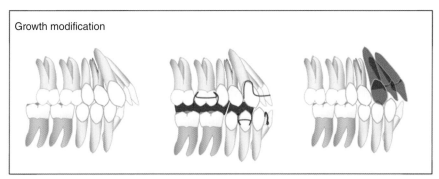

Growth modification

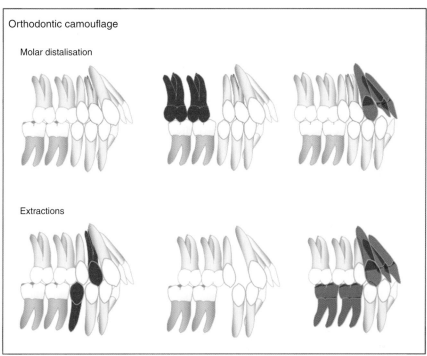

Orthodontic camouflage

Molar distalisation

Extractions

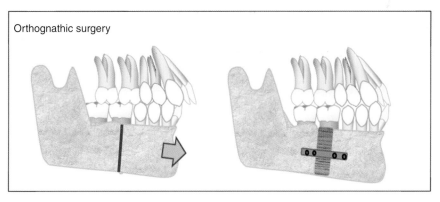

Orthognathic surgery

that the only long-term effects that may be attributed to treatment are changes in dentoalveolar relationships and primarily in the maxilla, where the appliances limit the ability of the maxillary dentition to follow the growing mandible.[9, 10] The highest-quality evidence is clear that functional appliances do not provide any additional long-term growth regardless of treatment timing.[4]

Orthodontic Camouflage

Alternatively, a camouflage approach can be taken, which means accepting the underlying skeletal pattern and managing the malocclusion alone, with the aim of correcting the post-normal occlusal discrepancy using fixed appliances. This might involve the use of fixed appliances on a non-extraction basis in conjunction with Class II traction, with extraction-based Class II mechanics or distalisation of the buccal segments, employing headgear, a distalising appliance (such as the Pendulum appliance) or with the aid of temporary anchorage device (TAD)-based fixed distaliser. In general, if there is any inherent growth potential a camouflage approach is reserved for those cases with a relatively mild skeletal discrepancy because the more severe cases are often more easily managed with an initial functional appliance. However, not all children will tolerate a functional appliance and in those cases with a less severe sagittal discrepancy, camouflage treatment with fixed appliances is often the best option, particularly if they are in the early permanent dentition. The non-growing post-pubertal or adult patient will also be amenable to camouflage treatment if the malocclusion is mild or moderate and this may take any of the forms described above, including the use of fixed-functional appliances; however, the use of these appliances, and indeed headgear in adults, can be problematic, particularly for molar distalisation because of poor compliance and the lack of growth.[11]

Orthodontics and Orthognathic Surgery

For the more severe cases that are non-growing and involve a significant skeletal discrepancy in the sagittal and/or vertical plane, a combination of orthodontics and orthognathic surgery will be required for definitive management within the goal of achieving occlusal correction in conjunction with the most harmonious facial features. This will involve a period of orthodontic decompensation using fixed appliances, aligning and coordinating the dentitions, and achieving normal inclination of the incisors prior to surgical correction. The process of levelling the dentitions will depend on the existing vertical dimensions but in Class II division 2 cases with a reduced lower anterior face height and increased curve of Spee, levelling of the lower arch is often achieved post-surgically, increasing the lower anterior face height with the mandibular advancement.

Growth Modification

Removable Functional Appliances

A short course of removable functional appliance therapy in a growing child is a very effective way to reduce a large overjet and correct the buccal segment relationship prior to definitive treatment with fixed appliances (Figure 18.3). This strategy has the advantage of significantly reducing anchorage need in the subsequent fixed appliance phase of treatment, allowing the orthodontist to focus on space requirements in what will now be a Class I malocclusion. Moreover, once established with a functional appliance, a child can be seen on a 10-weekly basis and generally requires only minimal adjustments as the overjet reduces and the buccal segment relationship corrects.

A wide variety of activator-type functional appliances have been described but in the UK, William Clark's Twin Block appliance is by far the most popular.[12] This two-component tooth-borne functional appliance is well tolerated and very effective at correcting a sagittal discrepancy. It can be individually modified to allow maxillary arch expansion, the addition of headgear and control mandibular buccal segment extrusion. It can also be used in conjunction with a simple upper fixed appliance if the maxillary incisors are significantly crowded or retroclined. A common feature of Twin Block therapy is rapid overjet correction but with a relatively slower rate of vertical compensation. The development of bilateral posterior open bites is therefore a common feature of treatment (Figure 18.4). It is possible to try to prevent the

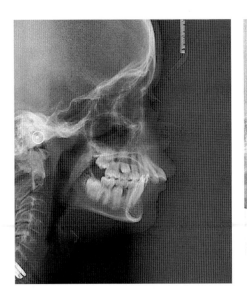 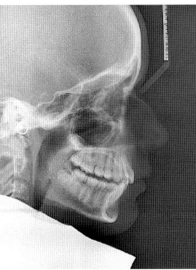

Figure 18.3 Cephalometric radiographs showing the correction of a Class II division 1 malocclusion after eight months of Twin Block functional appliance treatment. There has been retroclination of the upper incisors, some proclination of the lowers and favourable growth.

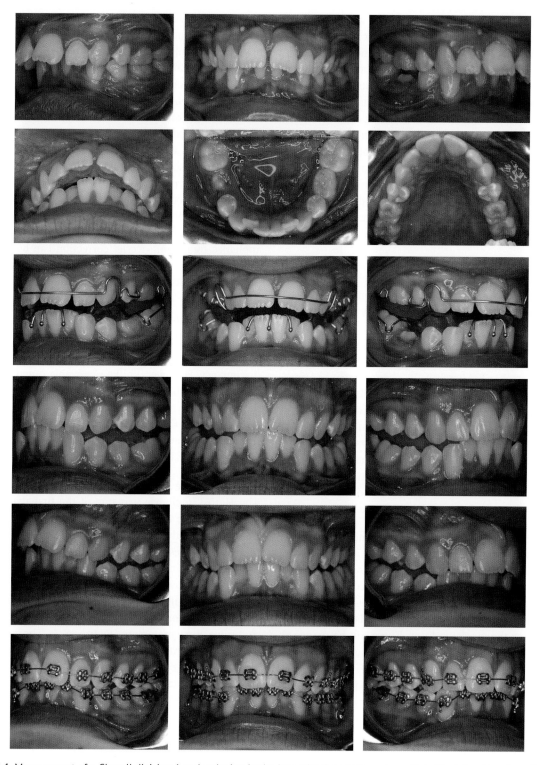

Figure 18.4 Management of a Class II division 1 malocclusion in the late mixed dentition using a Twin Block functional appliance. Overjet correction is usually achieved within six to eight months of full-time wear and this is followed by a few months of part-time wear to allow posterior open bites to close down before entering a fixed appliance phase. The upper six panels show the starting malocclusion in this 11-year-old girl, with subsequent panels (in groups of three, horizontally) showing the full-time Twin Block phase and then the part-time phase as the posterior open bites reduce, followed by the fixed appliance phase.

development of these open bites through selective grinding of the upper appliance buccal acrylic and avoiding cribs on the lower first molars but, in practice, a period of night-time and then alternate night-time appliance wear once the overjet has been corrected will usually be associated with effective closure of the open bites prior to fixed appliance therapy. A number of alternate activator-type functional appliances are available, including the Andreason Activator, Medium-Opening Activator or Bionator; however, the single block of acrylic and reduced retention associated with these appliances makes them more difficult to tolerate and their relative lack of adaptability means that the Twin Block remains the favoured generic functional appliance in the management of Class II cases.

Class II Division 2 Cases

In the management of Class II division 2 cases, the retroclined upper incisors and increased overbite can hamper mandibular advancement when using a Twin Block appliance. This problem can be overcome with a short period of removable or sectional fixed appliance therapy to increase the overjet prior to definitive treatment with the Twin Block (Figure 18.5). Alternatively, reverse curved springs or a small screw plate can be added to the Twin Block or a sectional fixed appliance can be used with the Twin Block to achieve concomitant incisor alignment and sagittal correction.[13] This strategy has the advantage of starting the functional appliance therapy as soon as possible, but can be associated with less significant initial mandibular advancement and more significant vertical opening, which can impact on ease of wear and compliance.

Managing the Transition from Removable Functional to Fixed Appliances

In a compliant growing individual who achieves full-time wear of a Twin Block, significant overjet reduction can be reduced in six to nine months. A characteristic feature of Twin Block therapy is the appearance of bilateral posterior open bites as the overjet reduces. These can be managed relatively easily by reducing wear of the appliance to night-time only and then alternate nights (Figures 18.4 and 18.5). This allows vertical development to proceed whilst maintaining overjet correction. Although selective trimming of the upper block can be undertaken, the strategy of reduced wear is easier and equally effective. Alternatively, the patient can discard the Twin Block whilst the open bites are present and transition to wearing a removable appliance with a steep anterior bite plane to allow lower buccal segment eruption whilst maintaining the corrected overjet.[14]

The post-functional fixed appliance phase of treatment usually occurs once the overjet and buccal segment relationship are corrected, any lateral open bites have closed down and the patient is in the permanent dentition. It is preceded by record-taking, including study models, clinical photographs and a cephalometric radiograph to ascertain the dentoskeletal relationships, particularly the degree of maxillary incisor retroclination and mandibular incisor proclination, which is often a significant contributor to overjet correction with functional appliance treatment. The need for extractions will be based on these relative tooth positions and existing space requirements, particularly lower incisor position. Some clinicians move into the fixed appliance phase of treatment before posterior open bites have closed down but generally it is thought that overjet correction is more stable in the presence of a stable buccal segment occlusion. During the early stage of fixed appliance treatment, overjet correction can be supported with the use of headgear, light Class II elastic wear and, if prescribed, choice of extractions (Figure 18.6).

Fixed Functional Appliances (Class II Correctors)

Fixed functional appliances or Class II correctors also posture the mandible forward to correct a Class II sagittal discrepancy. However, unlike removable functional appliances such as the Twin Block, these appliances are fixed permanently in the mouth during treatment. They can also be used in the mixed dentition as part of a two-stage treatment, but are increasingly used in conjunction with fixed appliances in the early permanent dentition.

Herbst Appliance

The Herbst appliance was one of the first fixed Class II correctors to be described, introduced in the early 1900s and subsequently popularised by Hans Pancherz.[15] The Herbst comprises a right and left telescopic arm with male and female components attached from the upper first molar to the lower first premolars. A fixed lingual and palatal arch unifies the maxillary and mandibular dentition with additional attachments on the lower first molars and upper first premolars (Figure 18.7). The mandible is postured forward to an edge-to-edge relationship, either in one step or in a progressive manner, depending on the size of the discrepancy.[16] The Herbst is usually placed during the circumpubertal growth stage to effect a greater initial skeletal response. However, it has also been utilised to compensate the dentition in adult Class II malocclusions, although the reported treatment time to address a Class II relationship without the assistance of growth is often extended.[17] There have been many modifications to the basic Herbst design, including the use of orthodontic bands, stainless steel crowns, cast frameworks and acrylic splint-type appliances. Moreover, more compact designs, such as the cantilever Herbst appliance, have also been reported.[18]

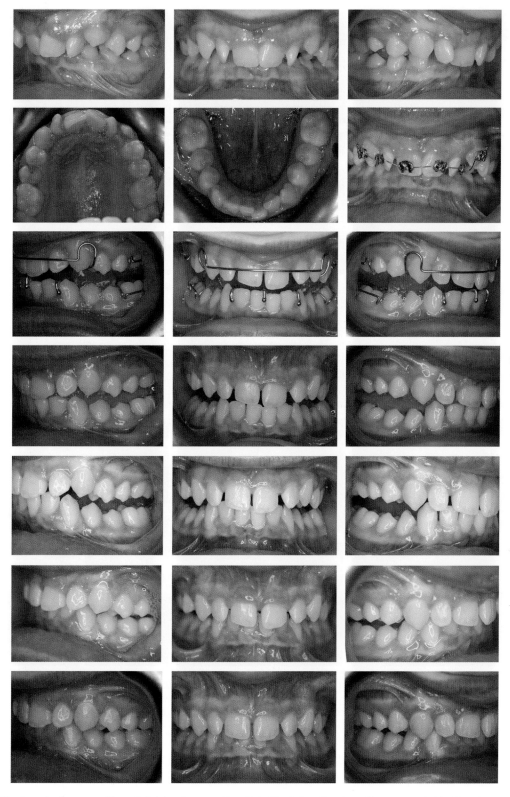

Figure 18.5 Treatment of a severe Class II division 2 case with a Twin Block functional appliance preceded by the placement of a simple upper sectional fixed appliance to correct the upper incisor position, create an overjet and allow the taking of a postured bite prior to fixed appliance removal and fitting of the Twin Block. The upper six panels show the starting malocclusion in this 12-year-old girl and placement of the upper fixed appliance, with subsequent panels (in groups of three, horizontally) showing the full-time Twin Block phase and then the part-time phase as the posterior open bites reduce. This case was associated with reduced vertical proportions and the formation of large posterior open bites during sagittal correction; however, they closed down during the part-time phase of functional appliance wear.

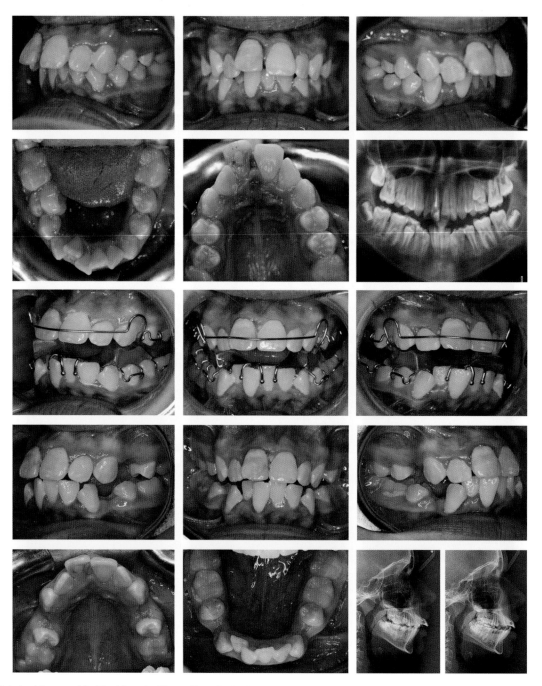

Figure 18.6 An 11-year-old girl with a significant Class II division 1 malocclusion associated with a large overjet, previous trauma to the UR1 and moderate crowding. The overjet was corrected with a Twin Block functional appliance with a decision to extract upper first and lower second premolars prior to the placement of fixed appliances. The extraction decision was based on the upper and lower incisor proclination and moderate crowding that was present.

The significant advantages of the Herbst appliance include minimal compliance requirements and an immediate improvement in profile at the time of insertion. It can be used in patients whose anticipated compliance with strict oral hygiene regimes may be questionable, particularly before comprehensive fixed appliances are placed. The appliance may be inserted to address the dental

relationship at the optimal time without the aforementioned concerns with poor hygiene and comprehensive multi-bracketed appliances. Treatment times with the Herbst appliance have been reported to average around nine months before fixed appliances are placed, with the combined treatment including fixed appliances significantly shorter than two-stage treatment with either

Figure 18.7 A 14-year-old male presented with a Class II division 1 malocclusion with increased overjet and upper arch crowding. The goals of treatment included addressing the Class II relationship by a combination of upper molar distalisation and mesial movement of the lower arch with any complementary growth of the mandible. An upper fixed edgewise appliance and a Herbst appliance with stainless steel crowns on the upper molars and lower first premolars were placed with associated palatal and lingual arches. After eight to nine months, the anteroposterior correction was achieved and the Herbst appliance removed. A lower fixed edgewise appliance was then also used, with archwires progressing from round to rectangular nickel titanium through to 0.019 × 0.025-inch titanium molybdenum alloy (TMA) to finalise tooth positions. The upper panels show the pretreatment facial appearance with subsequent panels organised in vertical pairs from left to right showing treatment progression.

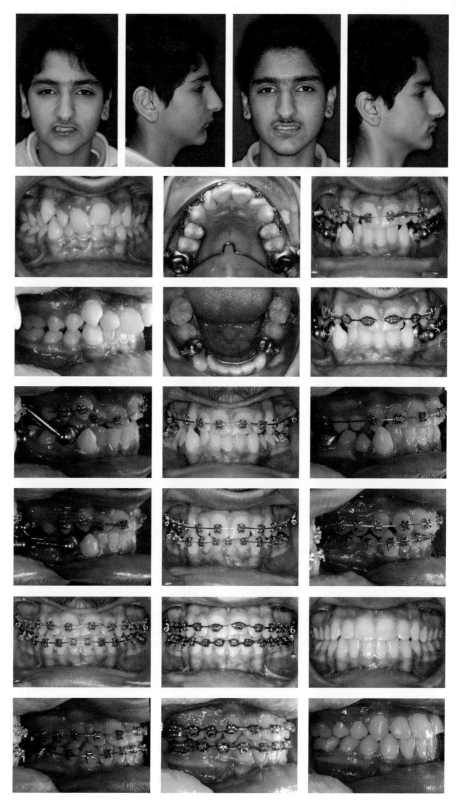

removable appliances or comprehensive fixed appliances alone.[19] Significant complications such as appliance breakage and short-term discomfort have been reported by some authors and may be the reason for a reluctance amongst some clinicians to universally accept this appliance. Moreover, the technical demands during construction are significant, with operator experience an important benefit. The necessity to have an experienced team available to handle complications cannot be understated.[20, 21] Long-term reports of patients treated with the Herbst appliance reveal outcomes similar to almost all functional appliances, with the only significant treatment effects represented by dentoalveolar compensation, reported to remain over 30 years of observation. When the effects of normal growth are taken into account, the long-term skeletal effects are of minimal clinical significance.[22]

Forsus™ Fatigue Resistant Module

The Forsus™ (Fatigue Resistant) module is one of the many commercially available Class II corrector devices that effect changes in the growing child analogous to other types of functional appliance. A combination of minor skeletal effects, related to the magnitude and direction of growth and dentoalveolar compensation, are routinely observed.[23] As with many fixed functional-type appliances, the significant advantage of the Forsus module is the ability of the clinician to combine alignment, levelling and arch coordination with fixed appliances and simultaneous anteroposterior correction. This has the potential to reduce treatment time and the need for prolonged patient compliance. Unlike rigid Herbst-type appliances, the Forsus module comprises right and left springs that are inserted into the headgear tube of the upper molar and a male rod that inserts into a nickel titanium spring (Figure 18.8). It has been suggested that the decreased impact of the flexible spring from the Forsus on positioning of the condyle may have a less deleterious impact on temporomandibular joint integrity than the more rigid Herbst appliance.[24, 25]

The combination of fixed appliances and Forsus module has been reported to effect significant changes in upper and lower incisor position and steepening of the occlusal plane.[26, 27] Technical modifications have been recommended to reduce these side effects and studies reporting effects are often complicated by these individual approaches. Positioning the male component of the module against the first premolar instead of the canine will reduce the rotational moment on the lower occlusal plane. Introduction of labial root movement in the lower incisors either by archwire bending or varying the third-order prescription of the lower incisor brackets have all been

suggested as mechanisms to control this perceived anchorage loss through lower incisor proclination (Figure 18.9). Placement of temporary anchors in the lower arch has also been reported to reduce the loss of lower incisor control.[28] Significant retraction and uprighting of upper incisor position has been reported and similar strategies have been suggested with the opposite goal to the lower by placing adjustments in the wire to effect palatal root movement or using high torque upper incisor brackets. There is insufficient evidence to draw any sound conclusion because of the absence of carefully considered studies. The Forsus module can be used to manage Class II division 1 (Figure 18.10) and Class II division 2 type malocclusions after multi-bracketed appliances have converted the division 2 into a division 1 (Figure 18.11). The Forsus module can also be utilised for correction of significantly crowded Class II problems combined with fixed appliances and premolar extractions (Figure 18.12).

The choice of Class II corrector should be based on the realisation of specific goals. These goals are often complex and should be carefully considered with the patient and parents. If the goals include compensation of the upper and lower teeth within the biological constraints and the patient is growing, then any of the multitude of removable or fixed functional appliances will have the same chance of satisfactorily treating most patients. The choice therefore becomes a practice management issue. If the patient or parents desire a significant change to the chin position, then combined surgery and orthodontics should be considered. If the goals of treatment are directed at retraction of the maxillary dentition, then either extractions or an upper arch distalising strategy are indicated.

Orthodontic Camouflage

Conventional orthodontic camouflage treatment for a Class II malocclusion utilising fixed appliances is an established technique in orthodontics. The incisor relationship and buccal segments can be corrected with Class II traction in milder cases, but for cases with increased anchorage requirements mid-arch premolar extractions are often prescribed to provide sufficient space for correction of the Class II relationship. A common extraction pattern involves the loss of upper first premolars and lower second premolars, which facilitates overjet reduction and molar correction through upper incisor retraction and forward movement of the lower molars (Figure 18.13). However, multiple extraction choices can be made, depending on the underlying malocclusion and prognosis of individual teeth (Figure 18.14).

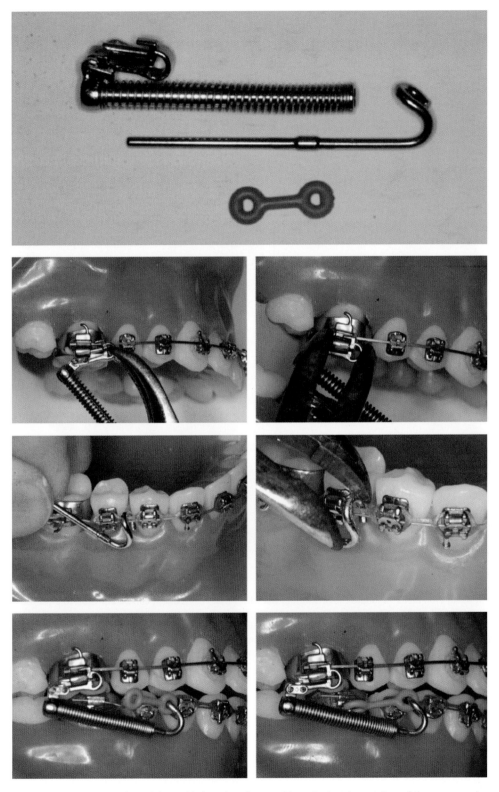

Figure 18.8 The Forsus™ module comprises right and left springs inserted into the headgear tubes of the upper molars and male rods that insert into these springs. The springs have a male component that clips onto the headgear tube using a utility plier and a male component that is crimped onto the archwire either between premolars or premolar and canine. The dumbbell elastomeric is attached from the anterior of the lower male component back to the first molar tube to minimise breakages of the premolar/canine brackets and prevent space from opening in the lower arch secondary to the mesial force on the anterior dentition.

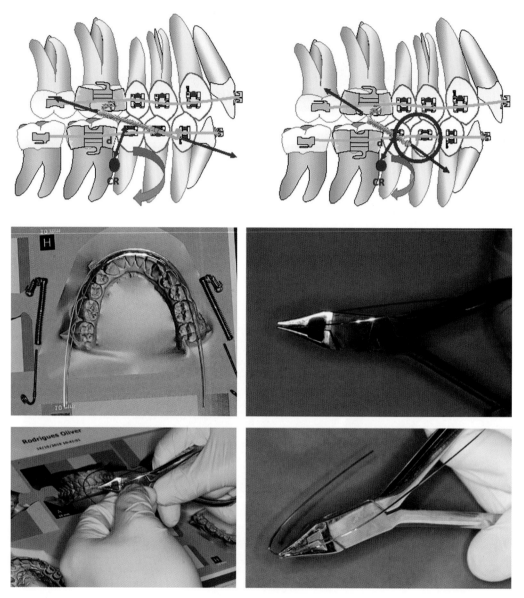

Figure 18.9 When using the Forsus™ module the position of the lower male component can be adjusted to alter the distance (d) of the centre of resistance (CR) of the protrusive force (upper panels). The archwires are prepared, coordinated and adjusted to add approximately 10–15° lingual root torque to the upper incisors (middle panels) and approximately 10° of labial root torque to the lower incisors (lower panels) to reduce the significant uprighting and proclination of the upper and lower incisors that occurs, respectively secondary to the anteroposterior forces generated with this appliance.

Molar Distalisation Strategies

Orthodontic camouflage can also be achieved using fixed appliances to selectively move the upper teeth distally with or without forward movement of the lower incisors. This has been demonstrated to be an effective strategy for Class II treatment.[29] However, once a Class I relationship had been established, the maxillary molars can move forward with residual mandibular growth, reflecting the underlying dentoalveolar compensatory mechanism.

A number of treatment strategies have been suggested that aim to move the upper molars distally, independent of the lower arch. Classically, headgear has been used either direct to molar bands on the upper sixes with or without a removable appliance (or Nudger) to help maintain molar correction[30] or direct to a removable appliance such as an en masse. The use of headgear has declined in recent years, largely due to concerns about safety, problems with compliance, a requirement for favourable growth and the emergence of alternative techniques to achieve successful molar distalisation. A number of non-compliant fixed distalising appliances have been described, including the Pendulum appliance and, more recently, the advent of TADs has introduced the prospect of more effective non-compliant predictable movement and control of the maxillary dentition.

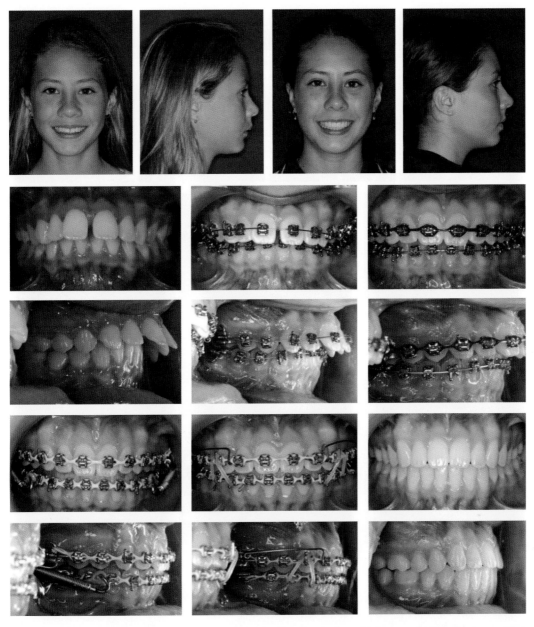

Figure 18.10 A 12-year-old female presented with a Class II division 1 malocclusion with increased overjet and upper incisor irregularity. The goals of treatment included addressing the Class II relationship by a combination of upper molar distalisation and mesial movement of the lower arch with any complementary growth of the mandible. Upper and lower fixed edgewise appliances were placed with archwires progressing from round to rectangular nickel titanium through to 0.019 × 0.025-inch TMA upper and 0.019 × 0.025-inch stainless steel lower. The upper arches were prepared with third-order adjustments to effect palatal root movement in the upper incisors and mild labial root movement in the lower incisors. A Forsus™ module was placed to the lower first premolars. A stainless steel wire is necessary in the lower arch to prevent fracture from the male arm of the module. After nine months, anteroposterior correction was achieved and the Forsus module removed, anterior seating elastics were worn at night and new 0.019 × 0.025-inch TMA archwires used to detail the occlusion. Differential 0.017 × 0.025-inch TMA intrusion springs were also used to manage a mild asymmetry. The upper panels show the pretreatment facial appearance with subsequent panels organised in vertical pairs from left to right showing treatment progression.

The Pendulum Appliance

The Pendulum appliance was first described in 1992 and is one of the most frequently used intraoral distalising devices.[31] A palatal acrylic button is bonded to the premolar teeth with two preactivated 0.032-inch titanium molybdenum alloy springs inserted into palatal attachments on upper molar bands (Figure 18.15). Molar distalisation of 2–6.4 mm has been reported, but a significant shortcoming

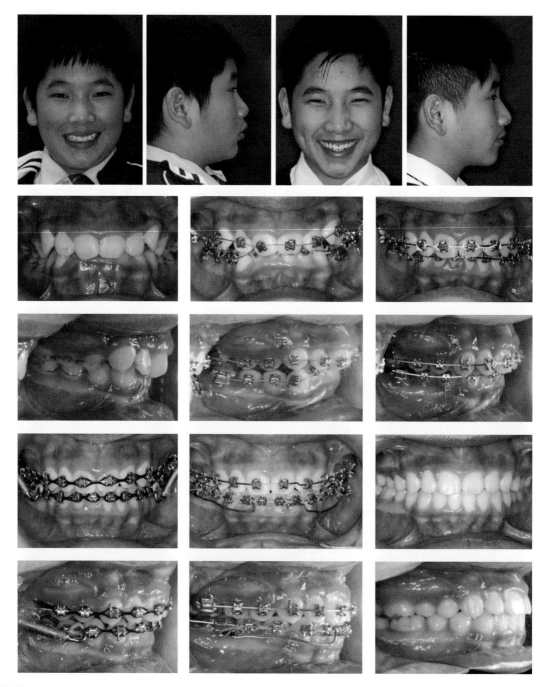

Figure 18.11 A 13-year-old male presented with a Class II division 2 malocclusion with increased overbite and upper incisor irregularity. The goals of treatment included addressing the Class II relationship by a combination of upper molar distalisation and mesial movement of the lower arch with any complementary growth of the mandible. Upper and lower fixed edgewise appliances were placed with archwires progressing from round to rectangular nickel titanium to place the upper incisors in a normal inclination. 0.019 × 0.025-inch TMA upper and 0.019 × 0.025-inch stainless steel lower archwires were prepared with third-order adjustments to effect palatal root movement in the upper incisors and mild labial root movement in the lower incisors. A Forsus™ module was placed to the lower first premolars. After 12 months, anteroposterior correction was achieved and the Forsus module removed, Class III elastics were worn at night to address the mild overcorrection and new 0.019 × 0.025-inch TMA archwires used to detail the occlusion. Differential 0.017 × 0.025-inch TMA intrusion springs were used to manage a mild asymmetry in the lower arch. The upper panels show the pretreatment facial appearance with subsequent panels organised in vertical pairs from left to right showing treatment progression.

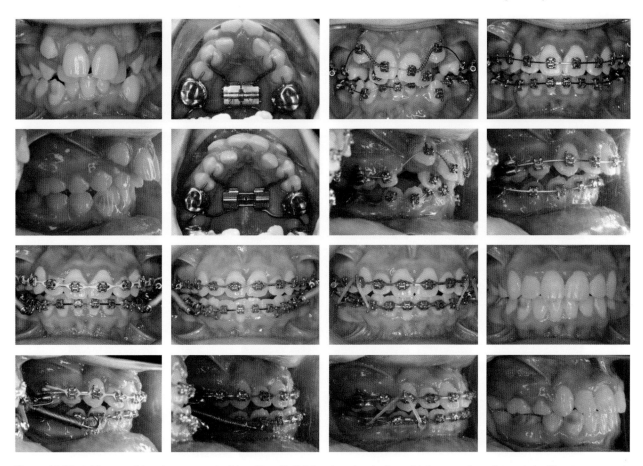

Figure 18.12 A 13-year-old male presented with a Class II division 1 malocclusion with increased overjet and significant upper and lower arch crowding and a narrow maxilla. The goals of treatment include expanding the upper arch, aligning the upper teeth and addressing the Class II relationship by a combination of upper molar distalisation and mesial movement of the lower arch with any complementary growth of the mandible. A maxillary expansion appliance was placed for approximately six months followed by extraction of the upper first and lower second premolars. Upper and lower fixed edgewise appliances were placed with archwires progressing from round to rectangular nickel titanium archwires to place the upper incisors at a normal inclination. Then 0.019 × 0.025-inch TMA upper and stainless steel lower archwires were prepared with third-order adjustments to effect palatal root movement in the upper incisors and mild labial root movement in the lower incisors. A Forsus™ module was placed to the lower canines. After 16 months, anteroposterior correction was achieved and the Forsus module removed, anterior seating elastics were worn at night and new 0.019 × 0.025-inch TMA archwires used to detail the occlusion. The panels show initial malocclusion and treatment progression and are arranged in vertical pairs from left to right.

of this appliance is the reported loss of anchorage, with the anchor teeth moving anteriorly and significant distal molar crown tipping of up to 14° (Figure 18.16).[32, 33] A number of clinicians have suggested modifications to the springs to help produce an uprighting effect, but this side effect is still difficult to overcome.[34] However, the loss of anchorage can be recovered during the retention stage by placing a Nance holding appliance to maintain molar position. The anteriorly displaced premolars predictably drift into the space secondary to the stretched gingival fibres, often resulting in the spontaneous improvement of anterior alignment (Figure 18.17).

TAD-assisted Molar Distalisation

The placement of various TADs in the palatal anchorage component of molar distalising appliances has also been suggested to help minimise anchorage loss; however, controlling the significant molar tipping effect still remains challenging, even with these appliances.[34–37]

Palatal Temporary Anchorage

TADs are now used routinely to deliver force systems directly from the device and/or prevent unwanted side effects of mechanotherapy by attaching screws indirectly to a range of appliances. The range of force application has

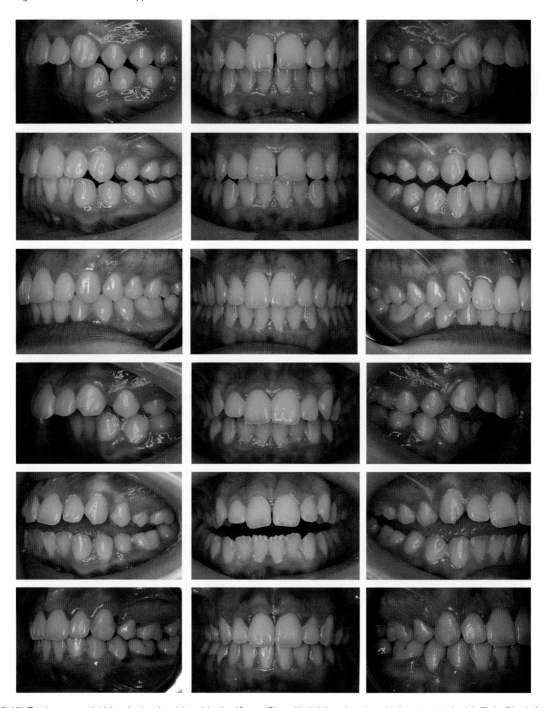

Figure 18.13 Twelve-year-old identical twin girls with significant Class II division 1 malocclusions treated with Twin Block functional appliances. In one of the twins, the response to the Twin Block was favourable, with rapid overjet reduction that was followed by non-extraction fixed appliance treatment to detail the occlusion (upper nine panels). In the other twin, the response to Twin Block therapy was less favourable and overjet reduction was poor. A decision was then made to treat the malocclusion with the loss of upper first and lower second premolars and fixed appliances (lower nine panels). Pretreatment malocclusion is shown in the upper three panels for each twin, with treatment progression in the panels below.

extended to all three dimensions, but is foremost in correcting Class II malocclusion, with patient compliance not required in the same manner as for traditional headgear. The relative stability of these devices makes it possible to

obtain complete anchorage to address the wide range of reciprocal forces in orthodontic mechanotherapy.

Intraoral distalising devices combined with microscrews placed in the palate have been reported and are frequently

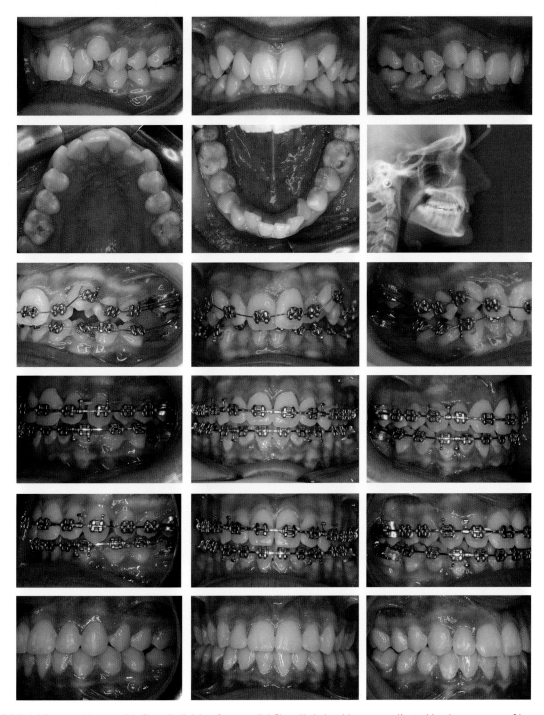

Figure 18.14 A 15-year-old case with Class II division 2 on a mild Class II skeletal base complicated by the presence of hypoplastic poor prognosis first permanent molars. Following extraction of these teeth, fixed appliances were used to correct the incisor relationship and close residual spaces. The upper six panels show the pretreatment malocclusion with treatment progression shown in groups of three panels moving downwards.

used to move posterior teeth distally or mesially, through a wide range of designs.[38, 39] Initially microscrews were placed in the dentoalveolar region, but this was associated with numerous complications including screw loosening, fracture, infection and damage to adjacent structures. In contrast, the placement of screws into the palatal region has been shown to exhibit much greater success. Palatal screws can be placed in the anterior palate under local anaesthesia with relative ease for both patient and operator. The bone quality and volume is important when selecting sites for

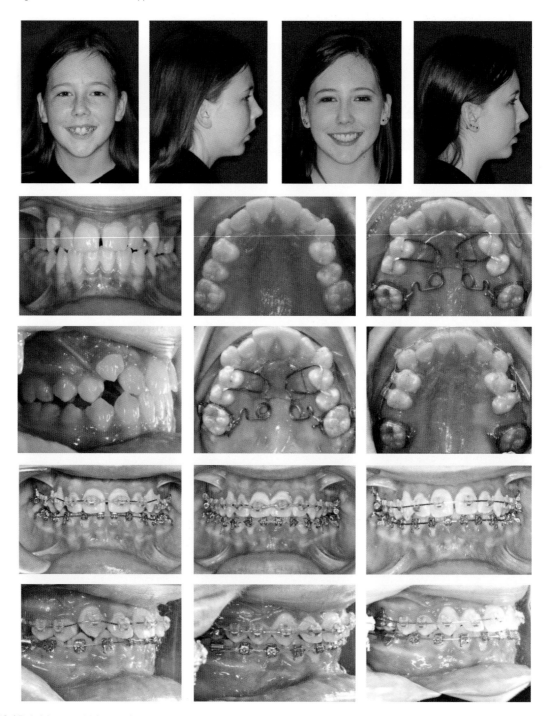

Figure 18.15 A 14-year-old female in the permanent dentition with a Class II malocclusion with upper crowding that may have been treated by either maxillary arch extractions or distalisation of the maxillary dentition. A fixed modified Pendulum appliance was inserted to move the upper molars distally. After correction of the molar relationship, fixed appliances were placed with archwires progressing from round to rectangular nickel titanium through to 0.019 × 0.025-inch TMA to finalise tooth positions. The upper panels show the pretreatment facial appearance with subsequent panels organised in vertical pairs from left to right showing treatment progression.

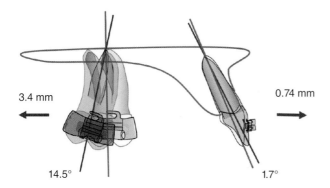

3.4 mm

0.74 mm

14.5°

1.7°

Figure 18.16 Average post-treatment displacement and angular changes following Pendulum appliance treatment. Source: modified from Byloff FK, Darendeliler MA. Distal molar movement using the pendulum appliance. Part 1: clinical and radiological evaluation. *Angle Orthod.* 1997;67(4):249–260.

implant placement.[40] Screws can be placed in the midline anterior to the premolars, posterior to the rugae or in paramedian locations at the level of the first premolars. Rapid progress in the development of microscrews using both animal and human models has resulted in more detailed comprehension of the bony microstructural implications in anchorage. The screws can be attached to the device by flowing light-cured acrylic over a custom-made framework, directly attaching the framework to the screws (Figure 18.18) or via an accurate impression or intraoral scan, precisely fit to a custom-made framework (Figure 18.19). This framework can be three-dimensionally printed or constructed on a model of the arch with associated compressed coils to produce the distalising force. Gurin-type locks are placed on the palatal arms of the framework to facilitate activation and reactivation of the coils. It is critical to extend the palatal attachments on the molar bands as high up in the vault as possible to direct the force through the centre of resistance of the molars, facilitating bodily-type movement. The upper molars can be independently moved distally until a slight overcorrection is achieved and the premolars left to drift distally secondary to the gingival fibre tension. Alternatively, fixed appliances can be placed whilst the molars are being moved and alignment coordinated with the placement of brackets. In some cases, the distalising appliance can be built into a mini-implant-supported expansion appliance (MARME). The expansion is performed first, then the distalising coil is activated by removing a component of the expansion (Figure 18.20). Once the teeth are aligned and retracted,

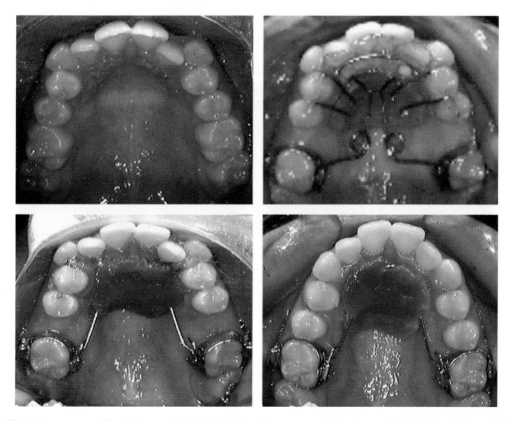

Figure 18.17 Typical sequence of Pendulum appliance effects. Panels are arranged from upper left to right and lower left to right: pretreatment maxillary arch; Pendulum appliance with TMA springs moving the molars distally over five months (note the premolars have moved anteriorly); a Nance holding device is constructed intraorally; after six months, the premolars have drifted distally to effect spontaneous improvement in incisor alignment.

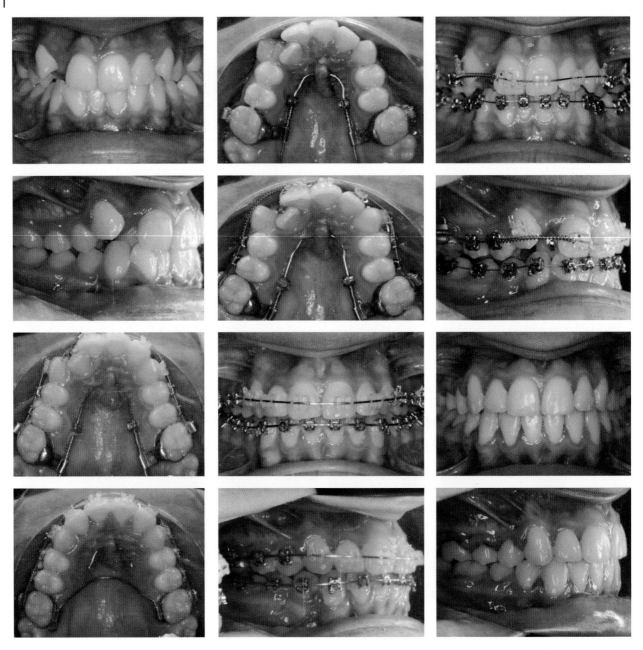

Figure 18.18 A 14-year-old female in the permanent dentition presented with a Class II buccal segment relationship and upper crowding that could be treated by either maxillary arch extractions or distalisation of the maxillary dentition. Two anterior midline palatal TADs were placed to anchor a distal-driving framework using compressed coils to the upper molars. After correction of the molar relationship, fixed appliances were placed with archwires progressing from round to rectangular nickel titanium through to 0.019 × 0.025-inch TMA to finalise tooth positions. Pretreatment and treatment progression are shown in paired vertical panels orientated from left to right.

the framework can be removed and inter-arch Class II elastics used in the finishing stages if required.

If treatment goals are limited to retraction of the maxillary dentition, then the use of TAD-supported molar distalisation is quicker, more direct and more effective when compared to headgear. Moreover, there is no significant effect on the position of the mandibular dentition, in contrast to fixed functional appliances.

Buccal Bone Miniplates

The success rate of intra-alveolar miniscrew temporary anchors has been reported to range from 37 to 94% and it is difficult to make valid comparisons, with significant uncertainty associated with sufficient bone quality to guarantee successful placement. Screw loosening, fracture, infection and damage to adjacent structures have all been routinely reported. Close screw–root proximity

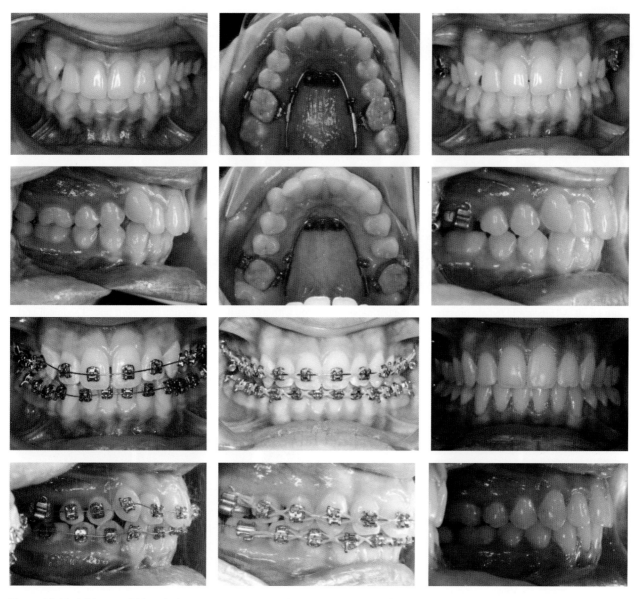

Figure 18.19 A 14-year-old female in the permanent dentition presented with a Class II type malocclusion and upper crowding that could have been treated by either maxillary arch extractions or distalisation of the maxillary dentition. Two paramedian palatal TADs were placed to anchor a distal-driving framework using compressed coils to the upper molars. After correction of the molar relationship, fixed appliances were placed with archwires progressing from round to rectangular nickel titanium archwires through to 0.019 × 0.025-inch TMA to finalise tooth positions. Pretreatment images and treatment progression are shown in paired vertical panels orientated from left to right.

has also been reported to reduce success by as much as one-third.

The first reported application of skeletal bone plates to assist in orthodontic tooth movement was by Jenner and Fitzpatrick in 1985.[41] Since then, a number of skeletal anchorage systems have been developed from titanium alloys that can be placed to facilitate distal movement of the upper and lower posterior teeth.[42–44] Miniplates have been suggested to overcome some of the limitations associated with alveolar placement of TADs. Placement is

more apical along the mandibular body or in the zygomatic buttress where bone quality is adequate and does not interfere with the path of most tooth movement. Several self-threaded titanium screws fix the bone plate to the zygomatic buttress, retromolar pad and along the mandibular body. Miniplates such as the Sendai Skeletal Anchorage (SAS) may also be indicated when root proximity limits the placement of miniscrews or when repeated failures may limit alternative locations. The arm of the miniplate exits transmucosally and may range from 10.5 (short) to

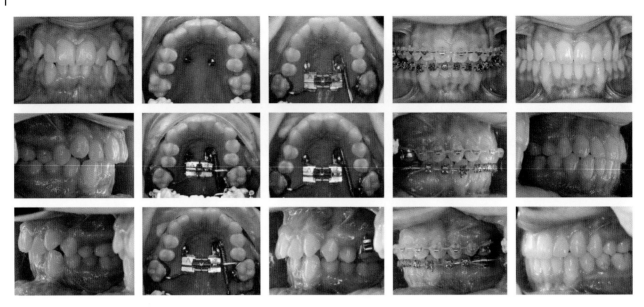

Figure 18.20 A 15-year-old female presented in the permanent dentition with a Class II malocclusion in the left buccal segment and a narrow, asymmetrical and crowded upper arch that could have been treated by either maxillary expansion and extractions or distalisation of the maxillary dentition. Two paramedian palatal TADs were placed to anchor a mini-implant-supported expansion appliance (MARME) modified with a distal-driving framework using compressed coils to the upper left molar. Initially a rigid strut was attached from the expansion screw to the upper left molar. On completion of the expansion, the strut was removed and the compressed coil released to effect a distal force on the UL6. After correction of the molar relationship, fixed appliances were placed with archwires progressing from round to rectangular nickel titanium archwires through to 0.019 × 0.025-inch TMA to finalise tooth position. Pretreatment images and treatment progression are shown in vertical panels consisting of three images orientated from left to right.

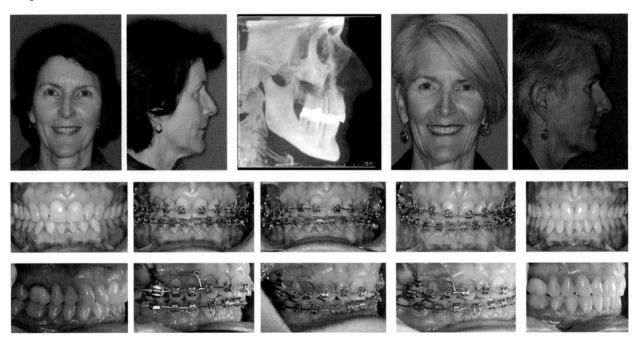

Figure 18.21 An adult patient presenting with a Class II division 2 type malocclusion and irregularity in the upper arch that could have been treated by compensatory tooth movement through upper arch extractions of distal movement of the upper arch. Bone plates were placed immediately lateral to the upper molars and archwires progressed through flexible nickel titanium to 0.019 × 0.025-inch TMA. Extension arms facilitated the placement of elastic force as close to the centre of resistance of the dentition to maximise translation of the entire maxillary dentition distally.

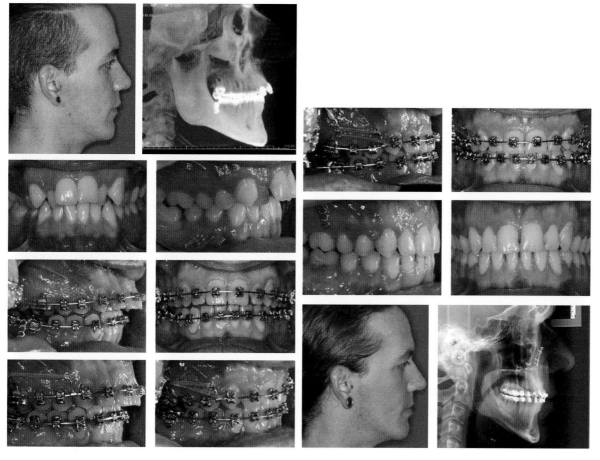

Figure 18.22 An adult patient presenting with a Class II division 1 type malocclusion and irregularity in the upper arch that could have been treated by compensatory tooth movements through upper arch extraction or distal movement of the entire upper arch. Note the lower arch asymmetry from earlier loss of the lower right first permanent molar. Bone plates were placed immediately lateral to the upper molars and the lower right second molar and archwires progressed through flexible nickel titanium to 0.019 × 0.025-inch TMA. Extension arms facilitated the placement of elastic force as close to the centre of resistance of the dentition as possible to maximise translation of the entire maxillary dentition distally. The lower right bone plate was used to protract the lower right quadrant forward to address the asymmetry. Pretreatment images are shown in the upper four panels with treatment progression shown in horizontal panels orientated in pairs moving downwards.

16.5 mm (long). The hook on the plate has a number of positions to provide various levels of force application, dependent upon the desired tooth movement. The body of the plate is positioned subperiosteally and is available in three different configurations (T, Y or I). Although some clinicians cite a lack of clinical guidelines and/or scepticism of the evidence, and are concerned with the need for a more invasive surgical procedure, miniplates provide a more predictable and highly successful option for a range of complex orthodontic movements. Moreover, greater forces can be applied in circumstances where whole arch retraction or protraction may be required.

There are some obvious concerns with placement of miniplates in growing children with the rate and extent of bony remodelling in the growing craniofacial region. It is important to note that even though studies report clinical

success, there can often be complications such as swelling, soft tissue hyperplasia, nerve damage, sinus perforation or infection. For miniscrews, these complications often result in mobility and failure of the screw but with miniplates, complications can usually be managed by excellent hygiene and topical application of antimicrobial agents or antibiotics. It is important to appreciate that experience in treatment planning, placement and managing any complication during treatment is necessary to ensure favourable outcomes with miniplates.

Efficient distal movement of the maxillary dentition can be achieved with the application of a miniplate placed lateral to the posterior teeth (Figures 18.21 and 18.22). Space can be created to align and/or retract protrusive upper teeth without the anchorage loss commonly reported with numerous fixed intraoral devices, even with the incorporation of miniscrews placed in the palate.[45–47] Although numbers vary, there is a body of evidence indicating high success rates with these anchors.[48] Although SAS offers several distinct advantages it is not common in anchorage reinforcement. A recent survey of orthodontists indicated that they infrequently considered skeletal anchorage, with many citing a lack of clinical guidelines and/or scepticism of the evidence.[49] Many operators desire information on success rates, risk factors and possible adverse effects of their treatment and more research is needed.

Orthodontics and Orthognathic Surgery

In those cases with a more significant skeletal discrepancy in the anteroposterior, vertical or transverse plane, then definitive correction of a Class II malocclusion will require a combination of orthodontics and orthognathic surgery. A detailed description of the orthodontic/surgical management of these cases is beyond the scope of this chapter but it almost always involves advancement of the mandible, either alone or in combination with maxillary repositioning. A key principle of presurgical orthodontic preparation is incisor decompensation, particularly uprighting of the lower incisors to overcome natural compensation for mandibular retrognathia and facilitate optimal surgical advancement. The advent of direct fixation and modern anaesthesiology has meant that whilst the core orthognathic surgical techniques have not changed significantly, the range and scope of surgical movements is now extensive. The advent of three-dimensional planning and printed wafers is also beginning to influence this area of Class II management.[50] Whilst the advent of fixed anchorage has increased the scope of orthodontic compensation for Class II malocclusion, the requirement for surgical correction still exists in a significant cohort of patients.

References

1 McNamara JA Jr., Components of class II malocclusion in children 8–10 years of age. *Angle Orthod.* 1981;51(3):177–202.

2 Bjork A. Prediction of mandibular growth rotation. *Am. J. Orthod.* 1969;55(6):585–599.

3 Johnston LE. Let's pretend. *Semin. Orthod.* 2014;20:249–252.

4 Batista KB, Thiruvenkatachari B, Harrison JE, O'Brien KD. Orthodontic treatment for prominent upper front teeth (Class II malocclusion) in children and adolescents. *Cochrane Database Syst. Rev.* 2018;(3):CD003452.

5 Johnston LE. Growing jaws for fun and profit. In: McNamara JA Jr (ed.). *Craniofacial Growth Series, Monograph 35. Center for Human Growth and Development*, Ann Arbor: University of Michigan, 1999.

6 Perinetti G, Primozic J, Franchi L, Contardo L. Treatment effects of removable functional appliances in pre-pubertal and pubertal Class II patients: a systematic review and meta-analysis of controlled studies. *PLoS One* 2015;10(10):e0141198.

7 Bishara SE. Mandibular changes in persons with untreated and treated Class II division 1 malocclusion. *Am. J. Orthod. Dentofacial Orthop.* 1998;113(6):661–673.

8 Solow B. The dentoalveolar compensatory mechanism: background and clinical implications. *Br. J. Orthod.* 1980;7(3):145–161.

9 Jakobsson SO. Cephalometric evaluation of treatment effect on Class II, *Division I malocclusions. Am. J. Orthod.* 1967;53(6):446–457.

10 Wieslander L. Long-term effect of treatment with the headgear-Herbst appliance in the early mixed dentition. Stability or relapse? *Am. J. Orthod. Dentofacial Orthop.* 1993;104(4):319–329.

11 Jambi S, Thiruvenkatachari B, O'Brien KD, Walsh T. Orthodontic treatment for distalising upper first molars in children and adolescents. *Cochrane Database Syst. Rev.* 2013;(10):CD008375.

12 Clark WJ. The twin block technique. A functional orthopedic appliance system. *Am. J. Orthod. Dentofacial Orthop.* 1988;93(1):1–18.

13 Dyer FM, McKeown HF, Sandler PJ. The modified twin block appliance in the treatment of Class II division 2 malocclusions. *J. Orthod.* 2001;28(4):271–280.

14 Sandler J, DiBiase D. The inclined biteplane: a useful tool. *Am. J. Orthod. Dentofacial Orthop.* 1996;110(4):339–350.

15 Pancherz H. Treatment of class II malocclusions by jumping the bite with the Herbst appliance. A cephalometric investigation. *Am. J. Orthod.* 1979;76(4):423–442.

16 Purkayastha SK, Rabie AB, Wong R. Treatment of skeletal class II malocclusion in adults: stepwise vs single-step advancement with the Herbst appliance. *World J. Orthod.* 2008;9(3):233–243.

17 von Bremen J, Bock N, Ruf S. Is Herbst-multibracket appliance treatment more efficient in adolescents than in adults? *Angle Orthod.* 2009;79(1):173–177.

18 Kanuru RK, Bhasin V, Khatri A, et al. Comparison of complications in removable mandibular acrylic splint

and cantilever Herbst for management of Class II mal-occlusion: a retrospective study. *J. Contemp. Dent. Pract.* 2017;18(5):363–365.

19 von Bremen J, Pancherz H. Efficiency of class II division 1 and class II division 2 treatment in relation to different treatment approaches. *Semin. Orthod.* 2003;9:87–92.

20 O'Brien K, Wright J, Conboy F, et al. Effectiveness of treatment for Class II malocclusion with the Herbst or twin-block appliances: a randomized, controlled trial. *Am. J. Orthod. Dentofacial Orthop.* 2003;124(2):128–137.

21 Schioth T, von Bremen J, Pancherz H, Ruf S. Complications during Herbst appliance treatment with reduced mandibular cast splints: a prospective, clinical multicenter study. *J. Orofac. Orthop.* 2007;68(4):321–327.

22 Pancherz H, Bjerklin K. The Herbst appliance 32 years after treatment. *J. Clin. Orthod.* 2015;49(7):442–451.

23 Zymperdikas VF, Koretsi V, Papageorgiou SN, Papadopoulos MA. Treatment effects of fixed functional appliances in patients with Class II malocclusion: a systematic review and meta-analysis. *Eur. J. Orthod.* 2016;38(2):113–126.

24 Aidar LA, Abrahao M, Yamashita HK, Dominguez GC. Herbst appliance therapy and temporomandibular joint disc position: a prospective longitudinal magnetic resonance imaging study. *Am. J. Orthod. Dentofacial Orthop.* 2006;129(4):486–496.

25 Aras A, Ada E, Saracoglu H, et al. Comparison of treatments with the Forsus fatigue resistant device in relation to skeletal maturity: a cephalometric and magnetic resonance imaging study. *Am. J. Orthod. Dentofacial Orthop.* 2011;140(5):616–625.

26 Hanoun A, Al-Jewair TS, Tabbaa S, et al. A comparison of the treatment effects of the Forsus Fatigue Resistance Device and the Twin Block appliance in patients with class II malocclusions. *Clin. Cosmet. Investig. Dent.* 2014;6:57–63.

27 Karacay S, Akin E, Olmez H, et al. Forsus Nitinol Flat Spring and Jasper Jumper corrections of Class II division 1 malocclusions. *Angle Orthod.* 2006;76(4):666–672.

28 Aslan BI, Kucukkaraca E, Turkoz C, Dincer M. Treatment effects of the Forsus Fatigue Resistant Device used with miniscrew anchorage. *Angle Orthod.* 2014;84(1):76–87.

29 Melsen B. Effects of cervical anchorage during and after treatment: an implant study. *Am. J. Orthod.* 1978;73(5):526–540.

30 Cetlin NM, Ten Hoeve A. Nonextraction treatment. *J. Clin. Orthod.* 1983;17(6):396–413.

31 Hilgers JJ. The pendulum appliance for Class II non-compliance therapy. *J. Clin. Orthod.* 1992;26(11):706–714.

32 Byloff FK, Darendeliler MA. Distal molar movement using the pendulum appliance. Part 1: Clinical and radiological evaluation. *Angle Orthod.* 1997;67(4):249–260.

33 Byloff FK, Darendeliler MA, Clar E, Darendeliler A. Distal molar movement using the pendulum appliance. Part 2: The effects of maxillary molar root uprighting bends. *Angle Orthod.* 1997;67(4):261–270.

34 Al-Thomali Y, Basha S, Mohamed RN. Pendulum and modified pendulum appliances for maxillary molar distalization in Class II malocclusion: a systematic review. *Acta Odontol. Scand.* 2017;75(6):394–401.

35 Kircelli BH, Pektas ZO, Kircelli C. Maxillary molar distalization with a bone-anchored pendulum appliance. *Angle Orthod.* 2006;76(4):650–659.

36 Polat-Ozsoy O, Kircelli BH, Arman-Ozcirpici A, et al. Pendulum appliances with 2 anchorage designs: conventional anchorage vs bone anchorage. *Am. J. Orthod. Dentofacial Orthop.* 2008;133(3):339.e9–17.

37 Sar C, Kaya B, Ozsoy O, Ozcirpici AA. Comparison of two implant-supported molar distalization systems. *Angle Orthod.* 2013;83(3):460–467.

38 Nienkemper M, Wilmes B, Pauls A, Drescher D. Multipurpose use of orthodontic mini-implants to achieve different treatment goals. *J. Orofac. Orthop.* 2012;73(6):467–476.

39 Tsui WK, Chua HD, Cheung LK. Bone anchor systems for orthodontic application: a systematic review. *Int. J. Oral Maxillofac. Surg.* 2012;41(11):1427–1438.

40 Baumgaertel S. Quantitative investigation of palatal bone depth and cortical bone thickness for mini-implant placement in adults. *Am. J. Orthod. Dentofacial Orthop.* 2009;136(1):104–108.

41 Jenner JD, Fitzpatrick BN. Skeletal anchorage utilising bone plates. *Aust. Orthod. J.* 1985;9(2):231–233.

42 De Clerck H, Geerinckx V, Siciliano S. The Zygoma anchorage system. *J. Clin. Orthod.* 2002; 36(8):455–459.

43 Sugawara J, Daimaruya T, Umemori M, et al. Distal movement of mandibular molars in adult patients with the skeletal anchorage system. *Am. J. Orthod. Dentofacial Orthop.* 2004;125(2):130–138.

44 Umemori M, Sugawara J, Mitani H, et al. Skeletal anchorage system for open-bite correction. *Am. J. Orthod. Dentofacial Orthop.* 1999;115(2):166–174.

45 Kinzinger G, Gulden N, Yildizhan F, et al. Anchorage efficacy of palatally-inserted miniscrews in molar distalization with a periodontally/miniscrew-anchored distal jet. *J. Orofac. Orthop.* 2008;69(2):110–120.

46 Liou EJ, Pai BC, Lin JC. Do miniscrews remain stationary under orthodontic forces? *Am. J. Orthod. Dentofacial Orthop.* 2004;126(1):42–47.

47 Sugawara J. Temporary skeletal anchorage devices: the case for miniplates. *Am. J. Orthod. Dentofacial Orthop.* 2014;145(5):559–565.

48 Lam R, Goonewardene MS, Allan BP, Sugawara J. Success rates of a skeletal anchorage system in orthodontics: a retrospective analysis. *Angle Orthod.* 2018;88(1):27–34.

49 Papageorgiou SN, Zogakis IP, Papadopoulos MA. Failure rates and associated risk factors of orthodontic miniscrew implants: a meta-analysis. *Am. J. Orthod. Dentofacial Orthop.* 2012;142(5):577–595.e7.

50 Cousley RR, Turner MJ. Digital model planning and computerized fabrication of orthognathic surgery wafers. *J. Orthod.* 2014;41(1):38–45.

19

Management of Class III Malocclusions

Grant T. McIntyre

CHAPTER OUTLINE

Introduction, 359
Treatment Timing for Class III Malocclusion in Relation to Facial Growth, 360
Comprehensive, Camouflage or Compromise Treatment for Class III Cases, 362
    Comprehensive Treatment, 362
    Camouflage Treatment, 364
    Compromise Treatment, 366
Managing the Class III Surgical/Orthodontic Patient with Fixed Appliances, 366
    Interceptive Treatment for Surgical/Orthodontic Cases, 367
Class III Malocclusion Occurring with Cleft Lip and/or Palate, 370
References, 370

Introduction

Class III malocclusion affects around 3% of the population.[1] Successful treatment of a Class III malocclusion with fixed appliances depends on a number of factors. These include patient cooperation, good dental health and the absence of significant medical problems, the severity of the underlying skeletal relationship, an understanding of the soft-tissue aetiological factors, and the nature and type of occlusal anomalies. Of these, motivation and good dental/medical health are obviously important, but the nature of any underlying skeletal discrepancy will determine if the case can be treated successfully on a non-surgical basis or if orthognathic surgery will also be required.

The skeletal relationships underpinning Class III malocclusions present as a spectrum of features, with a variable contribution of maxillary retrusion (Figure 19.1) and/or mandibular prognathism (Figure 19.2), variability in the vertical skeletal relationship (Figures 19.3 and 19.4) with dentoskeletal asymmetries (Figure 19.5).[2] Moreover, many developmental dentofacial abnormalities and syndromes present with a Class III malocclusion and Class III skeletal relationship.

Dentally, the nature and number of anomalies complicates the management of Class III malocclusion. Crowding,

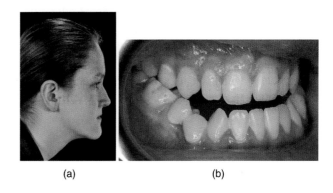

Figure 19.1 (a, b) Class III malocclusion associated with maxillary retrusion.

rotations, hypodontia/microdontia, impacted canines, crossbites, reduced overbite/anterior open bite, infraoccluded deciduous teeth, ankylosed teeth following trauma, hypoplastic and transposed teeth (Figure 19.6) all increase the need for careful treatment planning and sequencing due to the added complexities of treatment.

Whilst the soft tissues do not play as crucial an aetiological role in Class III malocclusion when compared to Class II division 1 and Class II division 2 malocclusion, they modify the severity of the case through dentoalveolar compensation. Mechanics that alter the interaction

Preadjusted Edgewise Fixed Orthodontic Appliances: Principles and Practice, First Edition. Edited by Farhad B. Naini and Daljit S. Gill.
© 2022 John Wiley & Sons Ltd. Published 2022 by John Wiley & Sons Ltd.

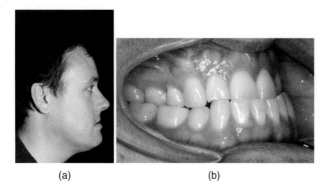

(a) (b)

Figure 19.2 (a, b) Class III malocclusion associated with mandibular prognathism.

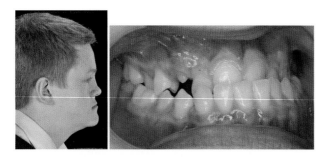

Figure 19.3 Class III malocclusion associated with reduced vertical facial height.

between the incisor positions/inclinations and soft tissues will jeopardise long-term stability (Figure 19.7). As such, retention should be considered at the outset of treatment and where there are any concerns about the establishment of a positive overbite and lip competence at the end of treatment, the clinician should include the need for indefinite retention in the informed consent process.

Treatment Timing for Class III Malocclusion in Relation to Facial Growth

The nature and extent of current and future growth should be considered for every patient with Class III malocclusion as anteroposterior, vertical and transverse growth are counterproductive (Table 19.1). Of these, the severity of the anteroposterior skeletal relationship is a key variable in treatment success and the integration of clinical and cephalometric information will help decide if further incisor compensation is possible or whether orthognathic surgery will be required. Even with less severe skeletal discrepancies, such tooth movements may lead to poor dentofacial aesthetics through undesirable consequences on the facial profile.

The nature of the vertical skeletal relationship also requires careful consideration. Class III cases with reduced

vertical proportions are unusual (Figure 19.3), but those with increased vertical skeletal relationships (Figure 19.4) are notoriously difficult to treat. Intrusion of the buccal segment teeth to improve an anterior open bite results in a closing mandibular rotation, worsening the anteroposterior skeletal relationship. Therefore cases with more than a mild increase in the vertical skeletal height may require surgical input.

Although dental asymmetries can be accommodated in comprehensive treatment, it is difficult to successfully compensate for any skeletal asymmetries which occur as part of a Class III case (Figure 19.5). Those that involve condylar pathology require careful diagnosis and management in conjunction with an oral and maxillofacial surgeon at an early stage. Condylar destruction rarely presents with a Class III malocclusion but condylar hyperplasia is almost always a unilateral phenomenon and associated with a Class III skeletal discrepancy. It requires to be diagnosed by nuclear medicine scanning using single photon emission computed tomography (SPECT), with the hyperplastic condyle being surgically reduced before any extensive skeletal growth and facial asymmetry and compensatory dental changes in the transverse dimension occur. Mandibular asymmetries arising from a functional mandibular shift should be determined during the diagnostic stage as failure to identify this will lead to inappropriate treatment.

As a general rule, however, cases with a negative ANB angle, an anterior open bite of skeletal origin, significant retroclination of the lower incisors,[3] or dentofacial asymmetry with a skeletal aetiology are unlikely to be successfully treated with non-surgical orthodontic treatment. Skeletal growth is at its peak in patients with Class III malocclusion between the ages of 14 and 17 years[2] (Figure 19.8) and patients and their parents generally prefer treatment to be undertaken at this age as it is more socially acceptable to wear fixed appliances. However, this presents a degree of diagnostic difficulty for patients with a Class III malocclusion as there is variability in the nature of skeletal growth, with a single lateral cephalometric radiograph being inappropriate for the prediction of future skeletal growth.[4] It should therefore be pointed out to patients and parents that whilst adolescent treatment of a Class III malocclusion may produce an aesthetically, functionally and stable Class I incisor relationship at the end of treatment, any final increments of mandibular growth may well lead to a return of the Class III malocclusion in retention, necessitating retreatment. Therefore, caution should be exercised in relation to planning non-surgical treatment for patients with Class III malocclusion where there is ongoing somatic growth. This is particularly important where extractions in the lower arch are planned

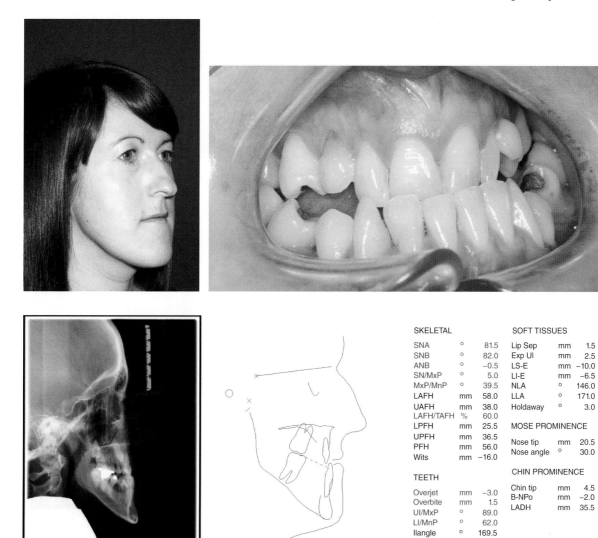

SKELETAL			SOFT TISSUES		
SNA	°	81.5	Lip Sep	mm	1.5
SNB	°	82.0	Exp UI	mm	2.5
ANB	°	−0.5	LS-E	mm	−10.0
SN/MxP	°	5.0	LI-E	mm	−6.5
MxP/MnP	°	39.5	NLA	°	146.0
LAFH	mm	58.0	LLA	°	171.0
UAFH	mm	38.0	Holdaway	°	3.0
LAFH/TAFH	%	60.0			
LPFH	mm	25.5	MOSE PROMINENCE		
UPFH	mm	36.5	Nose tip	mm	20.5
PFH	mm	56.0	Nose angle	°	30.0
Wits	mm	−16.0			
			CHIN PROMINENCE		
TEETH			Chin tip	mm	4.5
Overjet	mm	−3.0	B-NPo	mm	−2.0
Overbite	mm	1.5	LADH	mm	35.5
UI/MxP	°	89.0			
LI/MnP	°	62.0			
Iangle	°	169.5			
LI/APo	mm	0.0			
LI/NPo	mm	−1.0			

Figure 19.4 Class III malocclusion associated with increased vertical facial height.

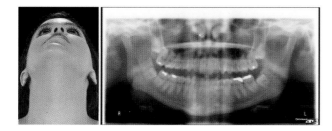

Figure 19.5 Class III malocclusion associated with facial asymmetry due to unilateral condylar hyperplasia affecting the left side.

at the start of treatment or lower incisor interproximal enamel reduction and extensive use of Class III inter-arch elastic traction are required during treatment to further compensate the lower incisor inclination. As a result,

where there is any concern that skeletal growth will be unfavourable, or where any family members exhibit a severe skeletal Class III relationship, it is prudent to delay the start of non-surgical treatment until at least 15 years of age (Figure 19.9).

Finally, where the clinician is in any doubt about the openness of the patient in relation to their concerns where there is an appreciable skeletal contribution to the malocclusion, it is usually wise to explore a combination of orthodontic treatment and orthognathic surgery along with other non-surgical options. Whilst the majority of patients seek a non-surgical solution, it may be that on reflection and further discussion, there are indeed aspects of dentofacial appearance that are of concern to the patient but not initially volunteered.

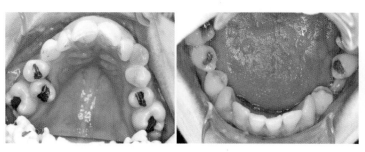
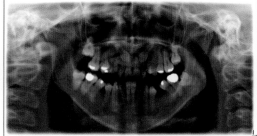

Figure 19.6 Crowding, rotations, spacing and impacted UR3, UL3 in a patient with a Class III malocclusion and Class 3 skeletal relationship (same patient as in Figure 19.4).

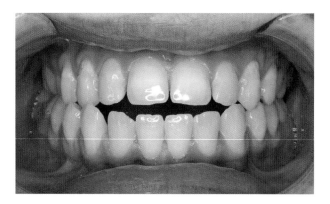

Figure 19.7 Class III malocclusion that had relapsed following treatment due to imbalance between lip and tongue pressures.

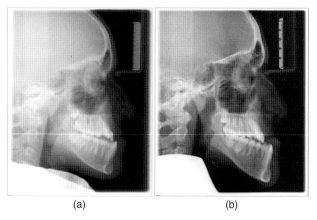

(a)   (b)

Figure 19.8 Growth in a patient with Class III malocclusion from age 14 (a) to age 17 (b).

Comprehensive, Camouflage or Compromise Treatment for Class III Cases

Orthodontic treatment for Class III malocclusions may be categorised as comprehensive, camouflage or compromise treatment (see Table 19.1), and these are discussed in turn in the following sections.

Comprehensive Treatment

Comprehensive treatment with fixed appliances aims to produce a Class I incisor relationship on a Class I skeletal base relationship. It is rare to find a Class III malocclusion occurring in a patient with a Class I skeletal base relationship and therefore comprehensive correction usually

Table 19.1 Factors involved in treatment planning decisions for Class III malocclusions.

	Anteroposterior skeletal relationship	Vertical skeletal relationship	Incisor relationship	Incisor inclinations	Overbite
Comprehensive	None[(a)]	None	Edge-to-edge	No compensation or proclined lower incisors and/or retroclined upper incisors	Normal or increased
Camouflage	Mild to moderate	None or mild	Minimal reverse overjet	No compensation or proclined lower incisors and/or retroclined upper incisors	Normal or only slightly reduced
Compromise	Moderate to severe	Moderate to severe	Marked reverse overjet	Incisor inclinations irrelevant	Amount of overbite irrelevant

(a) Following protraction facemask or surgical correction.

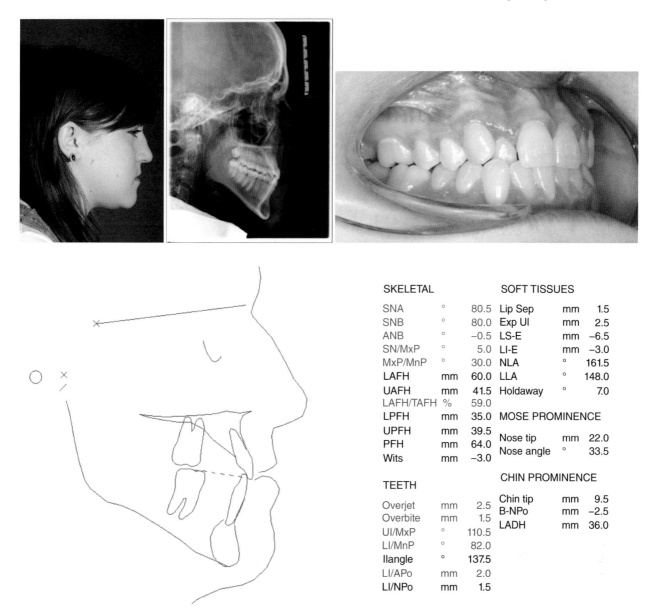

SKELETAL			SOFT TISSUES		
SNA	°	80.5	Lip Sep	mm	1.5
SNB	°	80.0	Exp UI	mm	2.5
ANB	°	−0.5	LS-E	mm	−6.5
SN/MxP	°	5.0	LI-E	mm	−3.0
MxP/MnP	°	30.0	NLA	°	161.5
LAFH	mm	60.0	LLA	°	148.0
UAFH	mm	41.5	Holdaway	°	7.0
LAFH/TAFH	%	59.0			
LPFH	mm	35.0	MOSE PROMINENCE		
UPFH	mm	39.5			
PFH	mm	64.0	Nose tip	mm	22.0
Wits	mm	−3.0	Nose angle	°	33.5
			CHIN PROMINENCE		
TEETH					
Overjet	mm	2.5	Chin tip	mm	9.5
Overbite	mm	1.5	B-NPo	mm	−2.5
UI/MxP	°	110.5	LADH	mm	36.0
LI/MnP	°	82.0			
Ilangle	°	137.5			
LI/APo	mm	2.0			
LI/NPo	mm	1.5			

Figure 19.9 A 15-year-old patient with a Class III malocclusion where further incisor compensation is possible.

requires adjunctive treatment with a facemask during growth, or at the completion of growth with orthognathic surgery. Surgical correction is discussed later but there is increasing evidence that skeletal protraction of the maxilla can be achieved with a facemask during skeletal growth.[5] This is best undertaken in the pre-adolescent years when maxillary protraction can be synchronised with subsequent fixed appliance treatment (Figure 19.10). The principles involved in the comprehensive treatment of Class III malocclusions with fixed appliances are detailed in Box 19.0 and in the text following.

> **Box 19.1 Principles involved in comprehensive/camouflage Class III orthodontic treatment**
>
> - Relief of crowding
> - Level and align arches
> - Increase overbite and overjet
> - Correct buccal segment relationships
> - Finish and detail occlusion
> - Plan retention

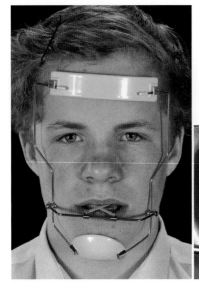
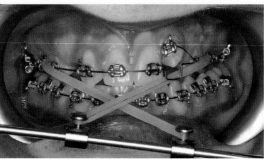

Figure 19.10 A 13-year-old patient with a Class III malocclusion and hypodontia affecting the upper permanent lateral incisors being simultaneously treated with preadjusted edgewise fixed appliances and protraction headgear to simultaneously align the arches, close space, correct the incisor relationship and align the upper left permanent canine, which required exposure earlier in treatment.

Camouflage Treatment

Camouflage treatment mechanics deliver a Class I incisor relationship but does not address the underlying skeletal relationship. The majority of non-surgical orthodontic treatment with fixed appliances falls into this category and the favourable prognostic factors for orthodontic camouflage are detailed in Box 19.1.

Box 19.2 Favourable prognostic factors for Class III orthodontic camouflage

- Patient past peak skeletal growth
- Mild to moderate skeletal Class III relationship: ANB angle greater than 0°
- Normal or slightly reduced overbite with either a normal or a mild increase in face height
- No pretreatment dentoalveolar compensation or proclined lower incisors and/or retroclined upper incisors
- The ability to achieve an edge-to-edge incisor relationship
- Once crowding and mandibular displacements corrected, molar relationship <0.5 unit Class III

Where future skeletal growth has been determined to be of no or minimal impact on either the treatment mechanics or outcome of treatment, the appliance prescription and sequencing of treatment mechanics should be considered at the treatment planning stage. These are outlined in Box 19.0. Some cases will also have a premature incisal contact and will slide forwards into a reverse overjet,

which makes the skeletal discrepancy appear worse than it actually is. These 'pseudo' Class III cases are therefore much simpler to treat, usually with camouflage biomechanics.

Which Fixed Appliance System?

There is no 'one size fits all' fixed appliance system that is suitable for effective treatment of every malocclusion and therefore the fixed appliance system and prescription should be determined in advance of the start of treatment (Table 19.2).

Cases that require proclination of the upper incisors should be treated with high torque values for the upper incisors (Bioprogressive, Tip-Edge), those that require lower incisor retroclination with a high negative torque value (MBT), and to avoid lower incisor proclination a low value for lower canine tip (MBT). The delivery of the prescription depends on not only the 'catalogue' values for the appliance but also on the manufacturing quality, wire dimensions used (which both influence 'play' between the wire and bracket) and the accuracy of bracket placement. Archwire bending can not only accommodate for anomalies in tooth morphology and bracket placement but can also help deliver additional tip and torque as dictated by the case. It is customary in Class III non-surgical fixed appliance treatment to swap the lower canine brackets to reverse the tip (Figure 19.11) and consequently reduce the propensity for lower incisor proclination. However, when using an appliance with a low value for lower canine tip such as the MBT appliance, the beneficial effect of this is limited and is likely to be negated by the resultant bracket placement error resulting from the poorer fit of the bracket bases.

Table 19.2 Tip and torque values for anterior teeth for common fixed appliance systems.

	Andrews		Roth		MBT		Bioprogressive		Damon Q		Tip-Edge	
	Tip	Torque	Tip	Torque	Tip	Torque	Tip	Torque	Tip	Torque	Tip	Torque
Upper central	+5	+7	+5	+12	+4	+17	+5	+22	+5	+15	+5	+22
Upper lateral	+9	+3	+9	+8	+8	+10	+8	+14	+9	+6	+9	+8
Upper canine	+11	−7	+13	−2	+8	0	+10	+7	+5	+7	+1	−4
Lower central	+2	−1	2	−1	0	−6	0	−1	+2	−3	+2	+1
Lower lateral	+2	−1	2	−1	0	−6	0	−1	+4	+3	+2	+1
Lower canine	+5	−11	+7	−11	+3	0	+5	+7	+5	+7	+5	−11

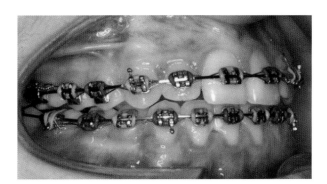

Figure 19.11 Lower canine brackets swapped to reverse tip values in a case being treated with preadjusted edgewise fixed appliances with the MBT prescription (note the cross-elastic being used to settle the buccal occlusion).

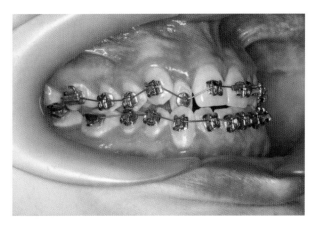

Figure 19.12 Self-ligating brackets being used for Class III camouflage treatment due to the benefit of secure robust engagement which is helpful for full engagement of the wires at the early stages of treatment. Note the button being used on the upper right lateral incisor as there was insufficient occlusal space to bond a bracket at the start (same patient as in Figure 19.9).

Whilst self-ligating systems do not appear to confer any advantages in terms of the appliance prescription, they allow secure robust engagement which is beneficial in aligning crowded arches on a non-extraction basis (Figure 19.12).

Camouflage treatment for a Class III malocclusion with fixed appliances can be augmented with auxiliaries including Class III intermaxillary elastics, possibly with interproximal enamel reduction.

Extractions

Relief of crowding frequently dictates that extractions are required (Figure 19.13). Any extraction space remaining after arch alignment can be strategically used for further incisor compensation. As a result, it is logical to extract the lower first premolars and either extract the upper second premolars or, where crowding is minimal, on a non-extraction basis with alignment being achieved by upper incisor advancement/proclination.[6] Transverse arch expansion in the upper arch for the correction of crossbites will also produce a small amount of space for relief of crowding and should be undertaken before any extractions. Interproximal enamel reduction in the lower arch rarely provides adequate space for alignment of the lower arch and further incisor compensation.

Elastics

Class III elastics (Figure 19.13) are frequently used to deliver the required amount of incisor compensation, usually with a full-dimension upper archwire for maximal torque expression. Where torque expression from a lower rectangular archwire would be undesirable for the correction of the incisal relationship, a round stainless steel lower archwire can be used to allow the lower incisors to be retroclined.

Intrude Upper Buccal Segments

Closure of any anterior open bite through incisor extrusion is notoriously unstable and therefore upper molar intrusion is advisable as this is more stable. However, as

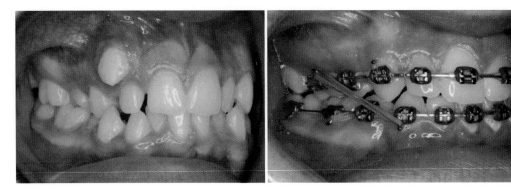

Figure 19.13 Class III case in the space closure stage following extraction of upper second premolars and lower first premolars. Class III intermaxillary elastics are being used to retract the lower labial segment.

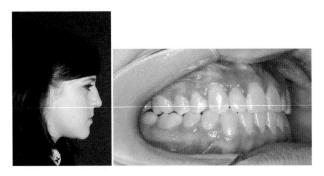

Figure 19.14 Class III patient at the end of camouflage orthodontic treatment. Whilst the positive overbite will help maintain stability of the correction of the incisor inclinations, long-term use of removable retainers will be needed (same patient as in Figures 19.9 and 19.12).

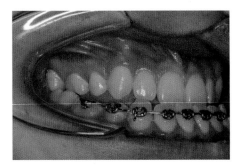

Figure 19.15 Compromise treatment with space closure being undertaken on a round stainless steel wire to maximise retroclination of the lower incisors. Indefinite retention will be necessary.

already mentioned, intrusion of the upper buccal segments results in a closing mandibular rotation, consequently worsening the anteroposterior relationship. Therefore, when correcting any open bite on a non-surgical basis, it is wise to use cephalometric software to determine the extent of the autorotation effect on the anteroposterior relationship before starting treatment in case the planned intrusive mechanics result in the case requiring surgery.

Retention

Retention should be planned at the start of treatment, taking into consideration the dental and skeletal changes that have occurred during treatment. Cases that have undergone incisor compensation, expansion, intrusive/extrusive movements and growth require particular attention to retention and long-term stability (Figure 19.14). There is no secret formula to retention for Class III cases and therefore the length of the retention period is more important than the type of retainers.

Compromise Treatment

Compromise treatment mechanics are used when it is not possible to deliver a Class I incisor relationship at the end of treatment and where the patient is unwilling to undergo orthognathic surgery. The patient needs to be aware that treatment will not address the underlying skeletal discrepancy and where upper arch extractions are required for relief of crowding, there is likely to be an increase in the reverse overjet. A round archwire is usually used in the lower arch to maximise lower incisor retroclination (Figure 19.15).

Managing the Class III Surgical/Orthodontic Patient with Fixed Appliances

Where it is expected that the growing patient will require orthognathic surgery at the completion of skeletal growth, it is useful for the patient to attend a joint orthodontic/orthognathic surgery clinic for a discussion of the objectives and timing of interceptive and comprehensive treatment.[7]

Interceptive Treatment for Surgical/Orthodontic Cases

Whilst skeletal growth during the adolescent years is being monitored, many patients will wish to have some treatment carried out to improve the alignment of the upper arch, which usually requires an upper fixed appliance and premolar extractions. As with all compromise options, this will result in an increase in the reverse overjet where extractions are required for the relief of crowding. Lower arch treatment should not be undertaken at this stage as retroclining the mandibular incisors following extractions compromises the prospects for full subsequent axial decompensation as part of the definitive orthodontic and orthognathic surgical phase, prejudicing optimal dentofacial harmony at the end of treatment (Figure 19.15). If the patient decided to pursue surgical treatment in the future, full decompensation would not be possible and extraction space would be re-created in the lower premolar region.

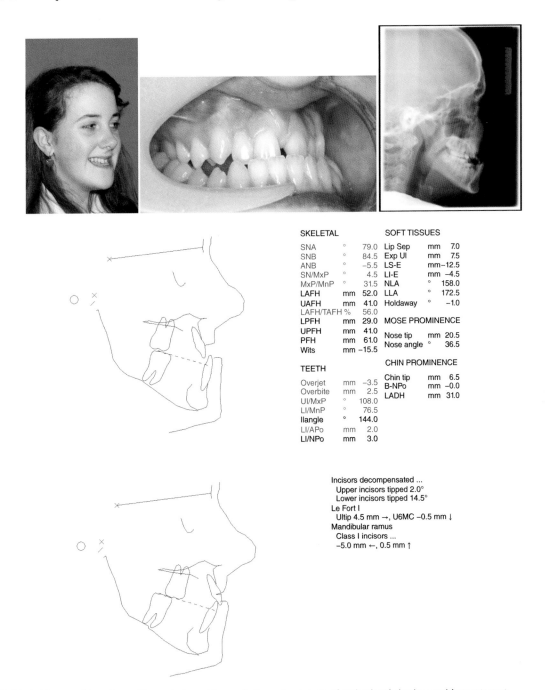

SKELETAL			SOFT TISSUES		
SNA	°	79.0	Lip Sep	mm	7.0
SNB	°	84.5	Exp UI	mm	7.5
ANB	°	−5.5	LS-E	mm	−12.5
SN/MxP	°	4.5	LI-E	mm	−4.5
MxP/MnP	°	31.5	NLA	°	158.0
LAFH	mm	52.0	LLA	°	172.5
UAFH	mm	41.0	Holdaway	°	−1.0
LAFH/TAFH	%	56.0			
LPFH	mm	29.0	MOSE PROMINENCE		
UPFH	mm	41.0	Nose tip	mm	20.5
PFH	mm	61.0	Nose angle	°	36.5
Wits	mm	−15.5			
			CHIN PROMINENCE		
TEETH			Chin tip	mm	6.5
Overjet	mm	−3.5	B-NPo	mm	−0.0
Overbite	mm	2.5	LADH	mm	31.0
UI/MxP	°	108.0			
LI/MnP	°	76.5			
Iiangle	°	144.0			
LI/APo	mm	2.0			
LI/NPo	mm	3.0			

Incisors decompensated ...
  Upper incisors tipped 2.0°
  Lower incisors tipped 14.5°
Le Fort I
  UItip 4.5 mm →, U6MC −0.5 mm ↓
Mandibular ramus
  Class I incisors ...
  −5.0 mm ←, 0.5 mm ↑

Figure 19.16 A 16-year-old patient with cephalometric prediction of outcome of orthodontic/orthognathic treatment.

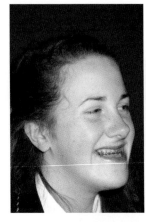
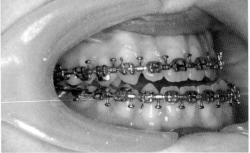

Figure 19.17 Patient on completion of presurgical orthodontics. Note the interdental ball hooks placed in preparation for surgery (same patient as in Figure 19.16).

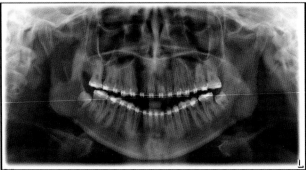
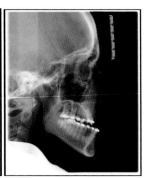

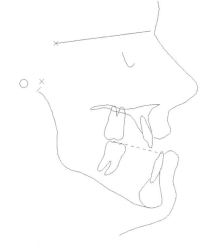

SKELETAL			SOFT TISSUES		
SNA	°	80.5	Lip Sep	mm	6.5
SNB	°	86.0	Exp UI	mm	5.0
ANB	°	−5.5	LS-E	mm	−11.5
SN/MxP	°	3.5	LI-E	mm	−3.0
MxP/MnP	°	29.0	NLA	°	147.5
LAFH	mm	59.0	LLA	°	152.5
UAFH	mm	42.5	Holdaway	°	−3.0
LAFH/TAFH	%	58.0			
LPFH	mm	35.5	MOSE PROMINENCE		
UPFH	mm	43.0			
PFH	mm	69.5	Nose tip	mm	26.0
Wits	mm	−15.5	Nose angle	°	40.5
			CHIN PROMINENCE		
TEETH					
			Chin tip	mm	12.5
Overjet	mm	−7.5	B-NPo	mm	−1.0
Overbite	mm	1.0	LADH	mm	32.0
UI/MxP	°	103.5			
LI/MnP	°	87.0			
Iiangle	°	140.0			
LI/APo	mm	5.0			
LI/NPo	mm	2.0			

At age 16, the patient should be reassessed on the joint orthodontic/orthognathic surgery clinic (Figure 19.16). The orthodontist and oral and maxillofacial surgeon should discuss the aims and objectives of treatment in relation to establishing a functional occlusion, optimal dentofacial aesthetics and predictable long-term stability and retention. This will require the patient and parents to be informed that presurgical orthodontic decompensation will result in an increase in the reverse overjet and therefore 'worsening' of the Class III malocclusion. This is achieved through the use of full dimension archwires frequently in combination with upper premolar extractions to provide space for upper labial segment decompensation. Whilst lower premolar extractions can usually be avoided as space is created for relief of crowding through lower incisor proclination, the clinician should assess the effect of lower incisor proclination in relation to the labial gingival biotype as part of the clinical decision process. Where this is problematic, lower arch extractions are required. The amount of crowding and pretreatment inclination of the upper labial segment are the primary determinants of which premolars are extracted but any differential

Figure 19.17 (*Continued*)

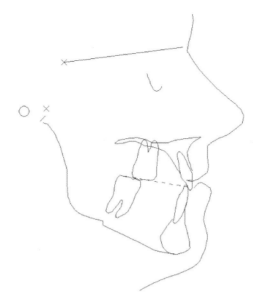

Le Fort I
  Choose all ...
  Ultip 4.0 mm →, U6MC
Mandibular ramus
  Class I incisors ...
  −6.0 mm ←, 2.5 mm ↑

impaction of the maxilla needs to be factored in to avoid the upper incisor inclination being adversely affected at the end of treatment. The other factor to consider during presurgical orthodontic treatment is the need for arch expansion to produce coordination.

The torque values of the bracket prescription are important in determining the amount of axial inclination for surgical cases. Prescriptions with high torque values for the upper labial segment (MBT, Bioprogressive, Damon Q) are preferred to minimise torque loss with upper labial segment decompensation, whilst a relatively high negative torque value for the lower labial segment (MBT) is counterproductive for delivering effective lower incisor decompensation. Where the required decompensation to enable the required surgical movements is not delivered by the appliance, additional torque can be delivered through third-order wire bending. The final important issue is that of arch form for surgical cases. Although arch form is normally selected in relation to the pretreatment arch form, this is less relevant for surgical cases where stability is primarily related to altered soft-tissue and bone relationships.

Following alignment, decompensation and arch coordination and closure of any remaining spacing, a set of 'check' models should be obtained to assess the planned occlusion at surgery and in particular to ensure the incisors and canines will be in a Class I relationship at the end of surgery. Interdental ball-hooks are then placed, a lateral cephalometric radiograph taken for computerised surgical planning and a facebow recording with final impressions for model surgery and surgical wafer construction (Figure 19.17). The combination of a clinical assessment on the joint clinic, computerised cephalometric planning and model surgery will determine the exact surgical plan, with many patients requiring a bimaxillary osteotomy.

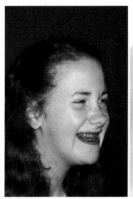
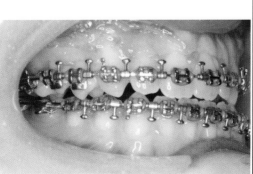
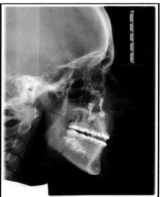

Figure 19.18 Patient following bimaxillary surgery with lateral cephalogram showing ideal maxillary–mandibular relationship and fixation plates in both jaws (same patient as in Figures 19.16 and 19.17).

Post-surgical orthodontic treatment should commence the day following surgery and while initial healing is taking place and intermaxillary elastic traction can begin to refine the new occlusal relationship, with dentoalveolar movement being accelerated due to the upregulation of bone turnover as a result of the healing response. The case is subsequently completed as for a non-surgical case and retention undertaken as normal (Figures 19.18–19.20).

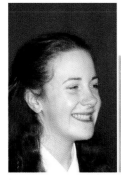
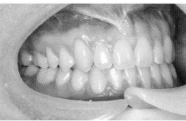

Figure 19.19 Patient on completion of post-surgical orthodontics (same patient as in Figures 19.16–19.18).

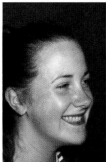
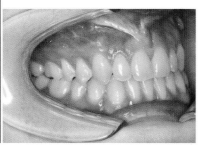

Figure 19.20 Patient at two years post surgery showing good stability (same patient as in Figures 19.16–19.19).

Class III Malocclusion Occurring with Cleft Lip and/or Palate

Cleft lip and palate is a heterogeneous condition ranging in severity from relatively minor lip clefts through incomplete and complete unilateral clefts of the lip and palate to the most severe form, complete bilateral cleft lip and palate (BCLP). Fortunately, Class III malocclusion is not a common association with BCLP and is a frequent presenting feature of all other clefting phenotypes. The orthodontic challenge for treating a Class III malocclusion in a patient with a cleft is not to be underestimated. This arises from the combination of the maxillary growth disturbance arising from the cleft and resultant surgery as well as dental anomalies, which are a frequent occurrence in patients with clefts. Following bone grafting where an alveolar cleft is present, adolescent arch alignment should proceed along the same lines as for a non-cleft patient, taking account of any anomalies and planning orthognathic care where appropriate along with other members of the cleft team (Figure 19.21).

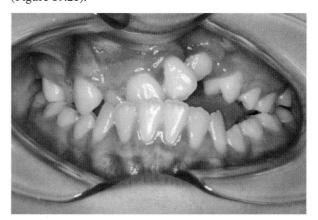

Figure 19.21 Class III malocclusion in a patient with unilateral cleft lip and palate.

References

1 Foster TD, Day AJ. A survey of malocclusion and the need for orthodontic treatment in a Shropshire school population. *Br. J. Orthod.* 1974;1:73–78.

2 Battagel JM. The aetiological factors in Class III malocclusion. *Eur. J. Orthod.* 1993;15:347–370.

3 Kerr WJS, Miller S, Dawber JE. Class III malocclusion: surgery or orthodontics? *Br. J. Orthod.* 1992;19:21–24.

4 Houston WJ. The current status of facial growth prediction: a review. *Br. J. Orthod.* 1979;6(1):11–17.

5 Mandall N, Cousley R, DiBiase A, et al. Early class III protraction facemask treatment reduces the need

for orthognathic surgery: a multi-centre, two-arm parallel randomized, controlled trial. *J. Orthod.* 2016;43(3):164–175.

6 Battagel JM, Orton HS. Class III malocclusion: a comparison of extraction and non-extraction techniques. *Eur. J. Orthod.* 1991;13(3):212–222.

7 Cunningham SJ, Johal A. Orthognathic correction of dento-facial discrepancies. *Br. Dent. J.* 2015;218(3):167–175.

20

Management of Deep Incisor Overbite

Farhad B. Naini, Daljit S. Gill, and Umberto Garagiola

CHAPTER OUTLINE

Introduction, 371
Aetiology, 372
   Skeletal, 373
   Soft Tissue, 373
   Dental, 373
Indications for Treatment, 373
Considerations in Treatment Planning, 374
   Age, 374
   Upper Lip to Maxillary Incisor Relationship, 374
   Incisor Relationship, 374
   Vertical Skeletal Discrepancy, 375
Methods of Overbite Reduction, 375
   Relative Intrusion of the Incisors, 375
   Absolute Intrusion of the Incisors, 375
   Proclination of the Incisors, 375
Appliances and Techniques for Overbite Reduction, 376
   Removable Appliances, 376
   Functional Appliances, 376
   Fixed Appliances (Continuous Arch Mechanics), 377
   Fixed Appliances (Segmented Arch Mechanics), 378
   Auxiliaries, 380
   Headgear, 380
   Absolute Anchorage, 381
   Orthognathic Surgery, 381
   Segmental Surgery, 381
   Conservative Management, 382
Stability of Overbite Correction, 382
Conclusion, 384
References, 384

Introduction

Incisor overbite may be defined as the degree of vertical overlap of the mandibular incisors by the maxillary incisors when the posterior teeth are in occlusion.[1] Overbite depth is usually measured perpendicular to the occlusal plane, either in millimetres or as the amount/percentage of the total crown height of the mandibular incisors that is overlapped by the maxillary incisors. An average overbite occurs when the maxillary incisors overlap the incisal third of the mandibular incisor crowns. In a Class I incisor relationship where the mandibular incisor tips occlude with the cingulum plateau of the maxillary incisors, the overbite depth is 2–4 mm on average (Figure 20.1). A normal incisor overbite is important for incising food, but also allows anterior guidance and disclusion of the posterior dentition in anterior excursion, which may help protect the posterior teeth from tooth wear and cuspal fracture.

Preadjusted Edgewise Fixed Orthodontic Appliances: Principles and Practice, First Edition. Edited by Farhad B. Naini and Daljit S. Gill.
© 2022 John Wiley & Sons Ltd. Published 2022 by John Wiley & Sons Ltd.

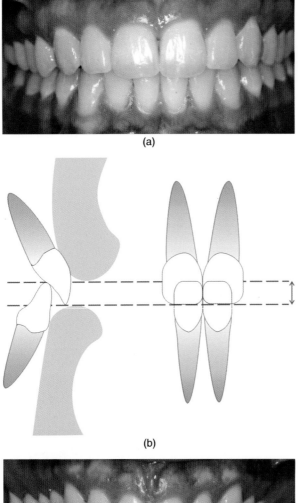

(a)

(b)

(c)

Figure 20.1 (a) A Class I incisor relationship with a normal overbite. (b) The maxillary incisors overlap the incisal third of the mandibular incisor crowns. (c) A deep anterior overbite with the maxillary incisors covering 100% of the mandibular incisor crowns.

Overbite is described in terms of its **depth** and **incisor contact**. Therefore, overbite may be:

- normal
- reduced (decreased)
- deep (increased)

and

- complete to dentition or palatal mucosa
- incomplete.

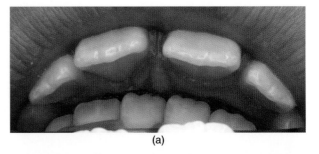

(a)

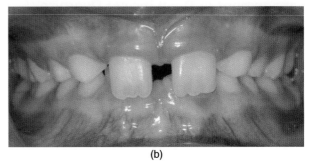

(b)

Figure 20.2 (a) Mandibular incisors impinging on the palatal mucosa. (b) Maxillary incisors impinging on the mandibular labial gingivae.

In addition, a deep overbite complete to the mucosa palatal to the maxillary incisors is known as an **impinging overbite** (Figure 20.2a). In some Class II division 2 malocclusions with minimal overjet the retroclined maxillary incisors may impinge on the gingivae labial to the mandibular incisors (Figure 20.2b). The incisal edges from impinging overbites often leave indentations in the mucosa. However, an impinging overbite *combined with poor oral hygiene* may cause irritation and discomfort, and occasionally lead to significant soft tissue damage, traumatic gingival stripping and recession palatal to the maxillary incisors or labial to the mandibular incisors; this is termed a **traumatic overbite** (Figure 20.3).

Aetiology

Deep incisor overbite problems may result either from an upward and forward (anticlockwise) rotation of the mandible during growth, or from excessive eruption of the incisor teeth, notably the mandibular incisors. Anterior teeth generally erupt until they make contact with the opposing anterior teeth, palatal mucosa or the resting tongue. The factors that contribute to an anterior deep overbite may be classified as (i) skeletal, (ii) soft tissue or (iii) dental.

Figure 20.3 (a, b) Traumatic overbite with mandibular incisors causing trauma to the palatal soft tissues and stripping of the gingivae palatal to the maxillary incisors. (c) Severe Class II division 2 malocclusion with maxillary incisors causing trauma and stripping of the mandibular incisor labial gingivae. (d) Following maxillary incisor proclination, orthognathic preparation and mandibular advancement surgery, the overbite has been corrected. The gingival stripping and recession labial to the mandibular incisors is evident.

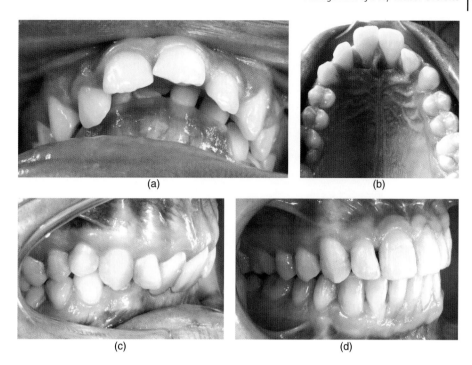

(a) (b) (c) (d)

Skeletal

Forward rotation of the mandible, in the direction of mouth closing, is due to increased posterior vertical facial growth compared with anterior vertical facial growth (Figure 20.4a).[2] Bjork[3] described seven structural signs found on a lateral cephalometric radiograph that may give an indication to the pattern of mandibular growth. The signs evident in forward growth rotators that can give rise to an anterior deep overbite are shown in Figure 20.4b.

Soft Tissue

An important aetiological factor in Class II division 2 malocclusion is a high lower lip line, which is thought to guide the maxillary and mandibular incisors to erupt in a more retroclined position. Patients with a reduced lower anterior face height, often described as short face individuals, may have increased mentalis muscle activity. This is sometimes referred to as a strap-like lower lip. Depending on the vertical height of the lower lip, this may cause retroclination of the mandibular incisors, or if a high lower lip position is also present, bimaxillary retroclination of the maxillary and mandibular incisors.

If there is a forward resting tongue position and/or an adaptive tongue to lower lip swallow pattern occurs, the overbite may be deep but just incomplete to the palatal mucosa.

Dental

Overeruption of the mandibular incisors often accompanies a Class II malocclusion. In Class II division 1 malocclusion with an increased overjet the mandibular incisors erupt until they contact the palatal mucosa, unless there is a forward resting tongue position and/or an adaptive tongue to lower lip swallow pattern as discussed in the previous section.

In Class II division 2 malocclusion the deep overbite is often the result of retroclination of the incisor teeth. The maxillary incisor cingulum plateau is often poorly defined. The maxillary incisors may also have an increased crown/root angle.

It is important to note that a deep overbite may be partly due to overerupted maxillary incisor teeth.

Indications for Treatment

Anterior deep bite may occur in the primary dentition. If so, it is often associated with a relatively short lower anterior face height, reduced mandibular plane angle and square gonial angles. That is, at this age it is primarily skeletal in nature. If the problem is treated in the primary dentition, it is likely to recur when the active treatment is discontinued. Therefore, at this stage of development, treatment is rarely indicated.

In the early permanent dentition, a deep overbite may need to be reduced if causing trauma to the soft tissues palatal to the maxillary incisors or labial to the mandibular incisors. It is important to note, however, that traumatic overbites are almost always associated with poor oral hygiene. The Index of Orthodontic Treatment Need (IOTN) is currently used within the UK National Health

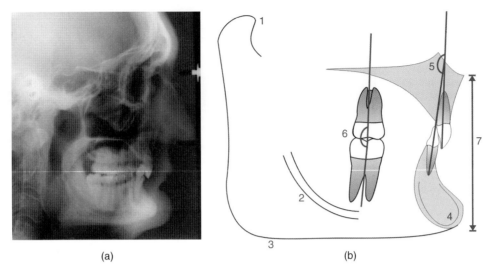

(a)   (b)

Figure 20.4 (a) Lateral cephalometric radiograph of a patient with a forward growth rotation of the mandible. (b) Bjork's seven structural signs indicating a forward mandibular growth rotation: 1, forward inclination of the condylar head; 2, an increased curvature of the inferior alveolar canal; 3, absence of an antegonial notch; 4, forward inclination of the mental symphysis; 5, increased interincisal angle; 6, increased intermolar (and interpremolar) angle; 7, a reduced lower anterior facial height.

Service to prioritise treatment by classifying malocclusions according to treatment need. Only patients with a deep overbite causing palatal or gingival trauma fall into the treatment need category (IOTN 4f).

Deep overbite is often associated with an increased overjet. During orthodontic treatment an increased overjet often cannot be fully corrected until the overbite has been reduced.

If the incisor overjet is not to be fully corrected and the overbite is not traumatic, there is no absolute necessity to reduce a deep overbite; in such situations, any overbite reduction may be unstable as the lower incisors may re-erupt following treatment.

Considerations in Treatment Planning

Age

A patient with a deep traumatic overbite is best treated while still growing, when correction may be relatively straightforward and before any long-term periodontal damage occurs. Growth modification using various functional appliances with capping of the mandibular incisors, or a simple upper removable appliance with an anterior bite plane may be used.

In non-growing patients any extrusion of the buccal segments tends to be unstable due to stretching of the pterygomasseteric sling. Therefore, true intrusion of the incisor teeth is required, and possibly surgical correction using a combined orthodontic and orthognathic approach.

Upper Lip to Maxillary Incisor Relationship

The amount of maxillary incisor exposure in relation to the upper lip at rest should be about 2–5 mm. In patients with reduced incisor exposure at rest it may be prudent to intrude the mandibular incisors rather than the maxillary in order to prevent an aged appearance to the smile. Conversely, in patients with increased gingival exposure ('gummy smile') it is better to intrude the maxillary incisors.

Incisor Relationship

- **Class II division 1 malocclusion**: a significant Class II skeletal pattern, depending on age, requires growth modification or mandibular advancement surgery. However, if the Class II division 1 incisor relationship is on a Class I or mild-to-moderate Class II skeletal pattern, then treatment will involve orthodontic mechanics to correct the inclinations and vertical position of the incisor teeth.
- **Class II division 2 malocclusion**: if the skeletal pattern is Class I or mild Class II, as is often the case, treatment will centre on levelling the lower arch and intrusion and palatal root torque of the maxillary incisors. If the skeletal pattern is a moderate-to-severe Class II, the incisor relationship may be converted to a Class II division 1 malocclusion by proclining the upper labial segment, and then depending on age requires growth modification or orthognathic surgery.
- **Class III malocclusion**: sufficient overbite is required at the end of treatment to maintain a stable incisor relationship. Examples include compensating for an

underlying mild Class III malocclusion by retroclining the mandibular incisors and proclining the maxillary incisors, and also in cases where a maxillary incisor is to be moved labially to correct an anterior crossbite. It is the presence of a positive overbite that will prevent relapse at the end of treatment.

Vertical Skeletal Discrepancy

- **Short face, low angle cases**: in growing patients, attempt to encourage extrusion of the buccal segments using anterior bite planes, functional appliances, bite turbos, cervical pull headgear or the Tip-Edge appliance. In this way the increase in lower anterior face height will improve the facial profile as well as helping to reduce the overbite.
- **Increased face height, high angle cases with deep bite**: it is important to avoid extrusive mechanics to the posterior teeth in order to avoid any further increase in face height.

Methods of Overbite Reduction

The method most suitable for each patient depends on the treatment objectives, which include the achievement of a stable end result. The dental movements required to reduce a deep anterior overbite may include one or more of the following:

- relative intrusion of the incisors (i.e. extrusion of molars and premolars)
- absolute intrusion of the incisors
- proclination of the incisors.

Relative Intrusion of the Incisors

This may be achieved by eruption, extrusion or distal crown tipping of the premolar and molar teeth. Vertical facial growth is required if the overbite reduction achieved in this way is to remain stable. Molar and premolar extrusion may be either passive (e.g. using an anterior bite plane) or active (e.g. using vertical elastics on fixed appliances).

When a reverse curve of Spee is used in the lower archwire, the incorporation of the second molars will help to extrude the first molars, with intrusion of the second molars. If the second molars are not included in the fixed appliance, intrusion of the first molar will occur with extrusion of the premolars. Therefore, effectively, incorporating second molars helps to extrude teeth further back in the dental arch, which theoretically produces greater hinge opening of the mandible and greater overbite reduction.

Absolute Intrusion of the Incisors

This can be difficult to achieve, and requires complex orthodontic mechanics. The mechanics tend to pit incisor intrusion against molar extrusion, thereby inevitably leading to some extrusion of the buccal segments as well as incisor intrusion. The only way to solely achieve true intrusion of incisors is with the use of implants for anchorage or orthodontic mini-implants/temporary anchorage devices (absolute anchorage).

Proclination of the Incisors

Overbite depth reduces as the incisor teeth are proclined. A useful two-dimensional geometric model has been described, stating that there is approximately 0.2-mm change in overbite for every degree of incisal angular change, e.g. 10° proclination leads to 2-mm reduction in overbite.[4] The converse should also apply, i.e. retroclination of incisors towards their correct inclination will tend to increase the incisor overbite (Figure 20.5). In clinical practice the actual change in overbite depth cannot be accurately predicted by this method alone due to other contributory factors, notably the intrusion or extrusion of the incisors and molars. It must be emphasised that in most cases the pretreatment labiolingual inclination of the lower incisors must be maintained for stability. Therefore, proclination of the incisors to reduce an overbite may only be used in select cases.

The other option is a combination of orthodontics and orthognathic surgery, in order to reduce a deep overbite surgically.

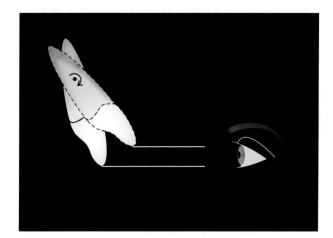

Figure 20.5 Retroclination of proclined maxillary incisors towards the correct inclination increases the overbite, and conversely proclination of normally inclined incisors reduces the overbite, as the teeth rotate around their centre of resistance. Source: modified from Naini FB. *Facial Aesthetics: Concepts and Clinical Diagnosis*. Oxford: Wiley Blackwell, 2011; reprinted with permission.

Appliances and Techniques for Overbite Reduction

The appliances and techniques that may be used for incisor overbite reduction are summarised in Table 20.1.

Removable Appliances

Anterior Bite Plane

This may be used on a simple upper removable appliance as a preliminary stage of treatment, and is ideally fitted in a growing patient as the permanent dentition is establishing. Clip-over anterior bite planes (Plint clip) may also be used with upper and lower fixed appliances, giving clearance for placement of lower anterior brackets in Class II division 2 deep bite cases. Overbite reduction occurs by preventing eruption of the mandibular incisor teeth, but allowing eruption of the posterior teeth (Figure 20.6). The lower anterior face height also increases. The addition of cold cure acrylic to the bite plane allows further reduction of the overbite during treatment. A very useful appliance in a Class II deep bite case is the Ten Hoeve appliance, also known as a 'Nudger' (Figure 20.7).[5] This appliance, used in combination with headgear, combines the benefits of an anterior bite plane with distal movement of the upper first molars to aid in Class II correction and bite opening.

Functional Appliances

These appliances are primarily indicated for correction of anteroposterior arch discrepancies in growing patients. However, capping of the mandibular incisors reduces mandibular incisor eruption while permitting buccal segment tooth eruption (the bite plane effect), thereby

Table 20.1 Appliances and techniques for overbite reduction.

Removable appliances	Anterior bite-plane (or clip-over bite-plane with fixed appliances)
	Dahl appliance (removable)
Functional appliances	Bite-plane effect, e.g. with activator-type appliances such as the Medium Opening Activator
Fixed appliances (continuous arch mechanics)	Preadjusted edgewise appliance: • Continuous heavy flat archwires, e.g. 0.019 × 0.025-inch stainless steel • Treating on a non-extraction basis, if possible • Banding second molars early in treatment • Placing an increased curve in the upper archwire, and a reverse curve of Spee in the lower archwire • 0.019 × 0.025-inch preformed counterforce nickel titanium archwires
	Tip-Edge appliance: anchor bends
	Lingual appliances
	Dahl appliance (fixed)
Fixed appliances (segmented arch mechanics)	Ricketts' utility arch
	Burstone's intrusion arch
Auxiliaries	Class II intermaxillary elastics
	Fixed bite-planes: • Bite turbos (turbo props) • Composite bite-planes (direct or indirect)
Headgears	Wedge effect with distal movement
	Cervical-pull headgear to maxillary first molars
	J-hook headgear to the upper labial segment
Absolute anchorage	Implant anchorage
	Miniscrew anchorage
Orthognathic surgery	Mandibular advancement to three-point landing
Segmental surgery	Lower labial segment set-down
	Mandibulotomy
	Upper labial segment impaction

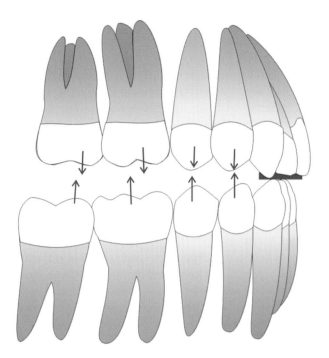

Figure 20.6 The anterior bite plane works by allowing eruption of the posterior teeth.

flattening an increased curve of Spee and reducing a deep overbite (Figure 20.8). Furthermore, the use of functional appliances causes an increase in the lower anterior face height.[6]

Fixed Appliances (Continuous Arch Mechanics)

Preadjusted Edgewise Appliance

Continuous Archwires Heavy flat stainless steel archwires may be used to level the occlusal plane, by a combination of mainly extrusion of posterior teeth and to a lesser extent intrusion of anterior teeth. The incorporation of the **second molar teeth** early in treatment will aid in arch levelling, but care must be taken to keep the tubes relatively occlusally positioned on the molar teeth for the maximum mechanical advantage (Figure 20.9). This allows for extrusion of the first molars and premolars as well as aiding incisor intrusion. Some patience on the part of the operator is required in allowing adequate time for levelling to occur.

When using preadjusted edgewise bracket systems, it is also important to remember that the angulation (tip) built into the canine brackets, particularly distally angulated maxillary canines, will cause the initial archwires to extrude the incisors (Figure 20.10a). As the angulation or tip is expressed, the incisors will re-intrude and the arch will level (Figure 20.10b). This is known as vertical 'round tripping'. To counter this phenomenon, it is possible to use

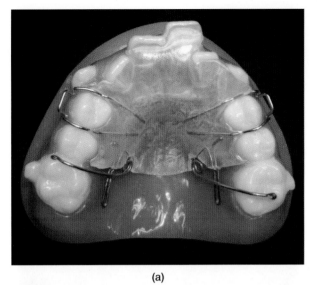

(a)

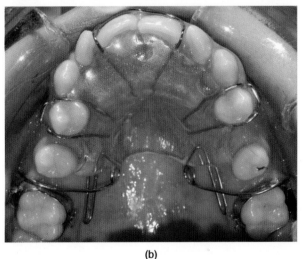

(b)

Figure 20.7 The Nudger appliance. Finger springs, in addition to headgear, aid in distalisation of the maxillary first molars. (a) A Nudger appliance showing degree of finger spring activation. (b) A Nudger appliance after three months of active wear.

reduced tip maxillary canine brackets, or to initially bypass the incisors in patients with very distally angulated canine teeth.

Another important biomechanical consideration is to avoid space closing intra-traction until the arch is level. This is because the space closing forces from the intra-traction in an arch that still has a curve of Spee will work against the forces in the archwire designed to level the occlusal plane (see Chapter 2, Figure 2.35).

Placing Curves in Archwires It is possible to sweep a reverse curve of Spee into a lower stainless steel archwire and an exaggerated curve in an upper archwire. This allows extrusion of the buccal segments, especially the premolars, and

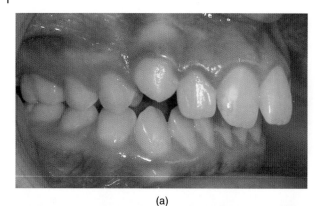

(a)

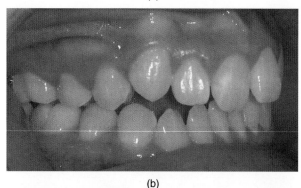

(b)

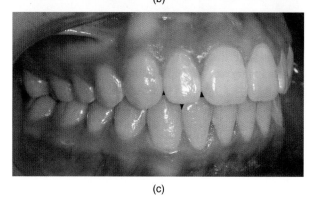

(c)

Figure 20.8 (a) Pretreatment Class II malocclusion with increased incisor overbite. (b) Following functional appliance treatment, the sagittal dental arch relationship has improved and the overbite has reduced. (c) Following fixed appliance treatment, with level arches and a normal overbite.

some intrusion of the labial segments. However, as the area of force application in the brackets is anterior to the centre of resistance of the mandibular incisors, there will be an often-unwanted tendency for proclination of these teeth.

Counterforce NiTi Archwires These rectangular nickel titanium archwires have built-in pronounced curves of Spee (Figure 20.11). The disadvantage with these so-called 'rocking chair' archwires is that they can cause distortion of the arch form if used for extended periods. Therefore, their use requires close supervision.

Tip-Edge Appliance

So-called 'anchor' or 'anchorage' bends used in the first stage of the Tip-Edge appliance system are extremely useful in overbite reduction. An intrusive force is applied to the labial segments, and an extrusive force to the molars. The premolar teeth are not incorporated at this stage of treatment. Therefore, the archwire acts as a lever arm, allowing light forces to be used over a relatively long range. The archwire of choice is a 0.016-inch round high-tensile stainless steel archwire. The use of Class II elastics in the Tip-Edge system greatly facilitates the bite opening effect of the anchor bends.

Lingual Appliances

The brackets in these appliance systems are bonded to the lingual aspect of the teeth, making the appliance more aesthetic than conventional fixed appliances. The anterior brackets in the maxillary arch may have a flat surface that occludes with the mandibular incisors, acting as an anterior bite plane in deep bite cases. The point of force application is also different to conventional appliances. An intrusive force directed through a lingual bracket in a normally inclined tooth will pass closer to both the centre of resistance and the long axis of the tooth, thereby theoretically producing intrusion with less proclination than labially positioned brackets (Figure 20.12).[7]

Dahl Appliance

Works along the same principle as the anterior bite plane and is often used to give occlusal clearance for anterior restorations in prosthodontics.[8]

Fixed Appliances (Segmented Arch Mechanics)

A systematic review and meta-analysis of true incisor intrusion attained during orthodontic treatment concluded that in non-growing patients, 1.5 mm of true maxillary incisor intrusion and 1.9 mm of true mandibular incisor intrusion was attainable with the segmented arch technique.[9] Segmented arch mechanics require greater chairside time for archwire fabrication and may potentially cause patient discomfort or soft tissue trauma if the wires impinge on the mucosa.

Ricketts' Utility Arch

This technique may be valuable in encouraging true intrusion of the incisor segment. The 'utility' archwire only engages the molar and incisor teeth, bypassing the premolars and canines (Figure 20.13).[10] It is stepped away from the buccal segment teeth, allowing better load deflection properties and reduced risk of archwire distortion during mastication. To reduce any extrusion of the molar teeth,

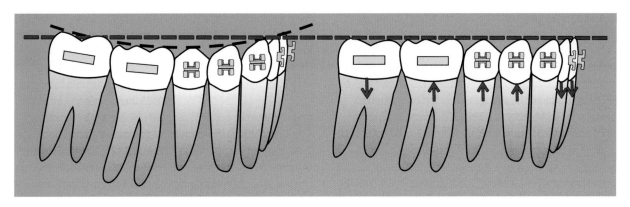

Figure 20.9 Banding the mandibular second molars to aid in arch levelling.

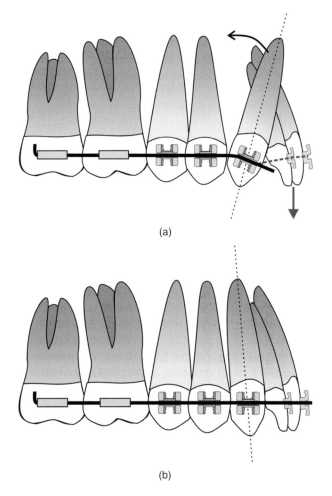

(a)

(b)

Figure 20.10 (a) If the canine teeth are distally angulated, engagement of the incisor brackets with the initial archwire (red dotted line) will extrude the incisors. (b) The arch will level as the canine angulation is corrected.

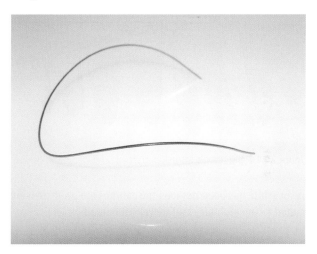

Figure 20.11 Counterforce nickel titanium archwire.

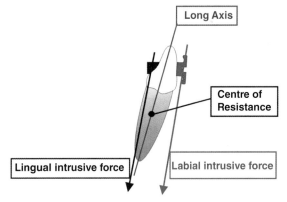

Figure 20.12 The relationship between an intrusive force to the centre of resistance and long axis of a tooth. Blue, lingual force; green, labial force. Source: Gill DS, Naini FB (eds). *Orthodontics: Principles and Practice*. Oxford: Wiley Blackwell, 2011; reprinted with permission.

double buccal tubes are used on the first molar bands, in order to allow use of a sectional archwire linking the buccal segments as well as the utility arch. In order to limit proclination of the mandibular incisor teeth, lingual crown torque must be built into the rectangular archwires used.

However, as the intrusive force on the incisors is anterior to their centre of resistance, some incisor proclination is inevitable unless a concomitant space closing force is also applied, though this will strain posterior anchorage. Once

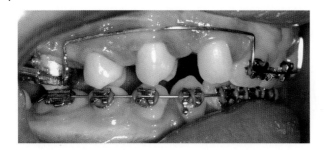

Figure 20.13 Ricketts' utility arch.

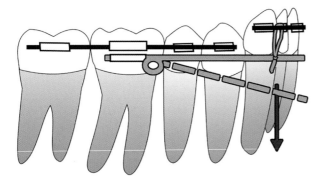

Figure 20.14 Burstone's intrusion arch.

the overbite has been reduced the canines are progressively ligated to the archwire and thereby intruded.

Burstone's Intrusion Arch

This appliance has been said to produce four times more incisor intrusion than molar extrusion. Prior to the introduction of microscrew anchorage, it was claimed to be the appliance of choice in adult patients where an increase in face height was not desired (Figure 20.14).[11] The anterior canine-to-canine region is aligned segmentally. The posterior molar and premolar teeth are also aligned as a segment and rectangular archwires as well as rigid palatal and lingual arches are placed, providing stable posterior vertical anchor units. The accessory rectangular archwire is vertically activated for labial segment intrusion by placing tip-back bends mesial to the molar tubes. It is placed in the additional buccal tubes on the first molar teeth and ligated to the canine region of the anterior segment archwire.

Auxiliaries

Class II Intermaxillary Elastics

These are used bilaterally from the anterior maxillary dental arch to the mandibular first or second molar teeth. They are used in the correction of Class II malocclusion and the reduction of overjet. An often-unwanted effect is the resultant vertical extrusive forces on the mandibular molar teeth. However, in low angle, deep bite malocclusion

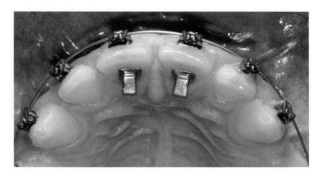

Figure 20.15 Bite turbos (turbo props) are bonded to the palatal aspect of the maxillary incisors.

the extrusion of the mandibular molars is beneficial in helping to reduce the anterior deep bite. An increased curve may be placed in the upper archwire to help reduce the unwanted maxillary incisor extrusion from the elastic force. However, the net effect of Class II elastics will be overbite reduction as the mandibular molars are closer to the condylar hinge axis than the maxillary incisors.

Bite Turbos and Composite Bite Planes

Bite turbos, also known as 'turbo props', are fixed anterior bite planes that are bonded to the palatal aspect of the maxillary incisors. They have a bite plane incorporated (Figure 20.15). These, as well as composite bite planes, may be used with conventional fixed appliances, giving the advantage of allowing the placement of upper and lower fixed appliances from the start of treatment. Composite bite planes may be made indirectly.[12]

Headgear

The direction of pull of the headgear largely depends on the patient's facial growth pattern. A combination-pull headgear or an Interlandi-type headgear may be used to provide straightforward distal movement of the maxillary molar teeth, causing the anterior bite to open. This is called the 'wedge effect' as the molar is moved distally and therefore closer to the condylar hinge axis. Cervical-pull headgear has an additional extrusive force on the maxillary molars, and is therefore ideal for use in low angle, deep bite Class II malocclusion (see Chapter 14, Figure 14.4).

In cases where the maxillary incisors have overerupted, a J-hook headgear may be attached to the anterior aspect of the maxillary archwire to provide an intrusive force directly to the maxillary incisors. This has the benefit of helping to reduce excessive gingival exposure; however, there are no safety features with this type of headgear and it may also place undesirably high intrusive forces on the maxillary incisor teeth. J-hook headgear is now rarely used.

Absolute Anchorage

Absolute vertical anchorage may be used to produce true intrusion of incisor teeth. If rigid endosseous dental implants have been placed for future restoration of missing teeth, they can be incorporated into a fixed appliance to allow intrusive forces to be placed on surrounding teeth. However, these implants cannot be placed until the end of active facial growth. They also need to be placed in exactly the correct position for the placement of future prostheses. Therefore, their use is restricted to skeletally mature adult patients and requires very precise joint planning between the orthodontist and prosthodontist.

Miniscrew anchorage (also termed microscrews, orthodontic mini-implants or temporary anchorage devices) on the other hand has a number of advantages over dental implants in that they are easier to place, cause minimal patient trauma and may be loaded immediately (as osseointegration is not required).[13] Their use effectively eliminates the problem of having to reduce or prevent the unwanted movement of anchor teeth. Because of their small size, they may be inserted into a number of locations allowing forces to be used in the required directions. Segments of teeth may therefore be intruded (see Chapter 12).

Orthognathic Surgery

Patients with a Class II division 1 or division 2 malocclusion often have an excessive curve of Spee. In patients with short faces, where an increase in the lower anterior face height is desired, the curve of Spee must be maintained prior to surgery by placing an increased curve of Spee in the mandibular archwires. When the mandible is advanced at surgery, there will be a three-point contact with the maxillary arch, in the incisor region and bilaterally in the terminal molar region. This is known as a three-point (or tripod) landing (Figure 20.16).[14] The lower arch is then levelled after surgery by extrusion of the premolars (Figure 20.17). It is important to note that a small amount of additional arch length is required for post-surgical levelling. This may be obtained by either maintaining some space in the lower arch before surgery, or allowing for some proclination of the lower incisors after surgery.[15]

Segmental Surgery

This may be considered for adult patients where levelling the curve of Spee by orthodontic mechanics is not achievable. In cases where a natural step exists in the mandibular arch, the arch may be aligned and levelled in segments, usually with an anterior segment from canine-to-canine and two posterior segments. The arch may then be levelled surgically.[16] This has the advantage that no increase in arch length is required. However, care must be taken to diverge the roots of the teeth where the surgical cuts are to be made.[17] If the lower anterior face height is to be maintained, a subapical osteotomy is undertaken to set down the lower labial segment (Figure 20.18a). If the face height is to be increased, a segmental osteotomy including the lower border is undertaken, sometimes referred to as a mandibulotomy (Figure 20.18b).[15]

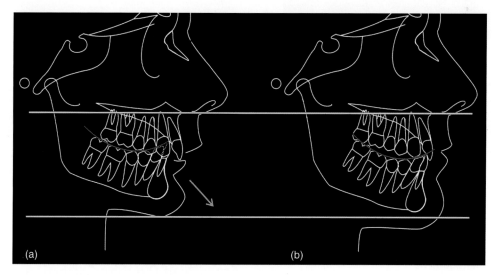

(a)   (b)

Figure 20.16 (a) Maintaining or creating an increased curve of Spee prior to mandibular advancement surgery. (b) Mandibular advancement to a three-point landing (incisors and terminal molars) occurs by a downward and forward vector of movement of the mandibular incisors. This will increase the lower anterior face height. The lateral open bites are closed orthodontically by extrusion of the mid-arch mandibular dentition postoperatively. Source: Naini FB, Gill DS (eds). *Orthognathic Surgery: Principles, Planning and Practice*. Oxford: Wiley Blackwell, 2017; reprinted with permission.

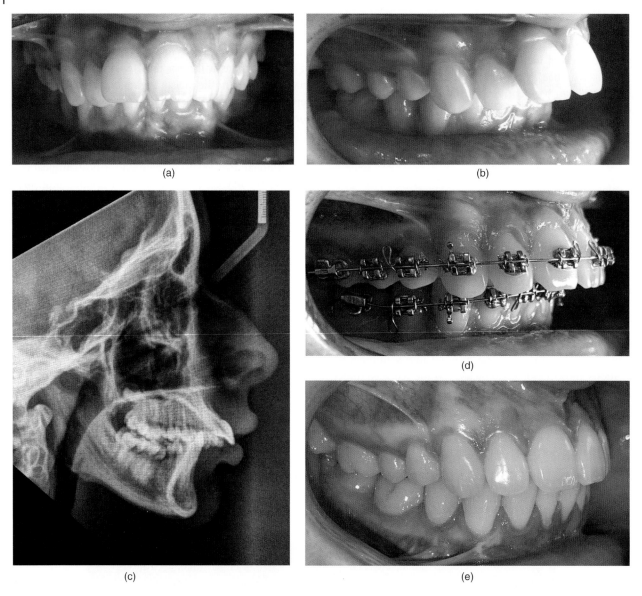

Figure 20.17 (a, b) Pretreatment photographs of a patient with a severe Class II division 1 malocclusion and a deep incisor overbite. (c) Lateral cephalometric radiograph shows a significantly increased curve of Spee. (d) Preoperative orthodontic preparation involved retroclination of the proclined maxillary central incisors, alignment and levelling of the maxillary dental arch, and maintenance of the mandibular curve of Spee. (e) Following mandibular advancement surgery to a three-point landing and closure of the lateral open bites, the arches are level and the overbite normal.

An anterior subapical maxillary segmental osteotomy may be undertaken to superiorly reposition the upper labial segment, particularly in cases of anterior vertical maxillary excess.[18]

Conservative Management

Some patients with heavily restored and/or compromised dentitions presenting with deep overbites and recurrent palatal trauma may not be good candidates for orthodontics or orthognathic surgery. These patients may be managed conservatively by improvement of their oral hygiene, particularly palatal to the maxillary incisors, and possibly the provision of a bite plate, which they can wear as needed, usually at night.

Stability of Overbite Correction

The stability of overbite reduction depends on a number of factors that must be considered from the treatment planning stage.

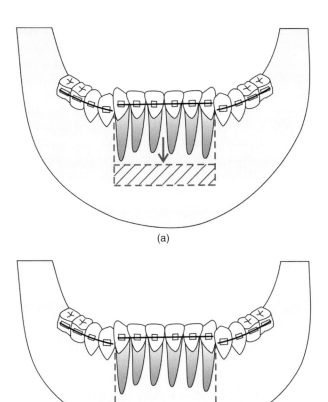

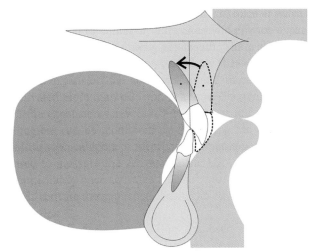

Figure 20.18 (a) Lower labial segment subapical setdown osteotomy. (b) Mandibulotomy. Source: (b) Naini FB, Gill DS (eds). *Orthognathic Surgery: Principles, Planning and Practice.* Oxford: Wiley Blackwell, 2017; reprinted with permission.

Figure 20.19 Incisor edge–centroid relationship. The dot in the maxillary incisor root is the centre of resistance. Note: Although the term 'edge–centroid relationship' is recognised and established in orthodontics, generally the term 'centre of resistance' is more accurate and thereby preferred to the term 'centroid'.

- **Good inter-incisal angle**: the inter-incisal angle must be corrected (average 135°) in addition to the overbite being reduced in order to prevent re-eruption of the incisors after treatment.[19]

- **Correct mandibular incisor edge–centroid relationship**: possibly the most important factor in overbite stability in all treated cases is correction of the relationship between the mandibular incisor edge and the maxillary incisor root centroid (Figure 20.19).[20] This is measured as the distance between the perpendicular projections of these two points on the maxillary plane (0–2 mm). This may be achieved by either retraction of the maxillary incisor root centroid using fixed appliances with palatal root torque, or proclination of the mandibular incisors to advance their edges. The decision depends on a number of factors including the facial profile and growth potential. If a patient has a retrognathic mandible, it is possible to procline the maxillary incisors and to either surgically advance the

mandible or in a growing patient to use a functional appliance to help advance the mandibular incisors. In a patient with good facial profile aesthetics, the treatment may be carried out with fixed appliances alone, so long as the palatal alveolar process is thick enough to allow retraction of the maxillary incisor root centroid. The crowns of the incisor teeth should also be maintained within the zone of soft tissue equilibrium between the musculature of the tongue and the lips.[21] An interesting proposition is that in Class II division 2 malocclusions it may be possible to intrude and torque the maxillary incisor roots palatally, allowing the mandibular incisor crowns to be proclined and hence occupy the position previously occupied by the maxillary incisor crowns, thus maintaining the incisor complex within the zone of soft tissue equilibrium.[22]

- **Avoid change in intermaxillary height in non-growing patients**: the extrusion of molars in non-growing patients is unstable, as the muscular forces from the pterygomasseteric sling will re-intrude the molars if the posterior vertical face height has not accommodated their extrusion.

- **Proclination of the lower labial segment in Class II cases**: this may still be unstable in the long term due to pressure from the lower lip.[23] Therefore, long-term retention may be required in such cases and must be discussed with the patient prior to treatment.

- **Vertical facial growth continues well into the late teenage years**: as the pattern of facial growth does not tend to change following treatment, it is prudent to place a bite plane on the maxillary removable retainer after the completion of orthodontic treatment. This may be worn on a part-time basis in order to maintain the corrected overbite until vertical facial growth has subsided.[24]

Conclusion

The correction of a deep incisor overbite requires a logical planning process in order to achieve the correct treatment objectives. The patient's age, pattern of facial growth, type of malocclusion and the respective clinician's skill are all factors that must be considered. Knowledge of the skills of prosthodontic and surgical colleagues is also vital if patients are to receive optimum treatment. For most patients, working through continuous archwires of increasing rigidity will level the dental arches and allow the clinician to attain a normal overbite. However, in more complex situations the other techniques discussed in this chapter will help to establish a normal incisor relationship.

References

1 Naini FB. Deep overbite malocclusion. In: Gill DS, Naini FB (eds). *Orthodontics: Principles and Practice.* Oxford: Wiley Blackwell, 2011.

2 Bjork A. Facial growth in man, studied with the aid of metallic implants. *Acta Odontol. Scand.* 1955;13:9–34.

3 Bjork A. Prediction of mandibular growth rotation. *Am. J. Orthod.* 1969;55:585–599.

4 Eberhart BB, Kuftinec MM, Baker IM. The relationship between bite depth and incisor angular change. *Angle Orthod.* 1990;60:55–58.

5 Cetlin NM, Ten Hoeve A. Nonextraction treatment. *J. Clin. Orthod.* 1983;17:396–413.

6 Naini FB, Gill DS, Payne E, Keel W. Medium opening activator: design applications for the management of Class II deep bite malocclusion. *World J. Orthod.* 2007;8:e1–e9.

7 Wiechmann D, Hepburn S. Lingual appliance techniques. In: Gill DS, Naini FB (eds). *Orthodontics: Principles and Practice.* Oxford: Wiley Blackwell, 2011.

8 Dahl BL, Krogstad O, Karlsen K. An alternative treatment in cases with advanced localized attrition. *J. Oral Rehabil.* 1975;2:209–214.

9 Ng J, Major PW, Flores-Mir C. True incisor intrusion attained during orthodontic treatment: a systematic review and meta-analysis. *Am. J. Orthod. Dentofacial Orthop.* 2005;128:212–219.

10 Ricketts RW. *Bioprogressive Therapy.* Denver, CO: Rocky Mountain Orthodontics, 1979.

11 Burstone CJ. Deep overbite correction by intrusion. *Am. J. Orthod.* 1977;72:1–22.

12 Philippe J. Treatment of deep bite with bonded biteplanes. *J. Clin. Orthod.* 1996;30:396–400.

13 Bae SM, Park HS, Kyung HM, et al. Clinical application of micro-implant anchorage. *J. Clin. Orthod.* 2002;36:298–302.

14 Naini FB, Witherow H. The three-point landing in mandibular orthognathic surgery: a modified technique. *Ann. R. Coll. Surg. Engl.* 2016;98:155–156.

15 Millett D. Specific considerations in the 'low angle' patient. In: Naini FB, Gill DS (eds). *Orthognathic Surgery: Principles, Planning and Practice.* Oxford: Wiley Blackwell, 2017.

16 Kole H. Surgical operations on the alveolar ridge to correct occlusal abnormalities. *Oral Surg.* 1959;12:277–288.

17 Naini FB, Gill DS. Preparatory and postoperative orthodontics: principles, techniques and mechanics. In: Naini FB, Gill DS (eds). *Orthognathic Surgery: Principles, Planning and Practice.* Oxford: Wiley Blackwell, 2017.

18 Shand JM, Heggie AA. Segmental surgery of the maxilla. In: Naini FB, Gill DS (eds). *Orthognathic Surgery: Principles, Planning and Practice.* Oxford: Wiley Blackwell, 2017.

19 Schudy FF. The control of vertical overbite in clinical orthodontics. *Angle Orthod.* 1968;38:19–39.

20 Houston WJB. Incisor edge–centroid relationships and overbite depth. *Eur. J. Orthod.* 1989;11:139–143.

21 Proffit WR. Equilibrium theory revisited. *Angle Orthod.* 1978;48:175–186.

22 Selwyn-Barnett BJ. Class II division 2 malocclusion: a method of planning and treatment. *Br. J. Orthod.* 1996;23:29–36.

23 Mills JRE. The stability of the lower labial segment. *Trans. Br. Soc. Study Orthod.* 1968;11–24.

24 Nanda RS, Nanda SK. Considerations of dentofacial growth in long-term retention and stability: is active retention needed? *Am. J. Orthod. Dentofacial Orthop.* 1992;101:297–302.

21

Management of Anterior Open Bite

Chung H. Kau and Tim S. Trulove

CHAPTER OUTLINE

Introduction, 385
Prevalence and Incidence, 385
Aetiology, 385
  Skeletal Origins, 386
Characteristics, 388
  Increased Lower Face Height: Long Face Syndrome, 388
  Anterior Open Bite, 389
Clinical Treatment, 389
  Concepts, 389
  Primary Dentition/Mixed Dentition, 389
  Late Mixed Dentition/Early Permanent Dentition, 389
  Late Permanent Dentition, 390
Retention and Stability, 394
Conclusion, 394
References, 394

Introduction

The anterior open bite (AOB) malocclusion represents one of the most challenging diagnostic and treatment decisions for an orthodontic practitioner. AOBs have multiple presentations and in many, but not all, cases there is a vertical component that is incorporated into the problem list. The aetiology of AOB is often multifactorial with inherited facial proportions, skeletal patterns, functional adaptations and other environmental factors contributing to the problem.

Prevalence and Incidence

One of the more reliable datasets to identify the open bite malocclusion comes from the US Public Health Service Survey 1988–1991. The authors found that of a sample population aged 8–50 years, those with a zero overbite comprised 9%.[1] Less than 5% of the sample had an AOB when the posterior teeth were in occlusion. The average open bite

for all persons having this condition was 1.1 mm and the average open bite was similar in both males and females. In all persons with AOBs, those in the younger 8–11 year age group had numerically greater average open bite (1.9 mm) than the 12–17 age group (1.0 mm) and the 18–50 age group (1.0 mm). This decrease may be related to growth and environmental influences such as oral habits. African Americans had a significantly greater average AOB than Caucasians and Hispanics (Table 21.1). While these data represent an American population, other similar studies in the Netherlands have shown that up to 60% of the adolescents in a population have an AOB. Furthermore, the data also showed that AOB occurred in 10–40% of adults.[2, 3]

Aetiology

The aetiology of the AOB malocclusion is multifactorial. The exact nature as to how the malocclusion occurs is subject to much controversy. It is accepted that environmental and inherited factors play an important role in

Preadjusted Edgewise Fixed Orthodontic Appliances: Principles and Practice, First Edition. Edited by Farhad B. Naini and Daljit S. Gill.
© 2022 John Wiley & Sons Ltd. Published 2022 by John Wiley & Sons Ltd.

Table 21.1 Average open bite for Americans aged 8 to 50 years, 1988–1991.

	Age groups (mean [SE] in mm)			
	All ages	8–11 years	12–17 years	18–50 years
All persons	(0.13)	1.9 (0.34)	1.0 (0.25)	(0.13)
Males	1.0 (0.17)	1.5 (0.42)	0.9 (0.42)	(0.19)
Females	1.2 (0.14)	2.1 (0.40)	1.2 (0.33)	1.0 (0.13)
Caucasians	0.8 (0.12)	2.1 (0.51)	0.6 (0.33)	0.6 (0.09)
African Americans	1.6 (0.16)	1.8 (0.42)	1.6 (0.36)	1.6 (0.19)
Hispanics	1.1 (0.09)	1.2 (0.19)	1.3 (0.26)	1.1 (0.13)

development of the abnormality that ultimately leads to the malocclusion.

Skeletal Origins

Growth-related Problems

Cranial Base Characterised by the Saddle Angle It has been shown that anatomical characteristics play an important role in defining an occlusion. The face and cranial base constitute a closed structure and the inclination of the anterior cranial flexure affects jaw orientation. In the 1970s, Björk popularised his view that a skeletal open bite was characterised by an increased flexure of the cranial base known as the saddle angle (Figure 21.1).[4] The larger the saddle angle, the longer the anterior face height and vice versa. It has also been found that the saddle angle is larger in blacks than whites (approximately 3° more on average).

The Mandible The shape and size of the mandible as well as its direction of growth have also been the subject of research. Björk and Skieller in their implant studies suggested that the mandible could be predictive of vertical growth pattern. They showed that the angulation of the lower border of the mandible, ramus inclination, ratio of the anterior face height to the posterior face height, hyperdivergent faces, amount of vertical molar movement during treatment, lower face height, amount of

Table 21.2 The seven features of backward rotators.

Aspects	Backward rotator
1 Inclination of the condylar head	Straight/slopes up
2 Curvature of the mandibular canal	Straight
3 Shape of the mandibular lower border	Notched
4 Inclination of the symphysis (anterior aspect below B point)	Slopes backward
5 Inter-incisal angle	Obtuse
6 Interpremolar or intermolar angles	Obtuse
7 Anterior lower face height	Tall

condylar growth and direction of condylar growth all were significant in identifying a vertical grower.[5, 6] In these patients, the growth of the condyle in patients with the long face syndrome and an increase in lower face height was more posteriorly directed. Table 21.2 summarises the seven criteria to assess a backward rotator (vertical grower).

It is important to note that information from the growth studies mentioned should be used cautiously. These 'predictors' were observed from samples that had extreme 'growers' in them and if these extremes were eliminated from the study, the prediction of mandibular growth would have been less accurate. Furthermore, many of the implants in these studies were lost as the patients grew, leading to doubts about the true findings of these implant studies as well.[8]

Short Mandibular Ramus In addition to the mandibular morphologies already mentioned, a short mandibular ramus predisposes a patient to an AOB. The shorter the ramus, the smaller the space available for the eruption of posterior teeth and the greater the chance the mandible will rotate downward and backward.[9]

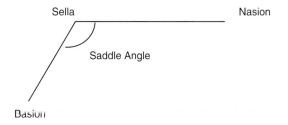

Figure 21.1 Saddle angle.

Maxillary Rotation The orientation of the maxilla also influences the vertical dental and facial relationships. Björk's implant studies show that rotation of the maxilla occurs during normal growth. The internal rotation of the maxillary core that occurs during growth is concealed by surface remodelling that maintains the orientation of the palatal plane. This maxillary rotation does not always occur in patients with vertical dysplasias.[4] If the maxilla is rotated down posteriorly, or up anteriorly, the amount of space for the eruption of the posterior teeth is reduced, space for the anterior teeth increases and there is a tendency towards an AOB.

Growth Rotations Not until the implant studies of Björk and Skieller was the idea of growth rotations appreciated. Issacson noted that in patients who had a vertical problem, differences are noted on the lateral cephalogram between the anterior face height and the posterior face height.[10, 11] This difference in height development leads to rotational growth or positional changes of the mandible and this affects the position of the chin. Therefore, patients with a larger than normal anterior face height versus posterior face height were more likely to have an increased face height.

Other Growth-related Specific Causes Other causative factors that are less commonly encountered include the following.

- **Muscular weakness syndromes**: in cases like these, the mandible is left open and there is no chance for the mandible to grow. The ramus does not lengthen normally as the mandibular elevator muscles are a major influence on growth of the ramus.[12]
- **Arthritic degeneration**: this can lead to injury to the mandibular condyle and prevents normal ramus growth. In recent years, authors have started to quantify arthritic problems in the adolescent. One such disorder is juvenile idiopathic arthritis. This debilitating disease is quantified by pain in the joints for more than six weeks. It often happens in the extremities but the temporomandibular joint may or may not present with pain, resulting in a difficult diagnostic problem.[13]
- **Total nasal obstruction**: this will cause the patient to adopt a posture where the mouth is open, and the mandible drops downward and backward.
- **True macroglossia**: this is very hard to diagnose. Certainly, if the tongue is truly large, it will occupy space and prevent a closing rotation of the mandible.

Functional Problems

Functional problems relate more to soft tissues and habits. Some of these functional problems can be classified as (i) sucking habits, (ii) tongue thrust and (iii) mouth breathing.

Sucking Habits Prolonged digit sucking, also referred to as non-nutritive suckling has been attributed to the development of the malocclusion. The effects of this habit on skeletal and dental development are usually not permanent if the habit ceases in the early stages. The amount of tooth displacement is dependent on the duration and also on the magnitude of the pressure. The effects of these habits on the developing occlusion have been well documented.[14, 15]

Tongue Thrust and Tongue Posture The tongue thrust as an aetiology of the anterior bite is controversial. Laboratory studies indicate that individuals who place the tongue tip forward when they swallow usually do not have more tongue force against their teeth than those who keep the tongue tip back; in fact, the tongue pressure may be lower.[16] In addition, the 'tongue thrust' is part of the normal swallowing pattern of children aged three to six years. Some adults maintain this feature, although this does not translate to an AOB for these patients. The modern viewpoint is that 'tongue thrust swallowing' is seen primarily in two circumstances.

- Younger children with reasonable normal occlusion in whom this represents only a transitional stage in normal physiological maturation.
- Individuals of any age with displaced incisors, in which the adaptation is to fill the spaces between the teeth.

A tongue thrust is thus considered an effect and not a cause of anterior occlusal problems. However, this does not imply that the tongue has no aetiological role in AOB. It is that the duration of the force on the incisors to sustain a substantial effect is just not sufficient to cause an AOB based on the equilibrium theory. If, however, a patient had a forward resting posture of the tongue, the duration of this pressure – even very light forces – could affect tooth position vertically and horizontally. It can therefore be concluded that the tongue posture at rest is the single most important factor in causing an AOB and not the actual action of the tongue thrusting forward.

Respiratory Pattern and Nasopharyngeal Obstruction Respiratory pattern has been attributed to the development of vertical problems repeatedly over time. This attribution is not without controversy. Solow and Kreiborg postulated that the relationship between obstruction of the airway and the position of the head on the cervical column was an important factor and that changes in the activity of certain muscles should lead to an extension of the head and maintenance of the airway. This alternatively should cause a stretching of the masticatory system and mimic muscles and soft tissue, including the skin. This stretching transmits to the periosteum and underlying skeletal structures. A prolonged obstruction will lead to remodelling of the bony units and a change in skeletal morphology. They call this the 'soft tissue stretching theory'.[17]

Other authors also favour the theory that nasopharyngeal obstruction and the subsequent sequelae play an important role in the development of the increased vertical dimension.[18] They carried out their own investigations after being convinced by Harvold's animal studies (where the experimental primates had changes to lower anterior face height after obstructions to respiratory function were carried out).[19] They reviewed possible causes of nasal obstruction and even suggested the removal of these obstructions as a means of treatment.

Characteristics

Described in this section are some features of the long face and the AOB.

Increased Lower Face Height: Long Face Syndrome

Increased lower face height, or the long face, is the manifestation of the elongation of the lower third of the face, leading to disproportions in facial height and width. A long face patient can be described as skeletal Class I rotated to Class II or as a Skeletal II or as a Skeletal III rotated into Class I. The excess face height makes anteroposterior mandibular deficiencies appear worse and prognathism appear better.

One other sign of excess facial height is lip incompetence, defined as separation of the lips at rest. Most of the time a 4-mm separation of the lips will be considered to be the outer limit of normal and anything beyond that will be considered as incompetent. Figure 21.2 shows a typical long face individual. Box 21.0 summarises the clinical and cephalometric characteristics of an increased vertical dimension.

Box 21.1 Clinical and cephalometric characteristics of an increased vertical dimension

Clinical examination

Extraoral

- Increased lower facial height
- Lip incompetence >4 mm
- Shallow mentolabial sulcus
- Convex profile
- Excessive gingival show on smiling

Dental characteristics

- Class II malocclusion
- Upright incisors
- Excessive eruption of posterior teeth
- Anterior open bite
- Narrow maxilla and posterior crossbite

Cephalometric evaluation

Skeletal characteristics

- Rotation of the palatal plane downwards
- Inferiorly tipped palatal plane
- Short mandibular ramus and posterior facial height
- Steep mandibular plane
- Increased height of the anterior mandibular alveolus
- Increased cranial flexure angle
- Increased maxillary and dentoalveolar height
- Increased anterior facial height

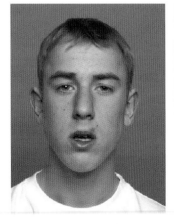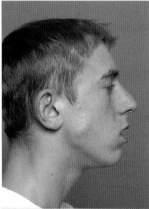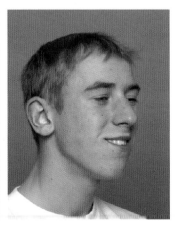

Figure 21.2 An 18-year-old male presenting with a typical long face (increased lower facial height, incompetent lips, high angle and AOB). Source: author's personal collection. Permission from the University of Wales, College of Medicine, 2001.

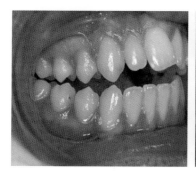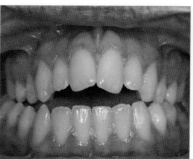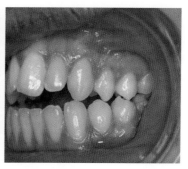

Figure 21.3 Same patient as in Figure 21.2 showing anterior open bite with an underlying skeletal entity. Source: author's personal collection. Permission from the University of Wales, College of Medicine, 2001.

Anterior Open Bite

The AOB can be classified as dental or skeletal. This classification depends very much on the original aetiological site. Figure 21.3 shows the AOB of the patient shown in Figure 21.2. This would indicate the patient has a skeletal open bite because of his underlying long face.

Clinical Treatment

Concepts

The principle of treatment for AOB is to understand the possibilities that can occur. These principles may be approached in a number of ways:

1. remove the aetiology (and wait for self-correction)
2. correct the dental malocclusion
3. correct the skeletal malocclusion (this is dependent on age).

The treatment of the vertical problem can be examined more specifically and chronologically.

Primary Dentition/Mixed Dentition

The presence of an AOB at an early stage should cause an orthodontist to look for prolonged and intense use of the fingers or thumb. When this is noticed, it might be necessary to resort to treatment measures that will stop the habit if patients are unable to do so on their own. In such cases the use of a maxillary palatal crib can be helpful. The concept of early treatment of patients is that deterioration of the occlusion is most pronounced during puberty, when growth intensity is greatest, but continues throughout the growth period. Patients with such tendencies should be treated early and the occlusion supported throughout the growth period. Retention, especially in the mandibular arch, should be maintained until mandibular growth is completed. Always try to assess the severity of the malocclusion, habits and/or skeletal problems. Attempts at growth modification and the control of posterior eruption can be helpful.

Late Mixed Dentition/Early Permanent Dentition

This stage of dental and skeletal development is considered by many clinicians to be an ideal time for interception as it presents a window of opportunity for growth modification. Some of the treatment modalities are discussed here.

High-pull Headgear with Occlusal Support

For minimal overbites and small AOBs, successful results can be achieved by careful control of the vertical dimension. Transpalatal bars can be used to prevent the dropping of the palatal cusps of the first molar. In addition, the use of high-pull headgear is claimed by some to intrude the first molars and is routinely used with the transpalatal bar. Occlusal splints together with high-pull headgear have also helped to control the vertical dimension (Figure 21.4).

Vertical-pull Chin Cup and Bite Splints

Extraoral anchorage using a vertical-pull chin cup (VPCC) with or without posterior occlusal coverage provided by bite splints has shown to be an effective method to control the vertical dimension during growth. Pearson demonstrated the effectiveness of the VPCC as an adjunct to orthodontic treatment with or without the use of fixed appliances. The VPCC has shown its ability to limit molar eruption with good patient compliance in the treatment of individuals with vertical growth problems.[20]

Bite Splints and Functional Appliances

Bite splints and functional appliances have been used more in European countries to manage open bites. The theory is that the open bite malocclusion is caused by the oral posture and is not skeletal in nature. These appliances combine a bite block effect with the freedom for incisors to erupt. Figure 21.5 shows a functional appliance with a modified Twin Block being used to treat an AOB.

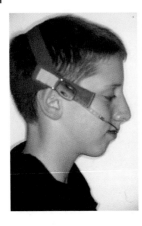
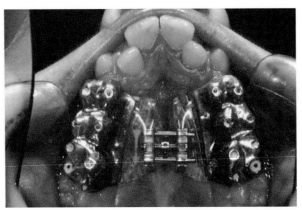

Figure 21.4 An 11-year-old patient with an anterior open bite. High-pull headgear with 'cap' splint rapid palatal expander. An attempt at correcting a dental open bite caused by thumb sucking. Source: author's personal collection. Permission from the University of Wales, College of Medicine, 2001.

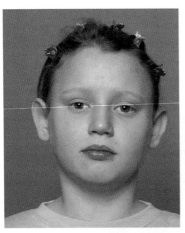
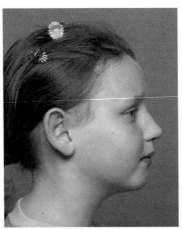
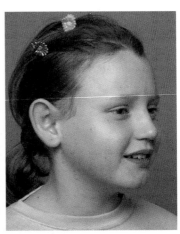

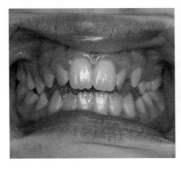
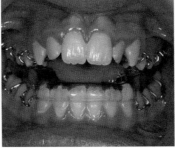

Figure 21.5 An 11-year-old patient with an anterior open bite. An attempt at correcting a dental open bite caused by thumb sucking. Source: author's personal collection. Permission from the University of Wales, College of Medicine, 2001.

Conventional Orthodontic Mechanics

When managing patients with conventional orthodontic mechanics, growth rotations should be remembered. It is advisable to manage these patients with the maximum control of the posterior teeth, especially when extractions are required. This will lessen the potential for backward and posterior rotation as a result of uncontrolled and undesirable molar extrusion as a result of treatment mechanics.

A Word of Caution: Growth versus Growth Modification

Unless treatment results obtained through growth modification are retained throughout growth, there is a high tendency for remaining growth to perpetuate the underlying skeletal problem. Van Der Liden states that particularly in the long face, suppression of vertical development during treatment is followed by an excessive increase in lower face height in subsequent years.

Late Permanent Dentition

There are three broad approaches to the treatment of AOB in the late permanent dentition. These may involve traditional fixed appliances with innovative additions to the biomechanical strategies or clear aligners. The following are some approaches.

Clear Aligners

Clear aligners play a significant role in orthodontic practice in the United States. At present, almost 300 000 new cases are started each year, with a significant number of cases using clear aligners. Invisalign (Align Technology, Inc., Santa Clara, CA, USA) is the major provider of custom-made aligners that sequentially treat malocclusions through a series of custom-made trays. The number of adults seeking orthodontic treatment has increased tremendously in the last two decades.[21] This shift in patient population might be directly linked to the introduction of clear appliances to the orthodontic marketplace. The trends in clear aligners has also increased amongst older adolesecents.[22] To many patients, clear aligners are perceived as more tolerable than ceramic and metal brackets.[23] Furthermore, adults using clear aligners are usually considered better-looking than adults wearing metal brackets.[24] These fundamental reasons have led to an increased acceptance and uptake of clear aligners in orthodontic practices.

Clear aligners have many advantages, including aesthetics, hygiene and time management in the orthodontic office.[25] These factors are particularly appealing for adults, since they have busy schedules and constantly have to present themselves on a social level. While there are many advantages to treatment with clear aligners, they have taken some time to be widely accepted. This is mainly due to the novel nature of the appliance and its many uncertainties. For example, in a 2005 systematic review of clear aligners, the authors were not able to find sufficient evidence to issue precise guidelines regarding Invisalign treatment because of the lack of published clinical trials.[26]

Even though clear aligners have not been shown to manage every malocclusion, it has been definitively shown that these appliances are very efficient in open bite management.[27] A recent study showed that clear aligners were successful in treating Class I and Class II malocclusions with AOBs. The peer assessment rating scores showed a similar improvement to the malocclusion as compared to controls.[28] One of the reasons why aligners are effective is that much of the biomechanical force from the plastic covering of the aligners is directed towards the posterior teeth, allowing for significant vertical control (Figure 21.6).

Contrary to this finding, Khosravi et al. reported a bite deepening of 1.5 mm on average in patients with AOBs treated with clear aligner therapy. Changes in incisor position were determined to be primarily responsible for the AOB correction. Only minimal changes in vertical molar position and the mandibular plane angle were noted in the treated sample.[29]

The MEAW Approach

In 1987, Young Kim presented the multiloop edgewise archwire (MEAW) as a resource to treat severe open bite without the benefit of surgical interventions. This technique used a combination of 0.016 × 0.022-inch stainless steel archwires and heavy anterior elastics to achieve molar intrusion and simultaneous incisor extrusion, resulting in closure of the AOB.[30]

The treatment effects of the MEAW appliance have been evaluated by various and found to be stable.[31, 32] Comparisons have been made to open bite groups and non-open bite groups. The appliance produces an increase in upper

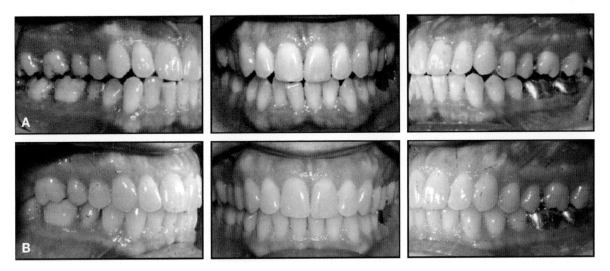

Figure 21.6 Patient with an anterior open bite treated with Invisalign therapy. Source: Kau CH, Feinberg KB, Christou T. Effectiveness of clear aligners in treating patients with anterior open bite: a retrospective analysis. *J. Clin. Orthod.* 2017;51(8):454–460.

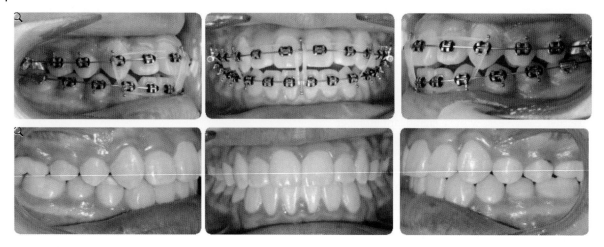

Figure 21.7 Patient with an anterior open bite. Reverse-curve nickel titanium wires placed conventionally. Crimpable hooks placed anterior and heavy elastics ($^3/_{16}$ inch, 4 ounces [113 g]) used in boxes and also anteriorly. Source: author's personal collection. Permission from the University of Alabama at Birmingham.

and lower dentoalveolar heights. No significant change was noted to the upper posterior dentoalveolar height, and the lower dentoalveolar height was significant decreased. Measurements have indicated that there was distal movement of the entire dentition. The inter-incisal angle also increased significantly. The appliance had a minimal effect in the skeletal pattern. Open bites are corrected by the altering the occlusal plane and distally uprighting the posterior teeth.

A simpler type of mechanics that has also been advocated would be to use reverse curve nickel titanium wires. These wires are placed conventionally to open the bite and 'crimpable' hooks placed in the anterior and canine regions. Heavy elastics are used to 'hold' the bite anteriorly and this intrudes the posterior segments.

Erdem and Kucukkeles[32] evaluated 18 patients treated with curved archwires and anterior elastics. Their cone beam study concluded that both maxillary and mandibular incisors extruded to increase the overbite. They also found no significant changes in the position of the posterior teeth. Figure 21.7 shows a patient that has these mechanics in place.

Temporary Anchorage Implants and Devices

Following on from Kim's idea of intruding posterior teeth, maybe attaining absolute anchorage in order to intrude posterior teeth would be an ideal solution.[33] With advances in osseointegration techniques, it is now possible to use implants as anchorage units. This idea has been exploited and clinicians have been successful in utilising intrusion mechanics in open bite malocclusions to prevent extrusion of posterior teeth (Figure 21.8).[34] These implants may be placed in the palate, buccal alveolus in the first

molar region and also the buccal shelves of the zygomatic arches.[35]

In addition to single tooth implants, skeletal anchorage systems using titanium manipulated plates temporarily implanted in the maxilla or mandible have been reported. These plates are implanted in the buccal cortical bone in the apical regions of the first and second molars and have been shown to produce as much as 3–5 mm of molar intrusion.[36]

Combined Orthodontic and Surgical Approach

Many surgical techniques have been suggested for the correction of the anterior skeletal open bite.[37, 38] The choice of procedure will be determined by a careful clinical and radiographic assessment.[39, 40] The combined approach to treatment should aim to improve the skeletal relations, masticatory function and facial aesthetics of the patient.[41] It is not our intention here to undertake an in-depth survey of surgical planning and techniques. Contemporary approaches to the surgical correction are planned around a Le Fort I osteotomy. This aims to correct any anteroposterior discrepancy while elevating the posterior maxilla and allowing mandibular rotation to close the bite (Figure 21.9).

However, if a skeletal open bite is characterised by a decreased posterior face height and a short mandibular ramus with steep gonial angle, then the theoretical ideal would be an osteotomy in the ascending ramus. Data from the University of North Carolina after a one-year follow-up showed that in single jaw surgery with the maxilla up only, there was a less than 1% chance for relapse (which represented no change). For five years and more, there was a 25% chance of the maxilla relapsing downward more than 2 mm and a 12–14% chance of a more than 2-mm change in overjet and overbite.[9] In a bimaxillary surgical procedure, after one year there was a 10% chance for clinical relapse

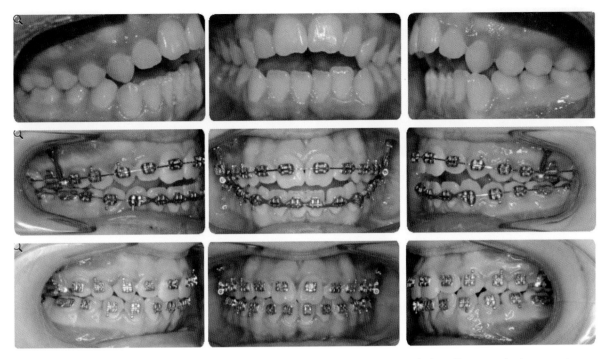

Figure 21.8 Management of a patient with anterior open bite using temporary anchorage devices. Source: author's personal collection. Permission from the University of Alabama at Birmingham.

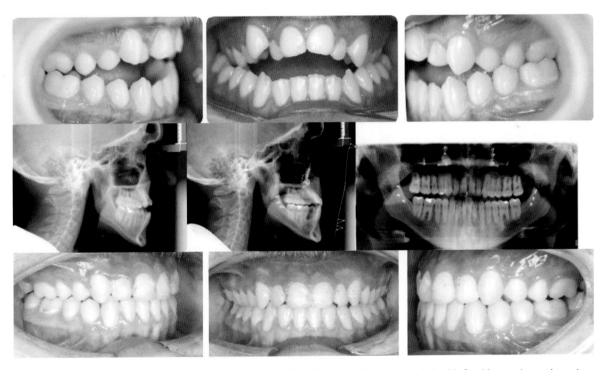

Figure 21.9 Adult patient with a skeletal and dental open bite. Maxillary dentition was bonded with fixed braces in sections. A three-piece maxillary osteotomy and mandibular bilateral sagittal split osteotomy (BSSO) was performed. Source: author's personal collection. Permission from the University of Alabama at Birmingham.

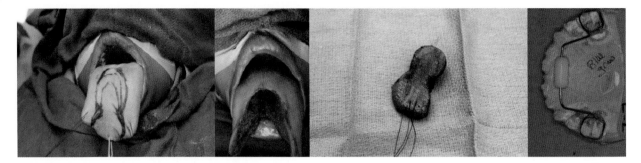

Figure 21.10 Surgical glossectomy of the tongue. Anterior open bite controlled thereafter with a 'blue-grass' appliance.

and after five years a greater than 20% chance of more than 2 mm of opening.

Surgical Reduction of the Tongue: Glossectomy

Finally, the large tongue or true macroglossia has been attributed as a causative factor of AOB. In such circumstances, partial reduction surgery may be a viable option. This leads to improved stability and prognosis of the corrected malocclusion (Figure 21.10).

Retention and Stability

After treatment, it is important to retain what has been achieved. Long-term studies of post-treatment retention have found a relapse rate of 35–42.9%.[42, 43]

The first requirement for an improved treatment outcome is to eliminate the cause. If the tongue posture is to blame, then appliances should be used to encourage more discipline in the tongue. Secondly, the application

of treatment mechanics that cause instability should be avoided. Teeth will tend to relapse after treatment, and therefore extrusion of incisors to achieve a positive overbite will tend to relapse into an open bite after treatment. If, however, this is anticipated, other compensations may be built into the system, for example overcorrection of overbite at the time of a Le Fort I surgical procedure. Lastly, the continued use of retention appliances, be they fixed or removable, is very much advised in most cases of AOB.

Conclusion

The treatment of AOBs is a challenging field in orthodontics. It is important when treating this problem to remember the aetiological factors, understand the problem through careful diagnosis, and finally treat the problem with the available mechanism based on patient expectations. Only in this way can the treatment and its outcome be rewarding and gratifying.

References

1 Brunelle JA, Bhat M, Lipton JA. Prevalence and distribution of selected occlusal characteristics in the US population, 1988–1991. *J. Dent. Res.* 1996;75 Spec No:706–713.

2 Burgersdijk R, Truin GJ, Frankenmolen F, et al. Malocclusion and orthodontic treatment need of 15–74-year-old Dutch adults. *Community Dent. Oral Epidemiol.* 1991;19(2):64–67.

3 Burgersdijk RC, Frankenmolen FW, Truin GJ, et al. [Dental characteristics and orthodontic treatment need of the Dutch adult population]. *Ned. Tijdschr. Tandheelkd.* 1989;96(9):422–425.

4 Björk A, Skieller V. Facial development and tooth eruption. An implant study at the age of puberty. *Am. J. Orthod.* 1972;62(4):339–383.

5 Björk A, Skieller V. Contrasting mandibular growth and facial development in long face syndrome, juvenile rheumatoid polyarthritis, and mandibulofacial dysostosis. *J. Craniofac. Genet. Dev. Biol. Suppl.* 1985;1: 127–138.

6 Skieller V, Björk A, Linde-Hansen T. Prediction of mandibular growth rotation evaluated from a longitudinal implant sample. *Am. J. Orthod.* 1984;86(5):359–370.

7 Pearson LE. Vertical control in treatment of patients having backward-rotational growth tendencies. *Angle Orthod.* 1978;48(2):132–140.

8 Leslie LR, Southard TE, Southard KA, et al. Prediction of mandibular growth rotation: assessment of the Skieller, Björk, and Linde-Hansen method. *Am. J. Orthod. Dentofacial Orthop.* 1998;114(6):659–667.

9 Proffit WR, Bailey LJ, Phillips C, Turvey TA. Long-term stability of surgical open-bite correction by Le Fort I osteotomy. *Angle Orthod.* 2000;70(2):112–117.

10 Isaacson RJ, Zapfel RJ, Worms FW, et al. Some effects of mandibular growth on the dental occlusion and profile. *Angle Orthod.* 1977;47(2):97–106.

11 Isaacson RJ, Zapfel RJ, Worms FW, Erdman AG. Effects of rotational jaw growth on the occlusion and profile. *Am. J. Orthod.* 1977;72(3):276–286.

12 Yogi H, Alves LAC, Guedes R, Ciamponi AL. Determinant factors of malocclusion in children and adolescents with cerebral palsy. *Am. J. Orthod. Dentofacial Orthop.* 2018;154(3):405–411.

13 Stoll ML, Kau CH, Waite PD, Cron RQ. Temporomandibular joint arthritis in juvenile idiopathic arthritis, now what? *Pediatr. Rheumatol. Online J.* 2018;16(1):32.

14 Popovich F, Thompson GW. Thumb- and finger-sucking: its relation to malocclusion. *Am. J. Orthod.* 1973;63(2):148–155.

15 Klein ET. The thumb-sucking habit: meaningful or empty? *Am. J. Orthod.* 1971;59(3):283–289.

16 Proffit WR. Lingual pressure patterns in the transition from tongue thrust to adult swallowing. *Arch. Oral Biol.* 1972;17(3):555–563.

17 Solow B, Kreiborg S. Soft-tissue stretching: a possible control factor in craniofacial morphogenesis. *Scand. J. Dent. Res.* 1977;85(6):505–507.

18 Woodside DG, Linder-Aronson S, Lundstrom A, McWilliam J. Mandibular and maxillary growth after changed mode of breathing. *Am. J. Orthod. Dentofacial Orthop.* 1991;100(1):1–18.

19 Harvold EP, Chierici G, Vargervik K. Experiments on the development of dental malocclusions. *Am. J. Orthod.* 1972;61(1):38–44.

20 Pearson L. Vertical control in full-banded orthodontic treatment. *Angle Orthod.* 1986;56(3):205–244.

21 Buttke TM, Proffit WR. Referring adult patients for orthodontic treatment. *J. Am. Dent. Assoc.* 1999;130(1):73–79.

22 Walton DK, Fields HW, Johnston WM, et al. Orthodontic appliance preferences of children and adolescents. *Am. J. Orthod. Dentofacial Orthop.* 2010;138(6):698.e1–12; discussion 698–699.

23 Ziuchkovski JP, Fields HW, Johnston WM, Lindsey DT. Assessment of perceived orthodontic appliance attractiveness. *Am. J. Orthod. Dentofacial Orthop.* 2008;133(4 Suppl):S68–S78.

24 Jeremiah HG, Bister D, Newton JT. Social perceptions of adults wearing orthodontic appliances: a cross-sectional study. *Eur. J. Orthod.* 2011;33(5):476–482.

25 Christou T, Abarca R, Christou V, Kau CH. Smile outcome comparison of Invisalign and traditional fixed-appliance treatment: a case-control study. *Am. J. Orthod. Dentofacial Orthop.* 2020;157(3):357–364.

26 Lagravere MO, Flores-Mir C. The treatment effects of Invisalign orthodontic aligners: a systematic review. *J. Am. Dent. Assoc.* 2005;136(12):1724–1729.

27 Schupp W, Haubrich J, Neumann I. Treatment of anterior open bite with the Invisalign system. *J. Clin. Orthod.* 2010;44(8):501–507.

28 Kau CH, Feinberg KB, Christou T. Effectiveness of clear aligners in treating patients with anterior open bite: a retrospective analysis. *J. Clin. Orthod.* 2017;51(8):454–460.

29 Khosravi R, Conhanim B, Hujoel P, et al. Management of overbite with the Invisalign appliance. *Am. J. Orthod. Denofacial Orthop.* 2017;151(4):691–699.e2.

30 Kim YH. Anterior openbite and its treatment with multiloop edgewise archwire. *Angle Orthod.* 1987;57(4):290–321.

31 Kim YH, Han UK, Lim DD, Serraon ML. Stability of anterior openbite correction with multiloop edgewise archwire therapy: a cephalometric follow-up study. *Am. J. Orthod. Dentofacial Orthop.* 2000;118(1):43–54.

32 Erdem B, Kucukkeles N. Three-dimensional evaluaton of open-bite patients teated with anterior elastics and curved archwires. *Am. J. Orthod. Denofacial Orthop.* 2018;154(5):693–701.

33 Chang YI, Moon SC. Cephalometric evaluation of the anterior open bite treatment. *Am. J. Orthod. Dentofacial Orthop.* 1999;115(1):29–38.

34 Prosterman B, Prosterman L, Fisher R, Gornitsky M. The use of implants for orthodontic correction of an open bite. *Am. J. Orthod. Dentofacial Orthop.* 1995;107(3):245–250.

35 Chang CCH, Lin JSY, Yeh HY. Extra-alveolar bone screws for conservative correction of severe malocclusion without extractions or orthognathic surgery. *Curr. Osteoporos. Rep.* 2018;16(4):387–394.

36 Umemori M, Sugawara J, Mitani H, et al. Skeletal anchorage system for open-bite correction. *Am. J. Orthod. Dentofacial Orthop.* 1999;115(2):166–174.

37 Kau CH, Almakky O, Louis PJ. Team approach in the management of revision surgery to correct bilateral temporomandibular joint replacements. *J. Orthod.* 2020;47(2):156–162.

38 Kau CH, Bejemir MP. Application of virtual three-dimensional surgery planning in management of open bite with idiopathic condylar resorption. *Ann. Maxillofac. Surg.* 2015;5(2):249–254.

39 Wang J, Veiszenbacher E, Waite PD, Kau CH. Comprehensive treatment approach for bilateral idiopathic condylar resorption and anterior open bite with customized lingual braces and total joint prostheses. *Am. J. Orthod. Dentofacial Orthop.* 2019;156(1):125–136.

40 Rahman F, Celebi AA, Louis PJ, Kau CH. A comprehensive treatment approach for idiopathic condylar resorption and anterior open bite with 3D virtual surgical planning and self-ligated customized lingual appliance. *Am. J. Orthod. Dentofacial Orthop.* 2019;155(4):560–571.

41 Veiszenbacher E, Wang J, Davis M, et al. Virtual surgical planning: balancing esthetics, practicality, and anticipated stability in a complex Class III patient. *Am. J. Orthod. Dentofacial Orthop.* 2019;156(5):685–693.

42 Lopez-Gavito G, Wallen TR, Little RM, Joondeph DR. Anterior open-bite malocclusion: a longitudinal 10-year postretention evaluation of orthodontically treated patients. *Am. J. Orthod.* 1985;87(3):175–186.

43 Denison TF, Kokich VG, Shapiro PA. Stability of maxillary surgery in openbite versus nonopenbite malocclusions. *Angle Orthod.* 1989;59(1):5–10.

22

Management of the Transverse Dimension

Lucy Davenport-Jones

CHAPTER OUTLINE

Introduction, 397
Crossbites, 398
Indications for Maxillary Expansion, 398
Removable Appliances, 399
 Upper Removable Appliance, 399
 Coffin Spring, 399
Functional Appliances, 400
Aligners, 400
Fixed Appliances, 400
 Headgear with Fixed Appliances, 400
 Archwires and Auxiliaries, 401
 Transpalatal Arch, 401
 Lingual Arch/Utility Arch, 401
 Cross Elastics, 401
 W-Arch/Porter Appliance, 401
 Quadhelix (Bihelix/Trihelix), 403
 NiTi Expanders, 404
Mid-Palatal Suture, 404
 Protraction Headgear, 404
 Rapid Maxillary Expansion, 405
Surgical Expansion, 409
 Surgically Assisted Rapid Palatal Expansion, 409
 Segmental Maxillary Surgery, 410
Retention, 411
References, 411

Introduction

The identification and treatment of transverse maxillary deficiency is a key consideration in planning orthodontic treatment. Transverse discrepancies are a commonly seen component of malocclusion, with a reported incidence of 7.5–22% in the mixed dentition and 10–14% in the permanent dentition.[1] However, inadequate diagnosis and insufficient treatment of transverse problems is common. Understanding the aetiology through careful clinical assessment, allows the clinician to identify the correct treatment to be provided. The aetiology can be dental, skeletal, functional or a combination.

Whilst some crossbites may resolve with habit cessation or interventions to improve breathing, most will not. The presence of a posterior crossbite has been linked to an increased incidence of temporomandibular joint dysfunction and facial asymmetry.[2]

Maxillary expansion can be at a slow or rapid rate, depending on the desired effect, and awareness of the stability of different techniques can aid the decision-making process. A range of appliances can be used to provide

Preadjusted Edgewise Fixed Orthodontic Appliances: Principles and Practice, First Edition. Edited by Farhad B. Naini and Daljit S. Gill.
© 2022 John Wiley & Sons Ltd. Published 2022 by John Wiley & Sons Ltd.

expansion. However, a Cochrane review in 1999 found no evidence for the advantage of using one technique over another.[3]

Whilst expansion of the mandibular arch can be achieved, it is likely to be less stable and only dental expansion or uprighting can be achieved. However, some studies have shown that expansion of the maxilla results in spontaneous expansion of the mandibular arch, possibly due to removal of the previous restriction of the mandible from the constricted maxilla.[4]

The majority of transverse problems are due to a narrow maxilla and implant studies have identified the mid-palatal suture as the most important factor in determining the width of the maxilla.[5] For cases undergoing dentofacial orthopaedics or orthognathic surgery, failure to identify a relative transverse deficiency can adversely affect the postoperative occlusion.

Expansion can be classified as slow or rapid with skeletal and dentoalveolar changes.

Crossbites

Orthodontic expansion is frequently undertaken during routine orthodontic treatment. It can be used for the relief of mild to moderate crowding and to eliminate a mandibular displacement associated with unstable crossbites. If a bilateral crossbite exists with no occlusal displacement, correction can lead to creation of an unstable unilateral crossbite; therefore, it is reasonable to accept bilateral crossbites in the absence of any other occlusal disturbance (Figure 22.1).

Multiple methods of maxillary expansion can be used, all of which transmit a force of varying magnitude directly across the mid-palatal suture. In younger children a removable appliance option may be used, but for patients in the permanent dentition fixed options are often better tolerated; for example, fixed appliances with adjuncts and rapid maxillary expansion (RME) is used when the transverse discrepancy is more severe. Lastly, surgical expansion techniques are used in patients where growth has ceased and the discrepancy is severe.

Indications for Maxillary Expansion

The following are clinical indicators for the use of maxillary expansion:

- Unilateral crossbite with displacement
- Distal molar movement
- Dental crowding

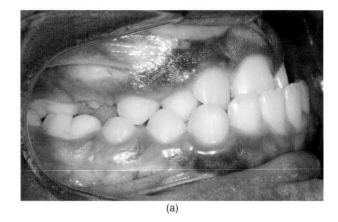

(a)

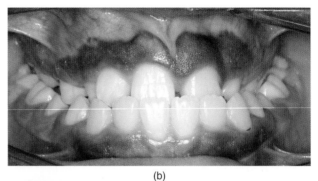

(b)

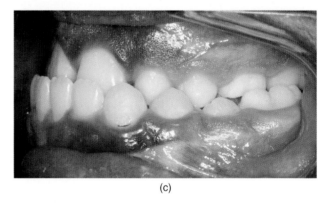

(c)

Figure 22.1 (a–c) A bilateral buccal crossbite with anterior crossbite, without displacement.

- Class II skeletal pattern requiring functional appliance therapy
- Early treatment of a Class III skeletal pattern as an adjunct to maxillary protraction
- Presurgical arch coordination for orthognathic surgery.

Contraindications to maxillary expansion include:

- High angle cases
- Anterior open bite (AOB) malocclusions
- Buccally flared posterior teeth
- Pre-existing buccal recession
- Reluctance to comply with planned retention.

Removable Appliances

Upper Removable Appliance

A removable appliance with a midline stainless steel expansion screw is a widely used device for maxillary expansion (Figure 22.2). It will provide an increase in intermolar and interpremolar width primarily by dental expansion and tipping. However, some orthopaedic effect may be demonstrated in very young patients. It is indicated for use when no more than 4 mm of expansion is required.

Orthodontic expansion with an upper removable appliance (URA) results in an increase in arch length and can be used to create space where crowding is mild to moderate. Any alignment is likely to remain stable if the intermolar expansion is limited to 2–3 mm.[6]

A small element of skeletal expansion may be achieved in younger children. The design of the appliance can be modified to provide symmetrical expansion, with a midline split in the acrylic baseplate, or asymmetrical expansion with the expansion screw placed nearer to the individual teeth requiring expansion. The baseplate split can be adapted to provide asymmetrical expansion with one large and one small segment providing an increased force to the teeth adjacent to the smaller segment, or a Y-pattern can be used to expand the maxillary posterior teeth as well as moving the incisors labially. Adams clasps can provide excellent retention as long as the teeth being clasped have enough of an undercut to retain the appliance.

The expansion screw is embedded in the acrylic baseplate with self-centring rectangular guides to provide controlled symmetrical or asymmetrical expansion and is activated by a quarter turn (0.2–0.25 mm activation) once or twice a week. This slow controlled expansion will provide expansion of 0.5–1 mm bilaterally per month. The width of the periodontal ligament is approximately 0.25 mm, and for dental expansion the appliance should therefore not be activated more than 0.25 mm at a time. The pitch or limit of the expansion screw is 0.8–1.0 mm per full revolution. Progress can be monitored by measuring the intermolar width with callipers or incorporating markers that can be used to measure the activation. The URA must be worn immediately once activated and care must be taken to not over-activate the appliance, which can adversely affect the retention.

Once the desired expansion has been achieved, the expansion screw can be blocked with composite or glass ionomer cement and URA wear continued for three to six months or until the next stage of treatment can be provided.

Removable appliances rely upon excellent compliance, which can be limited in some patients and may be reduced in all patients if the retention is not excellent. The retention of an appliance can be compromised in the mixed dentition with exfoliating teeth and erupting permanent teeth impacting on the fit. A noticeable reduction in the incisor overbite may be seen as the molars tip buccally and the palatal cusps move downwards.

Coffin Spring

Another example of a removable appliance is the Coffin spring (Figure 22.3), which utilises a split acrylic baseplate

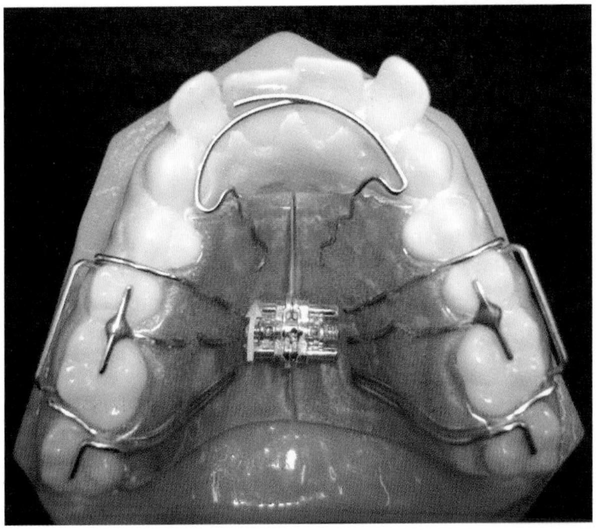

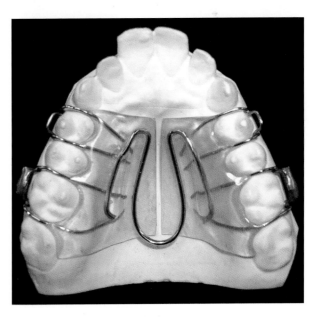

Figure 22.2 Upper removable appliance with a split acrylic plate and midline Hyrax expansion screw.

Figure 22.3 Upper removable appliance with a Coffin spring for transverse arch expansion.

and an embedded omega-shaped spring constructed using 1.25-mm diameter stainless steel wire and placed in the mid-palatal region. The spring is activated at the chairside by pulling the two sides apart manually with activation pliers. It provides slow and symmetrical expansion in the region of 1–2 mm per week. A labial bow can be added to the appliance for alignment of the anterior teeth.

Functional Appliances

The majority of functional appliances are used to improve moderate to severe Class II skeletal patterns in patients who are actively growing (Figure 22.4). The mechanism for incisor overjet correction is a combination of accelerated mandibular growth, restraint of maxillary growth, maxillary incisor retroclination and mandibular incisor proclination. Expansion of the maxillary arch is required to maintain good transverse coordination as the mandibular dentition is moved forward relative to the maxillary dentition. A guide to how much expansion is required can be determined by asking the patient to posture into a Class I incisor relationship and measuring the transverse discrepancy. This can also be assessed by using the same technique with the study models.

Different types of functional appliances use differing components for expansion, e.g. midline expansion screw, Coffin spring, buccal shields and a buccinator bow. With the Functional Regulator appliances, the use of buccal vestibular shields reduces the constrictive forces of the buccal musculature that have contributed to the narrowing of the maxilla. A Herbst-type appliance may incorporate a fixed banded RME component for concomitant expansion and sagittal correction (see Chapter 11, Figure 11.13).

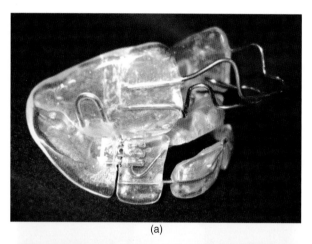

(a)

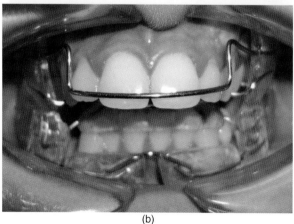

(b)

Figure 22.4 (a) A Function Regulator type II (FR-II) appliance, part of a group of functional appliances developed by Fränkel, may be used for anteroposterior dental arch improvement in growing Class II patients. (b) FR-II fitted intraorally.

Aligners

It has been shown that aligners have the least control on posterior teeth when correcting for transverse discrepancies.[7] The reported limits of expansion that can be achieved with aligners has been shown to be 2–4 mm.[8] Both three-dimensional model measurements and cone beam computed tomography (CBCT) have been used to assess the expansion that is achieved with clear aligner systems, which is mainly buccal translation and tipping of the molar teeth.[9] For patients requiring larger amounts of expansion, the activation should be reduced for each aligner to preserve periodontal health and the prescription should be adjusted with the addition of negative torque to support crown and root control. However, the efficiency of delivering expansion when compared to the predicted outcomes is 36%.[10]

Fixed Appliances

Headgear with Fixed Appliances

The use of retraction headgear remains a useful treatment option to increase arch length by distalisation of the maxillary molar teeth. As the posterior teeth are retracted, there is often a requirement for some expansion to coordinate with the wider part of the lower arch with which the retracted teeth will be occluding. Activation of the headgear facebow by expanding the inner bow will expand the intermolar width (Figure 22.5). This can also be undertaken with a fixed or removable expansion device concomitantly. There will inevitably be some buccal flaring of the molars using this technique, but this can be controlled with a rectangular stainless steel archwire and the addition of buccal root torque for control.

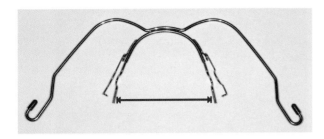

Figure 22.5 If headgear is to be used for extraoral anchorage or traction, concomitant expansion of the intermolar width may be achieved with placement of an expanded inner bow of the headgear facebow, which is inserted into the headgear tubes of the maxillary first molar bands. The hooks at the end of the larger outer bow attach to the headgear strap that produces the extraoral force of variable direction depending on the type of headgear. The inner bow of the facebow must have a safety locking mechanism and the headgear should have at least one and preferably two other safety features.

High-pull headgear is also useful for maxillary restraint during expansion in cases when the lower face height has a tendency to be increased.

Archwires and Auxiliaries

Expansion can be achieved in fixed appliances by the placement of overexpanded stainless steel archwires, particularly robust, large-dimension, rectangular archwires (e.g. 0.019 × 0.025-inch or 0.021 × 0.025-inch stainless steel archwires). The archwire can be expanded by one molar width or 10 mm, using the patient's study models or a wax bite registration as a guide. The use of a rectangular stainless steel archwire should reduce any buccal tipping of the maxillary molar teeth by maintaining torque control and additional buccal root torque can be added if required.

Auxiliary archwires can be added to the fixed appliances, such as jockey arches (Figure 22.6). These are constructed from large-dimension stainless steel archwires and can be 0.019 × 0.025-inch rectangular stainless steel or a larger-dimension round stainless steel archwire, such as 1.00–1.13 mm diameter. They slot into the headgear tubes on the molar bands and are then secured anteriorly with an orthodontic ligature to prevent the jockey wire from displacing. They should be cinched distally to secure in position and prevent ocular injury.

Auxiliary archwires are cheap and can be manipulated chairside to the desired dimensions whilst slotting into existing components of the fixed appliances. However, buccal flaring is likely, even with a large-dimension, rectangular, stainless steel base archwire. Buccal root torque can be added to the base archwire to reduce this effect.

Transpalatal Arch

The transpalatal arch (TPA) is a stainless steel wire connecting maxillary molars for anchorage reinforcement, described initially by Robert Goshgarian (see Chapter 11, Figure 11.5).[5] It is constructed using a 0.9–1.25 mm stainless steel wire, which is soldered, or inserted if removable, to molar and premolar bands that are cemented in place with glass ionomer cement. TPAs are often used to provide some anchorage in the transverse, vertical and anteroposterior dimension.[11] They are frequently used to retain the arch width following expansion with a quadhelix or RME, with extension arms on the palatal surface of the premolar teeth to maintain the expansion achieved (Figure 22.7).

If the TPA connector is expanded prior to fitting, it can be used as an active appliance to provide a small degree of expansion (3–4 mm) in a similar method to the use of a quadhelix. However, it is less flexible and adjustment can result in molar rotation. As with other fixed appliance components, oral hygiene must support the use of the TPA and regular review is required to ensure that the bands remain securely cemented in position.

Lingual Arch/Utility Arch

The use of a lingual arch (see Chapter 11, Figure 11.11) or utility arch (see Figure 11.20) can be considered. The lingual arch can be activated by opening the loops that are soldered mesial to the molar bands. Some degree of activation can be built-in to increase the arch width; these changes will occur from buccal flaring of the banded teeth.

Cross Elastics

To aid maxillary expansion, the use of cross elastics from the palatal attachment on the maxillary molar band to the buccal hook on the mandibular molar band can be used (Figure 22.8; see also Chapter 3, Figure 3.3c and Chapter 11, Figure 11.3). This is effective but can result in molar extrusion. The use of cross elastics should be for a short period and in younger patients whose growth should compensate for any extrusion. This extrusion can be reduced with rigid archwires and anchorage reinforcement, such as a TPA or high-pull headgear. Excellent patient compliance is required for the use of intraoral elastics to be successful.

W-Arch/Porter Appliance

The W-arch is a fixed modification of the Coffin spring and was described by Ricketts for use in the treatment of cleft patients.[12] A W-shaped, round, 0.9-mm stainless steel wire is soldered to molar bands, with extensions arms adapted along the palatal surface of the premolar teeth and

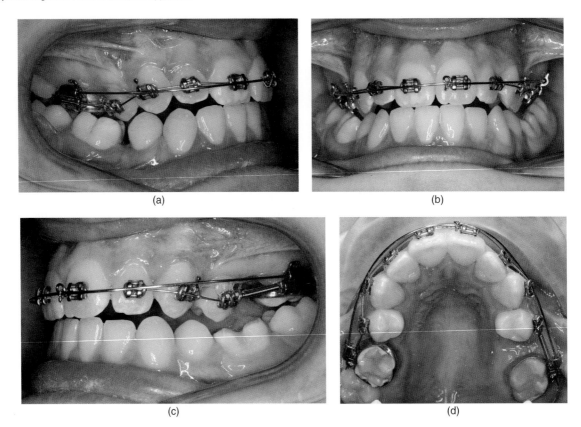

(a)

(b)

(c)

(d)

Figure 22.6 (a–d) A 1-mm diameter round stainless steel jockey arch *in situ* to maintain the arch form during orthodontic alignment. Note the circle loop anteriorly to allow ligation and prevent lateral migration of the wire.

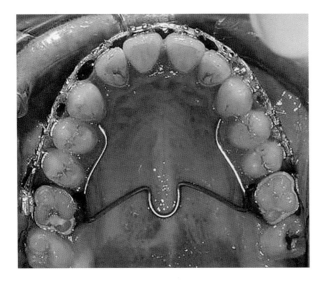

Figure 22.7 Transpalatal arch (TPA) with arms extended to the premolars.

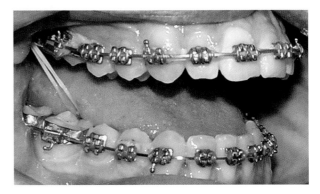

Figure 22.8 A cross elastic applied from the buccal hook of the upper right first permanent molar band to the lingual cleats on the lower right first permanent molar band.

the arch form continuing to form a palatal loop anteriorly (Figure 22.9).

It can be used in the primary and mixed dentition where mild to moderate expansion is required and compliance may be reduced. The W-arch is activated by opening the posterior apices, and the anterior section if required, with three-pronged pliers (Figure 22.10), which can incorporate both expansion and molar rotation,[12] and can be easily adjusted to provide more anterior or posterior expansion before cementation and can be removed for further activation as required. The 'W' wire is positioned 1–1.5 mm away from the mucosa to prevent trauma. The W-arch can be maintained in position for retention.

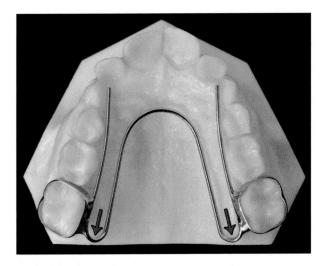

Figure 22.9 The W-arch (Porter expansion arch). The appliance may be activated, using three-pronged pliers, at the posterior apices and/or the anterior section.

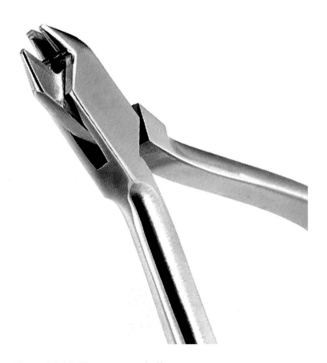

Figure 22.10 Three-pronged pliers.

Quadhelix (Bihelix/Trihelix)

The quadhelix device is a fixed expansion device first described by Herbst and later popularised by Ricketts,[13] using a modification of the Coffin W-spring to increase flexibility (Figure 22.11). The addition of four helices constructed from 0.9-mm stainless steel wire increases the flexibility and range of activation, whilst decreasing the force levels. The length of the palatal arms can be altered depending on which teeth are in crossbite for a more refined force application.

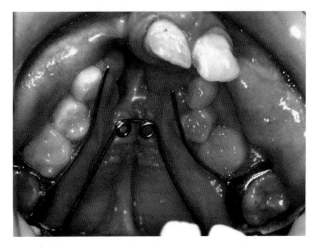

Figure 22.11 A quadhelix appliance in a cleft patient. The appliance has been soldered to the palatal aspect of the maxillary first molar bands.

The anterior helices can also be useful as a habit breaker for thumb or finger sucking and therefore used to correct anterior open bites. The posterior helices sit 2–3 mm distal to the first molars and are sloped parallel to the palatal surface. The wire structure is welded or soldered to the molar bands to form a fixed appliance, cemented *in situ* with glass ionomer cement.

The design can be modified to direct the expansion force to specific areas to move only one or two teeth and to rotate or torque the molar teeth. It is important to incorporate arms positioned palatal to the premolar teeth to ensure that they are expanded, along with the molar teeth. The quadhelix can be custom made or prefabricated using either stainless steel or, more recently, nickel titanium (NiTi) for a longer duration of force delivery. Also, it can be removable and insert into a palatal sheath with a friction lock onto the molar bands (Figure 22.12). The diameter of the wire used for construction can greatly influence the force delivered and the majority of the force will be transmitted in the molar region.

The quadhelix provides expansion primarily by buccal tipping of the maxillary posterior teeth, but some skeletal expansion may be achieved depending on the age of the patient. In prepubertal children the ratio of molar tipping to skeletal expansion has been shown to be 6 : 1.[14] A force level of 400 g can be achieved by an activation of approximately 8–10 mm or one molar width. As with other fixed appliances, patients are reviewed every six weeks. Initially the appliance may leave indentations on the tongue, but this will resolve once the appliance is no longer *in situ*.

Activation can be undertaken by either removal of the appliance and replacement with increased expansion by opening the anterior helices or whilst the quadhelix is

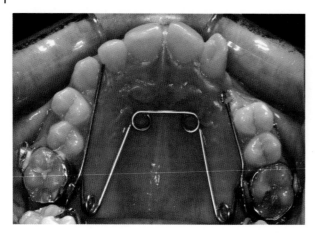

Figure 22.12 A removable quadhelix appliance. This appliance inserts into tubes on the palatal aspect of the maxillary first molar bands and may be ligated into position as shown on one side. The advantage of the removable quadhelix design is that it may be removed and reactivated more easily at the chairside.

in situ by the use of three-pronged pliers to expand the lateral arms.

As with many treatment options for expansion, overcorrection allows for some relapse once treatment is ceased. Expansion can be stopped once the buccal cusps of the maxillary molar teeth meet almost edge to edge with the buccal cusps of the mandibular molar teeth. However, research using three-dimensional imaging both before and after expansion with a quadhelix found that the palatal bone increased in thickness whilst the buccal bone decreased in both thickness and height in 30% of cases.[15] Dental expansion to skeletal expansion is 6 : 1 in prepubertal children; however, no difference has been demonstrated in the use of a quadhelix compared to a removable expansion device in terms of crossbite correction.[16]

The quadhelix appliance is frequently used alongside fixed appliances; once robust stainless steel archwires can be placed to maintain the acquired expansion, the quadhelix can be removed.

Bihelix or trihelix appliances can be used to treat cleft palate patients requiring expansion to correct anterior collapse and a narrow maxilla. The reduction in the number of helices allows placement in very narrow arches and can provide different vectors of force. They should be used in conjunction with planned alveolar bone grating and care should be taken to prevent fistula formation. Retention may be compromised by reduced clinical crown height.

NiTi Expanders

A fixed active NiTi expander can be used to direct a slow continuous force using thermoelasticity. It is constructed from 0.9-mm thermally activated NiTi and can be used simultaneously with fixed appliances and is retained by palatal sheaths on the molar bands. The use of ethyl chloride can increase the flexibility of the NiTi active component to aid fitting. It is then wrapped in gauze to maintain the low temperature to increase the working time during placement. Various sizes are available and expansion can be in the region of 3–5 mm. If more expansion is required, the NiTi expander will require replacing with a second larger size appliance once the initial expansion has been achieved. The NiTi appliance can also derotate and upright the posterior teeth during expansion.

Mid-Palatal Suture

The main area of resistance to any expansion is the mid-palatal suture. Skeletal expansion relies upon separation of the mid-palatal suture by distraction forces perpendicular to the suture line. Transverse growth is completed before anteroposterior and vertical growth and as with other craniofacial sutures, the mid-palatal suture becomes more tortuous and interdigitated as skeletal maturity progresses, thereby resulting in increased resistance to expansion as maturity continues.[17]

Skeletal maturity does not always correlate with chronological age, which can explain the reports of successful RME treatment in an older cohort of patients and why complications can occur in younger patients. The ideal time for non-surgical rapid expansion is during the pubertal growth spurt or in a patient less than 15 years of age.[18, 19]

Visualisation of the mid-palatal suture is by occlusal imaging with either an upper standard occlusal radiograph or three-dimensional CBCT,[20] and may provide more reliable information than chronological age. Following the pubertal growth spurt the interlocking and ossification increases to such an extent that skeletal expansion becomes impossible without surgical separation. Whilst non-surgical skeletal expansion may not be impossible for post-pubertal patients, it becomes far less likely.[21] Further resistance arises from the skeletal maturation of the junction between the maxilla and zygomatic complex.[17]

Protraction Headgear

In recent times, the use of RME along with facemask therapy to protract the maxilla is a commonly used protocol for the early management of skeletal Class III cases in prepubertal patients (see Chapter 3, Figure 3.11). RME is used to disrupt the maxillary suture system and promote maxillary protraction. The use of RME for expansion and its effect on the maxillary complex is covered in the next section.

Rapid Maxillary Expansion

Rapid maxillary expansion was first described by Emerson Angell in 1860,[14] and later redescribed by Haas. The aim is to provide more skeletal expansion than dental by transmitting heavy forces across the mid-palatal suture, resulting in a significant separation at the suture line, into which bone formation will occur. Evidence varies on the degree of skeletal to dental expansion but this is in the region of 25% skeletal expansion and 75% dental expansion.[22]

Clinical Management of RME

Clear verbal and written instructions on how to activate the expansion screw should be provided to the patient. The instructions should be to turn the screw a quarter turn twice a day (a.m. and p.m.). The exact magnitude of each rotation must be known as this can vary between manufacturers; most have 0.2–0.25 mm activation per quarter turn (0.8–1.0 mm per full revolution). NiTi expansion screws can be used and are claimed to provide a more controlled and continuous force application.

Unlike the URA, the RME appliance cannot be removed for activation and the use of a typodont for demonstration is a helpful chairside teaching tool. The activation key should be attached to a handle or tied to a piece of floss to prevent swallowing or inhalation, should it be released whilst turning. Alternatively, a swivel key can be used with a plastic handle extension (Figure 22.13). The swivel key will click after the end of a turn to signify the turn is complete. The key can also have an expansion counter indicator on the handle to record the number of turns undertaken. Alternatively, a printed table can be filled in to record the activation regime.

Once the magnitude of screw activation is known, a calculation must be made of the number of turns required to achieve the desired expansion and the review appointments planned accordingly. The clinician will decide on the desired regime, but two 90° turns per day is often used. Care must be taken to allow the soft tissues around the mid-palatal suture to adapt to prevent haemorrhage or tearing. The extent of the skeletal expansion depends on the patient's age and suture interdigitation. The activation holes within the screw head must be accessible and sufficient time is needed to demonstrate how to turn the screw

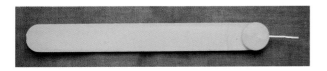

Figure 22.13 The activating key of an RME appliance may be attached to a handle to prevent swallowing or aspiration.

with the activation key, which will need to carried out by someone other than the patient.

Warning the patient and their parents about the formation of a midline diastema is very important. Whilst it will resolve following expansion, it can often be large in size and cause anxiety if the patient is not forewarned. The force produced across the mid-palatal suture with an RME appliance is high and can result in some discomfort and the use of analgesics may be required.

The patient should be reviewed one week following fitting and activation for clinical assessment and many clinicians will order an upper occlusal radiograph for confirmation of the bony separation at the mid-palatal suture (Figure 22.14). If a diastema is not visible or sutural separation felt not to have occurred, then the expansion must be stopped to prevent periodontal recession, loss of vitality of the incisor teeth and alveolar fracture.

An expansion measuring gauge can be used to verify the degree of separation at the screw thread and is easier to position than a probe and will provide a true horizontal measurement rather than the use of callipers on cusp tips, which may be buccally tipped rather than horizontally expanded.

Active treatment will continue until the desired magnitude of expansion has been achieved, which is often in the region of two to three weeks. Most clinicians will build in some overexpansion, resulting in the palatal cusps of the maxillary molars occluding with the buccal cusps of the mandibular molars. Once active expansion stops, the screw holes can be blocked with composite material, glass ionomer cement or an orthodontic ligature placed through the screw hole. The expansion device remains *in situ* for three to four months to allow for bony consolidation.

The force levels can accumulate following sequential activation and can be as high as 10 kg. If severe pain or discomfort, dizziness or severe pressure is experienced, expansion should be halted and the patient reviewed.

The total pitch of the activation screw can vary between manufacturers and should be known prior to active expansion to prevent the screw thread dislodging during active treatment. The pitch or maximum activation should be laser marked on the body of the screw along with a directional arrow and lot number. Some Hyrax screws deactivate when maximum expansion has been achieved to prevent overtreatment and the screw dislodging from the housing (Figure 22.15).

This sutural separation is non-parallel and triangular in its formation, with the maximum opening at the incisor region decreasing posteriorly along the suture. Therefore, the amount of space between the central incisors is not indicative of the expansion achieved more posteriorly.[23]

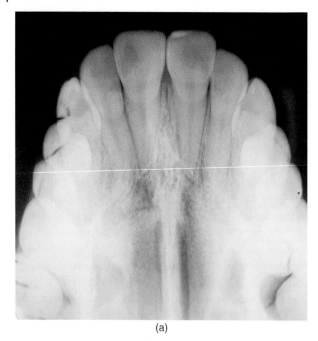

(a)

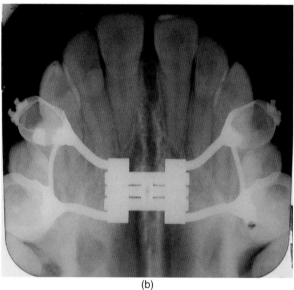

(b)

Figure 22.14 (a) Upper standard occlusal radiograph taken before treatment. (b) Upper standard occlusal radiograph taken following expansion, confirming the midline palatal split and symmetrical expansion.

The space that opens between the central incisors will resolve as the trans-septal fibres contract and some skeletal relapse occurs.

The mid-palatal suture separates supero-inferiorly with a pyramidal shape,[18] the base of which is on the palatal surface of the maxilla. The maxilla is often displaced in a downwards and forwards direction, which may increase the face height and rotate the mandible backwards.[24] The maxillary posterior teeth may tip buccally and extrude,

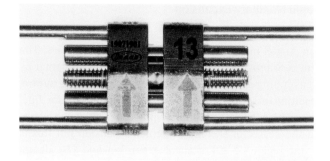

Figure 22.15 Hyrax screw with laser-marked directional arrow and maximum pitch visible on the body of the screw.

which can reduce the overbite. This increase in the width of the nasal cavity can result in an improvement in nasal breathing,[23] and a reduction in resistance to nasal airflow.

A systematic review found the long-term skeletal changes with RME to be 25% of the total dental expansion in prepubertal patients with no significant antero-posterior or vertical changes in either the maxilla or mandible.[25]

Along with the six indications for expansion RME described by Haas,[26] further indications for RME are:

- transverse discrepancy greater than or equal to 4 mm
- moderate/severe crowding
- maxillary molars already compensated for the skeletal discrepancy with a buccal inclination
- to facilitate maxillary protraction in Class III cases
- arch length problems
- cleft lip and palate cases
- patients who are in their prepubertal growth spurt
- Class II malocclusion where the incisor overjet is increased.

Other medical indications may include recurrent ear and nasal infection, and nasal stenosis.

Contraindications to RME treatment include:[27]

- poor oral hygiene
- skeletally mature patients
- single tooth crossbites
- pre-existing recession on the buccal aspect of the maxillary molar teeth
- poor compliance/attendance
- anterior open bite
- increased lower face height
- pre-existing root resorption
- periodontal attachment loss
- prognathic maxilla
- skeletal asymmetry of the maxilla
- nasal deformity
- temporomandibular joint pain or dysfunction.

Table 22.1 Comparison of slow and rapid maxillary expansion.

Slow expansion	Rapid expansion
Skeletal–dental change 1 : 4	Skeletal–dental change 1 : 1
Low force	High force
Longer duration of activation (3–6 months)	Shorter duration of active treatment (2–3 weeks)
Fixed or removable	Fixed
	Tooth-borne or bone- borne
Any age	Before fusion of mid-palatal suture
More stable	Less stable
Less frequent activation (0.5–1 mm per week)	More frequent activation (0.5–1 mm per day)

Diagnostic aids for RME treatment include:

- trimmed study models/digital scans in occlusion
- periodontal charting
- occlusal radiograph
- CBCT
- cephalometric tracing
- ENT assessment.

A comparison of slow and rapid maxillary expansion is provided in Table 22.1.

Banded RME

Following a short time with separators *in situ*, the molar and first premolar bands for the RME can be selected. They should be well fitting and match the anatomical contour of the teeth to be banded. An impression is taken with the bands in position and they are then removed and stabilised into the impression before sending to the laboratory. The separators are replaced.

The Hyrax (hygienic rapid expansion) screw activation mechanism is a non-spring-loaded jackscrew and is attached to large-gauge wire arms that are adapted to the palatal anatomy and soldered to bands on the molars and premolars (Figure 22.16). Alternatively, molar bands only are used and extension arms are adapted to cover the palatal aspect of the premolar teeth. The appliance should not contact the palatal mucosa and have a smooth housing design to prevent soft tissue irritation. Micro-expanders with a smaller body can be used when the maxilla is severely constricted.

The appliance is extremely rigid to allow heavy forces to be transmitted across the mid-palatal suture, exceeding the limit needed for tooth movement and sutural resistance. This results in compression of the periodontal ligament, bending of the alveolar process and opening of the mid-palatal suture (Figure 22.17).

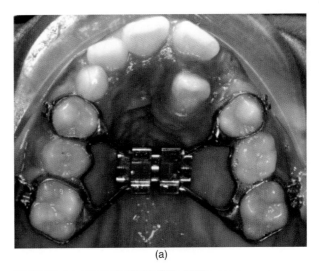

(a)

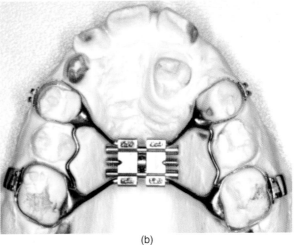

(b)

Figure 22.16 (a, b) A banded RME appliance on the working model and fitted intraorally. The palatal arms are closely adapted to ensure the premolar teeth are moved laterally during expansion.

Bonded RME

An alternative to banded RME is an acrylic splint covering the teeth that requires expansion with an embedded Hyrax screw. This appliance was described by Howe in 1982 and is useful for teeth that are crowded or tipped and a parallel path of insertion is not possible. The acrylic is extended over the occlusal, buccal and lingual tooth surfaces with clearance around the gingivae to allow for oral hygiene to be maintained.

Bonded RME eliminates the need for an appointment to place separators and potentially removes the error of bands being placed incorrectly within the impression. Bonded RME can also be used in both the primary and secondary dentition. In patients with an increased lower face height, or anterior crossbite, the acrylic can be built up to incorporate bite blocks and the capping helps to improve

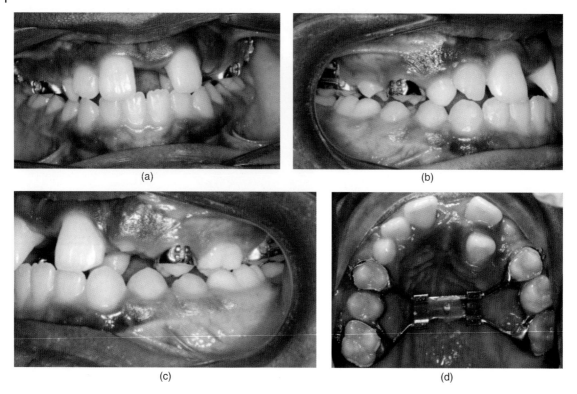

Figure 22.17 (a–d) The same appliance following three weeks of activation. The midline diastema is visible and the arch form broader. The screw hole has been blocked with composite to prevent further activation.

vertical control and prevent autorotation of the mandible downwards and backwards.

Bonding is undertaken using a light-cure composite resin, with only the buccal and palatal enamel being etched. Care should be taken to avoid using too much composite resin, which will make removal more time-consuming. Glass ionomer cement can also be used, but will have a reduced bond strength compared to composite resin.

Once expansion has been achieved and a period of retention completed, the bonded RME appliance can be removed with band-removing pliers or sectioned if required. The use of bonded RME to reduce the buccal tipping of the molars that occurs during expansion is discussed in the literature, but does not seem to be widely used, due to difficulties with bonding and debonding.

Bone-borne RME

The disadvantages of using a tooth-borne RME device have been well documented.[28, 29] Mommaerts described a bone-borne expander screwed directly into the palatal shelves. The use of bone-borne expansion devices (Figure 22.18) that are fixed with miniscrews and can be placed under local anaesthesia have been suggested

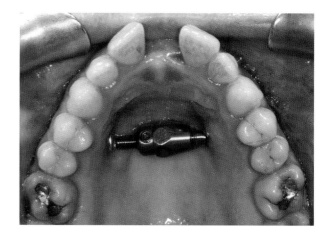

Figure 22.18 A bone-borne transverse palatal expander. Source: Naini FB, Gill DS (eds). *Orthognathic Surgery: Principles, Planning and Practice*. Oxford: Wiley Blackwell, 2017; reprinted with permission.

as resulting in more skeletal change and a reduction in unwanted dental changes, e.g. molar tipping, root resorption, a decrease in buccal bone thickness and crestal bone height.

There are many designs, from a jack-type design to a Hyrax screw soldered to 1.5-mm stainless steel wire to fully customised components, and all can be placed under local anaesthesia with titanium screws or arms to anchor to the palatal vault with the force transmitted across the mid-palatal suture. Many bone-borne expansion screws have a hexagonal body and are activated with a micro-spanner that fits snugly over the body of the screw. They frequently have a warning coloured thread that indicates that the screw is near the end of its maximum extension and should not be turned any further.

The degree of skeletal expansion has been shown to be similar with both tooth and bone-borne expansion devices; however, molar tipping and reduction in buccal bone height and thickness is more commonly seen with tooth-borne expansion devices.[30] For a patient in the post-pubertal growth spurt, bone-borne expanders produce greater skeletal change and less dental change when compared to tooth-borne RME, with significant buccal dehiscence and vertical bone height changes in the premolar region.[31]

The bone-borne expander can be left in position to act as a retainer during orthodontic alignment. A systematic review on the use of bone-borne expansion devices found limited data to support their use.[32] Complications can arise if the device becomes loose and gingival inflammation and ulceration occur or the pain experienced is severe.[33]

Surgical Expansion

In most orthognathic patients, if there is an element of transverse deficiency, expansion may be undertaken orthodontically with either fixed or removable appliances. In some cases, surgical expansion is indicated in order to ensure that a good postoperative occlusion is achieved to support postoperative occlusal stability. For post-pubertal patients with significant transverse discrepancies requiring correction, consideration can be given to surgical techniques. Both surgically assisted rapid palatal expansion (SARPE), sometimes referred to as surgically assisted rapid maxillary expansion (SARME), and segmental maxillary surgery are frequently used as adjuncts to conventional orthognathic surgery. Dental arch coordination is a key principle of presurgical orthodontics and if this cannot be achieved orthodontically, a surgical opinion should be sought.

Whilst transverse maxillary deficiencies can occur in patients with Class I skeletal patterns, they often occur in Class II skeletal cases with increased vertical dimensions, or in skeletal Class III cases where there is a three-dimensional deficiency of the maxilla. In the

hierarchy of stability for orthognathic surgical moves, maxillary expansion is the least stable.[34]

Surgically Assisted Rapid Palatal Expansion

Prior to undergoing SARPE the patient must be assessed by the multidisciplinary team (MDT clinic) and the space requirements for surgical access determined. Often a diastema between the central incisors must be created orthodontically, with space between the crowns of the central incisors as well as the roots, via adjustment to bracket position second-order bends in the archwire.

The indications for SARPE include:

- skeletally mature patient/fused mid-palatal suture
- V-shaped palate
- transverse skeletal narrowing discrepancy >5 mm
- excessive display of buccal corridors on full smile
- anterior crowding
- previous failure of non-surgical expansion.

The potential complications of SARPE include:

- inadequate mobilisation of the maxillary segments
- asymmetrical expansion
- loss of vitality of central incisor teeth
- loosening of appliance
- requirement for appliance replacement if maximum screw length is surpassed.

Prior to surgery, or intraoperatively, the archwire must be divided. The expansion device can be tooth-borne, which will have been fitted already by the orthodontist, or bone-borne, which must be available for fitting in the operating theatre. The archwire is divided anteriorly to allow for expansion between the two segments. Following the surgical cuts (Figure 22.19), the expansion device and screw are turned to check the separation is even across the suture.

As with RME, the main resistance to expansion at the mid-palatal suture is not the suture itself, but the surrounding structures, particularly the sphenoid and zygomatic buttresses, the pterygoid plates and the piriform aperture at the point of attachment to the maxilla.[35] During SARPE these attachments are surgically severed, removing resistance to expansion with the RME appliance. Identification of areas of resistance have resulted in the development of different osteotomy cuts to allow for maximum expansion. Some surgeons will separate all maxillary articulations whilst others will avoid pterygomaxillary disjunction to prevent injury to the pterygoid venous plexus.

SARPE can be carried out as a day surgery procedure, frequently at the same time as third molar removal. Following

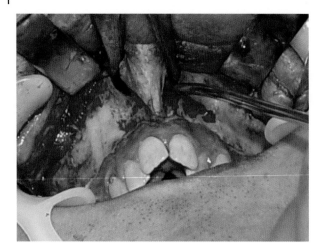

Figure 22.19 Intraoperative view of SARPE procedure.

SARPE the RME appliance is expanded at a rate of 0.5 mm per day (after a latency period; see below); as with conventional RME, the patient and parents must be warned about the creation of a large midline diastema (Figure 22.20). As with any expansion technique, stability is an issue and overcorrection has been advised.

SARPE is useful in patients who do not require further orthognathic surgery for coexisting skeletal anteroposterior or vertical discrepancies. SARPE is essentially osteogenic distraction across the mid-palatal suture. As with other types of distraction there is a latency phase in the immediate postoperative period. The latency phase allows for development of a fibrin callus and lasts for three to five days; the active distraction can then begin, as with RME,

by turning the screw twice daily one or two turns. During this time, bone matrix formation occurs along the collagen fibres with a fibrovascular bridge in the direction of the distraction force, this tension stimulating new bone formation. This active distraction phase normally lasts for 10–14 days depending on the magnitude of expansion required. It is followed by a consolidation phase, during which the callus calcifies. When the expansion is stopped the RME device remains *in situ* or is replaced by a robust TPA and rectangular stainless steel archwire for retention.

The stability of SARPE has been shown to be similar to that of RME,[36] with 50% skeletal and 30% dental relapse.[37] No significant difference has been demonstrated between tooth- and bone-borne appliances.[27]

Segmental Maxillary Surgery

With skeletal discrepancies, the transverse discrepancy can be absolute or relative. Absolute discrepancies demonstrate a true width discrepancy between the maxilla and mandible. Relative discrepancies may exist due to the anteroposterior skeletal pattern, but once this is corrected the transverse dimension does not require correction. Hand-held models or model surgery can identify whether the transverse problem is absolute or relative.

If concomitant orthognathic surgery is indicated, expansion can be achieved with a segmental approach to the maxillary surgical cuts (Figure 22.21). Along with the Le Fort I osteotomy, additional surgical cuts are made in

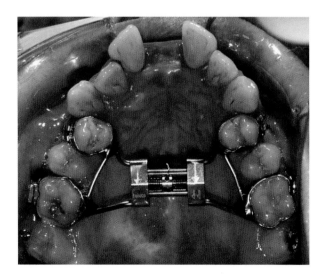

Figure 22.20 A large maxillary dental midline diastema occurs with the expansion following a SARPE procedure. Patients and parents should be warned about this temporary state to prevent unnecessary anxiety.

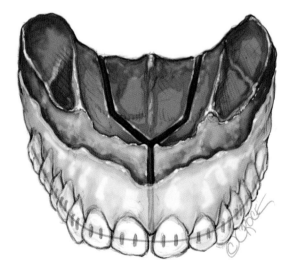

Figure 22.21 Segmental palatal osteotomies following a Le Fort I maxillary osteotomy. Source: Naini FB, Gill DS (eds). *Orthognathic Surgery: Principles, Planning and Practice.* Oxford: Wiley Blackwell, 2017; reprinted with permission.

the palate and along the mid-palatal suture as required. The segments are separated and then fixed into the planned position. As with SARPE the relative inelasticity of the palatal mucoperiosteum limits the degree of expansion that can be achieved and care must be taken to preserve the blood supply to the segments.

If anteroposterior or vertical skeletal discrepancies coexist, then segmental surgery is indicated to correct the transverse discrepancy in the same procedure. The maxilla is segmented during the Le Fort I procedure with osteotomies and bone grafting directly into the expanded suture can be carried out to aid stability.

Retention

No clinical consensus exists for the optimal retention regime following maxillary expansion. A systematic review found that the retention period ranged from 5 to 16 months with a variety of different appliances being used for retention and relapse rates of 0–27%.[38]

Understanding the stability of expansion is challenging when many studies use different anatomical landmarks as reference points and overcorrection is often a desired treatment outcome. However, overcorrection may not be necessary and relapse without overcorrection may be as low as 1.6%.[39] A longer retention phase following maxillary expansion and maintaining the RME appliance *in situ* for more than seven months has demonstrated less relapse.[40] More relapse has been noted when treating older patients, up to 27% of intermolar distance.[22] Six months of either fixed retention or 24-hour wear of removable Hawley-style retainers is thought to be sufficient to avoid relapse; however, as with the correction of other elements of malocclusion, lifelong retention should be planned based on the presenting aspects of the malocclusion.[38]

References

1 Jonsson T, Arnlaugsson S, Karlsson KO, et al. Orthodontic treatment experience and prevalence of malocclusion traits in an Icelandicadult population. *Am. J. Orthod. Dentofacial Orthop.* 2007;131(1): 11–18.

2 Petrén S, Bondemark L, Söderfeldt B. A systematic review concerning early orthodontic treatment of unilateral posterior crossbite. *Angle Orthod.* 2003;73(5):588–596.

3 Harrison J, Ashby D. Orthodontic treatment for posterior crossbites. *Cochrane Database Syst. Rev.* 2001;(2):CD000979.

4 Gianelly AA. Rapid palatal expansion in the absence of crossbite: add value? *Am. J. Orthod. Dentofacial Orthop.* 2003;124:362–365.

5 Bjork A, Skieller V. Growth in the width of the maxilla studied by the implant method. *Scand. J. Plast. Reconstr. Surg.* 1974;8(1–2):26–33.

6 Lee RT. Arch width and archform: a review. *Am. J. Orthod.* 1999;115(3):305–313.

7 Clements KM, Bollen AM, Huang G, et al. Activation time and material stiffness of sequential removable orthodontic appliances. Part 2: dental improvements. *Am. J. Orthod. Dentofacial Orthop.* 2003;124(5):502–508.

8 Boyd RL. Esthetic orthodontic treatment using the Invisalign appliance for moderate to complex malocclusions. *J. Dent. Educ.* 2008;72(8):948–967.

9 Tong H, Enciso R, Van Elslande D, et al. A new method to measure mesiodistal angulation and faciolingual inclination of each whole tooth with volumetric cone-beam computed tomography images. *Am. J. Orthod. Dentofacial Orthop.* 2012;142(1):133–143.

10 Zhou N, Guo J. Efficiency of upper arch expansion with the Invisalign system. *Angle Orthod.* 2020;90: 23–30.

11 Gill D, Naini F, McNally M, Jones A. Management of transverse maxillary deficiency. *Dent. Update* 2004;31:516–523.

12 Ricketts RM, Bench RW, Gugino CF. *Bioprogressive Therapy.* Denver, CO: Rocky Mountain Orthodontics, 1979: 93–126.

13 Ricketts RM. Growth prediction: Part 2. *J. Clin. Orthod.* 1975;9:340–362.

14 Frank SW, Engel AB. The effects of maxillary quad-helix appliance expansion on cephalometric measurements in growing orthodontic patients. *Am. J. Orthod.* 1982;81:378–389.

15 Corbridge JK, Campbell PM, Trayvon R, et al. Transverse dentoalveolar changes after slow maxillary expansion. *Am. J. Orthod. Dentofacial Orthop.* 2011;140:317–325.

16 McNally MR, Spary DJ, Rock WP. Randomized controlled trial comparing the quadhelix and the expansion arch for the correction of crossbite. *J. Orthod.* 2005;32(1):29–35.

17 Zimring J, Isaacson R. Forces produced by rapid maxillary expansion: III. Forces present during retention. *Angle Orthod.* 1965;35:178–186.

18 Bishara S, Staley R. Maxillary expansion: clinical implications. *Am. J. Orthod. Dentofacial Orthop.* 1987;91:3–14.

19 Melsen B. Palatal growth studied on human autopsy material. A histologic microradiographic study. *Am. J. Orthod.* 1975;68:42–54.

20 Angelieri F, Franchi L, Cevidanes LHS, et al. Cone beam computed tomography evaluation of mid-palatal suture maturation in adults. *Int. J. Oral Maxillofac. Surg.* 2017;46:1557–1561.

21 Wertz R, Dreskin M. Midpalatal suture opening: a normative study. *Am. J. Orthod.* 1977;71:367–381.

22 Lagravère MO, Carey J, Heo G, et al. Transverse, vertical, and anteroposterior changes from bone-anchored maxillary expansion vs traditional rapid maxillary expansion: a randomized clinical trial. *Am. J. Orthod. Dentofacial Orthop.* 2010;137(3):304.e1–12.

23 Gray LP. Results of 310 cases of rapid maxillary expansion selected for medical reasons. *J. Laryngol. Otol.* 1975;89(6):601–614.

24 Haas A. The treatment of maxillary deficiency by opening the midpalatal suture. *Angle Orthod.* 1965;35:200–217.

25 Lagravere MO, Major PW, Flores-Mir C. Long-term skeletal changes with rapid maxillary expansion: a systematic review. *Angle Orthod.* 2005;75:1046–1052.

26 Haas A. Long-term posttreatment evaluation of rapid palatal expansion. *Angle Orthod.* 1980;50:189–217.

27 Koudstaal MJ, Smeets JBJ, Kleinrensink G-J, et al. Relapse and stability of surgically assisted rapid maxillary expansion: an anatomic biomechanical study. *J. Oral Maxillofac. Surg.* 2009;67:10–14.

28 Northway WM, Meade JB. Surgically assisted rapid maxillary expansion: a comparison of technique, response and stability. *Angle Orthod.* 1997;67:309–320.

29 Matteini C, Mommaerts M. Posterior transpalatal distraction with pterygoid disjunction: a short-term model study. *Am. J. Orthod. Dentofacial Orthop.* 2001;120:498–502.

30 Moon H-W, Kim MJ, Ahn HW, et al. Molar inclination and surrounding alveolar bone change relative to the design of bone-borne maxillary expanders: a CBCT study. *Angle Orthod.* 2020;90(1):13–22.

31 Liu S, Xu T, Zou W. Effects of rapid maxillary expansion on the midpalatal suture: a systematic review. *Eur. J. Orthod.* 2015;37:651–655.

32 Verstraaten J, Kuijpers-Jagtman AM, Mommaerts MY, et al. A systematic review of the effects of bone-borne surgical assisted rapid maxillary expansion. *J. Craniomaxillofac. Surg.* 2010;38:166–174.

33 Ramieri G, Spada M, Australia M. Transverse maxillary distraction with a bone-anchored appliance: dento-periodontal effects and clinical and radiological results. *Int. J. Oral Maxillofac. Surg.* 2005;34:357–363.

34 Bailey L, Tanya J, Cevidanes LHS, Proffit WR. Stability and predictability of orthognathic surgery. *Am. J. Orthod. Dentofacial Orthop.* 2004;126:273–277.

35 Bishara SE, Staley RN. Maxillary expansion: clinical implication. *Am. J. Orthod. Dentofacial Orthop.* 1987;91(1):3–14.

36 Sokucu O, Kosger HH, Bicakci AA, Babacan H. Stability in dental changes in RME and SARME: a 2 year follow up. *Angle Orthod.* 2009;79:207–213.

37 Altug-Atac AT, Karasu H, Aytac D. Surgically assisted rapid maxillary expansion compared with orthopedic rapid maxillary expansion. *Angle Orthod.* 2006;76:353–359.

38 Costa J, Galindo T, Mattos T, Cury-Saramago A. Retention period after treatment of posterior crossbite with maxillary expansion: a systematic review. *Dental Press J. Orthod.* 2017;22(2):35–44.

39 Petrén S, Bjerklin K, Bondemark L. Stability of unilateral posterior crossbite correction in the mixed dentition: a randomized clinical trial with a 3-year follow-up. *Am. J. Orthod. Dentofacial Orthop.* 2011;139(1):e73–e81.

40 Cozzani M, Guiducci A, Mirenghi S, et al. Arch width changes with a rapid maxillary expansion appliance anchored to the primary teeth. *Angle Orthod.* 2007;77(2):296–302.

Section V

Appendices

Appendix 1

Orthodontic Instruments

Farhad B. Naini and Daljit S. Gill

This is not an exhaustive list, but shows the most commonly used instruments in an orthodontist's armamentarium. Other instruments have been described in the appropriate chapters of the book and may be found using the index.

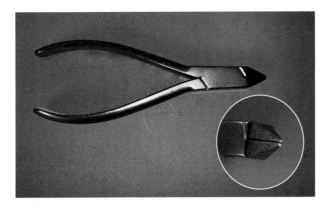

Figure A1.1 Adams pliers. Also known as universal pliers, these were designed by the orthodontist Philip Adams. They are used for bending heavy-gauge wires and adjustment of wires on removable appliances.

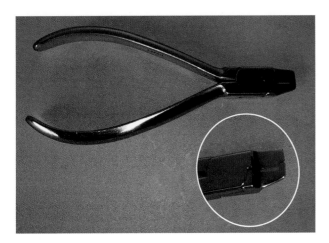

Figure A1.2 Band crimping pliers. These are designed to crimp the gingival margins of orthodontic bands.

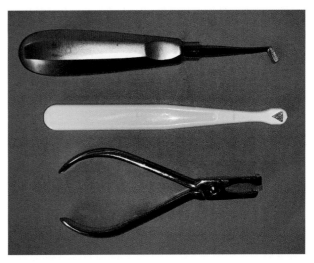

Figure A1.3 (*Top*) Band pusher. Developed by the orthodontist John Valentine Mershon, the rectangular serrated (to minimise slippage) tip is used to seat bands by carefully applying pressure to the edges of the bands to pass them through the contact points of adjacent teeth. They are also used for adapting the edges of the band round the tooth after seating. (*Middle*) Band seater; also known as a band biter. Consists of a plastic handle and bite shelf, with a triangular-shaped serrated metal part on one side that engages the occlusal edge of a band, whilst the patient bites on the opposing side of the bite stick to help seat a band. (*Bottom*) Band-removing pliers. Used to remove bands from posterior teeth. The longer beak carries a plastic cap that is placed on the occlusal surface of the tooth and the shorter beak engages the gingival band margin. Occlusal-directed pressure is applied to remove the band.

Preadjusted Edgewise Fixed Orthodontic Appliances: Principles and Practice, First Edition. Edited by Farhad B. Naini and Daljit S. Gill.
© 2022 John Wiley & Sons Ltd. Published 2022 by John Wiley & Sons Ltd.

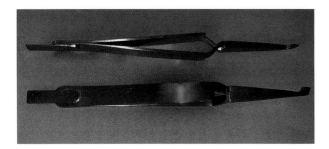

Figure A1.4 Bracket placement tweezers. Used to hold, position and place brackets. The thin opposing end may be placed in the horizontal or vertical slot of twin brackets to help position and seat them.

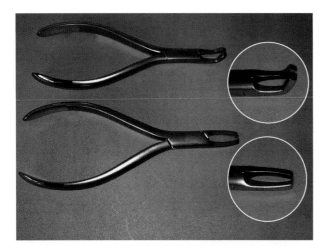

Figure A1.5 Bracket-removing pliers. Anterior bracket-removing pliers have a straight tip. Posterior bracket-removing pliers have a curved tip permitting easier access to the buccal surfaces of the posterior teeth.

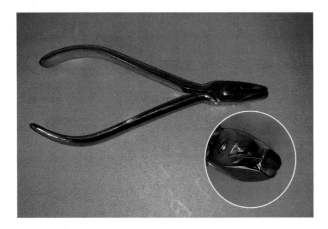

Figure A1.6 Contouring pliers. A convex tip fits into an opposing concave tip, which allows the subtle contouring of adaptable archwires (as well as contouring and adaptation of stainless steel orthodontic bands). The size and shape of the tips varies by manufacturer. They are also referred to as hollow chop contouring pliers. See also De La Rosa pliers (Figure A1.9).

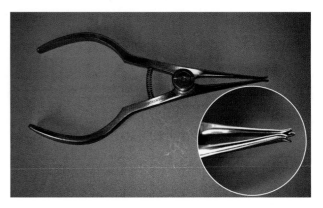

Figure A1.7 Coon's ligature locker. These pliers tie a metal ligature with the initial twist placed directly at the bracket and subsequent twisting of the instrument twists the ligature wire away from the bracket. Therefore, the fit of the ligature is tighter round the bracket, hence the term 'ligature locker'. These pliers have reverse action, i.e. squeezing the handles increases the separation of the tips. The forked blunt tips touch when the instrument is passive. Compressing the handles spreads the tips. See also Figure 14.23.

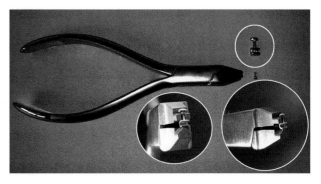

Figure A1.8 Crimpable hook pliers. These are used to hold, position and crimp (i.e. tightly press) crimpable hooks onto an archwire.

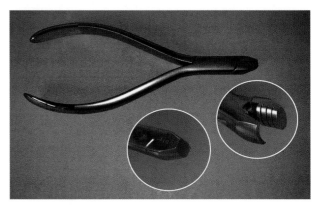

Figure A1.9 De La Rosa contouring pliers with grooves. These may be obtained with or without grooves. They are used for subtle contouring of adaptable archwires (e.g. stainless steel). When present, the grooves allow contouring of archwires of different sizes without inadvertent torquing of the wire. The grooves usually measure 0.016 inch (0.4 mm), 0.018 inch (0.45 mm) and 0.022 inch (0.55 mm).

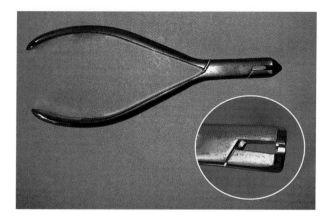

Figure A1.10 Distal end cutter. This useful wire cutter has its cutting edges set at right angles to the long axis of the instrument. The inner part of the cutting end cuts the wire whilst the outer part holds the distally cut end of the wire. The cut distal end of a wire is thereby safely gripped after having been cut and removed from the mouth. A full-thickness rectangular archwire (0.022 × 0.028 inch) or round archwire up to 0.020-inch stainless steel may be cut with this instrument.

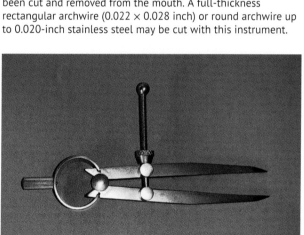

Figure A1.11 Dividers. This is a type of compass with two pointed arms joined at one end. It may be used to measure the size of tooth crowns or intraoral distances (e.g. intercanine width), used together with a dental ruler. Alternatively, it can be used to measure such distances on dental study models.

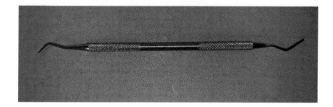

Figure A1.12 Flat plastic. This instrument is designed for placing and contouring pliable restorative materials, e.g. placement and contouring of glass ionomer cement on the occlusal surfaces of posterior teeth to open the anterior occlusion.

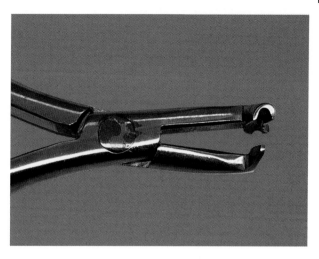

Figure A1.13 Hammerhead NiTi distal end bend back pliers. These may be used to bend back the distal ends of nickel titanium archwires.

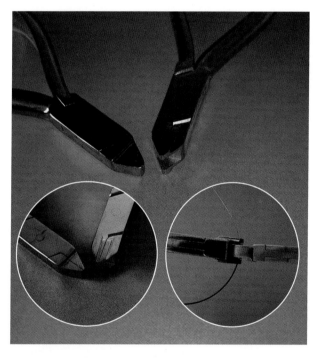

Figure A1.14 Individual torquing pliers. A pair of pliers with one fitting round the other, both holding the section of rectangular archwire from opposite sides. Twisting one relative to the other places torque into the small section of the archwire being held without distorting adjacent sections of the archwire. See also Figure 14.64.

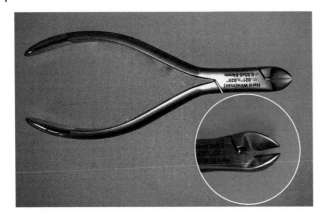

Figure A1.15 Ligature cutter. This wire cutter has two tapering pointed opposing beaks, which terminate in sharp cutting edges. They are used to cut stainless steel ligature wires. They should not be used to cut larger-diameter wires.

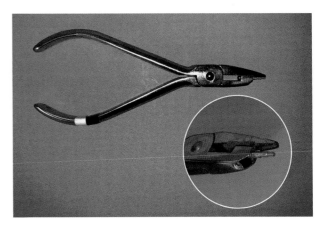

Figure A1.18 Loop-forming pliers. These were developed by Charles Tweed. They have opposing beaks, one concave and the other round in cross-section. The round beak is stepped in three sections of different diameter, allowing the formation of reproducible loops in archwires.

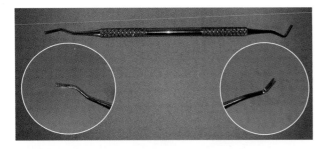

Figure A1.16 Ligature director (tucker). This instrument has a straight tip and the opposing end has an angled tip, both carrying a notch used to engage archwires and direct them into position. They are also used to tuck ligature ends under bracket wings.

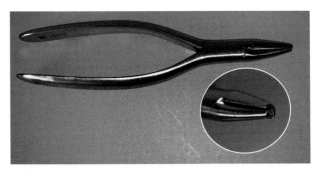

Figure A1.19 Loop-forming pliers (large). These larger loop-forming pliers are useful for bending and adjusting heavy-gauge wires, such as Coffin springs, omega loops on transpalatal arches and U-loops on heavy archwires.

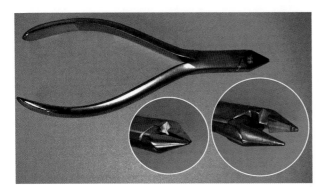

Figure A1.17 Light wire pliers. These have a round beak and opposing pyramidal beak. A similar instrument with shorter beaks is referred to as bird beak pliers. They are used to form loops in archwires (usually round archwires), as well as to place first- and second-order bends in archwires.

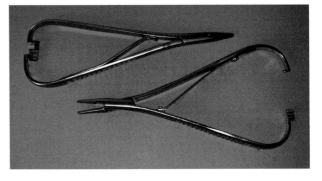

Figure A1.20 Mathieu pliers. These are used predominantly to hold and tie stainless steel ligatures. The handles have a positive locking ratchet and spring, enabling the tips to open and close almost instantaneously.

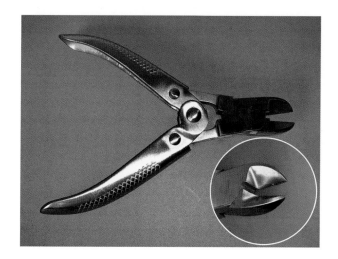

Figure A1.21 Mauns wire cutter. These relatively heavy-duty wire cutters are used to cut wires up to 1.0 mm in diameter outside of the mouth. They are predominantly used when constructing removable appliances.

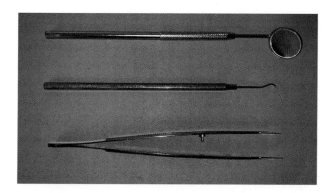

Figure A1.22 Mirror, probe and tweezers. A dental mirror, dental probe (normal or short tip) and college tweezers are prerequisite instruments to a fixed appliance adjustment kit.

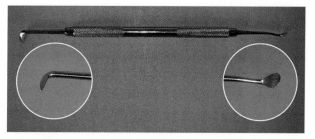

Figure A1.23 Mitchell's trimmer. This versatile instrument was developed by the dentist William Mitchell (c. 1899).

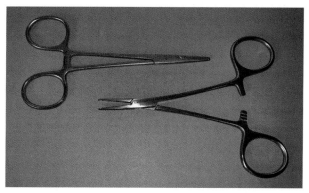

Figure A1.24 Mosquito pliers. Also termed haemostats or mosquito forceps, these pliers have a mechanical locking mechanism located between the handles, enabling the tips to open and close almost instantaneously. They have serrated tips, which may be straight or curved. Some designs have a notch at the tip, to better hold an elastomeric ligature. They are used predominantly for placement of elastomeric ligatures. Two may be used in conjunction to place separator elastics between the contact points of adjacent teeth to create space for later band placement.

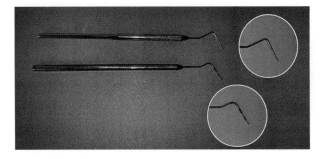

Figure A1.25 Periodontal probe. (*Top*) This graduated pocket-measuring periodontal probe has a long, thin and blunt tip, used to assess gingival health, bleeding on probing and periodontal pocket depths. The most commonly used periodontal probe is shown, which has Williams markings with circumferential lines at 1, 2, 3, 5, 7, 8, 9 and 10 mm for measuring the depth of periodontal pockets. The orthodontist may also use the tip to measure small distances and lengths intraorally as required. (*Bottom*) In 1978 a meeting of the World Health Organization (WHO) in Geneva published the WHO Technical Report Series 621. This led to the development of the Community Periodontal Index of Treatment Needs (CPITN) and a specific periodontal probe termed the WHO-621 Trinity probe. It has a smooth ball end of diameter 0.5 mm, a first coloured band at 3.5–5.5 mm and another coloured band at 8.5–11.5 mm. The CPITN was intended to provide a global standard for clinical practice and research, although several different periodontal screening tools were adapted from it. All these methods use the WHO 621 probe. The Basic Periodontal Examination (BPE) is the technique recommended by the British Society of Periodontology since its introduction in 1986. It is a screening tool to quickly obtain a rough picture of the periodontal condition of a patient, although it does not provide an exact periodontal diagnosis. For the purposes of a BPE, the mouth is divided into sextants, namely the second molar to first premolar in each quadrant, and the upper and lower canine-to-canine regions (third molars are excluded). At least two teeth must be present in a sextant for it to be scored. If only one tooth is present in a sextant, the tooth is included in the adjoining sextant. The probe is gently walked round measuring the depth of the gingival sulcus or periodontal pockets with a force of approximately 10–20 g. Six sites on each tooth are explored and the worst score per sextant is the BPE score. The BPE is usually recorded in a simple six-box chart. Ideally, the gingival sulcus should be no more than 3 mm in depth with no bleeding on probing. There should be good gingival health with no bleeding on probing if orthodontic treatment is contemplated.

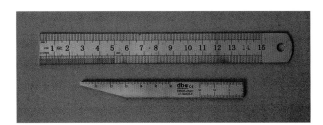

Figure A1.26 Ruler. (*Top*) A metal ruler is useful for measuring facial (e.g. lower anterior face height) and dental parameters, sometimes together with dividers. (*Bottom*) An overjet ruler is useful for clinical measurement of the incisor overjet.

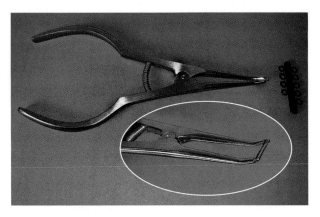

Figure A1.27 Separator pliers. These pliers have two long angled beaks connected with a circular hinge. The beaks carry blunt grooved tips, which hold elastomeric separating modules. Squeezing the handles increases the separation of the beaks, allowing interdental placement of the separating elastics.

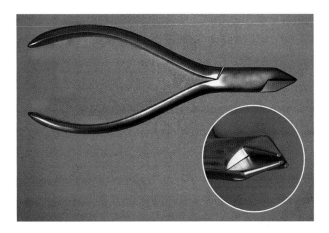

Figure A1.28 Triple beak pliers. Also termed three prong pliers, these have a double beak opposed by a single beak meeting between the double beak, allowing placement of sharp bends in an archwire.

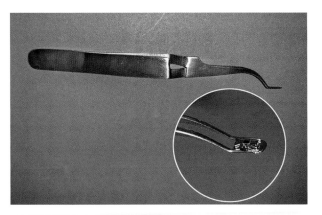

Figure A1.29 Tube placement tweezers. Used to hold, position and place molar tubes. The tip is curved to aid visualisation and placement of tubes on the buccal aspect of molar teeth.

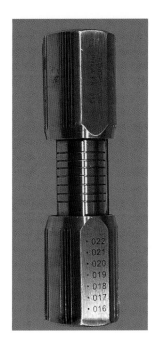

Figure A1.30 Turret. Also known as a torquing turret, this tubular metal device has a number of grooves of different calibrated sizes. It may be used to shape a straight length of orthodontic wire into an arch form. Some of the grooves may also be used to place torque into sections of a rectangular archwire.

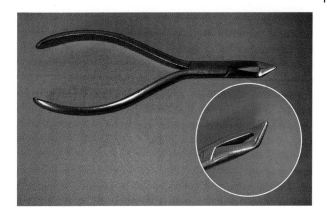

Figure A1.32 Weingart pliers. These pliers have long slender beaks usually set at an angle to the long axis of the instrument. The beaks are serrated, allowing an archwire to be gripped firmly when being directed into or removed from molar tubes. They may also be used to place bends in an archwire or squeeze crimpable stops onto an archwire.

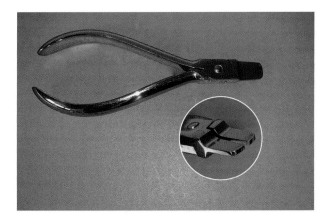

Figure A1.31 Tweed torquing pliers. They are also termed Tweed arch-forming, arch-bending or arch-adjusting pliers. These pliers are used as a pair. They were developed by the orthodontist Charles Tweed specifically for adjusting square or rectangular archwires. They may hold an archwire from opposite sides, with the flattened sides of the blades in contact, whereby twisting one relative to the other places a twist in the archwire in the third order, i.e. torque. See also Figure 14.66.

Appendix 2

Orthodontic Elastics and Elastomeric Materials

Farhad B. Naini and Daljit S. Gill

CHAPTER OUTLINE

Introduction, 423
Intraoral Elastic Configurations, 423
  Intra-arch Elastics, 423
  Inter-arch Elastics, 423
Points of Application, 424
Instructions for Use of Intraoral Elastics, 424
Elastomeric Materials, 425
  Elastomeric Modules, 425
  Elastomeric Chain, 425
  Elastomeric Thread/String, 425
  E-links, 425

Introduction

When orthodontists refer to 'elastics' at the chairside, the reference is to intraoral elastic rings of variable diameter and capable of exerting different force levels for orthodontic tooth movement, rather than to other elastomeric materials, such as elastomeric modules or chains.

Orthodontic elastics have an internal lumen diameter usually measured in inches. They may also be described in relation to their lay flat length, width and thickness (Figure A2.1). However, orthodontic elastics are predominantly described in relation to their internal diameter (Table A2.1) and amount of force exerted in use, usually measured in ounces or grams of force (Table A2.2). The standard force index employed by manufacturers indicates that when *stretched to three times the original lumen diameter*, elastics exert the force stated on the package. A force gauge may be used to check the elastic force at the chairside.

Elastics are usually presented in packets containing 100 elastics and each manufacturer uses a different method to indicate the force of the elastics in each set of packets, e.g. some are colour coded, whereas others are identified using the names of different animals, countries, sports or other forms of identification.

Elastic forces may be measured at the chairside using a force gauge, e.g. a Correx (Figure A2.2) or Dontrix (Figure A2.3) tension gauge. The elastic may be applied to one of the points of force application, e.g. molar tube hook, and then stretched towards the other point of force application, e.g. a canine bracket hook, using a force gauge.

Intraoral Elastic Configurations

Intraoral elastics may be used in different configurations, either within a dental arch or between the maxillary and mandibular dental arches.

Intra-arch Elastics

These are used within a dental arch. When intra-arch elastics are used for space closure between the posterior and anterior dental units, they are also referred to as **Class I** elastics.

Inter-arch Elastics

These are used between the maxillary and mandibular dental arches. The most common configurations are as **Class II**

Preadjusted Edgewise Fixed Orthodontic Appliances: Principles and Practice, First Edition. Edited by Farhad B. Naini and Daljit S. Gill.
© 2022 John Wiley & Sons Ltd. Published 2022 by John Wiley & Sons Ltd.

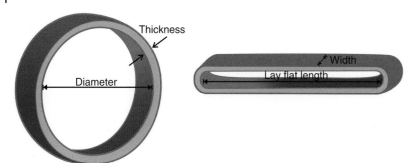

Figure A2.1 Orthodontic elastics may be described in relation to their internal lumen diameter (usually measured in inches) or their lay flat length, width and thickness.

Table A2.1 Internal diameter of intraoral orthodontic elastics.

Lumen diameter (inches)	Lumen diameter (mm)
1/8	3
3/16	4
1/4	6
5/16	8
3/8	10

Points of Application

Elastics may be applied to a variety of regions of a fixed appliance. For example:

- Integrated hooks on a bracket or tube
- Hooks soldered or crimped onto archwires
- Kobayashi stainless steel ligatures tied round any bracket
- Loops bent into archwires (e.g. circle or U-loops)
- Orthodontic mini-implants/temporary anchorage devices.

or **Class III intermaxillary (maxillomandibular) elastics**. These may be **short** (e.g. from a mandibular premolar to the maxillary canine region) or **long** (e.g. from the mandibular second molar to the maxillary canine region).

Alternatively, the configuration may be **diagonal**, e.g. an anterior diagonal elastic from the mandibular right to the maxillary left canine may be used to promote dental midline correction; or **cross elastics**, which are from the buccal side of one arch to the lingual side of the opposing arch, usually used to correct a dental crossbite. They may also be vertical in direction, as in extrusive or **settling** elastics, which may be configured in box, rectangle or triangular shapes. Vertical elastics combined with flexible archwires can encourage interdigitation of the dentition in the final stage of occlusal detailing.

Instructions for Use of Intraoral Elastics

Intraoral elastics are placed and changed by the patient. As such, the clinician is reliant on the patient's cooperation. It is thereby essential that patients understand why they are being asked to wear elastics, in order to maximise the likelihood of their compliance. Patients are often under the misapprehension that elastics are just an add-on, and that not wearing them will make little difference to their progress. This is understandable as most intraoral elastics are light and their force cannot always be readily felt by the patient. Therefore, the clinician's explanation of the requirement for elastics is paramount. The clinician should provide an explicit explanation of their importance, particularly emphasising that the archwires have done

Table A2.2 Force exerted by intraoral elastics in use (i.e. when stretched to three times their original lumen diameter).

	Force												
	Very light		**Light**				**Medium**					**Heavy**		**Very heavy (orthopaedic)**
Ounces	0.5	1	2	3	4	5	6	7	8	9	10	11	12	12 +
Grams	14	28	57	85	113	142	170	198	227	255	283	312	340	340 +

Note: 1 ounce = 28.3 grams.

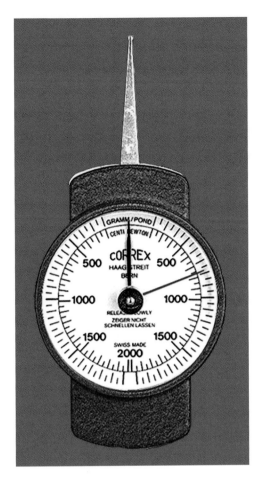

Figure A2.2 Correx bidirectional tension gauge.

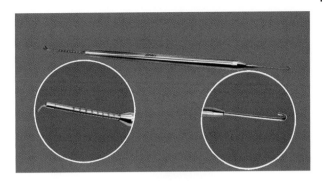

Figure A2.3 Dontrix tension gauge.

Elastomeric Materials

Elastomeric materials are used commonly with orthodontic fixed appliances, predominantly to apply forces to move teeth along archwires.

Elastomeric Modules

These are predominantly used to hold archwires within brackets (see Chapter 14), but may also be used in conjunction with a stainless steel ligature to apply space closing forces (see Chapter 15).

Elastomeric Chain

This is a chain of connected elastomeric rings used for sliding mechanics and space closure. They may be open (the rings are connected by a horizontal piece of elastomeric material, with various available lengths) or closed (with the rings next to one another without any inter-ring space) (Figure A2.4).

Elastomeric Thread/String

Also described in Chapter 14 is a stretchable thread used to apply forces to move teeth, and is available in various cross-sectional thicknesses (Figure A2.5).

E-links

Elastomeric E-links® are provided in 10 graded lengths. They are stamped from latex-free material and remain active for a considerable period of time, usually between 6 and 12 weeks (Figure A2.6). As such, they can be useful for intra-arch space closure. They are opaque white or grey in colour. They are usually placed from the buccal hook

much of their job, and that the elastics are now the primary motive force. For example, the clinician may convey this information to the patient as follows: 'The wires have now accomplished most of what we desired from them. The force moving your teeth is now entirely from these elastics. So, if you're not wearing the elastics, nothing is happening!'

Patients should be provided with two packets of elastics, and instructed to keep one packet with them at all times, e.g. at school or work, allowing immediate replacement in case of breakage or loss. Routine replacement is usually once every 24 hours and patients should be asked to change their elastics at the same time each day, e.g. in the evening before sleep. Elastics should only need to be removed for brushing the teeth and other forms of oral hygiene maintenance. Progress should be monitored and the importance of elastic wear re-emphasised at each appointment.

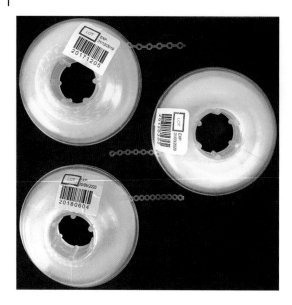

Figure A2.4 Elastomeric chain.

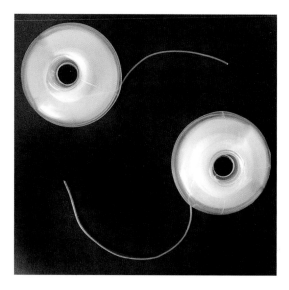

Figure A2.5 Elastomeric thread/string.

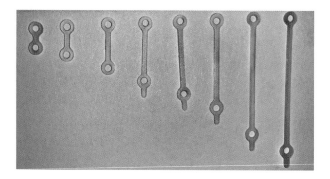

Figure A2.6 Elastomeric E-links®.

on the first molar tube to the canine hook or an anterior archwire hook (Figure A2.7). In premolar extraction cases, an E6 is often an appropriate size, though an E5 may be required once most of the space has been closed. The larger sizes (E5–E10) have a small extension tail that allows locking round archwires. These can be cut off with ligature cutters if not required, or alternatively placed as the distal link, which will conceal the tail behind the molar hook.

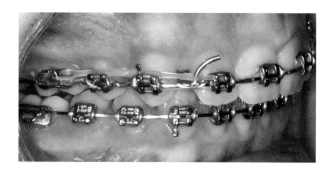

Figure A2.7 An elastomeric E-link placed from the buccal hook on the maxillary first molar tube to the anterior archwire hook.

Index

a

absolute anchorage 61, 381
absolute intrusion, of incisors 375
active self-ligating brackets 69
active unit 58, 71, 251, 307
Adams pliers 415
adhesive pre-coated (APC) brackets 133
adjunctive surgical interventions 292
aesthetic archwire 185–187
aesthetic-centred *versus* occlusion-centred planning 11–13
aetiological factor 333
ageing process 323
Alexander vari-simplex prescription 124–125
aligners, transverse dimension management 400
alignment 257–258
  accelerated tooth movement 292–293
  archwire ligation methods 267–269
  archwire removal 273–277
  archwire size and material 263–264
  bracket positioning variations 258
  cinching *versus* bend backs 269–271
  crossbite correction 282–283
  diastema closure and frenectomy 287–288
  ectopic and impacted canines and incisors 283–286
  impacted mandibular second molars 286
  initial alignment 258–263
  intrusion of overerupted maxillary second molars 286–287
  lacebacks placement 264–267
  in non-extraction cases 278
  pain from initial archwires 291–282
  space creation and redistribution 277–281
  step-by-step archwire placement 271–273
  treatment mechanics 249
  wire bending 288–291
alignment errors 312–313
allergic reactions 87
alternative treatment options 22
alveolar bone, frontal resorption of 257
anaesthetic complications 87
anchorage 57–58
  adjunctive methods for 73
  assessment 61
  classifications 61–62
  clinical orthodontics 58
  conservation 58
  control with fixed appliances 62–73
  creation 73–74
  direct *versus* indirect 223–226
  elastics 203–204
  extraoral traction 207–208
  headgear 207–208
  importance 58
  intermaxillary traction 203–204
  lingual arches and space maintainers 205–207
  loss 74
  palatal arches 204–205
  preparation 64, 250–255
  requirements 250–255
  terminology 58–59
  value 59–61
anchorage loss 58, 219, 252
anchorage reinforcement 20, 59, 252–255, 280
anchorage unit 63–71, 251, 307
anchorage value 59–61, 251
anchor unit 251
Andrews, Lawrence 299
Andrews' standard prescription 123
Andrews straight-wire appliance 118–121
Angle, Edward H. 114–117
Angle's Edgewise appliance 117
Angle's molar classification 312
ankylosis 285
anterior bite plane 376
anterior open bite (AOB) 385–389, 394
anteroposterior anchorage 228
APC (adhesive pre-coated) brackets 133
apically repositioned flap 285
Appareil de Schangé 114, 115
appliance factors 308
appliances and techniques, for overbite reduction 376–382
arch form 255–256
arch length 71–72
arch stops 71
archwire 68, 175
  aesthetic 185–187
  aligning 191–192
  arch form 179–180
  beta-titanium 184–185
  binding 258
  clearance 259
  cobalt chromium 181
  fatigue 187–188
  fixed appliances 401
  friction 258
  intrusion 212, 214
  ligation method 267–269
  metal alloys corrosion 188–191
  migration 261
  nickel allergy 195–197
  nickel titanium 181–184
  ovoid 256
  pain from 192–194
  piggyback 216–217
  placement of, step-by-step 271–273
  precious metal alloys 180
  preformed 255
  properties 176–179
  protection from masticatory forces 265

Preadjusted Edgewise Fixed Orthodontic Appliances: Principles and Practice, First Edition. Edited by Farhad B. Naini and Daljit S. Gill.
© 2022 John Wiley & Sons Ltd. Published 2022 by John Wiley & Sons Ltd.

archwire (*contd.*)
  removal   273–277
  root resorption from   194–195
  sectional   214
  sequence   191–192
  shape   179–180
  size and material   263–264
  stainless steel   180–181
  utility   212, 214
  working (*see* working archwires)
archwire bends   64
archwire cinching   72
archwire ligation   134–135
arthritic degeneration   387
asperities   51
autonomous model   21–22
auxiliaries   65–66, 380
  anchorage and space management   203–208
  Class II correction   208–211
  fixed appliances   401
  tooth movement   211–217
auxiliary slots   132
axis of rotation   37

b

band crimping pliers   415
'Bandeau' arch   58
banded RME   407
banding technique   145
band-removing pliers   415
base contour   132
base surface   132
Basic Periodontal Examination (BPE)
    scores   236, 238
bearing points   50–51
Begg appliance   117
bend backs   269–271
beta-titanium   184–185, 264
bihelix appliances   403–404
binding   52, 69
  archwires   258
biocompatible   176
Bioforce archwires   184
biohostability   176
biological factors   69–71
biomechanics   29
bite splints   389
bite turbos   380
bite wafers   193
blue lights   154
bodily movement   256
body image disorder   4
Bolam test   103

Bolitho test   103
bonded retainers
  adhesives   157–158
  defined   322
  maintenance of   326–327
  problems and complications with   326
  types   157
bonded RME   407–408
bond failure rate   154
bonding
  additional uses   158
  adhesives   152–154
  after enamel etching   150–151
  to artificial substrates   151
  bracket types   148
  effectiveness of adhesives   154–156
  enamel preparation   148–150
  future possibilities   158
  health risks associated with   154
  history   147–148
  indirect   151–152
  of molar tubes   154–155
bone anchorage   72–73
bone-borne RME   408–409
Bonwill-Hawley arch form   255
bowing effect   225
bracket design   113–135
bracket positioning   128–129, 258, 259
bracket prescription   65
bracket-removing pliers   416
brackets   68–69
  auxiliary features   139
  bonding   148
  convenience features   140
  design features   137–140
  direct bonding technique   141–142
  direct *versus* indirect bonding   140–141
  fracture   167
  groove   239
  height gauges   129
  indirect bonding technique   142–143
  to maximise efficiency of treatment
      and   318
  molars and premolars bands   143–145
  placement tweezers   416
  primary design features   138
  selection tips   145–146
  size   260
  slot siting features   138–140
bracket slot deformation   312
bracket torque options   127

bracket width   48
buccal bone miniplates   352–356
buccolingual inclination   312, 316–317
burns   171
Burstone's intrusion arch   380

c

camouflage treatment mechanics   364–366
canine guidance   312
canine retraction   265
capillary pressure   256
carbon dioxide (CO_2) lasers   168
Cartesian coordinate system   39
casein phosphopeptide amorphous
      calcium phosphate (CPP-ACP)
      242, 244
catapult injury   254
catenary curve   255
centreline (dental midline)   314
centre of mass   33
centre of resistance   33–34
centre of rotation   37
ceramic brackets   131–132, 166–167
cervical vertebral maturation (CVM)
      method   8
chamfered corners   134
changing tooth inclination, by root
      movement   47
Chasles, Michel   40
chemically cured glass ionomer   153
chemically cured no-mix composite   152
chemotherapeutic cleaning   240–241
chewing gum   193
The Children Act   102
cinching   269–271
circumferential supracrestal fiberotomy   324
Class I elastics   423
Class I malocclusions   17
Class II correctors   338–342
Class II division 2 cases   338
Class II division 1 malocclusion   374
Class II division 2 malocclusion   374
Class II elastics   423–424
Class II intermaxillary elastics   380
Class II malocclusion   17, 208–209
  fixed Class II correctors   211
  growth modification   336–342
  Herbst appliance   209–211
  options   334–336
  orthodontic camouflage   342–356
  orthodontics surgery   356

orthognathic surgery 356
Class III camouflage treatment 145
Class III cases 362–366
Class III intermaxillary (maxillomandibular) elastics 424
Class III malocclusion 17, 360–362, 370, 374–375
Class III surgical/orthodontic patient 366–370
clear aligners 391
clearance, archwires 259
clear plastic retainers 328
closed exposure 284–285
coated metal archwires 185–186
coatings 190
cobalt chromium 181
Coffin spring 399–400
composite bite planes 380
composite polishing techniques 170
composite stop 261, 262
compound contoured bases 129
comprehensive orthodontic correction 81–82
compromises 22
cone beam computed tomography (CBCT) 222, 283, 400
consent 79
    clinical predictions 89
    costs of treatment 81–82
    damage to teeth 84–85
    dental health 83–84
    effective communication 88–89
    expected compliance 81
    family and friends involvement 89
    implied 80
    key factors 82–83
    occlusal function 84
    orthodontic treatment 100–102
    pain and discomfort 86–87
    patient information leaflets 88
    periodontal damage 85–86
    principles 80
    psychosocial benefits 84
    rare and unusual injuries 87
    relapse 87–88
    retention protocol 81
    smile aesthetics 83
    for treatment 80, 81
    treatment benefits 83–84
    types 80
    unfounded claims 84
    valid 80–81
    verbal 80

websites 88–89
    withdrawal 81
    written 80
conservative management 382
contact angle (θ) 52
contemporaneous documentation 109
continuous arch mechanics 377–378
contouring pliers 416
controlled space closure
    anchorage classification 299
    completion of alignment and levelling 298
    monitoring 308–309
    objectives during 298–299
    types of 299–300
controlled tipping 46
conventional orthodontic mechanics 390
Coon's ligature locker 416
copper NiTi (CuNiTi) wires 183
correct mandibular incisor 383
corrosion 188–191
cortical anchorage 72–73
couple 35–37
crevice corrosion 189
crimpable hook pliers 416
crimpable split tubes 261
critical contact angle, for binding 52
crossbite correction 282–283
cross elastics 401, 424
crown angulation 118, 312
crown inclination 118, 312
curve of Spee 119
cytotoxicity, of adhesives 154

d

Dahl appliance 378
Damon Clear brackets 168
Damon prescription 126–127
Data Protection Act 98
debanding injuries 171
debonding
    band removal 169, 170
    ceramic brackets 166–167
    composite resin removal 169, 170
    demineralisation lesion management 156
    efficient and safe 165
    electrothermal 168
    finishing techniques 169–171
    iatrogenic damage 171
    laser 168–169
    lingual appliances and bite turbos 168

particulates 171–172
patient appraisal 156
    preparation 166
    procedure and enamel damage 156, 157
    risks 156
    self-ligating brackets 168
    solvent use 168
    stainless steel brackets 166
    tooth colour change 156
deep incisor overbite 372–384
definitive treatment plan 5, 23–26
degree 16–17
De La Rosa contouring pliers 416
dental, aetiology of deep bite 373
Dental Complaints Service 93–94
dental extractions 279
dental midline 314
    correction 265, 424
dental pain 87
dental plaque biofilm control methods 238–241
dentist responsibilities 329
dentogingival fibres 323
depth, overbite 372
DERHT. *see* direct electric resistance heat treatment (DERHT)
detailing, of teeth 250
determinate 47–48
diamond finishing bur 169
diastema closure and frenectomy 287–288
dietary control 244
digit sucking habits 8
direct anchorage 223, 225
direct bonding 141–42
direct bone anchorage 73, 74
direct electric resistance heat treatment (DERHT) 184
direction of movement 30
direct visualisation 128
displacement of rigid bodies 39–41
distal-end bend back 269
distal end cutter 417
dividers 417
DMFT scores 237
dry field 149
duty of candour 107–108
duty of care 103

e

E-arch appliance 115–116
ectopic and impacted canines and incisors 283–286

ectopic tooth 283
edge-centroid relationship 383
edgewise straight-wire appliance,
      preadjusted 117–121
effective anchorage 220
elastics
   anchorage 203–204
   forces 423
   settling 424
elastomeric chain 265, 425
elastomeric ligatures 134, 267
elastomeric materials 425–426
elastomeric modules 273-276, 425
elastomeric string 285, 425
elastomeric thread 285
elastomeric traction 224
electrothermal debonding 168
E-links 425–426
emotional costs of treatment 22
enamel 169–170
   decalcification 84
   etching 149–151
   fracture 85
   fractures 171
   preparation 148–150
enamel surfaces 241–244
en masse retraction 49, 305–306
equal molar/incisor movement 300
erbium-doped yttrium aluminium
      garnet (Er:YAG) laser 168
Euler, Leonhard 39
extension arms/hooks 301
external (extrinsic) motivation 4
extractions 20
extraoral anchorage 61, 66, 252
extraoral traction 252
extrusive elastics 424

f

facemask 66
facial axis of the clinical crown (FACC)
   120
facial axis (FA) point 120–121, 138
facial soft tissue form and thickness 16
fatigue 187–189
fibre-reinforced composite archwires
   186–187
figure-of-eight configuration for
      elastomeric modules 271
figure-of-eight ligation method 267
finishing techniques 169–171, 250
fixed appliances
   archwires and auxiliaries 401
   continuous arch mechanics 377–378

cross elastics 401
   headgear with fixed appliances
      400–401
   lingual arch/utility arch 401
   NiTi expanders 404
   quadhelix (bihelix/trihelix) 403–404
   segmented arch mechanics 378–380
   transpalatal arch 401
   transverse dimension management
      400–404
   W-arch/Porter appliance 401–402
fixed appliance treatment 236–245
fixed retainers 322
   advantages of 325
   disadvantages of 325
   maintenance of 326–327
   placement of 325–326
   problems and complications with
      326
flat plastic 417
flexible timing of anchorage 220
force 30
   generation 306
   levels 304
   relaxation 267
   systems 47–48
force application method 303–304
Forsus™ appliance 211
Forsus™ (Fatigue Resistant) module
   342
frame of reference 30, 31
fretting corrosion 189
friction 51, 68
   archwires 258
frictionless mechanics 299, 301,
   306–308
frontal resorption, of alveolar bone 257
fully twisted tie-back/laceback 265
functional appliances 376–377, 400
functional occlusion 14
function regulator type II (FR-II)
   appliance 400

g

galvanic corrosion 189
GDPs. *see* general dental practitioners
   (GDPs)
General Dental Council (GDC)
   Standards 93
general dental practitioners (GDPs) 93,
   99
Gillick-competence 102
Gingival Bleeding Index 236
gingival recession 86

gingivitis 86
glossectomy 394
gold chain attachment 285
good inter-incisal angle 383
gram force-millimetre (gf-mm) 35
growth chart 8
growth estimation 21
growth-related problems 386–388

h

hammerhead NiTi distal end bend back
      pliers 417
handicapping malocclusions 8
Hawley, Charles 255
Hawley-type retainer 327–328
headgears 66, 73
   anchorage 207–208
   anchorage reinforcement with
      252–255
   appliances and techniques, for
      overbite reduction 380
   extraoral traction 252
   with fixed appliances 400–401
   protraction 404
   safety with 254
health 14
health of teeth 17
Herbst appliance 209–211, 338–342
high-pull headgear 66
   with occlusal support 389
home cleaning 237–240
Hooke's law 306
horizontal parallax technique 283
hyalinisation 257
hydrogen absorption 188
Hyrax screw activation mechanism
   407
hysteresis 183

i

immobilisation, of teeth 251
impacted mandibular second molars
   286
impacted tooth 283
impinging overbite 372
implied consent 80
0.018-inch slot 132, 300
0.022-inch slot 132, 300
incisal edge recontouring 318
incisor contact, overbite 372
incisor relationship 374–375
incisor retraction 300
incisor segment, retraction of 49
inconveniences 22

indeterminate 48
Index of Orthodontic Treatment Need (IOTN) 4
indirect anchorage 223, 225
indirect bonding 142–43, 151–152, 318
indirect bone anchorage 72–73
indirect visualisation 128
individual torquing pliers 417
informed consent 21–23
initial alignment 258–263
initial consultation 94–97
insertion torque (mini-implants) 221
Insignia software 128
inter-arch elastics 423–424
inter-arch relationships 118
interbracket span 48, 260
interdental enamel reduction 279
interdental fibres 323
intergranular corrosion 189
interim wire 293
intermaxillary anchorage 62–63
internal (intrinsic) motivation 4
interproximal contacts (spacing) 314
interproximal enamel reduction 318
intra-arch elastics 423
intraoral anchorage 61
intraoral distalising appliances 74
intraoral elastics 424–425
intraoral musculature 71
intrusion archwires 212, 214
intrusion of overerupted maxillary second molars 286–287
inverting brackets 127
ion implantation 185

k

Kloehn-type headgear 252
Kobayashi ligatures 134–135

l

labiolingual inclination 312
lacebacks 70–71, 264–267
Lang brackets 117
laser debonding 168–169
lasers 169
late permanent dentition 391–394
Law of acceleration 38
Law of action and reaction 38
Law of inertia 38
Le Bandeau 113–114
levelling 293–294
Lewis brackets 117
ligation 69
  archwire 267

ligature, archwire 267
ligature cutter 418
ligature director (tucker) 418
light continuous force 258
light-cured composite 152
light-cured glass ionomer 153–154
light-curing units 155–156
light force 257
light wire pliers 418
line of action 30
lingual appliances 378
lingual arches 71, 205–207
  fixed appliances 401
lip–incisor relationship 16
load-deflection characteristics 307
long axis of the clinical crown (LACC) 138, 139
long face syndrome 388
long ligatures 135
loop designs 307
loop-forming pliers 418
loop mechanics 52–54, 299, 301
loss of vitality 87
low flexural rigidity 258
low-level laser therapy (LLLT) 193
low-profile bracket wings 134
low-pull (cervical) headgear 66

m

macro-mechanical bracket bases 132
magnitude 30
malocclusion 17
marginal ridge height discrepancies 313–314
Mathieu pliers 418
Mauns wire cutter 419
maxillary expansion 398
maxillary lateral incisor 145, 146
maxillary sinus floors, perforation of nasal and 221
maximum anchorage 62
MBT versatile+prescription 126
mechanical cleaning 237–240
mechanical injury 85–86
mechanics 29
mental capacity 14
metal alloys corrosion 188–191
metal brackets 129–131
metal casting 130
metal injection moulding (MIM) 130–131
microbiologically influenced corrosion 189–190
micro-mechanical bracket bases 132

microscrews 381
mid-palatal suture 404–409
milled 129–130
Miller's classification of gingival recession 236, 239
mini-implants 221, 252
minimal anchorage 62
miniscrew anchorage 381
miniscrew implants 219
missing teeth 20
Mitchell's trimmer 419
moderate anchorage 62
modified Bass technique 239
moisture-insensitive primer (MIP) 153
molar bands 143–145
molar distal movement 20
molar mesial movement 20–21
molar protraction 300
molar relationship 312
moment 34–35
moment arm 35
moment of the couple 43
moment of the force 42
moments, generation of 307
moment-to-force ratio 42–44
monitoring space closure 308–309
monocrystalline alumina 131–132
monocrystalline alumina brackets 167
Montgomery *versus* Lanarkshire Health Board 100
mosquito pliers 419
mouthguards 245
multidisciplinary care 15
multifluted tungsten carbide bur 169, 170
multiloop edgewise archwire (MEAW) approach 391–392
multistrand stainless steel 264
muscular weakness syndromes 387
mutually protected occlusion (MPO) 312

n

Nance palatal arch 72
nasopharyngeal obstruction 387–388
need for retention 22
neurovascular tissues, damage to 221
Newton's Laws of Motion 38–39
Newton's Third Law 251
Newton's Third Law of Motion 38, 58
nickel allergy 195–197
nickel titanium (NiTi) 181, 258
  coil springs 211–212
  fixed appliances, expanders 404

nickel titanium (NiTi) *(contd.)*
  martensitic stable 182
  superelastic austenitic active 182–183
  thermodynamic martensitic active 183–184
  wire 65
nickel titanium copper chromium alloys 183
non-axial loading 299
non-extraction cases 278
non-retentive bases 132
non-steroidal anti-inflammatory drugs (NSAIDs) 192
non-surgical methods 287
notching 69
Nudger appliance 376

o
occipital-pull headgear 252
occlusal contact discrepancies 313–314
occlusal correction, comprehensive orthodontics for 81–82
occlusal forces 69
occlusal relationship 317
occlusion 71
occlusion-centred approaches 13
OMI-cortex interface 222
one-couple force system 48
one-way shape memory effect 183
open exposure (of canines) 283–284
optimal force 30
optimum force 30, 59, 251
organic solvents 168
orthodontically induced external root resorption (OIERR) 194
orthodontic biomechanics
  basic concepts and principles 30–38
  clinical applications 47–54
  definition 29-30
  displacement of rigid bodies 39–41
  Newton's Laws of Motion 38–39
  static equilibrium 39
  tooth movement 41–47
orthodontic camouflage 335–356
orthodontic camouflage treatment 13
orthodontic discomfort management 244–245
orthodontic elastics 423–426
orthodontic finishing 312, 317–318
orthodontic instruments 415–421
orthodontic mini-implants (OMIs) 219, 381
  advantages 220

anchorage from 221–223
clinical and radiographic planning 226
disadvantages 220
explantation 227
failure 220
force application 227
insertion 226–227
  predictable treatment outcomes 220
  pre-insertion preparation 226
  reduced treatment times 220
  root divergence 226
  success rates 223
  usage with fixed appliances 226–227
orthodontic pain 244–245
Orthodontic Plaque Index (OPI) scores 236, 238
orthodontic retainers 322–329
orthodontics alone 15
orthodontics surgery 81, 356
orthodontic treatment
  advertising 94
  complaints 93–94, 108–109
  consent 81
  dentolegal issues 99–100, 102–106
  duty of candour 107–108
  ethical issues 99–100
  initial consultation 94–97
  non-attendance 105–106
  non-compliance 105
  non-payment of fees 106
  obtaining consent 100–102
  pretreatment records 97–99
  relapse 107
  retention 106–107
  supervision of orthodontic therapists 106
  transfers 105
orthodontist responsibilities 329
orthognathic surgery 356, 381
overbite reduction methods 375
overjet relationship 317
ovoid, archwires 256

p
pain
  and discomfort 86–87
  from initial archwires 291–282
  non-pharmacological management 193–194
  orthodontic mini-implants (OMIs) 221
  pharmacological management 192
palatal arches 204–205

palatal temporary anchorage 347–352
parallelogram method, force vectors 31
partially engaged, archwire 267
passive self-ligating brackets 69
paternalistic model 21
patient burden 23
patient-related factors 308
patient responsibilities 329
patient's presenting complaint 22
Pendulum appliance 345–347
penetrating eye injury 87
peppermint oil 168
pericision 324
periodontal disease 86
personal protective equipment (PPE) 166
phase transformation 182
Physiological Anchorage Spee-wire System (PASS) 65
physiological spacing 287
piggyback (overlay) archwire 216–217, 260
pin and tube appliance 116
pitting corrosion 188–189
plastic brackets 132
point of application/origin 30
polycrystalline alumina brackets 131, 167
porcelain 171
Porter appliance 401–402
positioners 328–329
posterior segment, protraction of 49
post-manufacturing finishing 190
post-treatment changes 323–324
power arms 301
powerscope 2™ appliance 211
preadjusted edgewise appliance,
  overbite reduction 377–378
  continuous archwires 377
  counterforce NiTi archwires 378
  Dahl appliance 378
  frictionless mechanics with 306–308
  lingual appliances 378
  placing curves in archwires 377–378
  sliding mechanics with 300–306
precious metal alloys 180
precise localisation 283
predictable treatment outcomes 220
presence of teeth 17
prevention or reduction of canine mesial crown tip 264–265
primer 152–153
proclination 38
  of incisors 375

of lower labial segment in Class II
cases 383
professional cleaning 240
ProTorque Latin/Hispanic and
Sugiyama evidence-based Asian
(SEBA) prescriptions 127
protraction 37–38
protraction headgear 404. *see also*
facemask
pseudoelastic behaviour 182
pulpal injury 171
pure rotation 37, 47
push-coil 282
push-pull mechanics 282

q

quadhelix 228
(bihelix/trihelix) fixed appliances
403–404

r

rapid maxillary expansion (RME) 282,
407–409
ratcheting movements 41
reactivation 183
reactive (anchor) unit 58, 251
reciprocal anchorage 59
rectangular NiTi, interim wire 293
rectangular stainless steel 293
redistribution of space 18
reduce corrosion 190–191
reduced treatment times 220
regional acceleratory phenomenon
(RAP) 292, 308
reinforcing sleeves 260
relative intrusion, of incisors 375
removable appliances 376, 399–400
removable functional appliances
337–338
removable retainers 325–329
residual moments 307
resistance to sliding (RS) 67
resultant force 31
retention protocol 82
retentive bases 132
retraction 37–38
retractor 250
retroclination 38
reverse-engineering brackets 318
reverse-pull headgears. *see* facemask
'reversing' (using contralateral) brackets
127, 259
rhomboid shape 128, 133
ribbon arch appliance 116–117

Ricketts' Bioprogressive prescription
125–126
Ricketts' utility arch 378–380
risk/harm/cost *versus* benefit
considerations 22
rocking-chair archwires 378
rollercoaster effect 121, 225
root angulation 315–316
root divergence 226
root movement 46–47
root parallelism 315
root/periodontal damage 220
root resorption 85
root uprighting 47
rotation-oscillation brushes 238
electric toothbrush 240
rotations 118
Roth prescription 123–124
round nickel titanium (NiTi) 255, 293
round stainless steel, interim wire 293
Royal London Hospital space analysis
18

s

sacrifices 22
saddle angle 386
saliva 69
scalers 169
second molars incorporation 304–305
second molar teeth 377
sectional archwires 214
segmental maxillary surgery 410–411
segmental surgery 381–382
segmented arch mechanics 308,
378–380
self-etching primer (SEP) 154
self-ligating brackets 135, 168, 267
separate canine retraction 49
separators 143–144
shape memory effect 183
shared decision-making 22–23
short mandibular ramus 386
short 'quick lig' ligatures 134
simple tipping 46
single photon emission computed
tomography (SPECT) 360
single *versus* double wing, bracket
tie-wings 133
site of crowding 16–17
Six Keys of Occlusion 312
skeletal 373
sliding mechanics
advantages of 52
friction 299, 301

with preadjusted edgewise appliance
300–306
for space closure 49–52
social costs 22
soft tissue
aetiology 373
irritation 86–87
problems 221
space analysis 16, 17–21, 297
space closure
categories 49
with closing loop mechanics 52–54
with sliding mechanics 49–52
space creation 277–281, 283
space maintainers 205–207
space planning 17–21
spatial planes 30, 31
special needs orthodontics 6
split stop 269
square, archwires 256
stability 16
stability of overbite correction 382
stages of treatment errors, finishing
312–317
stainless steel 129
0.018-inch or 0.017 x 0.025-inch
302–303
0.019 x 0.025-inch 300–302
archwire 180–181
brackets 166
ligatures 134, 267
static equilibrium 39
static occlusion 13
step-by-step archwire placement
271–273
stopped arches 280
storage of records 98–99
straight-pull headgear 66, 252
straight-wire appliance 121–123
archwire ligation 134–135
auxiliary slots 132
bracket base 132–133
bracket material 129–132
fully customised 128
non-customised 123–127
optimal bracket positioning 128–129
semi-customised 127–128
slot dimensions 132
standard, auxiliary, headgear and lip
bumper tubes 133
tie-wings 133–134
straight-wire technique 300
stress corrosion 189
subsurface demineralisation 235

superelasticity   182
superelastic nickel titanium   264
surgically assisted rapid maxillary
     expansion (SARME)   409
surgically assisted rapid palatal
     expansion (SARPE)   228,
     409–410
swapping brackets   127–128

t
TAD-assisted molar distalisation   347
tapered, archwires   256
tear-out injuries   171
teeth translation   40–41
temporary anchorage devices (TADs)
     219, 381
  implants   392
temporary bite opening   262
Ten Hoeve appliance   376
therapeutic diagnosis approach   16, 278
thermally active nickel titanium   183,
     264
thermoelasticity   183
three-dimensional anchorage
     applications   228–231
three-point (tripod) landing   381
tie-wing ligation   134
tie-wings   133–134
tight contacts   119
tip   38
Tip-Edge appliance   117, 378
Tip-Edge system   65–66
tipping   38
  movement   256
titanium   131
titanium molybdenum alloy (TMA)
     258, 264
titanium niobium   185
T-loop   307–308
tongue posture   387
tongue thrust   387
toothbrushing   239
tooth, impacted   283
tooth movement
  accelerated   292–293
  ballista spring   217
  centre of resistance   41–42
  closing loops   212, 213
  control   41
  extension hooks   41–42
  hooks   216
  nickel titanium coil springs   211–212

piggyback archwires   216–217
  with preadjusted fixed appliances
     256–257
  resistance to undesirable   251
  sectional archwires   214
  torquing spurs   214–216
  types   44–46
  utility and intrusion archwires   212,
     214
tooth reduction, and enlargement   18
tooth size discrepancy (TSD)   18, 20,
     317–318
topical fluoride agents   241–242
topical non-fluoride agents   242–244
torque   38
torque-in-base   129, 133
torquing spurs   214–216
total nasal obstruction   387
transition temperature range (TTR)
     183
translation   46
transpalatal arch (TPA)   228, 252
  fixed appliances   401
transverse anchorage   231
transverse dimension management
     404–409
  aligners   400
  crossbites   398
  fixed appliances   400–404
  functional appliances   400
  maxillary expansion indications   398
  mid-palatal suture   404–409
  removable appliances   399–400
  retention   411
  surgical expansion   409–411
traumatic overbite   372
treatment burden   23
treatment mechanics   249
  alignment   249
treatment planning   3–4
  age   374
  aims   11–14
  definitive   5, 23–26
  extractions   15–16
  general dental health   6–7
  handling patient expectations   4, 6
  incisor relationship   374–375
  mechanics   23
  medical history   6, 7
  non-extraction   15–16
  options   14–15
  patient concerns   4

patient motivation and compliance
     4
  previous orthodontic   7
  problem list   9–11
  timing   7–9
  upper lip to maxillary incisor
     (lip-incisor) relationship   374
  vertical skeletal discrepancy   375
treatment timing   7–9, 22
treatment with limited objectives   15
tricalcium phosphate   242
trifocal ellipse (Brader)   255
trihelix appliances   403–404
'true consent,'   23
true macroglossia   387
tube-shift/parallax technique   283
turbo props   380
Twin Block therapy   336
two-couple force system   48–49
two-stage space closure   305–306
tying-in, archwire   267

u
ulceration   244
undermining resorption   257
uniform attack   188
upper lip, to maxillary incisor
     relationship   374
upper removable appliance (URA)
     399
utility arch   401
utility archwires   212, 214

v
valid consent   23, 80–81
vector   30–32
verbal consent   80
vertical anchorage   228–231
vertical facial growth   383–384
vertical parallax technique   283
vertical-pull chin cup (VPCC)   389
vertical round tripping   377
vertical skeletal discrepancy   375

w
Wagon wheel effect   121
W-arch appliance   401–402
websites, patient education   88–89
white spot lesion   235
wire bending   288–291
written consent   80